MW00334322

THE SEARCH FOR MIND-BODY ENERGY

Meditation, Medicine, and Martial arts

JOHN BRACY

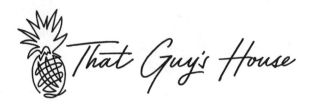

Copyright © 2020, Mind Body Energy International LLC

All rights reserved. No part of this publication may be reproduced, distributed or transmitted in any form or by any means without permission of the publisher, except in the case of brief quotations referencing the body of work and in accordance with copyright law.

ISBN: 978-1-913479-41-1

Book Design by Michael Maloney

Cover Design by Cathy's Cover

First edition published in 2020

That Guy's House

London

Dedicated to those who, with passion and an open mind, also search...

Contents

Conclusion

Acknowledgements

Few large works are ever the product of one person, and this is certainly true in the case of the present offering. This project could not have come to fruition without the kind attention and support of many individuals who helped make it possible.

It is with the deepest appreciation that I express my gratitude to the teachers and mentors who have inspired and guided my work over the last four decades. I am thankful for my Taiwan acupuncture professor, "Sunny" Ho, as well as my late internal martial art teachers, Ho Shen-ting and Chang Shr-jung. I am equally grateful to my Beijing master and fourth generation formal lineage holder, the late Liu Xing-han, and my *kung fu* "family" in Beijing. I also feel the deepest of gratitude towards the Yi Family, my adopted *kung fu* brethren in Taiwan, who through formal ceremony, accepted me as an "inner door initiate" of their tradition. I am also grateful to my late Beijing "Uncle," Liang Kequan, who was so fond of "tree shaking." I am also extremely grateful to my first formal *qi gong* teacher, the late Dr. Tim-Fook Chan, who was my supervisor at Feng Chia University in Taiwan, and the first to formally teach me to how to harness the body's energy through the yogic breath control.

I am also deeply appreciative of James Feld, MD and Huy Hoang, MD, for providing me with venues through which I was able to research and personally witness some of the ways that "energy work" can be helpful to pain patients.

I am also appreciative of those who helped me forge the manuscript. This work would not have been possible without the kind support of a number of individuals. First and foremost among those is Peter J. Miller. Other important contributors are Roger Niez, Richard Gall, Garold L Johnson, Frank Wuco, Brent Werner, Mike Junge, and many other individuals who have contributed generously. I also wish to thank Tom Greensmith for his review, and in particular his comments on the sections covering Tibetan Buddhism and the transliteration of Tibetan script. In this regard, a special note of appreciation also goes to Kunzang Dechen Chodron for her help and suggestions on Buddhist *tantric* material.

Special thanks also go to Columbia University *professor emeritus* Craig Richards, for the comments and suggestions that guided the development of the manuscript; to Frank Van Gieson, for his suggestions and comments on the body-mind in terms of speculative physics; to Tony Costa, for his expertise and recommendations on subjects relating to physiology; to Huy Huang, MD, for his review of the sections covering physiology and electrophysiology; and to Sheralyn Winn, DC, LAc, for her review of sections covering traditional Chinese medicine.

Most importantly, I wish to thank the many patient and loving students and friends who have supported the present work over the decade and more that it took to complete the material, especially my good friend Camille, and her Whispering Pines Writer's Retreat.

How Chinese words / phrases are transliterated in the present work

To the frustration of scholars and those familiar with the Chinese language, I ask for a great degree of forgiveness for my failure to adhere solely to one standard method of transliterating Chinese characters into Romanized form.

There are several ways to transliterate Chinese. In mainland China, the *pinyin* system is used, and, as of the 1970s, this method has increasingly become the standard accepted by scholars, replacing the previously preferred Wade-Giles system. There are also other, lesser known methods, such as the James Legge and Yale systems.

The following work is not intended as an academic text. It is neither written by, nor for, a sinologist. It is intended for a wider audience, comprising anyone who is interested in reading about subjects such as the use of the mind, *qi (ch'i), ki,* and *prana,* and how these might fit into their meditation, healing, martial arts, and yogic practices. Thus, in general, my choice of Chinese Romanization in any particular instance is based on the easiest and most accessible meaning for the casual reader, who is likely unfamiliar with Chinese language and transliteration systems.

As an example, the Wade-Giles representation of *t'ai-chi ch'üan* is more accessible to the average reader than its *pinyin* counterpart, *taijiquan.* However, the way a Westerner would read *baguazhang* is closer to the pronunciation of the art's name, as opposed to the Wade-Giles form, *pa-kua chang.* Similarly, Beijing is more familiar to the Western reader than the older, and Wade-Giles, transliteration of the "Northern Capital," Peking.

Note on pinyin compound words / phrases

Again, the present work is not intended to be a scholarly text, and some *pinyin* translations of Chinese words are rendered in a way that make them more accessible to readers unfamiliar with *pinyin* transliterations. For example, *nei qi* — for "inner *qi*" — is used instead of *neiqi.* However, this practice of separating compounds is not universal. Consider, for example, how *neiguan* — referring to a type of Taoist passive yoga — is rendered. The list of transliterations used herein can be found in the "Glossary of Chinese Terms," near the back of the book.

Disclaimer

The information presented in this book includes no medical claims. The Material presented is for research, discussion, and investigational purposes only. The case histories included are also for research and discussion only, and they should not be construed as medical advice. Furthermore, no one should attempt any of the exercises or training protocols described in the pages that follow without first consulting their licensed health care professional.

Foreword

I was an "inner door" student of John Bracy for ten years. Along that path, I earned a black sash in kung fu, an instructor's license in *baguazhang,* lineage in *bagua's* sixth generation, *taijiquan* teaching certification, and I opened my own Chinese Internal Arts training program at my university, The Claremont Colleges. Most important of all, I transformed from a mid-career heart attack candidate to a healthy and happy human being. For that, I will always be grateful to John.

While I cannot claim to have mastered all of what is contained in this book, I have certainly experienced it. My reactions (and those of the others I've observed) varied from, "Wow!" to "Oh my God, how is this possible?" John has an intuitive command of the human body that is way off the charts, grown from his own experiences and through working with others, and combined with an unusual ability to impart knowledge to his students. While few readers will have occasion to work directly with John, those of us who have can provide an insight into his method. I, for example, will never forget going to John with cramps in my spine muscles, which my MD merely gave me pain pills for. John, on the other hand, massaged the front of my spine and totally released what had been intractable pain. I will leave most of it to your imagination, but I stress that he did this from the *front*. In the cases of many of my Claremont students that John worked with, doctors were unable to diagnose a problem, whereas he used his understanding of the body and its subtle energy inter-connections to identify and address the conditions that they presented. While John has Chinese medical training, it is his intuition that guides his understanding. When I worked with him directly, he would come into every private session with a new insight and a way to teach it. If I asked, he would say it was something that he was working with on himself recently.

For many, simple exercises that cure problems will be enough. For myself, understanding of "why" and "how" has always been equally important. In these chapters, you will find at least a state-of-the-art explanation (and I think one that pushes the envelope) of human life energy *(qi)* and its connections to the body, mind, and health. In the ten years since I last had a face-to-face relationship with John Bracy, I have used his insights to continue to improve my health and well-being, addressing new problems and conditions with non-intrusive methods.

So, read on and get well. I have.

Donald Crone
Professor Emeritus
Politics and Asian Studies
Scripps College

Foreword

John Bracy is one of a handful of people who have permanently changed my life for the better. When I was in my early 20s, he guided me on a journey that proved to be one of extraordinary healing and training, and which irrevocably changed who I was and how I existed in my own body. Bracy is uniquely gifted in the development of conscious control of fascia and energy for fighting, healing, and for me, the art of distance running.

Shortly after I graduated from UC San Diego in 2009, Bracy offered to help me after observing the gray pallor of my face and excessive kyphotic curve of my spine. As a budding sponsored marathoner, I jumped at the opportunity to receive extra help on my journey towards the Olympic Trials. Knowing that Bracy had trained my father to the point of being an excellent *taiji* and *bagua* instructor, I knew he had many unique skills and understandings that I'd be unable to find anywhere else.

Over the course of two intensive years of training and hands on work, my body transformed into a highly integrated and graceful machine. To understand how impressive this was, I'll just add that my high school running coach informed me that I had by far the worst running form of anyone who ran at my level. I lumbered along like a tank, essentially willing my way to first place in distance races. By the time John and I ended our period of training together, due to me moving on to pursue graduate studies in Counseling Psychology, I received the ultimate compliment: a professional dancer saw me running by and stopped me to offer praise for my flawlessly efficient form.

On the way there, Bracy trained me to a level of physical and energetic awareness so high, I would have scoffed had he claimed that I'd reach such a point beforehand. I discovered how, when running, the effortless flicking of my arms could pull the rest of my body through each step, thanks to a dynamic physical connection which John specializes in teaching. Buoyed by new energetic exercises and the highly impressive results that they delivered, my running goals quickly elevated from small improvements to aiming straight for the Olympic Trials. Unfortunately, however, the chances of a perfect ending to this story were undermined by my own emotional maturity and self-awareness, which were not quite up to that particular task when I was a young twenty-something.

I became a certified instructor through his program, and then, in testament to that, became the *InTensional* Running Coach by training, among other things, the power of fascial and energetic awareness to interested runners.

The details, nuances, and conceptual framework that Bracy provides in this book, as well as in his classes and one-on-one training sessions, is fertile ground for a wide variety of people -- from those wishing to be free of pain, to anyone wanting that extra edge in performance. If you are looking for a change in a practical and ever-deepening way, you are in the right place.

Timur Crone
Creator of InTensional Running™
Chi Arts Association Instructor
MA Counseling Psychology
Certified Massage Therapist (CAMTC #78225)
USATF Certified Coach
Certified Strength and Conditioning Specialist

Section I

The root of the way of life, of birth and of change is qi; the myriad things of heaven and earth all obey this law. Thus, qi in the periphery envelops heaven and earth; qi in the interior activates them. The source wherefrom the sun, moon, and stars derive their light, the thunder, rain, wind, and cloud their being, the four seasons and the myriad things their birth, growth, gathering and storing: all of this is brought about by qi. Man's possession of life is completely dependent upon this qi.

— The Yellow Emperor's Classic of Medicine [1]

Introduction

*D*uring a 1980s acupuncture class in Taiwan, our teacher asked for a volunteer. As a classmate made his way to the front, I had no idea that we were about to take part in one of the most amazing demonstrations of internal energy, which the Chinese call *qi* (also transliterated as *ch'i*), I would ever witness. Our small group gathered to watch as our teacher, Professor "Sunny" Ho, asked the volunteer to look away so that he couldn't watch what was going on. Holding an acupuncture needle in his hand, Sunny then aimed the instrument at the *hegu* point in the webbing between the thumb and index finger of the volunteer's hand.[2]

The teacher held the needle as if he were about to insert it, yet it never came closer than an inch or so from the student's hand. This was extremely interesting. No one uttered a sound as the teacher focused on the needle and its target. A few moments later, the targeted point began to pulse and turn red. In short order, the red spot transformed into a pulsing mound, producing the same kind of effect one might expect if a needle had actually pierced the skin.

No verbal cues had been given to the volunteer. Later, he told us that he believed the needle had actually been inserted into the acupoint. Was this evidence of the mysterious energetic force the Chinese call *qi*, or was it merely a demonstration of the power of belief and the mind-body's response to subtle suggestion? For me, it would become one of many demonstrations I would witness over the next four decades that convinced me of the reality of the yet-to-be-defined mysterious force known to the Chinese as *qi*, to the Japanese as *ki*, and to practitioners of yoga as *prana*. However, personal experience and belief are one thing. Proving the existence of an undefined and willfully directed *force of nature* is an entirely different kind of challenge altogether.

Qi, prana, "subtle energy," and "internal energy" are a few among many terms for the enigmatic force. In **The Search for Mind-Body Energy**, we will consider to what extent the life energy known to the Chinese culture as *qi* might be identical, or at least similar, to the life-spiritual force that the indigenous people of the northeast Americas refer to as *manitou*. In that culture, shamans have long described *manitou* as the invisible webbing between the visible world and a transcendental part of reality. For them, *manitou* is the link between the physical and spiritual realms.

Tibetan Buddhists call the life-spiritual force that moves through the *tsa* energy channels *lung* or "wind." Practitioners of the Tibetan tantric traditions believe that when willfully directed within the body, the invisible lung energy awakens psychic powers that can lead to enlightenment. The famous eleventh-century Buddhist scholar, Pandit Naropa, strongly believed in the power of *lung-wind* energy to induce higher knowledge in the practitioner. Consequently, and based on this insight, he taught an entire set of yoga-meditation-energy practices to further *tantric* disciples on their path to spiritual enlightenment.

For many young people, both in the East and the West, their introduction to an invisible life force was through the Japanese anime television series *Dragon Ball Z*, wherein the main characters activate their *ki* energy to empower their martial arts practices. Likewise, since the 1970s, an entire generation became aware of the power of an invisible and willfully directed energy through George Lucas's *Star Wars*. The story centers on the sagas of a spiritual-warrior clan, the *Jedi*, who must learn to master their relationship with the *Force*.

My Personal Introduction

My introduction to the principles of energetic medicine was a weekend seminar presented by Dr. Stephen Chang in 1979. However, it wasn't until I studied acupuncture in Taiwan that I became immersed in, and began to have personal experience with, the energetic life energy known in Chinese culture as *qi*; and it was around this point that things were about to get a little strange.

Around that time, I began to have curious tactile and visual experiences. I would come to identify these as representations of "internal energy." As I started to try to make sense of these strange, sometimes unsettling experiences, it was a challenge. What was the meaning of the visual "energy" that I was seeing around people? Gradually, though, some of these impressions started to make sense. Sometimes I would see dark spots in or around a person, which represented some sort of disease or imbalance. In rare cases, I observed sparkles of light floating around a person's head — a presentation that is very revealing of a person's spiritual life path. I still don't understand the meaning of many impressions, but I do have some ideas about how my ability to perceive these kinds of things came about. Let me return to that in a moment.

In Taiwan, my experience with *qi* was becoming increasingly strange, as I continued to study and experiment with more nuanced aspects of "energy." I learned that while some patterns of energy in or around a person were connected to an injury, other configurations indicated conditions of blocked energy. Learning to distinguish between different energy patterns helped in my study of healing, energy practices known as *qigong* (*ch'i kung*), and martial arts. Eventually, I was able to identify the exact location of a blocked acupuncture point or pain pattern, not only through the memorization of acupuncture charts and the elaborate rules that come with the Chinese healing arts, but through a kind of visual perception. Many of those perceptions are similar to the experiences described by the nineteenth-century Prussian scientist Carl Von Reichenbach. I will go into more detail on Reichenbach's "energy" research in Chapter One. However, at this point, I should say something about the way I use the word "energy."

A *Force of Nature*

To the great annoyance of a generous editor who provided comments and suggestions on the early stages of this work, sometimes, when I discuss subtle energy or internal energy, I place quotation marks around the word "energy." An example might be the discussion of how a particular master uses his "energy" to heal. Other examples include how a martial arts master utilizes his or her "energy" to weaken an opponent, or, in another example, to describe how a Taoist meditator manages the flow of "energy" within his or her body. However, in these usages, it is presumptive to assume that the "energy" we are talking about is the natural and accepted force that we typically refer to as "energy." At this juncture, it is unknown if these phenomena and sensory experiences represent a form of "energy" at all. It is important to keep in mind that they may be of an entirely different class of phenomena. It is my impression that some writers on these subjects sometimes forget the fact that, at least for the moment, "internal or subtle energy" has not been scientifically established as a "force of nature."

The overly liberal use of the term "energy" can be misleading, since currently no such "energy" has been accepted by mainstream science. In many examples, there may be an energy that can be willfully directed, but it is also possible that the observed effect or sensation described as "energy" could be due to something else that has nothing to do with "energy" at all. Perhaps non-contact healers, such as those described in Section IV, really do have the power to extend an invisible force and thereby influence a patient's healing. I do think it is possible for some gifted individuals to influence the healing of another person, but here, in the form of speculation to make a point, all we can say for certain is that a gifted individual may be able to attain a particular mind-body state, which allows them to influence a patient through some unknown mechanism.

In support of this point, let us imagine that one day in the future it is discovered that a person, upon attaining a particular mental state, is able to either heal a patient completely, or to at least increase the rate of healing. Assume then, for the moment, that said healing was discovered to be effected, not through the direction of an invisible force, but instead through the way the patient's brain "tunes into," and positively responds to, the healer's positive intentions. If such a discovery were made, would it mean that all those who had previously focused their search for proof of an **invisible emitted energetic force** were wrong?

Pertaining to the possibility of an invisible directed human force, it is a challenge to assign meaning to observed laboratory phenomenon, such as the very large electromagnetic and infrared field emissions that sometimes occur when an "energetic" healer projects healing intent to a patient. Examples of this kind of phenomena are included in Section IV.

Some models describing the relationship between a person's ability to extend an energetic force, as in non-contact healing, rely on a cause and effect way of looking at things. However, in the example of non-contact healing, there are two problems with that proposed explanation.

The first has to do with measurements of non-contact healers. In those kind of studies, sometimes the assumption is made that high electromagnetic (EM) and other measurements, such as infrared field emissions emitted by a healer's hands or fingers, are evidence of *qi*, or "internal energy." Keep in mind that measurements like these are **correlations**, not proof of an internal energy such as *qi*. In other words, they may occur simultaneously with a healer's ability to project energy, or these may be examples of something else that occurs at the same time. Although there may be a high correlation, it is presumptive to say that this observation represents a form of what the Chinese refer to as the mysterious *qi*. My instinct is that, when more clearly understood, *qi* will be described as something far greater than EM or infrared radiation. For example, as covered in Sections IV, VIII, and XII, these kinds of "energy healing" effects may be at least partly explained in terms of *information* that joins with minute amounts of emitted EM or infrared emission, rather than a one-day definable "energy."

"Seeing" Energy

The most easily observed of the "energy" patterns around the body appear like waves of heat, similar to those one sometimes sees rising from a hot surface. At other times, and for some reason especially around large old trees, the energy appears in a series of sinewave-like patterns that emit outwards from the source, and which can extend over a surprising distance. Many people can "see" energy fields. Over the past decades, I have taught many classes where participants learned to perceive these subtle fields visually. Nearly anyone with an open mind can learn to see and work with these normally invisible patterns of energy that exist in and around the body, and often around other living things, especially in nature and, for some reason, even more so around trees.

Some larger, healthier trees radiate especially interesting energy patterns. One morning, shortly after I suffered a serious back injury, I limped to the place where I would meet a private student in a small park. At the park's center stood a grand old tree, and as I waited for the client to arrive, I sat in silent amazement, watching the harmonious sinewave-like energy patterns around it. I felt that if I could ever fully understand the meaning of these impressions, I should be able to transform them into an immediately accessible and powerful healing force that I could instantly tap into and take advantage of. I am still working on that one.

After returning from my first year in Taiwan, the ability to "see" energy imbalance in and around a patient's body became helpful in my work as a therapist and trainer. I was fortunate to be able to apply and hone this skill when I assisted Dr. James Feld in his practice of treating chronic pain patients.

Years later, I would apply what I had learned in new ways while working with patients at the Natural Health Medical Center in Los Angeles. During that later period, I concentrated on methods of helping patients relieve pain and rehabilitate without drugs or surgery, through combinations of Taoist yoga and *qigong*.

Sometimes, the results obtained from working with alternative methods like these were impressive, and these remain a testimony to the effectiveness of a complementary healing system that joins conventional medicine with prescriptive "energy work." One standout case occurred when the center's director, Dr. Hoang, advised a prospective back surgery patient not to undergo his scheduled procedure. In that case, an intervention via a simple, non-invasive technique succeeded, and, on the advice of Dr. Hoang, the patient was recommended to avoid surgery. This was a result that wouldn't have been possible without my ability to sense the patient's patterns of energy blockage, and then design a simple exercise that would be helpful to him.

All cases aren't so dramatic, but another stands out. In this example, the UCLA surgeon of a woman who was scheduled for carpal tunnel surgery saw such improvement after only five sessions of Taoist yoga and *qigong* energy therapy, that the scheduled procedure was thus canceled. That intervention was especially remarkable, as when I first saw the patient, her pain was so debilitating that she was unable to lift either of her two young children.

Learning to "See" and Work with "Energy"

I am sometimes asked about how I was able to perceive and work with these subtle energy fields. I offered a possible explanation in an article published in 2002, in *Qi: The Journal of Traditional Health and Fitness*.[3] There, I shared my understanding of how these unusual abilities came about. The story involves an old guru from India.

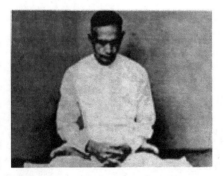

Photo I-1
Sri Surath

As I discussed in the article, my ability to perceive and work with subtle energies manifested shortly after meeting with Sri Surath (Photo I-1), when one of his senior disciples asked if I might work with the *Bhakti* yoga master. The problem was that, although Sri Surath suffered from Parkinson's disease, he refused medication. His American devotees were desperate to find anything that might help alleviate the symptoms, but before I could have physical contact with the *Brahmin*, I would have to be interviewed and approved.

I was interviewed by Sri Surath, and subsequently received permission to work with him. Later, during our scheduled therapy session, I applied traditional bodywork to the guru. Afterward, Sri Surath and I, along with some of his disciples, shared a meal that had been prepared by members of the group, and ever since that day, I have wondered whether something strange might have taken place, of which I was completely oblivious. I felt nothing out of the ordinary at the time, but later, as the master left the room, one of the disciples told me that a kind of initiation had taken place. This had something to do with the master's extension of subtle energy, known as *shakti*. Apparently, everyone present, except for me, was aware of the exceptional *shakti* in the room. Not long afterward, I began to have strange experiences that I would trace back to that moment and my interaction with Sri Surath.

The Meaning of Internal Energy

Citing both lore and scientific investigation, the present work considers the meaning of "internal energy" from various viewpoints and traditions. It is the life force referred to by the Chinese as *qi*, by the Koreans as *gi*, by the Japanese as *ki*, and by the Hawaiian shamans as *mana*; while in Sanskrit, it is called *prana*. As explained in the following pages, some scientific investigators have referred to it as "influence" or "information." The present work is not intended as a comprehensive or scholarly presentation, but rather an introduction and cross-cultural discussion of the subject.

The possibility of a mysterious, invisible force that can empower body and mind is both intriguing and controversial. Some of us are attracted to the personal empowerment and healing potential associated with developing strong "internal energy." Practices such as yoga, *qigong*, meditation, and Chinese forms of martial arts and moving meditation such as *t'ai-chi chüan*, are centered on the idea that, within those traditions, life energy pervades the mind-body. In some traditions, the balance of one's energy flow is the definition of health and vitality, while others believe that its mastery leads to spiritual advancement. In considering the meaning of these theories and practices, we will ask if there is an objective way to measure this enigmatic life force. We will also consider how it might be possible that mastery of one's energy flow can promote spiritual development.

Entire disciplines have been designed for the purpose of learning to access and gain conscious control over subtle or internal energy. Categories of practice devoted to the study of internal energy fall within the purview of the energy healer, *t'ai-chi* master, Taoist alchemist, Tibetan lama, yogi, and many others. Despite the fact that within each of these disciplines, the study of subtle energy life force is viewed differently, there are enough similarities to warrant a discussion of the shared meaning of subtle or internal energy. This point speaks to the primary intention of the present work, namely, to initiate a larger conversation concerning the commonalities among the aforementioned disciplines.

One aspect of the present work considers whether techniques such as "energetic meditation," non-contact healing, acupuncture, and sexual yoga can awaken the power of the *life force*, and if so, whether it is the same "energy" tapped into by the Tibetan holy man high in the Himalayas.

Along with Western protocols, some hospitals in China today offer the therapies of non-contact healing specialists, who believe they can direct *wai qi* (external *qi*) healing to treat cancer and other illnesses. In this vein, one study cited in Section IV describes a non-contact healer's ability to annihilate bacteria in a Petri dish through the application of his internal energy and intention. In another study cited in the same chapter, one researcher distinguishes between the energy that has a deadly effect on bacteria, which he calls "negative energy," and a separate kind of healing energy he calls "positive energy."

Accessed by focused consciousness and directed through intention, many different techniques are devoted to the conscious control and direction of the invisible life force. The pages that follow include not only descriptions of the methods used to direct the life force external to the body, but also the various means concerned with mastering the flow of life energy within the body. Moreover, this work also includes the views of experts on the subject that might account for energetic healing, and how mastery of the energy flow within the body can function to initiate mystical-spiritual knowledge. In other applications, a person's ability to direct conscious control over subtle energy is sometimes cited as the explanation for uncanny human abilities, ranging from telekinesis (moving objects without physical contact) to control over the weather and, as some believe, the ability to read another person's thoughts.

In some forms of martial arts, the highest skill is said to be related to mastery of one's internal energy. In those examples, a master's ability to sustain a heavy blow without injury or remaining unharmed while allowing a heavy vehicle to run over his midsection, is also credited to control over his internal power. Thus, we also consider whether this might be the same force that a *t'ai-chi* or other kind of martial arts master can direct against an opponent.

Explanations for the way an energetic vibration is said to move through the body are intriguing. Some traditions, like those of the Tibetan *tantric* yogi, are especially compelling because of the way "energy practice" is associated with the development of enlightened consciousness. As discussed in the sections on *kundalini*, Tibetan *tantra*, and Taoist energetic meditation, the expert practitioner is said to develop greater understanding and awareness, not only through subjective cognitive processes, but also through controlling the flow of energy throughout the body, and in particular, the movement of energy in or around the genitals, tailbone, perineum, and spinal corridor.

As described in ancient Indian, Chinese, and Tibetan teachings, the transmutation and migration of "subtle energy" in the body is believed to trigger a kind of evolutionary change in the practitioner's brain structure, which in turn awakens new psychic potential. Although explained in terms of theoretical constructs that vary between traditions, when this occurs, new insights, increased creativity, and realization of an advanced stage of being emerges. If these were only stories from an ancient culture, they would be intriguing. However, reports like these persist into modern times, and, if only possessing a thread of truth, the methods of those ancient cultures in describing the benefits derived from one's mastery of internal energy hold a promise of human potential that is too powerful to be ignored.

Lending itself to documentation and objective study, some aspects of subtle human energy are increasingly measurable. Consider the research described in Section IV. There, one study documents how some energetic healers can project a large and measurable electromagnetic field from their palms. Commenting on the observation, one scientist involved in this kind of research describes this type of bioenergetic evidence as quite "robust" and easily measurable.

Kundalini

While some aspects of the internal or subtle force phenomenon are becoming increasingly easy to measure, other, more enigmatic forms remain elusive and resist objective study. *Kundalini* is an example of the more mysterious side of our adventure. In Section VI, *kundalini* is described as an aspect of internal energy that, although a powerful and potentially life-changing phenomenon, resists objective measurement.

Kundalini stands apart from other forms — what might be considered frequencies — of internal energy, due to the way that the force can take over the body of those who dare activate this most potent aspect of their "energy." Reports included in Section VI explain the effects of *kundalini* on the practitioner, with experiences ranging from ecstasy to extreme and incapacitating physical pain, as well as psychological instability and hypersexuality. Such reports suggest that some forms of "internal energy" have both advantages and disadvantages.

Although the names for the subtle life force differ across cultures — *lung* energy of Tibetan Buddhism, *nei qi* of Chinese yogic and healing traditions, and prana of various Indian yogic traditions — descriptions of this *énergie vital*, or life force, are closely related, if not identical.

Perhaps it was luck, or perhaps fate — what the Chinese call *yuan-fen* (缘分) — that brought me to my teachers in Taiwan. When I was at Feng Chia University in the early 1980s, my martial arts instructor was Professor Yi Tien-wen. He taught me as part of a group of eight Western students that were assigned to him as part of a graduate student exchange program at the university. Yi was a professor at the university, and the son of the grandmaster of his family's martial arts style. Later, I was honored to be initiated by Grandmaster Yi as an "inner door" disciple, and then licensed to teach the martial arts of the formerly secret society. Over the next two decades, I would train with younger and older masters of the family style, both in Taiwan and at our southern California studio.

I am forever grateful to Sifu Yi, his father, Grandmaster Yi, and my other teachers in Taiwan and Beijing. I am also grateful for my acupuncture teacher, Sunny Ho, who also happened to be a member of the same formerly secret Yi clan. I must also thank my program supervisor at Feng Chia University, as well as my first formal *qigong* teacher, Dr Tim-fook Chan.[4] Other teachers that I want to thank include the late master Chang Shr-jung, retired Chinese Republic of China air force general, Ho Shen-ting, and my teachers in Beijing, Liu Xinghan and Liang Kequan. I am fortunate and honored to have been able to grasp a little bit of the *pi mao* (皮毛), "skin and hair," or superficial level, of their rich and invaluable traditions.

Endnotes

1 Adapted from a quote from the Yellow Emperor's *Classic of Internal Medicine*, cited in Steven Chang's *The Complete Book of Acupuncture*, Celestial Arts, 1976.

2 David Chan, former classmate in Taiwan and currently professor at Emperor's College of Traditional Medicine in Santa Monica, was also present and witnessed this demonstration.

3 Bracy, John, "Internal energy in the martial arts," *Qi: The journal of traditional health and fitness*, Summer 2002. www.qi-journal.com.

4 The father of my former Taiwan classmate David Chan, who was mentioned in Endnote 2.

Chapter 1

The Quest for Internal Energy

*T*his is a detective story. The pages that follow detail a search for clues to the meaning of "internal energy." In our search, we will ask questions that pertain to the mind-body energetic force known to the Chinese as *qi*, to Koreans as *gi*, and to the Japanese as *ki*. We will consider scientific research that investigates this phenomenon, and, as good analytical sleuths, we will compare and contrast various methods by which many believe this power — this "life force" — can be accessed.

Our detective story looks for clues to a mystery that can be traced back to the earliest recorded times and cultures. The pages that follow include evidence that will help us answer questions such as: is "internal energy" real or imagined? Can mental power influence the strength of one's life force? Can the power of internal energy in the healing arts be attributed to belief? Related concerns will also be addressed. For example, we will consider whether aspects of the enigmatic force can be scientifically measured. We will also look at how this yet-to-be-named energetic force can be consciously directed through the power of intention, and to what extent it can cure diseases. We will ask if it possesses the power to restore youth and promote longevity. What exactly is this *life force?*

Some clues are found in the domain of the acupuncturist and the energy worker (energy healer), while others are provided through the work of the sports trainer and martial artist. There are also hints about the meaning of the life force to be found in the traditions of energetic meditation and yoga.

Our investigation will consider ancient sources and their descriptions of "internal energy." Moreover, our quest will also include newer, often controversial questions. For example, the pages that follow include new proposals for defining the meaning of the meridians / channels* — those energy pathways of the body that are the cornerstone of traditional Chinese medicine, yoga, and energetic meditation. These controversial proposals include expanded, and in some cases brand-new, explanations of how those channels can be accessed more effectively, to deepen the practices of meditation, *qigong* healing, and martial arts like *t'ai-chi chüan*. [1]

* In traditional Chinese medicine (TCM), the current standard translation of the body's *jing luo* (経絡) energetic lines is, increasingly, "channel."

Formerly, the term "meridian" was favored. However, in the present work, the reader will notice both terms, sometimes used in conjunction with the adjective "myofascial." The reason for this is that a heterodox description of these lines is presented, first in Section II and later in Section XII. There, it is proposed that the meridians / channels function as much more than simply conduits of energy. In those chapters, they will also be described as demonstrable **physical structures** that play a *physical* (as opposed to only a theoretical, or energetic) role in health maintenance and healing. Second, in later chapters, speculation will be presented that they operate as "embedded antenna structures." When used, the term meridian is chosen because it more accurately describes the multiple functions that these structures are hypothesized to exhibit.

> Tantric: Involving the practices of *tantra*. In Buddhism called *Vajrayana*, *tantra* is often described as "esoteric Buddhism," the "Diamond Way," or the "Thunderbolt Way."

Box 1-1 Definition of tantric and tantra

One of the questions that will be asked is whether, and to what extent, the "energy" described by the Chinese as *qi* (also written *ch'i*) might be the same as, or indeed differ from, the invisible life force that in Sanskrit is called *prana*, and in the Tibetan *tantric* tradition is called *lung*, or "wind" (རླུང་) (See Box 1-1).

A central question presented in many of the chapters that follow addresses whether or not descriptions of the flow of internal energy within the body, as described by Tibetan yogis and Chinese *neidan* meditators, is actually a yet-to-be-named force of nature, a product of their imagination, or a representation of the energetic meditator's ability to interact with another dimension. Other challenging questions will be asked, such as: is there really an "energy" that can be projected by a healer to produce non-contact healing? If so, and as it pertains to non-contact healing, what *is* the real source of the *qi* master's ability to heal? It will also be asked if there is the possibility of internal energy in the martial arts.

The notion of a subtle energetic force that animates body and mind pervades traditional Eastern culture. In the search for a more complete definition of subtle or internal energy, Eastern notions of a subtle energetic force will also be compared with the beliefs of Western indigenous peoples, as well as the notion of a life-spiritual force described in esoteric Christianity. In the later chapters, these will also be compared to current Western research, and the investigation of the power of intention.

Later chapters will look at the link between traditional Eastern descriptions of life energy, known as *qi, ki,* and *prana,* among other terms, as well as Western studies of the power of intention. In this light, our discussion will also include details of this fascinating area of investigation now being undertaken in highly controlled Western scientific studies. As mentioned in the Introduction, the goal of the present work is to begin a broad conversation that compares concepts such as *qi, prana, lung, thigle,* and *kundalini* in the East, with the understanding of the life force as described in indigenous cultures of the West, such as those of the Native Americans and Hawaiians.

Traditional Chinese Medicine: Subtle Forces and Subdivisions

The concept of *qi* forms the basis of traditional Chinese medicine (TCM). In that tradition, the term *nei qi*, literally "internal energy," serves as an umbrella phrase for a range of subtle bio-energetic forces that fall within the purview of TCM. This ancient form of healing includes numerous subdivisions that govern the conversion of different kinds of qi within the body, and the energetic force's relationship to body fluids, visceral organs, and life processes. These subdivisions include *yuan qi* (元気 [2], primordial or original *qi*), *wei qi* (衛気, the defensive *qi* that protects the body from external pathogenic influences), *ying qi* (営気, nurturing *qi)*, *gu qi* (谷 気, the *qi* that is extracted from the food we eat), ancestral or inherited *qi* (宗気), and *zhen* (真), or true *qi*.

Beyond an Eastern Phenomenon

Although the energetic life force serves as the foundation of most forms of traditional healing and both Chinese and Indian yoga practices, as well as some forms of martial arts, the belief in an animating life force is not limited to Asia, but is found in most, if not all, traditional cultures. Parapsychologists in the former Soviet Union studied the life force they called "bio-plasma." They believed bio-plasma was "a fourth state of matter," other than liquid, solid or gas, and speculated that bio-plasma energy accounted for the glowing energy patterns around living things observed with Kirlian photography.[3] The Hawaiian shaman knows the sacred life force as *mana*. Indigenous Americans in the northeastern United States — the Algonquian people — speak of the life force as *manitou*, the omnipresent subtle energetic force believed to manifest everywhere.[4]

According to James Mayor and Bryon Dix, in their study of the natural magnetic fields of New England, the indigenous Americans' description of *manitou* can be compared with the *qi* force that falls within the purview of the Chinese *feng shui* geomancers. [5] For both of these indigenous peoples, the earth's flowing currents of invisible energy lie in an intermediary space that connects the mundane to the supernatural. In *The Manitou: The Supernatural World of the Ojibway*, Johnston Basil informs his readers of the nature of manitou, which is characterized as "mystery, essence, substance, matter, supernatural spirit, anima, God, deity, godlike, mystical, incorporeal, transcendental and invisible reality." [6]

However, the present discussion is not limited to Native American, European, or Chinese traditions, nor to ancient texts or even traditional views of subtle bio-energy. The discussions that follow also include a review of the scientific literature on the phenomenon. Each of these diverse sources of information contributes, in its own way, to our discussion of the meaning of internal or subtle energy life force. Further to this, each source yields a particular set of clues, which, when taken together, reveal a larger view, or mosaic, of the internal energy puzzle.

As I mentioned earlier, some of the views presented here are controversial, as they are not fully understood scientifically, or even fully perceptible due to the limitations of human physical senses and intellect. In the opening paragraph, I promised you a mystery, and I believe that mysteries are to be embraced, even if they are not yet fully understood. Prominent among the more controversial views is the notion that, for most purposes, the phenomenon identified as subtle energy is indistinguishable from what in current scientific investigations is known as the power of "intention," or psi*. To briefly introduce a point in support of this statement, consider that regardless of whatever the force or action of *nei qi, prana,* or *lung* may actually be, when it becomes more fully understood, it will be revealed not as an Asian phenomenon, but a *human phenomenon*. For example, if the *qi* energy of acupuncture and other healing arts is "real," it is not a specifically Chinese or Asian phenomenon, but an aspect of life that both pervades and surrounds all biologic forms.

> *According to parapsychologist Mario Varyoglis: "*Psi* is the 23rd letter of the Greek alphabet and first letter of the word 'psyche.' It is the term parapsychologists use to generically refer to all kinds of psychic phenomena, experiences, or events that seem to be related to the psyche or mind, and which cannot be explained by established physical principles." [7]

Eastern vs. Western

It informs the discussion to consider the different ways that what might be called internal or subtle energy is dealt with in the East compared to the West. Keep in mind the earlier statement that, at this point, it is impossible to state objectively that something called internal or subtle energy *actually exists*. However, we have subjective reports by those who engage in subtle energy practices concerning the bodily sensations that they identify in terms of sensitivity to, or control over, internal energy. These reports include electrical-like sensations throughout the body, especially in the hands and fingertips.

Let us consider a report on psychic phenomena by one of the most respected scientists of the late nineteenth century, Sir William Crookes. Crookes (1832-1919) was a chemist, physicist, and member of the Royal Society. He discovered thallium and invented the radiometer, as well as the Crookes Tube, and was a pioneer in the development of vacuum tubes. Crookes agreed to take up an examination of the (at the time) popular psychic phenomenon then referred to as Spiritualism. Consider his list of tactile experiences associated with the presence of the "psychic force" during *séance*. Documented by an assistant, Dr. Crawford, Crookes's partial list included:

- The sensation of cool breezes, generally over the hands
- The sensation of a slight tingling in the palm of the hands and fingertips
- The sensation of a sort of current throughout the body
- The sensation of a "spider's web" contacting the hands and feet, and other parts of the body

Using this example, consider how tactile experiences like those listed above are dealt with differently in the East and West. In other words, might there be an unconscious cultural bias in Eastern culture that tends to influence researchers to perceive and explain phenomena in terms of *qi* or *ki?* In general, a traditional Eastern approach to explaining the experience of the aforementioned sensations might be to make some kind of yoga, *qigong (ch'i kung)*, or meditative practice based on the practitioner's attention to these kinds of sensations. An example of one's attention placed upon the body's subtle sensation is found in the teaching of Padmasambhava (a.k.a. Guru Rinpoche), who is most famous for revealing the *tantric* yogas of Tibetan Buddhism.

It is interesting, and perhaps an important clue, that in the case of the mind-body sensations that Guru Rinpoche taught his devotees to pay attention to, many were much like the ones described by Crookes. The instructions left by Guru Rinpoche served as markers, designed to inform the practitioner that they were on the right track. In this example, sensitivity to sensations became the tool that might lead the Rinpoche's disciples to enlightenment. Thus, sensitivity to, and even exaggeration (by mental attention), of tactile sensations became a hallmark of these practices. For example, Guru Rinpoche taught that mastery of *tantric* yoga, involving attention to these kinds of sensations, would lead the practitioner to Buddhism's ultimate goal: realization of the nature of the mind. In the same manner, the Taoist alchemists believed that their conscious control of sensations identified as *nei qi* could unveil the ultimate secrets of life, including the path to immortality.

For practitioners of Eastern traditions, experience was the essence. By comparison, in Western-style investigations, objectivity in research is prioritized, and the individual's subjective experiences are secondary, or even unimportant. To demonstrate this point, once again, let us consider the studies by Crookes.

Crookes, as a Western scientist interested in documenting the phenomenon of a yet-to-be-identified energy, made extensive notes on the sensations that occurred during his investigation of psychic phenomena. Crookes, like Western scientists in general, was less interested in the philosophical explanation of what might be causing these sensations, such as the *Tao, qi,* or *prana*, or as-yet-named "life energy," but instead focused on what could be empirically verified and, in the end, reliably predicted.

It may be for these reasons that the individual's subjective experience of the movement of electrical-like sensations through the body — warmth in the palms of the hands, tingling in the fingertips, and so forth — are to this day often studied differently by Eastern and Western scientists. A good example of these culturally biased approaches is found in the studies of non-contact healers presented in Section IV. Citations there include observations by Drs. Akira Seto and Chikaaki Kusaka, who, using an electromagnetic (EM) field detector, documented how some energetic healers could intentionally emit an extraordinarily large bio-magnetic field from their hands. Through their statements, it is clear that Seto and Kusaka believed their measurements not only identified the source of emissions as *qi* or *ki,* but that they were close to identifying the secret of *qi* or *ki* as a biological phenomenon. Seto and Kusaka studied thirty-seven individuals who, according to the published study, met the following requirements:

1. Persons who insisted they could emit the external *Qi*

2. Persons who [were] thought to have the ability to (sic)

Observations like those included in the Seto and Kusaka study are very important, and serve to contribute to the discussion of subtle/internal energy phenomenon. However, to illustrate how researchers in the East sometimes allow cultural bias to influence their assumptions, investigators in the Seto and Kusaka study, which included university researchers, medical doctors, and physiologists, assumed beforehand that something they call *qi* energy both exists and can be emitted. However, this assumption is problematic, since "*qi*" has not yet been defined, or in other words, it is not yet scientifically accepted that something called *qi* exists. Secondly, they describe the emission of the EM field by some individuals in their study as examples of them being able to "emit *qi.*" Despite there being no definitive, irrefutable evidence that "emitting *qi*" is genuinely possible in our physical reality, some scientists, like those in the Seto and Kusaka study, presume that the detected EM radiation from subjects in their experiment demonstrates an ability to intentionally emit qi. Consider the title of their paper:

> "Detection of extraordinary large bio-magnetic field strength from human hand during external **qi** *emission*" [emphasis added] [8]

Again, results like those obtained from the Seto and Kusaka study are intriguing, and perhaps even invaluable in their contribution toward arriving at a meaningful understanding of internal subtle energy (*qi, ki,* etc.). However, I must stress again how drawing the conclusion that a person's ability to emit an impressive, force of nature-like bio-electrical field is proof of the existence of *qi* is presumptive. Furthermore, it may be misleading. Perhaps such an emitted field is synonymous with internal energy, but perhaps it is not. It is more probable that when *qi, ki, prana,* or internal energy by another name is eventually verified, it will be shown to be much more than only the emission of a bio-electrical field. For example, as will be covered later, it is possible that one day, what is now referred to as an energetic life force will be established as an *informational,* and possibly even a multi-dimensional, phenomenon linked to human intention.

Now, contrast the Seto and Kusaka investigation with that of a leading Western scientist's study of the power of intention. Dr. William Tiller has conducted numerous experiments on the power of human intention to interact non-physically with, and exert influence over, the physical environment. In one of those studies, Tiller documented how a person physically separated from a device could non-physically cause the device to register an electrostatic charge. Of significance, is the fact that the experimental subject producing this mysterious effect had to first attain a specific mind-body state, and then *intend* to interact with the device. The experiment was conducted under strict laboratory conditions, and the results were later confirmed by outside laboratories.[9] The study, described in more detail in Section VII and again in later sections, offers compelling evidence suggesting that it *is* possible for a person who has attained a particular mind-body state to initiate a physical effect from the exertion of human intention alone. Results like these suggest that human intention *can* act as a subtle, but no less real, natural force.

It is instructive to consider Western vs Eastern approaches to this kind of human non-contact influence research. In a Western-style study of intention, such as Tiller's, the researcher informs the reader that they are conducting experiments to test and document whether intention might be able to influence the external environment. These scientists do not seek to prove intention exists as something quantifiable, and they do not label the "force" per se; rather, they are interested in studying the phenomenon of intentionality. Moreover, they seek to elicit the subjective experience of a person engaged in the requisite mind-body state necessary to cause this subtle human influence, such as the individual's experience of "an inner electrical equilibrium." One must then ask, if the same study was conducted in the East, wouldn't a person's experience of "electrical equilibrium" be identified as *qi*?[10]

Are Psychic Phenomena Related to *Qi / Ki / Prana*?

In the search to arrive at a meaningful definition of subtle or internal energy, it is also important to consider whether a relationship exists between subtle (internal) energy and psychic phenomena. In other words, at least in some cases, might "energy" subjects and psychic phenomena be identical, or at least related? Let us revisit the points noted by Dr. Crookes's assistant, concerning the participants' tactile experiences during a *séance*. In many ways, their sense experiences seem to be identical those of *qigong* masters and other energy practitioners when they manipulate subtle energy in and around their bodies. For example, where participants in Dr. Crookes's studies reported sensations such as feeling a "cool breeze" flowing over the hands, *qigong* practitioners likewise report similar sensations, such as tingling, or "electrical-like" magnetic sensations, over their hands in meditation, healing, and martial arts. Similarly, these sensations are also concentrated in the palms of the hands and fingertips.

In the same vein, where Crookes reported sensations of a current moving through the bodies of his psychic subjects, a similar sensation is also common to intermediate and advanced practitioners of many forms of yoga, meditation, *qigong*, and *t'ai-chi*. Compare these subjective experiences to those of individuals in the study of intention conducted by Tiller, and once again there are similar reports by individuals, who, after attaining an ordering of their biological rhythms called "entrainment," or "internal coherence," also report the experience of an "electrical equilibrium" throughout their bodies.[11] At this juncture, it is impossible to say whether the feeling of an "electrical current" and electrical equilibrium are the same, but the similarities between these reports seem too close to ignore. The commonalities between these disparate regimens and their respective reports are strong, and worthy of consideration as to what extent these kinds of experiences might be *eodem fonte*, or from the "same source."

When evaluating the meaning of sensations reported by the yogi, the Taoist *neidan* alchemist, the Tibetan *tantric* practitioner, lama, or the *t'ai-chi* master, it is important to take note of how the sensations they experience during practice produce biofeedback signals that inform the practitioner that they are "getting in touch" with their internal energy. The Tibetan lama relies on cues like these to initiate control over the movement *lung-wind* (internal energy) within his or her body. Likewise, for the energetic healer, the meditator, or the internal martial arts master, subtle signals like these serve as valuable markers that inform the adept that they are making appropriate progress.

In examples from ancient times, those skilled in perceiving the flow of subtle energy in and around the body sometimes drew maps over representations of the human frame, to illustrate the pathways and energy centers they perceived while in a state of deep meditation. For Chinese inner alchemists, the energy lines they became aware of flowed like rivers through their bodies, and contributed to the foundation of traditional Chinese medicine. Their perceptions of the mapping of energy pathways became the first charts of the acupuncture points and channels (Figure 1-2).

Subjective Evidence

Some of the chapters that follow consider the subjective experiences of practitioners and their interaction with what they identify as subtle life energy. Whether from the perspective of a shaman, Tibetan Buddhist lama, Taoist meditator, internal martial artist, or yogi, it is important to keep in mind that such reports are highly subjective, and do not offer empirical evidence to support the claim that a subtle, but no less profound, force of nature exists.

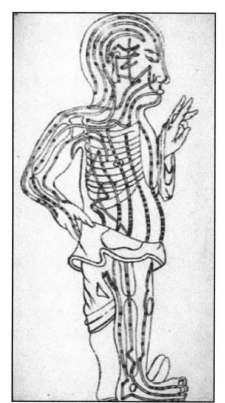

Figure 1-2

Ancient Acupuncture Channel Chart

Source: Wikipedia commons

Nevertheless, this does not mean that subjective reports of personal experience lack value. The energetic healer's description of the way non-contact *wai qi* (external *qi*) energy influences the patient, the *tantric* yogi's report of the sensation of subtle *lung-wind* as it travels through invisible tsa energy channels, and the *t'ai-chi* master's explanation of how the co-influences of *qi* and mind can merge to help defeat an opponent, all possess valuable clues that help us reveal the nature of the mysterious life energy force.

The importance of differentiating between a subjective feeling and claims that one is harnessing an undefined force of nature will be emphasized in Section VII. There, the remarkable reports by early *t'ai-chi* pioneers and their revolutionary approach to practicing martial arts, based on *qi* and mind, are discussed. No doubt, those practitioners observed and systematized something profound. Whether or not the sensations they linked to their practice were actually evidence of *qi* is unclear. However, what is clear was their ability to articulate their newfound skills and link them to the importance of paying attention to, localizing, and mapping sensations they identified as *qi*.

Correlates of the Internal Energy Experience

As stated above, reliable measurement of subtle or internal energy is presently elusive. Adding to the problem is the fact that the meaning of "subtle" or "internal' energy is not yet clearly defined. However, there is a great deal of information about the phenomenon's correlates, e.g., electrical-like feelings in the body, increased warmth, and blood flow to certain areas.

Keep in mind that correlates are events that occur simultaneously, or near simultaneously. However, although these are often confused with cause-and-effect events, it is important to remember that correlation does not imply causation. For example, when a person actuates a light switch, the lights go on. However, unless they have personally inspected the wiring and possess personal knowledge of the room's lighting connection to the electrical grid, it cannot be said with certainty that flipping the wall switch causes the lights to go on. Without more detailed knowledge and inspection, it could be that someone in an adjacent room switches the light on from his side of the wall whenever the individual meddles with the dead switch on the other side. Without intimate knowledge derived from inspection of the wiring, all you can say with certainty is that there is a high correlation between your flicking the light switch and the room being illuminated. In other words, normally it is impossible to say that flipping a light switch actually turned the lights on.

Some of the correlates — those things that occur simultaneously — when a non-contact healer "externalizes" his or her subtle energy are described in Section IV. Observations made through scientific inquiry also noted there include a healer's ability to emit an extremely large and measurable bioelectrical field, and the presence of a large infrared radiation that registers on the palm of the healer's hand. Again, these types of observations are extremely valuable; they contribute to understanding the meaning of directed human subtle energy as a type of healing life force. However, it would be a mistake to suggest that measurements like these, which sometimes include large and measurable electrical fields radiated from a practitioner, are either synonymous with, or define, internal energy.

Is it Possible to "See" Energy?

Another controversial question pertaining to the discussion of internal energy is whether or not it is possible to *see* it. Some individuals from both the East and West claim to be able to attune to visual cues associated with what is often called strong *qi* energy. As discussed in Section VIII, most people, even the most skeptical, if they possess an open mind, can learn to see *something* that *might* be "energy". Again, this is subjective, as the person claiming to have "eyes on" a visible rendering of something that is otherwise invisible has no method or means to record and present as evidence what they claim to have seen. Such is the frustration of persons throughout history with heightened sensory perception.

The ability to visually perceive such "energy fields" is common to many spiritual-healing-energetic traditions in both the East and West. Visually, the appearance of subtle energy around the body is most often reported as an *aura*. However, at least for energetic practitioners who have learned to visually attune to the human energy field, the phenomenon presents as a smoky-white coloration around the palms of the hands, or sometimes as faint, yet still distinct, flashlight projections that extend from the fingertips.

One early Western scientist, the Prussian Carl von Reichenbach (1788-1869), believed that "energy" could be seen, and what was being observed acted as a "force of nature." Von Reichenbach, a highly respected chemist, metallurgist, and geologist was famous for his discovery of paraffin and creosote. As a member of the Prussian Academy of Sciences, von Reichenbach tried to convince his fellow scientists of the reality of a force he named *Od*, or *odic force*, after the Norse god Odin. For years, he tried in vain to prove through his scientific experiments that there was actually an extremely subtle magnetic fluid that could be directed by the mind and force of will. Here he introduces us to his *odic force:* [12]

> How unbounded its influence is on the whole of humanity, and even on the whole animal and vegetable kingdom, will be proved shortly. Od is, accordingly, a cosmic force that radiates from star to star, and has the whole universe for its field, just like light and heat.[13]

This is a good juncture to introduce the notion of a what appears as the fascinating relationship between two attributes. These concern a person with "high internal energy" and high sexual energy. Section VI is dedicated to the discussion of internal energy as it relates to sexual energy, because, in many traditions found in both East and West, the subject occupies an important place along the continuum of human energetic forces, which includes sexual energy. It is noteworthy that the relationship between a person's high-level internal energy, or psychic force, and sexual energy has been noted throughout history. For example, Reichenbach also observed this relationship and, according to the famed psychic spy, and the man oft-cited as the father of "remote viewing," Ingo Swann (1933-2013):

> Von Reichenbach observed that a strong Odic force correlated with sexual arousal, noting that some female "sensitives" refusal to work in the proximity of a "horny male" because of the "disturbing nature of their odic energies." [14]

For von Reichenbach, his principal informants in investigating the *"Odic force"* were psychics, then called sensitives, who made observations about subtle life energy while in darkened rooms. In his essay, *The Laws of Odic Light*, von Reichenbach describes the glowing luminescence around living bodies, and his research also included photographs of the Odic force.[15] Through reports of what these sensitives observed, von Reichenbach documented how various parts of the body, particularly the fingertips, hands, and feet emitted a glow. To Reichenbach, this was evidence of a human-emitted energetic force, and it is interesting to consider whether this might be the same energy that is described by Chinese masters as *qi*. Reichenbach described the appearance of the body's energy field in the following way:

> In a somewhat shaded light, say in a room where the brilliancy of day has become enfeebled by the sky being overcast, or in evening candle-light, let a man hold his hand before his eyes at ordinary seeing distance. Then let him look at his fingertips, holding them against a dark background, distant a step or two.
>
> Most men will see nothing unusual under such circumstances. But there will be a few among them everywhere who make an exception. On their attention being drawn to the matter, will, by looking narrowly, make out over the tip of each finger an extremely delicate current, colourless, non-luminous, like air, subject to motion, a few lines ... It is not smoke, nor vapor [Duft], nor steam [Dunst]; it looks like a fine flame, resembling — but notably more delicate in appearance than — an ascending body of heated air.[16]

On the appearance of the Odic force around flowers, he writes:

> Take a good middling or a good high-sensitive into the dark [to observe] ... a pot of flowers in bloom. After a couple of hours have gone by, you will hear strange stories. The flowers, so you will be told, will come forth out of the gloom and grow visible. First of all, they will distinguish themselves from the black night of the general darkness in the form of a vaguely defined grey cloud. In this, later on, clearer spots will be formed. These

will finally separate from *each other definably*; the individual blooms will become distinguishable. [17]

One challenge to arriving at a concise definition of subtle or internal energy is the multifaceted use of the term. Consider that, while in one context, *qi* internal energy refers to the invisible force underlying the mechanisms of acupuncture, the term simultaneously applies to the art of Asian calligraphy. In this context, internal energy describes the unseen force that animates the brush strokes delivered by a master calligrapher and conveys the expert's vital energy reflected through the inked strokes applied to canvas or paper. Consider the placement of pagodas on the Chinese landscape. The exact location of the very old pagodas was determined by geomancers conversant in the art of *feng shui*, the art of "wind and water." In this example, the pagoda acts as a precisely placed acupuncture needle on the terrain, which thereby influences the local *qi* of the environment.

If the diverse meanings of the term "internal energy" seem difficult to fathom, we are not the first to have been challenged in this way. Perplexed by the broad range of definitions attributed to the enigmatic and invisible force, Harvard's Professor of Medicine David Eisenberg, who early in his career as one of the first American medical exchange students studying in China, encountered a range of phenomena purported to be demonstrations by various masters of their apparently conscious control over *qi* energy.

Dr. Eisenberg's list of applications attributed with mastery over the *qi* force includes: the healing power of acupuncture, demonstrations of a master bending iron rods with bare hands, demonstrations of "protective *qi*" that prevented a performer from becoming injured while concrete blocks were smashed against his body, yogic self-healing exercises, manipulation of invisible internal energy outside the body, manipulation of subtle energy inside the body, manifestation of psychic powers such as telepathy, energetic massage, light strikes that seemingly enabled a performer to break rocks with his hands, and at least one demonstration of a performer effortlessly breaking rocks by smashing them against his skull.[18] Although in each of these examples the practitioner claimed that their demonstration represented mastery over their internal *qi*, one must wonder if all these demonstrations of skill really are evidence of a subtle or internal energy force.

The Magnetists

Early Western investigations of subtle energy as a natural force can be traced to the magnetists. During the Renaissance, the magnetists, who among their members counted prominent early scientists such as Jan Baptist van Helmont (1577-1644), promoted the notion that a "vital effluence" radiated from every object in the universe, and through this influence, all objects exerted a mutual influence on one another. Here, van Helmont shares his "great secret":

> I have hitherto avoided revealing the great secret –– that the strength [of the vital fluid] lies concealed in man, [and that] merely through suggestion and power of the imagination to work outwardly, [this force can] impress this strength on others, which then continues of itself, and operates on the remotest objects.[19]

Van Helmont, a physician, chemist, and natural philosopher — famous for his discovery of carbon dioxide and the classifier of gases as a distinct physical state — firmly believed that man possesses a life force constituted by the merging of earthly and heavenly/cosmic fields:

> Material nature draws her forms through constant magnetisms from above and implores for them the favor of heaven; as heaven, in like manner, draws something invisible from below, there is established a free and mutual intercourse, and the whole is contained in an individual.[20]

No doubt the inspiration behind the film *The Men Who Stare at Goats*, van Helmont believed that the human mind was so powerful that, when properly focused, it could kill. He speculated that psychic power, expressed through the medium of "mutual magnetic influence between living creatures," if excited to a heightened state he called "ecstasy," was able to "kill animals by staring at them for a quarter of an hour."

The notion that highly-focused psychic energy has the power to kill or cause disease is an old belief, prevalent in traditional cultures. In Spanish, it is called *mal ojo*, and although often translated as "the evil eye," according to the *curandera* Avila Elena, a more accurate translation is "illness caused by staring." [21] As Elena explains, "Our eyes are always sending energy to what we are staring at." [22]

Contemporaneous with van Helmont, there were other magnetists that fall into the category of "magnetic healers." One remarkable energy healer during this period was Valentine Greatlakes (1628-1682), an Irishman who, following instructions revealed to him in a recurring dream, began a healing practice he called "magnetic stroking." Greatlakes, a Protestant in predominantly Catholic Ireland, became well-known as a healer in both his native land and later in London. He was noted for his ability to successfully cure epilepsy, paralysis, deafness, ulcers, and diverse nervous disorders. A book documenting the veracity of the Greatlakes' cures, which included many signed testimonials confirming healing by magnetic stroking, was published in 1666. [23] [24]

However, most famous of the magnetic healers was the French physician and scientist, France Mesmer (1733-1815). Mesmer, whose work is often confused with the early form of hypnosis known as mesmerism, studied the effects of magnetic influences on the human body. At first, he used magnets to generate cures, but later abandoned this after he realized it was the human body itself that generated the healing influence.

Based on the actions of what he perceived as the body's magnetic field, Mesmer believed a subtle energetic exchange took place between both animate and inanimate objects. He called this energy "animal," meaning "animated," *magnetism*. Mesmer theorized that a physician was able to transfer his more abundant animal magnetism to the patient, which the physician could then replenish.

Mesmer conducted his healing sessions in a darkened room, and during treatment, his patients would sometimes enter a trance state. It was due to his use of these trance states that the association was made between hypnosis and what was then called mesmerism. It is interesting that some writers have compared Mesmer's work to *qigong* non-contact healing, like that discussed in Section IV. [25]

Although their research interests were often discredited, leading to them being exiled to the fringes of their profession, other scientists continued searching for proof of the subtle life energy well into the twentieth century. Notable among these was William Reich (1897- 1957). Trained in psychiatry under Sigmund Freud, Reich believed he had discovered the vital energy of living organisms, which he named "orgone." He even built devices called "orgone collectors," that he believed could concentrate and preserve orgone energy for healing and other purposes (A larger version of one of these is shown in Section IV, see Photo 4-1). Here, Reich introduces us to his belief in a "universal life energy,"

> I am well aware of the fact that the human race has known about the existence of a universal energy related to life for many ages. However, the basic task of natural science consisted of making this energy usable. This is the sole difference between my work and all preceding knowledge.[26]

Early Western scientists accepted the notion of an invisible magnetic fluid surrounding the body at least until the rise of the French philosopher and scientist Rene Descartes (1596-1650). For better or worse, Descartes laid down the rules of scientific investigation, and principle among these was the doctrine that the mind and body were completely separate entities. This, of course, ignored the requirement that there might be an invisible intermediary between mind and body, which could also interact with the external environment. An interesting footnote regarding Descartes is that he did believe in the existence of a "life fluid." However, according to his writings, the life fluid was embedded in the blood, where he believed "animal (animated) spirits" resided. [27]

Psychic Energy and Spiritualism

Between the late 1800s and 1930s, the primary investigators of energetic phenomena in the United States and England were the Spiritualists. Most often remembered for the *séance* and their attempts to communicate with the dead, the actual concerns of the Spiritualists were much broader. The study of Spiritualism included the movement of objects without physical contact — telekinesis — and the study of biological phenomena, such as increasing the growth rate of plants. They were also interested in developing the ability to perceive auras, the subtle energy believed to radiate from living things.

Until the mid-to-late-1800s, the quasi-scientific approach of the Spiritualists was widely rejected by more modern-minded scientists of the period. Their rejection was based on the Cartesian assumption that nothing inside the body, including thought and intention, could exert an influence on anything outside the body. However, this a priori assumption became problematic when human bio-electric fields began to be measured outside the limits of the physical body, a discovery proving that humans could interact in a non-physical way with their environment. This discovery was the proverbial fly in the ointment for nineteenth-century scientists. On this point, Swann writes:

> Faced with these phenomena, at about 1858, early researchers began to recognize that the human organism was somehow bound up with a "force" that operated beyond the periphery of the physical body — and yet had an impact on physical matter.[28]

The Ancient Chinese

To the ancient Chinese, *nei qi* (internal energy) was as an animating force and an invisible link between the human being and nature. In many Asian traditions, man's possession of *qi* was believed to affect every aspect of health and personal power. This model proposes that bountiful and balanced *qi* energy is the source of a rich and healthy life, while *qi* deficiency results in loss of personal power and ill health. However, their theory of life energy was not limited to human beings, and was understood to pervade all of the natural world, postulating that plants have *qi* energy, as do mountain ranges. In traditional Chinese society, one who studied these forces in the natural world became the *feng shui* geomancer; one who studied it in the body became the traditional physician; and one who taught man how to live in harmony with the forces of nature fulfilled the exalted role of philosopher-sage.

In Chinese culture, it was the inner alchemists of the *neidan* tradition who distinguished the varieties of internal energy. In seeking to refine the inner *qi*, or *nei qi*, their goal was to attain immortality by transmuting the gross seminal *jing qi* into refined *shen qi*, or spiritual *qi*.

The *feng shui* master is concerned with the flow of *qi*, which passes like an invisible river through the hills, garden, and house or business. According to traditional belief, the balance of *feng shui* forces ensures success, but by the same token, failing to consider the proper rules that govern the flow of *qi*, such as by misplacing building entrances, or not recognizing the relationship between a window and a garden pool, invites disaster. Whether or not one considers that in these modern times such beliefs are only superstitious relics of the past, today even the most educated and influential classes of Chinese businessmen still hire the services of skilled *feng shui* experts to ensure that the "wind and water" is correct before a new office building is considered fit for habitation. They believe it is a good practice to appease the gods and nature spirits — just in case they are real.

Above are just a few of the diverse meanings for what the Chinese call *qi*. In written or spoken Chinese, when combined with the preface for heaven or sky, *tian qi* refers to the weather. In other uses, it refers to the emotion of anger. In this book, *qi* most often refers to *nei qi,* the subtle energy of the body's channels, the *qi* of energetic meditation, the *qi* of sexual alchemy, and the *qi* that some suggest is the hidden power of martial arts, such as *t'ai-chi* and *aikido,* as portrayed in fantasy media like *Dragon Ball Z.*

In the East, internal energy is traditionally credited as the energetic force empowering acupuncture and energetic healing. Practitioners of "energetic" traditions, such as energetic yoga, *qigong,* and non-contact forms of Chinese healing called *wai qi* ("externalized" *qi*) believe that control over their body's subtle bio-energetic force is the key to both self-healing and the ability to heal others. Others believe that active or passive forms of "energetic" meditation can endow practitioners with the secrets of enlightened consciousness.

The pages that follow are notes from a journey that explores the practices of the Hawaiian *kahuna,* the energy arts of the Chinese alchemists, the traditional acupuncturists, and the mind-body disciplines of *tantric* yoga. We consider the lore of the *t'ai-chi* master and the science of non-contact energy, together with the power that is awakened when a person learns to harmonize their own internal rhythms. The common theme is the quest for a deeper understanding of the yet to be fully described phenomenon of the *life force*, in a way that embraces both Eastern and Western paradigms.

Endnotes

1 As described in the introductory pages, although the majority of the present work relies on *pinyin* style Romanization, there are a few exceptions. In this chapter, the Wade-Giles Romanization is used for *t'ai-chi ch'üan,*

2 The Chinese characters in this paragraph are the simplified (current mainland China usage) versions, since these are the forms most cited in acupuncture and traditional medical texts.

3 Electromagnetic plate-induced photography of coronal discharges around hands and fingertips. Named after Semyon Kirlian, who discovered the phenomenon in 1939.

4 According to the subject's entry in Wikipedia, *Manitou* is described as:
"The spiritual and fundamental life force understood by Algonquian groups of Native Americans. It is omnipresent and manifests everywhere: organisms, the environment, events, etc. Aashaa monetoo = 'good spirit,' otshee monetoo = 'bad spirit.' The Great Spirit, Aasha Monetoo, gave the land, when the world was created, to the Natives (in particular, the Shawnee)."

5 As noted by Paula Gunn Allen in the introduction to Ingo Swann's *Psychic sexuality,* Panta Rei, [Crossroads Press digital edition] Retrieved from Amazon.com Kindle Reader.

6 Basil, Johnston, *The manitous: The supernatural world of the Ojibway,* New York Harper Collins, p. 242.

7 Mario Varyoglis, "What is Psi? What isn't?" http://archived.parapsych.org/what_is_psi_varvoglis.htm

8 Seto, et al., "Detection of Extraordinary Large Bio-magnetic Field Strength" *Journal of Acupuncture and Electro-Therapy Research,* Vo. 17, pp. 75-94.

9 Covered in more detail in Section VII, in his research, Tiller investigated the power of intention to influence the external world via a gas discharge device experiment. The gas discharge device was designed to investigate *intention* as a real-world force of nature (as opposed to theoretical or conceptual). Tiller and fellow investigators found that when a practitioner was next to the device while in a state of biological harmony, and then *intended* to interact with the device, the device registered the intention. Tiller et al conducted numerous tests with multiple individuals between 1977 and 1979.

See William Tiller, *Science and human transformation,* pp. 5-7.

10 Tiller, William A, *et al,* "Cardiac coherence: A new, noninvasive measure of autonomic nervous system order" *Alternative Therapies,* Vol. 2, No. 1, January 1996 *p.* 64.

11 Tiller, p. pp. 52-65, 1996.

12 F.D. O'Byrne, Translator and author of the Introduction, *Reichenbach's letters on od and magnetism:* Published for the first time in English, with extracts from his own works, so as to make a complete presentation of the Odic Theory. London, 1952, p.39.

13 O'Byrne, p.23

14 Swan, Ingo, *Psychic sexuality: The bio-psychic "anatomy" of sexual energies,* Panta Rei/Crossroads Press, 1998/2014 Psychic *sexuality,* Panta Rei, [Crossroads Press digital edition] Retrieved from Amazon.com Kindle Reader location 1174.

15 F.D. O'Byrne, Translator and author of the Introduction, *Reichenbach's letters on od and magnetism:* Published for the first time in English, with extracts from his own works, so as to make a complete presentation of the Odic Theory. London, 1952 From the introduction, p. xxxii.

16 O'Byrne, p. lii.

17 Ibid., p. 30.

18 Eisenberg, David, MD, *Encounters with Qi: Exploring Chinese medicine,* Norton & Norton, New York, NY, 1985.

19 Swann, Ingo, *Psychic sexuality: The bio-psychic "anatomy" of sexual energies,* Panta Rei/Crossroads Press, 1998/2014 Psychic *sexuality,* Panta Rei, [Crossroads Press digital edition] Retrieved from Amazon.com Kindle Reader location 951.

20 Smith, Suzzy, *ESP and Hypnosis,* Excel Press, iUniverse, Lincoln, NE, p. 17.

21 Avila, Elena, *Woman who glows in the dark: A curandera reveals traditional Aztec secrets of physical and spiritual health,* Penguin Putnam, New York, 2000, p.58.

22 Avila, p.60.

23 David Robertson writes in his article "From Epidauros to Lourdes: A history of healing by faith" about an Irishman named Greatlakes: As cited in "Healing in the reformation period: 1400 -1700," http://www.voiceofhealing.info/02history/reformation.html

24 See also Swann, Ingo, *Psychic sexuality," Amazon* Kindle, location 96.

25 See https://en.wikipedia.org/wiki/Franz_Mesmer

26 Wilhelm Reich, Archives of the Orgone Institute.

27 Coopersmith, Jennifer, *Energy, the subtle concept: The discovery of Feynman's blocks from Leibniz to Einstein,* Oxford University Press, pp. 19-22.

28 Swann, Ingo, *Psychic sexuality: The bio-psychic "anatomy" of sexual energies* Panta Rei/Crossroads Press, 1998/2014 Psychic *sexuality,* Panta Rei, [Crossroads Press digital edition] Retrieved from Amazon.com Kindle Reader location 1349.

Section II
Internal Energy in Traditional Medicine

The Traditional, the Controversial,

and the Innovative

Those who disobey the laws of Heaven and Earth have a lifetime of calamities while those who follow the laws remain free from dangerous illness.

— The Yellow Emperor's Classic of Medicine [1]

II

Internal Energy in Traditional Chinese Medicine

The Traditional, the Controversial, and the Innovative

Introduction to Section II

*I*n our search for clues that might reveal the meaning of "internal energy," numerous approaches will be considered. Many of those involve the individual's ability to direct conscious control over their subtle life force, or "internal energy." For example, attention directed to cues in the body might be employed as a biofeedback technique. Relying on that feedback, practitioners believe they can control their flow of internal energy. Their aim is to direct that energetic force for self-healing, energetic meditation, energetic yoga, and other purposes. Other sections will consider the influence of one's posture on energy. There, through yogic posture and exercises, such as "standing practice," it will be considered whether one's physical orientation might influence the flow of "energy" within the body.

In the present section, our focus is on the unconscious governing of the body's internal energy. This aspect of our quest considers the body-mind energy management that falls within the purview of traditional Chinese systems of healing. These systems are concerned with the "energy" that is known in Chinese as *qi* (氣).

Both the principles and techniques that comprise traditional Chinese medicine (TCM) provide numerous clues to the meaning of internal energy. The traditional TCM literature describes how *qi* energy transforms and flows within the body to govern one's lifespan and vitality. For these reasons, TCM provides an excellent hunting ground for investigating the meaning of the *life* force.

Some of the material that follows is controversial. Although classical models of TCM will be covered, we will also challenge some of its primary assumptions. For example, we will consider alternative ways to think about the meaning of meridians, which is the TCM term for the energetic pathways that are said to flow both deep within and on the surface of the body.

As we think about the meaning of internal energy within the TCM framework, alternative, and potentially controversial, questions will be considered. For example, we will ask whether it might be possible that acupuncture — the technique of inserting fine needles into specific points on the body — may have developed independently and outside of China.

Later, we will look at new proposals that might more accurately describe the body's acupuncture meridian network. * There, it will be considered whether the meridians might be understood, not only as imaginary lines that conduct electrical current, but as physically real myofascial structures. According to the model described there, the meridian "channels" will be considered as definable piezoelectric "pathways" that can be demonstrated through dissection.

* See note on the mixed use of the terms "channel" and "meridian" that is included in Chapter One.

The conventional narrative will be challenged in other ways. For example, we will also consider to what extent these myofascial tracks might function as gateways to advanced consciousness and, perhaps, higher dimensions. As the reader may infer, many of these proposals push against the accepted boundaries of science. Similarly, and conversely, we will attempt to connect the esoteric and immeasurable to established scientific phenomena. For too long, many practitioners of both modern medicine and TCM have been reluctant to synthesize and harmonize causal and correlative paradigms in their respective practices.

TCM is a health maintenance and therapeutic system with ancient roots. The art's comprehensive approach includes an energetic model that describes health and illness. It also includes prescriptive measures to employ when a person falls ill due to an imbalance in their internal energy. In TCM, health is viewed as the relative balance between various natural influences. Chief among these influences are *yin* and *yang* — terms for opposing energetic forces — and the traditional five element theory, a classification system based on the relationship between the elements of fire, earth, metal, water, and wood.

Yin and Yang:

Shade - Sunny

Female - Male

Winter - Summer

Box 2-1 Attributes of *Yin and Yang*

Chapter 2

Overview of Traditional Chinese Medicine

*T*he TCM canons offer explanations for the role of internal energy in every life process. Some of these describe how food is converted into *qi* within the body, others are concerned with the management of body fluids and blood,[2] and there are those that describe how a traditional physician is able to influence the flow of subtle energy in order to heal body and mind.

However, TCM's central theme is balance. As described in ancient medical manuals, a person's health and longevity are dependent on the proper balance between energetic forces within the body, and one's energetic balance can become destabilized as a response to external (exogenous) or internal (endogenous) forces. In the language of TCM, potentially destabilizing influences that can disturb one's energetic balance include: excess heat, false heat, deficient *yin*, excess *yang*, cold, wind invasion, and dampness. In these cases, the individual's unconsciously managed energetic balance has been disturbed and requires an intervention. The role of the TCM healer is to help the patient restore their energetic balance.

There are many tools available to the TCM practitioner to accomplish this goal. These include balancing the patient's energy through acupuncture, the use of suction cups to draw excess heat from the body, massage and prescriptive yoga to influence the therapeutic flow of internal energy, and the use of medicinal herbs.

The treatises defining TCM also describe how the visceral organs consume, assimilate, and transform nutrients and air into bodily fluids and internal *nei qi* (內氣). The traditional language describing the relationships between visceral organs is metaphorical, and models the relationships between the emperor, his ministers, and court officials. For example, the heart is traditionally viewed as the "emperor organ," which is protected by the *xinbao,* or pericardium, and which is classically regarded as the heart's (emperor's) ambassador. Likewise, the lung is considered the prime minister, the liver the general, and the stomach, the minister of granaries, and so forth. The following description of organ relationships from the 200 BCE classic *Guanzi* captures the flavor of the traditional organ system:

The heart is the emperor of the human body. Its subordinate officers are in charge of the nine orifices and their related functions. As long as the heart remains on its rightful path, the nine orifices will follow along and function properly. If the heart's desires become abundant, however, the eyes will lose their sense of color, and the ears will lose their sense of sound. Thus, it is said: "Keep your heart empty -- this is the art of the heart through which the orifices can be mastered." [3]

Overview of Foundational Theories

TCM is comprised of three main components: 1) a complex explanation of life processes, 2) theory of disease, and 3) therapeutic interventions that address imbalance. Of the foundational theories, the aforementioned *yin* and *yang* is the most prominent. As suggested by the contrasts presented in Box 2-1, the *yin-yang* (陰阴) school considers all phenomena to be representations of a particular mix between *yin* and *yang*. In this scheme, *yin* is female, which expresses itself as receptivity, and *yang* as male, or active. Distinctions between *yin* and *yang* can be understood in terms of contrast. For example, topographical features of the earth, such as valleys *(yin)* and mountains *(yang)*, can only manifest because of their relationship to one another. The second-century BCE philosopher Tung Chung-shu informs us how the principles of *yin* and *yang* influence the weather as well as an individual's health and behavior:

> When Heaven is about to make the *Yin* rain down, men fall sick; that is, there is a movement prior to the actual event. It is the *Yin* beginning its complementary response. Also, when Heaven is about to make the *Yin* rain down, men feel sleepy. This is the *qi* of the *Yin*. There is (moreover) melancholy which makes men feel sleepy, this is the effect of *Yin* on *Yin*; and there is delight which keeps men fully awake, this is the *Yang* attracting the *Yang*. At night (the *Yin* time) the waters (a *Yin* element) flood more, by several inches. When there is an east wind, (fermenting) wine froths up more. Sick men are very much worse at night. When dawn is about to break, the cocks all crow and jostle one another; the morning's *qi* invigorates their *jing*. Thus, it is that *Yang* reinforces *Yang*, and *Yin* reinforces *Yin*, and accordingly the (manifestations of the) two *qi* whether *Yang* or *Yin*, can reinforce or diminish each other.

> Heaven has the *Yin* and *Yang*, and so has man. When the *Yin qi* of Heaven and Earth begins (to dominate), the *Yin qi* of man responds by taking the lead also. Or if the *Yin qi* of man begins to advance, the *Yin qi* of Heaven and Earth must by rights respond to it by rising also. Their *Tao* is one. Those who are clear about this (know that) if rain is to come, then the *Yin* must be activated and its influence set to work. If the rain is to stop, then the *Yang* must be activated and its influence set to work. (In fact), there is no reason at all for assuming anything miraculous (lit.,

connected with spirits), *shen* about the causation and onset of rain, though (indeed) its rationale is profoundly mysterious. [4]

Thus, through the lens of *yin* and *yang,* life is the interplay between opposing forces. Applied to traditional medicine, when *yang* becomes too dominant in the body, it manifests as an imbalance of *yang* health issues, such as excessive "liver heat" and restlessness. In contrast, other conditions represent a deficiency of *yin,* such as kidney *"yin deficiency"* that manifests as night sweats and chronic urogenital infections. Alchemist-philosopher Ko Hung's *Pao Po Tzu* states,

> Actually, the best of the *Yin-Yang* techniques can cure minor diseases, and the least of them can prevent debilitation and exhaustion, but that is all it amounts to. There are obvious natural limits to these principles. How on earth could they enable one to summon spirits and immortals, or to turn misfortunes into blessing? [5]

Adopted from the principle of *yin* and *yang* balance in nature, the influence of *yin* is evidenced in winter and represented in both softness and cold. In contrast, the influence of *yang* is evidenced in summer and represented by hardness and heat. Explained by the classical model, life is sustained by the delicate balance between *yin* and *yang*. Too much cold and you'll die; too much heat and you'll die. Thus, the traditional model is one concerned with homeostasis of body-mind.

Five Elements

Another ancient cosmological theory employed in philosophy, medicine, and Chinese martial arts is the *wu xing* (五行), or "five-elements." Sometimes translated as the "five phases," the five-elements are symbolic correlations that date to the earliest written accounts of Chinese philosophy. In many ways, they substitute for what we would today refer to as "cause and effect", and they were most likely derived from, or associated with, magic and superstition.[6] Sinologist Joseph Needham suggests the five-elements served as a "symbolic correlation system," which ancient Chinese shaman relied upon to "carry out their operations that were based on 'coordinative' or 'associative' thinking." This intuitive-associative system developed its own causality and logic. [7]

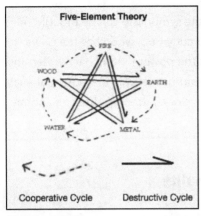

Diagram 2-2

Star-shaped representation of the *wu xing* (五行) or *"Five-Elements."*

Five-Element Theory

As the term suggests, *wu xing* theory comprises five-elements — or phases — that interact through creative and destructive cycles to form the earliest Chinese explanation for how phases ("elements") of nature work together to create the life cycle and other phenomena. Thus, five-element theory describes life as a transformative process from birth to decay and death to rebirth; a cyclic process of "the five types of *qi* dominating at different times." These are represented by symbolic interactions between the elements of water (水), wood (木), fire (火), earth (土), and metal (金), and expressed as either creative or destructive relationships by the five-pointed star configuration shown in Diagram 2-2. Although initiated as a philosophy in ancient times, the five-element theory remains current in many Chinese traditions, from the grouping of foods and tastes (eg, "the five tastes"), to martial arts techniques, and the combinations of acupuncture points that might be selected for treatment.

In some ways comparable to the interplay of the cosmological forces *yin* and *yang,* each element of the five phases either works together with or competes against another to effect "creative" or "destructive" patterns. Represented by the outer line circling the star-shape in Figure 2-2, the creative cycle progresses through the following sequence: fire creates earth, which creates metal, which creates water, which creates wood, which creates fire. The symbolism that forms the five-elements "creative cycle" of causality can be thought about in the following way: fire produces ash (earth), and then, from deep in the earth, metal is produced; from the bowels of the earth, water springs forth and is driven to the surface, which in turn gives birth to the wood of the plants and trees; thus, the wood of the tree becomes tinder for fire, which restarts the cycle.

In contrast, the five-element theory also includes a "destructive" cycle within its cosmology. Illustrated by the solid arrows forming the star shape in Figure 2-2, the destructive path illustrates the interaction between hostile forces. In the context of five-element cosmology, the symbolism can be thought of in the following way: metal can be made to cut wood, wood has the power to bind and hold the earth, earth possesses the power to hold back water, and water has the power to quench fire. This order reveals the potential each element possesses to produce a destructive or controlling effect on another.

The Five-Elements and Personality

An interesting application of the five-element theory is its use as a psychological diagnostic-treatment based on **five seasons**. In this context, the theory purports to explain personality based on five types that correspond approximately to the four seasons as normally understood, but with an additional season that falls between late summer and early fall, that is sometimes called "Indian summer."

Demonstrating how the seasons contribute to personality, the theory offers interventions based on what is traditionally seen as the intimate link between one's psychological balance relative to the "seasons," and how, in turn, this relates to the viscera and organs. These relationships are described in the classic traditional medical text, *The Yellow Emperor's Classic of Medicine:*

> Not so long ago, there were people known as achieved beings who had true virtue, understood the way of life, and were able to adapt to and harmonize with the universe and the seasons. They too were able to keep their mental energy through proper concentration.[8]

More details of the five-element theory applied to personality and emotions is provided in Appendix A.

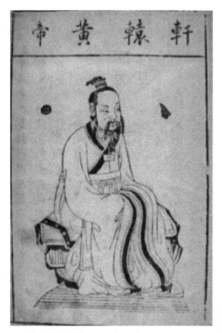

Figure 2-3

Cover of the Yellow Emperor's *Classic of Medicine*

The *Huangdi Neijing*

The Yellow Emperor's Classic of Medicine, or *Huangdi Neijing* (黄帝内経), is considered the single most important canon of acupuncture and traditional medicine (Figure 2-3). The text includes the earliest description of psychosomatic medicine, and it explains how excessive emotions lead to physical disease, even though such an understanding of how one's psychology could impact physical health did not emerge in the West until the 1950s.[9][10] Contributing a description of how *qi* transforms in the body, as well as providing a system of diagnosis and discussion regarding the nature of acupuncture points, the *Classic* is attributed to the legendary first, or "Yellow," emperor of China, Huangdi. The text purports to be a record of the discussion of medicine between the emperor and his minister of medicine, Qi Bo. Due to its importance as a medical text, both historically and currently, it is useful to devote a few paragraphs to the work.

Often abbreviated as the *Neijing*, scholars disagree as to the dating of the *Classic*. Some popular sources date the text at around 5,000 years, while others, including the renowned sinologist Joseph Needham, trace the origins of the text to around the first century CE. Another scholar, James Curran, writing in the *British Journal of Medicine*, describes the Yellow Emperor Huangdi as a semi-mythical figure, and argues that the text is most likely a compilation of several authors. Incidentally, Curran believes that the text was written around 300 BCE.[11]

Regardless of the works provenance, the description of *qi* energy and the therapeutic methods outlined in the *Neijing* have since become foundational to TCM. Primary among the guidelines that the *Classic* offers is the instruction that it is best to address a problem before it manifests as a disease. As Needham points out, many of the analogies contained in the text juxtapose the role of the physician with that of a political leader. For example, it advises that disharmonies, whether political or physical, are best nipped in the bud. These principles are expressed through the perennial wisdom of the physician-sage, who "treats illness before, not after, it has arisen." The principle is reflected in the *Neijing's* admonishment, "to administer drugs after the illness has developed, or to impose order after disorder has developed, is like digging a well when one feels thirsty, or casting daggers in the midst of battle. Is that not too late?"[12]

The *Neijing* includes a description of how the *qi* travels through acupuncture meridians, or *jing luo* (経絡). It also informs the reader that *jen qi,* (真氣) or "true *qi*" is the *qi* of one's innate constitution. Among other notable points presented in the *Neijing* is the description of *wei qi* (衛氣), or "protective *qi*." This form of *qi* circulates along the body surface during the day and inside the body at night. Furthermore, the main purpose of *wei qi* is to provide an outer protective layer for the body, which serves as a protection against pathogens, particularly those of the *exogenous* class.

The Organ System

As described in TCM, the body's visceral organs, although classified as *yin* or *yang*, are further divided into categories of *zang* or *fu*. *Fu* organs are *yang* in nature; they are considered "hollow," and are concerned with the digestion of food and the elimination of waste. The *fu* organs are the urinary bladder, gallbladder, stomach, large intestine, small intestine, and an "organ system" that doesn't have correspondence in conventional physiology, referred to as the "triple warmer."

In contrast, *zang* organs are *yin* in nature; they are considered "solid" and are concerned with the regulation of *qi* and blood. *Zang* organs are the heart, kidney, spleen, lungs, liver, and the pericardium (often referred to as the "heart constrictor", and also considered an "organ" in the Chinese system). Each *zang* organ is assigned a specific task related to transformation and governance of the body's *qi* energy and blood. TCM describes the function of the *zang* organs in the following way: the heart is the "emperor organ" and dominates the heart and mind, while the pericardium is considered the ambassador and "protects the heart." The spleen works with the stomach to digest food and maintain physical strength, and the liver promotes the movement of *qi* in the body. The role of the kidneys is to control reproduction and store sexual essence, while the lungs control dispersal and "descent" of *qi*.

Diagnosis

TCM includes novel ways of diagnosing imbalances. Principle among these is the reading of the "pulses." TCM diagnosis includes six locations for palpating the pulse, with three on each wrist. The nature of each pulse informs the diagnostician of the conditions of the patient's internal organs and *qi* status. Pulses are evaluated based on twenty-nine different types and qualities, such as "floating," "deep," "hidden," "knotted," "slippery," and so on.

An additional diagnostic method employed by TCM practitioners involves observing the tongue, on the basis that its appearance, along with other associated symptoms, is useful when diagnosing. For example, if the patient presents a pale complexion, pasty white tongue, and weakness in the extremities, these are indications of *yin*-deficiency disease.

Acupuncture and Other Energetic Treatments

After the patient is diagnosed in terms of *yin* and *yang*, along with the other axes of diagnosis (inner vs outer, hot vs cold, full vs. empty), various therapies are applied to restore balance. In some cases, acupuncture -- the placing of micro-thin needles into "acupuncture points" -- might be used to "move the *qi*" or to "release stagnant liver energy." (An ancient drawing of acupuncture needles is included in Figure 2-4.) In addition, herbal remedies are often used to help the patient regain harmony and balance. In some cases, other approaches, such as moxibustion might be used to "increase *yang*." [13]

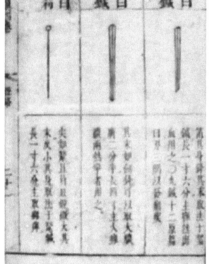

Figure 2-4
Ancient Drawings
of Acupuncture Needles,
Source: *Wikipedia Commons*

Meridians

According to traditional theory, internal energy in the form of *zang-fu qi* — the internal energy of the organs — travels through the body along pathways called *meridians* or "channels." ** As evidenced by silk books discovered in a famous archeological dig of what became known as the *Mawangdui* tombs, the meridians have been present in Chinese medicine practices since ancient times. In that discovery, it was revealed that these aspects of TCM date back to at least the second century BCE. [14]

** See the note concerning the use of "channel" and "meridian," and sometimes the adjective "myofascial," included in Chapter One.

Theory of Disease

According to TCM, a disease can be either "external" or "internal." External causes, called *exogenous,* are those that arise from the environment. Examples of exogenous influences are wind, cold, dryness, and heat. By contrast, a disease originating from internal sources is considered *endogenous*. Diseases in this category are generated from emotional imbalance.

According to TCM theory, excessive or imbalanced emotions harm the organ associated with that particular emotion. Examples of excessive emotions harming one's health include the idea that excess joy or giddiness can damage the heart, grief can damage the lungs, fear can damage the kidney, dwelling (obsession) can damage the spleen, and anger can damage the liver.

Viewed from the perspective of traditional theory, each of the "solid" organs has specific responsibilities related to the manufacture and governance of the body's *nei qi* internal energy, and this is one aspect of a broad description of the body's energetic physiology that has no equivalent in Western physiology. Consider the "*qi* of the kidneys," which relates not only to the subtle bio-energy involved in the organ proper, but also to the body's general vitality, including healthy sexual function. However, the influence of kidney energy goes beyond organ and sexual function, and includes aspects of physiology far removed from the organ itself. For example, in Chinese medical terms, "weak kidney function" could present (particularly in males) as chronic knee "coldness," and general weakness or pain. It could perhaps even manifest as dysfunction in hearing, all of which may be diagnosed in terms of kidney *qi* deficiency. In this scenario, weak kidney *qi* could have a pernicious influence on the knees, but also lead to chronic problems with the lower back and hip. Demonstrating the relationship between a problematic knee, lower back pain, and other symptoms associated with kidney *qi* deficiency, it is not uncommon for the root cause to be attributed to excessive sexual release.

Chapter 3

Acupuncture and the Energy Channels

*T*here are a number of TCM therapeutic interventions, including herbal prescriptions, massage, and moxibustion (the burning of the herb mugwort on targeted acupuncture locations). However, acupuncture remains the most well-known.

TCM therapies, such as acupuncture and massage, are designed to interact with the body's energetic channels. Their purpose is to promote or inhibit the flow of *qi* within the visceral organs and /or energetic pathways. Depending on how they are counted, there are either twelve main channels and eight extra channels, † or fourteen main channels and six extra vessels. Diagram 2-6 illustrates the lung channel.

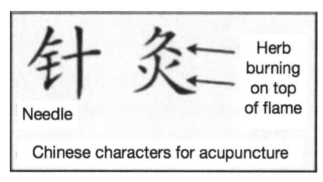

Needle

Herb burning on top of flame

Chinese characters for acupuncture

Box 2-5

† The "extra channels" circulate the *jing* essence throughout the body, and form what Maciocia calls a "genetic blueprint" for the body. Thus, they serve as the connection between *xian tian earlier* heaven and *ho tian later* heaven *qi* energy. (More on pre- and post/earlier and later heaven in Section V) [15]

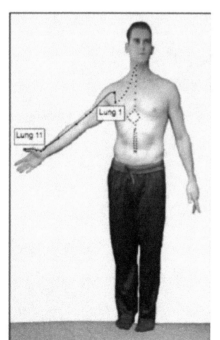

The Body's Bio-energetic Network

Today, acupuncture is popular all over the world, and regarded by many as an effective, low risk, and low-cost method of managing pain and rebalancing the body's "energy." Part-art and part-science, acupuncture involves the placement of micro-thin needles into specific locations on the surface of the body, referred to as *xue* (穴) (diagram 2-7) or "acupoints," that lay along the energetic meridian lines.

Diagram 2-6

**Deep and Surface Aspects
of Lung Channel**

What is an Acupuncture Point?

The traditional medical text *Lingshu Jing* (靈樞經) describes the nodal (acupuncture) points as places where spirit and energy may enter or leave.[16] Arising from their interest in parapsychology, some scientists in the former Soviet Union studied the body's energy system in the context of what they termed bio-plasma. Their research documented the existence of acupuncture points through their use of a low-resistance measuring device called a Tobioscope. Subsequent investigators were able to obtain similar objective evidence to support the existence of acupuncture points, based upon electrical conduction and resistance at the designated locations.

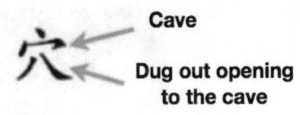

Diagram 2-7

Deconstruction of the Chinese character for "Location," or an Acupuncture Point

Evidence for Acupuncture Points

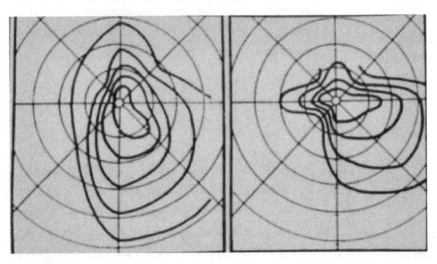

Figure 2-8

Mapping the conductivity of acupuncture points

Borrowed from Robert Becker, MD, *The Body Electric*

A milestone for researchers demonstrating that acupuncture had "an objective basis in reality" was Robert Becker's documentation of the environs surrounding acupuncture points. Suggesting that acupuncture was based on more than simply belief or placebo, Becker was the first in the West to demonstrate that acupuncture points possessed distinctive differences in polarity compared to their surroundings, and that the acupuncture meridians conducted currents. Becker also demonstrated that meridians conducted a direct current flow of bio-electrical energy into the central nervous system.

Becker describes his observations of acupuncture points and meridians:

> Our readings indicated that the meridians were conducting current,
> and its polarity, matching the input side of the two-way system we'd
> charted in amphibians, showed a flow into the central nervous system.

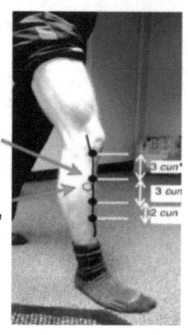

Traditional location of acupuncture point St-36 (Stomach 36)

Approximate location of OT36 (Omura's True 36) About 1.5 cm from traditional St-36

Diagram 2-9
Lower Aspect of the Stomach Acupuncture Channel / Meridian

Each point was positive compared to its environs, and each one had a field surrounding it, with its own characteristic shape. We even found a fifteen-minute rhythm in the current strength at the points, superimposed on the circadian ("about a day") rhythm we'd found a decade earlier in the overall DC [direct current] system. It was obvious by then that at least the major parts of the acupuncture charts had, as the jargon goes, "an objective basis in reality." [17]

Since Becker's early work supporting the objective reality of the meridians and their points, acupuncture has been subjected to extensive scientific investigation in both the East and West. To date, thousands of clinical trials have been conducted examining the efficacy of acupuncture and moxibustion. Noteworthy is the investigation by a biophysicist, Maria Reichmanis, who demonstrated that the meridians possessed measurable bio-electrical attributes, and that acupuncture lines acted as low-resistance pathways for the flow of electricity. [18] [19]

Acupuncture Point Characteristics

Relying on a sophisticated variation of muscle testing, Yoshiaki Omura, MD, PhD, studied acupuncture point characteristics, making use of an applied kinesiology technique that he himself developed, known as the "Bi-digital O Ring Test" (BDORT). [20] Omura reports that most points contain high concentrations of neurotransmitters and hormones, including acetylcholine, methionine-enkephalin, beta-endorphin, Adrenocorticotropic hormone, secretin, cholecystokinin, norepinephrine, serotonin, and GABA. [21]

Point Location Controversies

At this juncture, it is useful to consider that there are sometimes different descriptions of acupuncture point locations, and sometimes major differences between acupuncture charts that map the acupoints. This is especially true of older illustrations, as there wasn't an organized attempt at standardizing acupuncture charts until after China's communist revolution, when the new government focused on standardization.

As an example of variation in point descriptions, consider the location of one of the body's most studied acupuncture points, Stomach 36 (St-36). Shown in Diagram 2-9, the point lies laterally and below the knee. Compare this traditional location to the point that can be referred to as Omura's Stomach 36, or OTS-36 (Omura's True Stomach 36). The following is part of a discussion on the apparent disparity between these two locations for St-36, from an article published in the *Journal of Acupuncture and Electrotherapy Research*:

> At the anatomical location of ST 36 described in traditional textbooks, Omura found there is no acupuncture point. However, in the close vicinity, there is an acupuncture point which he named as true ST 36 in the mid-1980s, but it is generally known as Omura's ST 36. When the effects of the acupuncture on these 2 locations were compared, Omura's ST 36 produced very significant well-known acupuncture beneficial effects including improved circulation and blood chemistry, while in the traditional ST 36, the effects were small. [22]

The Meridians: The Body's Energy Pathways

Some researchers propose that the meridians function to unify the body's bio-electric network. For example, James Oschman, in *Energy Medicine*, describes the body's acupuncture meridian system as a "continuously interconnected semiconductor electronic network."[23] This proposal suggests that the body operates as a "hard-wired" system that is not only very fast and extensive within the body, but also possesses a form of intelligence necessary to manage "traffic" within the system.

Two attributes define the meridians; these are the deep and surface aspects. The surface aspects are those lying near the surface of the skin, which can be accessed through acupuncture and massage. The image shown in Diagram 2-6 illustrates the complete lung meridian, including both deep internal lines (broken lines), along with the surface aspect of the meridians (solid lines). Note that although the diagram depicts only the right side of the lung meridian, the twelve meridians are all located bilaterally.

In Diagram 2-6, the surface aspect of the lung meridian is represented by the solid line, which begins under the clavicle (Lung 1) and travels down the inside of the arm to the thumb (Lung 11). Deeper pathways of the meridian, indicated by broken lines in the drawing, reflect the meridian's pathway, which begins in the stomach and then descends to the small intestine, before reversing direction to ascend and enter the lungs (from which the name of the pathway is derived). From there, the lung meridian in the core of the body continues its upward journey to the side of the throat, and then descends to the surface of the body to the previously described point Lung 1.

Studying the interaction between the surface and sub-surface route of the lung channel provides an insight into why some points on the surface of the meridian have uses unrelated to the depiction of the line shown on surface-only charts. For example, pricking, or sharp pressing, of the medial aspect of the thumb next to the inner cuticle (Lung 11) is a reliable treatment -- and at an early stage, often provides immediate relief -- of acute lateral sore throat.

While this application would not make sense if one were only to consider the surface aspect of the channel, the deeper aspect of the meridian justifies the intervention.

"Energy Transfer" During Acupuncture Treatment?

Since traditional Chinese medicine is based on the notion of *qi* energy, it is natural to ask whether it might be possible for an acupuncturist, or another therapist, to augment a patient's energy by donating their own. One dramatic study suggesting that this might be possible has been undertaken by Professor Myeong Soo Lee.

In Lee's study, investigators compared the results of acupuncturists using bare hands in needle application to those using electrical shielding gloves. The study involved the Stomach 36 acupuncture point, and the results showed that acupuncture applied by therapists with non-shielded hands produced significantly higher immune system responses in the patient. In the published paper, Lee suggested that what he calls "bioenergy *(qi)* transfer" acts as an "electromotive force, which is purported to remove the stagnation or blockage of energy and restore an equilibrium state." [24]

The Origin of Acupuncture

Several popular Chinese stories describe the genesis of acupuncture, one of which concerns a Chinese general on an ancient battlefield. According to the story, at a crucial moment during a battle, the general's arm was pierced at a specific acupoint, and, to his amazement, his toothache was cured. Thus, the art of acupuncture was born.

Despite being associated chiefly with the ancient Chinese, acupuncture was also practiced in ancient Egypt. Dating back as far as 1,500 BCE, [25] Egyptian literature describes the placing of needles as a form of medical intervention. When also taking into account the "golden needle" technique of ancient Tibetan culture, it appears an argument could be made that the use of acupuncture points and meridians did not originate in Asia, and that other ancient cultures possessed the ability to intuit the subtle energy lines, or "channels", on the surface of the body, and had knowledge of the therapeutic use of acupoints. Examples of acupuncture-like techniques found elsewhere include the Bantus of Africa, and in particular those of South Africa, who practice a healing art that involves scratching specific areas of the skin to treat illness. There is also at least one Brazilian tribe that is known to treat illness by shooting tiny arrows from a blowpipe at specific locations on the patient's body. [26]

Perhaps the most famous evidence supporting a non-Chinese genesis of acupuncture emerged with the discovery of the "Ice Man." The mummified remains of the Ice Man, named Oetzi by archeologists, were found in an alpine valley between Austria and Italy in 1991, after his remains were revealed by a melting glacier. Researchers examining Oetzi's corpse found tattooed marks on what experts determined to be significant acupuncture points, as the markings, made by a mixture of charcoal and crystal, were placed on locations relevant to stomach and back disorders. Further evidence of the markings acting as location points came in the form of x-ray results, which suggested that the Ice Man had suffered from ailments for which the marked points would have been appropriate treatments.[27]

Multiple and Competing Theories

Acupuncture is largely thought of as a monolithic system handed down from a single source, but in reality, acupuncture medicine, much like traditional Chinese martial arts systems, derives from hundreds of family lines, many of which hold conflicting theories. In the twentieth century, the Communist government of Mainland China began to standardize traditional medicine into its present form, a process described by Dr. Henry McCann in an article published in the *Journal of Chinese Medicine*:

> The seemingly homogenous model of Chinese medicine known as "Traditional Chinese Medicine" (TCM) is the product of a twentieth-century synthesis of many approaches to Chinese medicine that was created in response to many factors, including the near decline of Chinese medicine under the Kuomintang government, ‡ the needs of administering inexpensive medical care to a vast Chinese population after the Communist revolution, and the People's Republic of China's (PRC) desire to have TCM mimic modern western scientific models of research design and education.[28]
>
> > ‡The Kuomintang (KMT), also called the Nationalist Party, is a political party founded in 1912 by Sun Yat-sen. From 1927 to 1948, it was led by Chiang Kai-shek, and played a major role in Mainland China's history. After losing the Civil War to the forces of the Communist Party (CCP), it retreated to Taiwan, where it was the ruling party until 2016, when the presidency was won by Tsai Ing-wen of the Democratic Progressive Party.

Acupuncture Comes to the West

Literature describing acupuncture as a healing art is generally considered to have been introduced to the West by the French Jesuits in the 1600s. However, it is interesting to note that the first mention of acupuncture in Western literature is not provided by the Jesuits, but by the Portuguese adventurer Fernand Mendez. In 1542, Mendez, writing in his journal, *Fingimentos*, made reference to the practice while documenting his voyage to Japan. However, the first monograph on the subject was indeed authored by the Jesuits, and published in France in *Secrets de la Medicine des Chinois* (1771). [29]

When modern Western medicine first encountered acupuncture, early attempts at defining the art's mechanism for relieving pain focused on the technique as a placebo, with explanations that ranged from psychological suggestion to hypnosis.[30] [31] In the 1960s, Wall and Melzack's "gate theory" of pain was widely applied as an explanation for acupuncture's ability to moderate pain through analgesia brought about by the interaction of competing neurons.

In the 1970s, researchers proposed a new model to account for at least some of the benefits of acupuncture, explaining those in terms of endorphin release.[32] In the same decade, another researcher, Dr. David Bressler, Director of UCLA's Acupuncture Research Project, reported that his clinic had administered acupuncture to more than 18,000 patients, employing the technique as the "sole analgesic agent" in major surgeries. Furthermore, the technique was successfully used to treat conditions from bronchial asthma to hearing loss, and even as an intervention to mitigate addiction to heroin and smoking. Bressler reports that the therapy has a normalizing effect – raising when low and lowering when high – on leukocytes and lymphocytes (different types of white blood cells). Acupuncture was also used to great effect in the treatment of horses, cats, and dogs, yet still its underlying mechanism remained a mystery.[33] In a 1975 paper, Bressler states:

> Although most informed observers now acknowledge the fact that acupuncture is a highly effective technique for treating acute and chronic pain and other disorders, there remains a great deal of disagreement as to the procedures necessary for achieving effective therapy results.

Dr. Bressler supported his point with examples of the kinds of research his team conducted at UCLA:

> [Our research is based on] the results of over 18,000 patient treatments by traditional Chinese, modern Chinese, Korean, Japanese and Western acupuncturists. We have performed several major surgical procedures using acupuncture as the sole analgesic agent and have investigated its usefulness in the treatment of bronchial asthma, sensoral-neural hearing loss, obesity, cigarette smoking, and heroin addiction.[34]

In the same report, Bressler details how his UCLA clinic had, with the participation of veterinarians, conducted studies on the effectiveness of acupuncture in the treatment of a "wide variety of disorders in dogs, cats, and horses." However, despite the impressive results that these studies produced, an "energy" explanation that might reveal why the technique is sometimes so effective was not forthcoming.

In the 1980s, two of the most promising explanations for how acupuncture worked were gate control theory, and the suggestion that the analgesic effects of acupuncture could be understood in terms of endorphin release. These were explained to me first-hand when I assisted with the treatment of pain patients under Dr. James Feld. During a period that I was working at Feld's office in Southern California, I met a young medical doctor who would visit and assist with patients as part of his residency training. During the period, we would often discuss acupuncture and how the technique worked. On one particular day, his interest was especially piqued. He excitedly told me about how (at the time) new theories of endorphin release seemed to explain the underlying mechanism of needling therapy. However, when I asked him how these might account for some of the rehabilitation applications of acupuncture, he appeared to be at a loss. As chance would have it, a particular patient arrived for an appointment at just that moment.

The patient, an architect by profession, had some years before suffered a traumatic spine injury, which affected his ability to walk normally. Unable to effect an orthodox walking gait, he moved by stepping one foot forward and dragging his weaker leg behind. This patient's arrival was the perfect opportunity to demonstrate what I meant by the rehabilitation benefits of acupuncture, and I invited the visiting physician to observe as I began the session.

The acupuncture treatment involved a few classic leg-strengthening points, and, as was typical of this particular patient, it immediately triggered a leg shaking spasm that continued for several minutes. As he watched on, the young doctor seemed to grow increasingly perplexed, and his apparent confusion only intensified at the conclusion of the appointment, when the formerly foot-dragging architect hopped off the exam table and walked out of the room *sans drag*. Neither gate control nor endorphin theory could explain the rehabilitation effect that the young doctor had just witnessed, I don't recall him saying another word to me for the rest of the morning.

The gate control and endorphin theories that were described by the doctor are just two of many proposed explanations that have been put forward over the last four decades, as researchers have attempted to uncover the mechanism that might explain why the technique has been so effective in some cases. In the published paper cited earlier, Bressler includes a list of some of the other methods that were investigated by the UCLA research project:

> Traditional [energy and] meridian [channel] notions, gate control [theory of pain] simple reflex notions, neurophysiological interference theories, holographic theories,[35] autonomic theories, a variety of biochemical explanations, and a host of psychological theories (including hypnosis explanations). [36]

Later, Bressler discusses what remains a perennial frustration for investigators searching for a meaningful description of acupuncture's underlying mechanism. He writes: "These theories do not provide a comprehensive rationale for achieving effective therapeutic results, and the practitioner is often left mystified." [37]

Since there continues to be a lack of an explanation for "energy technologies," it is time to consider new theories that might begin to explain the elusive, sometimes powerful, underlying healing principle that enables acupuncture and other "energetic" practices to work.

Chapter 4

Ether and an Expanded Physics

*R*ecently, some investigators have speculated that the body's "energy," and its interaction with energetic meridians, might be understood in the context of a theoretical substance called *ether*. For example, physician Richard Gerber, MD, who uses "energy medicine" in his medical practice, believes that "energetic meridians play a role in connecting the etheric body with the physical body," forming what Gerber calls a "physical-etheric interface." In other words, he sees a link between the physical body and the intangible aspects of consciousness and intelligence.[38]

In Western medicine, use of the term *ether* can be traced to the sixteenth century Swiss physician Paracelsus (1493 – 1541), who believed that humans were connected to the heavens through a "subtle pervasive fluid." Paracelsus believed that *ether* possessed magnetic qualities, and he described the subtle fluid as a vital force that was not contained inside an individual, but, rather, radiated around them "like a luminous sphere which could be made to act at a distance." [39]

The most well-known Western physician to employ techniques designed to address the body's *etheric* subtle energy field was Franz Mesmer. As a famed pioneer of hypnosis, Mesmer believed that a universal fluid, which he referred to as *fluidum*, filled the universe and acted as an invisible connection between individuals.[40]

Harold Burr (1889-1973) was another who offered scientific evidence to support the idea of an etheric field. In the 1940s, Burr discovered, first with plants and later with salamanders, that an electric field surrounded all living things, and he documented several fascinating aspects of the "etheric" energy field in his research. For example, he observed that the electrical field of plant seedlings did not resemble the seedling itself, but the adult plant.[41] This discovery was later supported by Semyon Kirlian's "electrographic photography," which lead to the development of Kirlian photography and the ability to photograph the "energy fields" around living things.[42] Here, Gerber discusses the "etheric body" further:

> In the metaphysical literature, the energy field that surrounds and pen-
> etrates living systems is referred to as the "etheric body." It is said the
> etheric body is one of many bodies contributing to final expression of

the human form. The etheric body, in all likelihood, is an energy interference pattern similar to a hologram.[43]

The Meridians Considered in Light of Expanded Physics

Now our search for clues into the nature of "internal energy" takes a more extreme turn toward the theoretical, as we push against the boundaries of accepted science. This chapter considers the possible role of meridians as an "embedded antenna network," and as a possible link to other dimensions.

Recent modeling of the physics of acupuncture points and meridians by Stanford University *Professor Emeritus* William Tiller suggests new ways of thinking about the meridians, and two aspects of Tiller's models are introduced here. The first proposes that acupuncture points and meridians operate in concert with a special form of bio-electricity, while the second posits that acupuncture points and meridians may function as an embedded antenna array.

The first of these proposals is the radical theory that the functionality of acupuncture points and meridians can be explained through their interface between known and yet-to-be-identified forms of electromagnetic (EM) energy. Tiller suggests that this unidentified form of electromagnetism exists beyond Maxwell's four linear partial differential equations; the equations that currently define EM field properties.

Tiller's proposal is explained through what he calls an *expanded gauge symmetry*. He suggests that the bio-electromagnetism of humans, and perhaps all vertebrates, may be quite different from EM as normally considered where, according to Tiller, "the magnetic monopole charge is experimentally accessible." [44] He describes the theoretical modeling of an acupuncture point in the following way:

Diagram 2-10

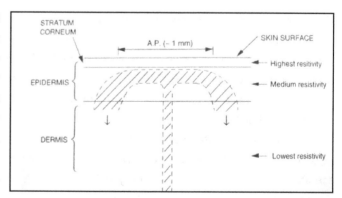

Schematic illustration of ion pumping along the meridian locus via chi-induced A(t) field followed by a fountain-like broadening of excess ions at the skin surface. Tiller explains this broadening of high conductivity zone at the acupuncture point (AP) satisfies the conditions needed for an antenna transmission / reception at the AP.

Subtle energy wave flow along the etheric meridians yields a transduced flow of magnetic vector potential, * A, waves along the physical locus of these meridian channels (sometimes nerve fibers).

Such A-flow means an electric field, E, is generated along this channel, which pumps ions along the channel[45] and, if large enough, produces electrolytic dissociation of water (H20 ⊠ H+OH) to greatly increase the ionic conductance of the channel and increase the electrical conductivity of the AP at the skin surface (as is observed).

Because the surface of the skin blocks the continued outward passage of ions, they must fan outwards in a radial direction, much like a fountain, and then work their way back into the sub-epidermal tissue while recombining (H+ + OH→ H2O), since they are no longer in the high field region.

The size of the charge fountainhead is appreciably larger in diameter than the channel of charge feeding into the surface, so the conditions needed for EM radiation emission and reception are fulfilled by the AP, and the charge patterns will certainly function as a monopole antenna with overtones of helical character, ** depending upon the detailed shape of the fountainhead.

From William Tiller, William, Science and Human Transformation

* Transduced flow of magnetic vector potential. Note the principle of transduction is described in Section XII.

** Pertaining to a characteristic helix shape

As Tiller explains, gauge theory represents "a new synthesis of quantum mechanics and symmetry, wherein gauge invariance is recognized as the physical principle governing the fundamental forces between all elementary particles. Such invariance must be satisfied for all observable quantities to ensure that any arbitrariness A and [electrical potential] do not affect the field strength." [46]

Tiller suggests that a presently undetectable bio-electromagnetism may be associated with acupuncture points and meridians, and, as introduced above, that the function of acupuncture points and meridians can be better understood as an **interaction** between a known and a hitherto undocumented form of electromagnetism.

The idea that a special kind of bio-electromagnetism might exist, and that it could one day contribute to our understanding of "energetic" healing, such as acupuncture, is compelling. If proven accurate, the theory could account for observations that researchers have long noted concerning the unusual relationship between *qigong (ch'i kung)* / internal energy masters, and electricity.

One account of the sometimes strange relationship between electricity and *qi* was documented by David Eisenberg. As a medical exchange student in China, Eisenberg described his interaction with a particular *qi* master, telling of how the master provided him with a roasted pork lunch, which was prepared right in front of him. Shockingly, Eisenberg says, the master cooked the lunch while holding bare and live electrical wires in his hands, and yet suffered no apparent injury. [47]

---

† Dr. Tiller defines ether in the following way:
Ether: Sanskrit akash. Though not considered a factor in present scientific theory on the nature of the material universe, ether has for millenniums been so referred to by India's sages. Paramahansa Yogananda spoke of ether as the background on which God projects the cosmic motion picture of creation. Space gives dimension to objects; ether separates the images. This "background," a creative force that coordinates all spectral vibrations, is a necessary factor when considering the subtler forces - thought and life energy (prana) – and the nature of space and the origin of material forces and matter.

William Tiller, Science and Human Transformation

The Interface Between Bio-physics and the Etheric

The second part of Tiller's proposal suggests that the acupuncture meridians function as an embedded antenna system. Arguments in support of this idea are extrapolated from the known attributes of acupuncture points, which, according to Tiller, possess the requirements necessary to function as an antenna (Diagram 2-10).

Tiller proposes that the acupoints and meridians function as an interface between known bio-physics and an "other-dimensional," undefined "etheric" energy. Tiller writes that the acupuncture and meridian system "are located at the etheric † substance level rather than at the physical substance level to explain the lack of major histological difference between A.P.s and surrounding tissue."

Another Perspective on the Meaning of "Balance"

Dr. Tiller describes the electrical resistance properties of acupuncture points:

It is now well known that an electrical resistance of about 50,000 ohms exists between any two A.P.s [acupuncture points], while, over the same length of normal skin, the equivalent resistance is a factor of [about] 20 times higher. Most of this resistance is in the outer surface of the skin (called the stratum corneum ....) This A.P. resistivity changes strongly with hypnogogic state [the state just before falling to sleep], increasing by a factor of [about] 2-3 during sleep and, in the case of emotional excitation, the [resistance of the] points are observed to increase in the area. . . (As Helms points out),[48] A.P.s are situated in the surface depressions located along the cleavage planes between two or more muscles. They are located in a vertical column of **loose connective tissue** which is surrounded by the thick and dense connective tissue of the skin... ‡

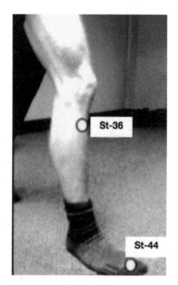

Diagram 2-11
Stomach Meridian Acupuncture Points Stomach 36 and Stomach 44
No significant histological differences have been discovered between acupuncture points

‡ Emphasis added. Note the description of acupuncture points being located in "loose connective tissue." This is an important point that will be returned to later in our discussion of myofascial meridians.[49]

As introduced earlier, since they are known to conduct current, the energetic meridians have long been established as having a "basis in physical reality." However, researchers have been unable to discern significant differences between each acupuncture point, which might explain why, for example, while one acupuncture point has one effect, a different point along the same meridian could work in a completely different way. To illustrate, consider two points along what is referred to as the stomach meridian, shown in Figure 2-11. (Another portion of the stomach meridian is illustrated in Figures 2-9.)

These examples demonstrate that there remains no explanation to account for why a point below and to the outside (lateral) of the knee (Acupoint St-36 in Diagram 2-11) is effective for acute stomach/digestion disturbances. Likewise, it is not known why a point along the same channel, located in the webbing between the second and third toe (St-44 on the diagram), is effective for the treatment of acute lateral knee pain. As Tiller explains, other than their location, there is no significant histological difference between the two points. There are hundreds of examples like this, and, at present, knowledge of this kind of body-energy-point information is still predominantly transmitted from one generation to the next through "family" lineages.

However, if Tiller's proposal that acupuncture, along with other energetic healing modalities, operate as an interaction, or exchange, between known EM and EM-like forces and the *ether*, then it is conceivable that these undefined elements may contain sufficient data or "information" to account for differences between various acupuncture points. This subject is explored further in Section XII.

The Acupuncture Meridians and Pathology

Another clue as to the nature of acupuncture points is the way they sometimes respond during needling. Occasionally, during the course of an acupuncture treatment, a therapist inserting a needle into an acupoint will observe that the needle "sets" in the point in a way that "locks," or holds it tightly, in position. Tiller's thoughts on this phenomenon provide more insight into the nature of acupuncture points, their therapeutic use, the body's energetic meridians, and the goal of treatment to establish "energetic balance." In commenting on how pathology affects a particular point in this way, and in light of the proposed new physics of acupuncture points, he describes the phenomenon in terms of a "holding force" that is responsive to the imbalance of "acupuncture circuitry."

> When an acupuncture needle is placed in the appropriate point, a suction-like force holds the needle in place so that, if one tries to withdraw it, the skin pulls up around the needle and it is not easily withdrawn. However, after the needle has remained in the point for the proper length of time so as to bring about a temporary balance to the

circuit, the needle may be withdrawn with no effort and the skin does not pull up around the needle. This suction force, which is probably due to the osmotic pressure difference, ΔP, between the points, seems to be proportional to $\Delta R...$.[50]

Tiller's view supports the traditional TCM concept of health in terms of "energetic balance." He points out how pathology, or "imbalance," in parts of the body's organ and meridian systems results in a *differential* between the left and right sides of the body. He describes the phenomenon in the language of mathematics, where Δ ("delta") refers to **change** in the body's EM field. On this, Tiller observes:

> When measuring the electrical resistance between symmetrical points on the left and right sides of the body, one often finds that the resistance is different in the forward direction (R) than when the electrodes are reversed (R^1) **When a person is healthy relative to the organs associated with that meridian, these two resistances will be the same ($R = R^1$). However, if pathology is developing in one or more of these particular organs, R will be different than R^1.** ($\Delta R = R - R^1 > 0$). * As the degree of pathological advancement increases, the magnitude of ΔR increases. This difference has been called the semiconductor effect which is the electrical correlate of the well-known heat response time difference between APs when pathology is present. [Bold emphasis added] [51]

> *In this formula, Δ = DELTA/ change. *R* = *Resistance* in terms of DC polarity of forward direction of the meridian.

> R^1= *Reverse of direction.* Thus, the formula, $\Delta R = R - R^1 > 0$ variation of resistance, which represents the pathology of the meridian and/or organ system.

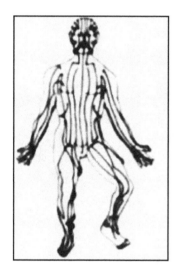

Figure 2-12

William Tiller's Modeling of the Body's Meridian System as an Antenna Array

From William Tiller, *Science and Human Transformation*

Implications for Tiller's Model of Acupuncture Points

Tiller concludes this section of his thesis by describing how the expanded physics of acupuncture points and the meridian network function as an "antennae array."

Accordingly, conventional EM and yet-to-be-observed EM-like *(etheric)* fields together comprise the *antenna array-meridian network* (Figure 2-12). This model suggests that the "external EM and subtle energy environment [presumably the proposed *ether* field] communicate with the internal physical and 'subtle substance' of the body via a network of points on the surface of the body." [52] In other words, the conjectured physics behind acupuncture -- and by extension, other "energetic technology," such as energetic healing, yoga and meditation -- involves a relationship between known and unknown cross-dimensional interactions.

The model proposes that the meridians operate as a mechanism that communicates between / interacts with the EM and the subtle "etheric" energies outside and inside the body. [53] Furthermore, the notion of the meridians as a sending / receiving system suggests that they may operate as an energetic mechanism which has a healing effect on the patient. More discussion of the meridian network as an antenna array is included in Section XII.

Chapter 5

Fascial Networks — Physical Structures that Form the Meridians

More clues to the meaning of internal energy are revealed through the study of the meridians. Also called "channels," one set of clues relates to the characteristics of meridians as physical structures. Earlier cited studies, such as those by Becker, Reichmanis, and Tiller, demonstrate that meridians exist in a measurable way, e.g., conduct current, yet there is little evidence that verifiably defines the network of meridians as anatomical structures. However, a new view of the meridians may change that perception.

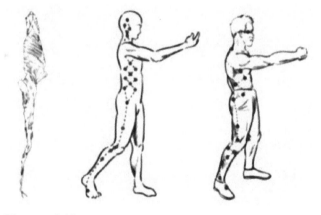

Diagrams 2-13

Three Comparisons: Illustration based on Thomas Myer's "lateral line" from Cadaveric Dissection (left), Illustration of the "Lateral Line" placed on a Human Form (center) and Illustration of the Surface Aspect of the Gallbladder Meridian (right)

Left and center illustrations based on images from Thomas Myers, Anatomy Trains. Illustrations by Sergio Verdeza

A new hypothesis suggests that, at least for the majority of the body's surface meridians, the energetic channels can be understood as networks of fibrous fascia. This proposed description of the meridian system as a myofascial network has been advanced by Peter Dorsher, MD. Dorsher's proposal is based on comparisons between acupuncture meridians and myofascial track dissections made by Thomas Myers, MT. In comparing the traditional acupuncture meridians with myofascial networks, which Myers calls "anatomy trains," Dorsher found that a high correlation exists between the myofascial structures and the traditionally described meridian pathways.

Standard anatomy textbooks define fascial lines as "bands of sheet connective tissue, primarily collagen, beneath the skin that attach, stabilize, enclose, and separate muscles and other internal organs." [54] Fascia can be thought of as the stretchy layers of conductive material that in some ways can be compared to plastic wrap, stretched and interlaced throughout the body. Fascia is stretchy, transmits *strain,* and is *piezoelectric.* Piezoelectric refers to the way pressure or stress, when applied to specific structures, generates an electrical discharge, and this will be particularly relevant to the information discussed in this chapter.

Referring to the body's fascial network, Myers defines the myofascial anatomy trains as _anatomical pathways that transmit strain and movement._ [55] Myers is a therapeutic massage and bodywork specialist, certified in Structural Integration (Rolfing). In his analysis of human cadaver dissections, he demonstrated how the body is supported by an interconnected web of fascia, tendons, and ligaments that he calls a "connective tissue matrix." His description of the body's support and movement function in terms of a fascia _matrix_ provides a broader understanding of the role of connective tissue than what is generally understood. Accordingly, Myers explains these in terms of "anatomical grids postulated as integral to the support and function of the locomotor system." [56]

Comparing Myers's description of _anatomy trains_ with acupuncture meridians, Dorsher observed that in eight of nine comparisons, "there was substantial overlap in the distributions of the anatomically derived myofascial meridians with those of the principle acupuncture meridian distributions." [57] In other words, the myofascial lines identified by Myers have a high correspondence with the long-speculated physical evidence of the body's energetic pathways, known in TCM as meridians / channels. Diagrams 2-13 provides three comparisons: an illustration based on Myer's dissection of the "lateral line," an illustration based on his drawing of the lateral line, and, for comparison, the path of the traditional "gallbladder meridian," superimposed over an illustration of a boxer.

As Dorsher explains, the "strong correspondence of the distributions of the acupuncture and myofascial meridians provides an independent, anatomic line of evidence that acupuncture principal meridians likely exist as myofascial networks within the human body." [58] Dorsher's observation of Myer's myofascial lines as acupuncture meridians advances our understanding of these systems. Diagrams 2-14 below offer two additional comparisons between Myer's myofascial lines and acupuncture meridians.

Citing an earlier study by Yangevin and Yando, who reported that 80% of the twenty-four acupuncture points in the anatomical sections of a cadaveric arm entered intermuscular or intramuscular tissue planes,[59] Dorsher explains that, "Myofascial meridians are postulated to occur along body paths where connective tissues (including myofascia, tendons, and ligaments) not only have anatomical continuity, but also exhibit a gradual change in tissue orientation (ie, direction / depth of connecting fiber structures) along entire pathways." [60]

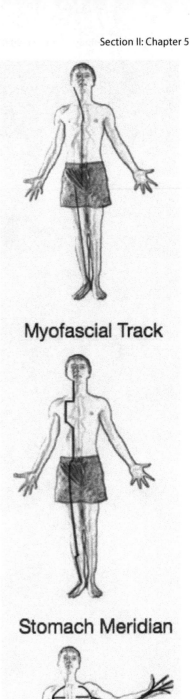

Myofascial Track

Stomach Meridian

Myofascial Track

Pericardium Meridian

Diagrams 2-14

Comparisons Between Myer's Myofascial Meridians and Acupuncture Meridians

Drawings based on representations in Peter Dorsher, MD's,

"Myofascial Meridians as Anatomical Evidence of Acupuncture Channels." [62]

As Dorsher explains, the "anatomical configuration conceptually allows strain to be transmitted across the structure in a given myofascial meridian." [61] Although an individual myofascial meridian may attach at skeletal sites along its course to anchor these pathways (i.e., "bony stations"), a portion of its fibers continue onward to the next part of the myofascial track "meridian." In regard to incorporating this view of the meridian system in an approach to pain therapy, Dorsher suggests that what might be an "optimal pain treatment" would not only require attention on the site of the patient's presenting pain, but also to other potential musculoskeletal problem areas along the myofascial meridians that course through the entire region. For example, a patient may present with recurrent posterior neck pain despite frequent neck manipulations. However, the same patient might be found to have untreated hamstring and plantar fascia restrictions. Treatment of those musculoskeletal issues (especially on the same myofascial meridian) in conjunction with localized neck pain therapy may lead to durable improvement of the patient's neck pain.

Two Aspects of the Meridians as a *Connective Tissue Matrix*

There are two advantages to working with the body's energetic meridians as physical structures. The first is as a pain management and rehabilitation technique, and the second applies to the training of athletes.

As a pain management and rehabilitation tool, a therapist (or self-healer) who learns to work with meridians not as imaginary energy lines, but rather as anatomical structures, can enhance and add new depth to therapies like chiropractic, physical medicine, or massage. Whether in one's own self-healing or through intervention by a therapist, approaching the meridians as stretchy physical pathways supports the principle that pain and rehabilitation in the body is rarely just a local issue.

As an enhanced training method for athletes, learning to become aware of the meridians as piezoelectric fascial networks adds another dimension to physical conditioning. For example, in their analyses, Myers and Dorsher illustrate how a myofascial tensional band runs from the hip to the neck, from the lower back to the back of the neck, and from the index finger to the side of the head. This model reveals the body as a reflexive, interconnected system, a view that can be hugely valuable in the training of athletes. The model also suggests a rationale for some innovative treatment and training approaches. For example, in some cases, a slight and gradual stretching of the little finger in just the right way can enhance athletic potential by inducing healthful strain along the entire myofascial / meridian line.

Furthermore, the interconnected myofascial network approach also provides another layer of meaning to energetic exercise like *qigong*. As the practitioner learns to direct beneficial tension along a meridian, this provides an additional source of feedback, allowing the individual or therapist to better engage the entire myofascial system (an example of this principle is illustrated in the "Look at Moon" posture presented in Section III).

An example of how directing tension to specific meridians can benefit athletic training came to me in the form of a *qigong* and energetic martial arts teacher, who asked me to help him increase the combat effectiveness of his practice. Although he trained regularly in a graceful and fluid way, he felt that he could not apply effective force in a real close-combat situation. In response, I developed a training regimen for him based on working with the body's fascial network in ways that would increase tension during practice, with the assumption being that this would allow him to generate more physical power. To accomplish this, his new goal was not to concentrate only on the feeling of *qi* through his body, which previously had been the center of his practice, but to also add to the sense of resistance in his body by consciously engaging the myofascial meridians.

The importance of learning to work with the bouncy-stretchiness of the myofascial meridian system as physical structures cannot be overstated. In my experience as a coach and therapist, it is one of the most valuable lessons I can offer to students and clients in order to help them access the power of their "connective tissue matrix" and have it become the cornerstone of their training.

This approach allows them to grasp the interstitial merging between "energy" and "structure," as through greater conscious access to their body's myofascial network, "mind" and "intention" merge with their physical skill. Applied to an athlete, a physical technique becomes more effective because the (fully activated) piezoelectric nature of the meridian allows "mind" and "intention" to integrate with bio-mechanics. Through this approach, a pain patient learns to appreciate how changes applied to the way they walk can relieve years of chronic neck pain. Likewise, a martial artist or boxer learns how the conscious triggering of a punch or strike by a twitch of their finger can access deep structures that enable them to down an opponent with the slightest touch.

The theme of the myofascial system as a piezo-electric approach to training will be returned to throughout the present work. It is the basis of the physical *dao yin* yogas that will be discussed in Section III, and the new model of working with the body's antenna structures that will be forwarded in Section XII. Furthermore, it also forms the basis of "source point" work that is covered in the next chapter.

Chapter 6

Outer Nourishes Inner — A New Look at "Source Points"

*I*n some applications, the stimulation of key acupoints along a myofascial track can trigger the release of healthful influences in the body. This is because *stress*, when directed to those specific locations, can affect an entire meridian. Examples of these point-distal target relationships include treatment for knee pain by pressure applied to the webbing between the second and third toes (St-44), treatment of stomach disorders by stimulation of a point below and lateral to the knee (St-36), and treatment of acute sore throat by pressure to the medial aspect of the thumb (Lu-11). However, some aspects of the meridians also travel deep into the body's core and interact with the viscera. Thus, stimulation directed to a category of points called "source points" (原穴), can also influence the visceral organs.

Significantly, the application of beneficial stress applied to source points can be either conscious or unconscious. This chapter looks at how stimulation directed to key locations can induce these positive health influences deep in the body's core. These discussions are based on the dovetailing of two threads of previously introduced information.

The first of these threads concerns the discussion of the meridians provided by Peter Dorsher, MD. There it was described how Dorsher, relying on Myer's definition of anatomical trains (myofascial tracks), defines the meridians as anatomical pathways that transmit strain and movement.

The second thread has to do with the characterization of acupuncture points by Tiller (citing Helms), as "situated in the surface depressions along the cleavage planes between two or more muscles," and "located in a vertical column of [unless otherwise stressed] loose connective tissue." The merger of those two discussions suggests ways in which an individual can more effectively self-heal and self-empower.

In ancient times, acupuncture points were not resting idly on a plane of connective tissue. They did not wait for their value to be discovered by a shaman, who one day decided to stick a shard into the locus; they were situated where they were because they provided an important function, and their location contributed to that purpose. Thus, read this as an example of **the unconscious management of the body as a subtle energy system**.

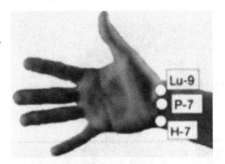

A New Way of Looking at the Body's *Yuan*, or "Source Points"

Is it possible that healthy visceral organ function depends on a regular jolt of piezoelectric charge through the meridians? Although acupuncture points are naturally stimulated through movement, the targeted application of stress is especially efficacious when it initiates through *yuan*, or "source points," associated with a particular organ.

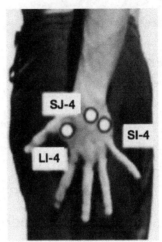

In acupuncture, there are twelve traditionally described source points, each playing a powerful role in terms of their relationship to the organ from which the meridian derives its name. Located near the wrists and ankles, source points are places where the energy of the meridian is said to "pool." [63]

Source points are shown in Diagram 2-7. Those strategically placed locations are situated in just the right way to interact with and transmit a piezoelectric charge to the associated organ.

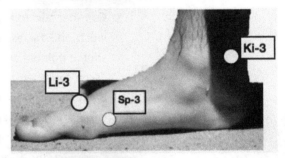

An example of the potent interaction between a source point and its assigned organ is seen in the relationship between the heart meridian source point and the heart organ. The point, *shen men* (H-7, see Diagrams 2-15), is located on the inner side of the wrist, at the crease, and in line with the little finger. Translated into English as "spirit gate," the point is used to treat heart palpitations, sleep disorders, and psychological disturbances. [64] In TCM theory, the "heart meridian" addresses not only heart issues, but also psychological concerns.

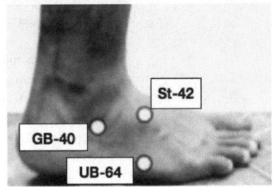

Diagrams 2-15

(Yuan) Points Located Near the Wrists and Ankles: Important Locations for Diagnosis and Treatment of Organ Dysfunction

Source points of the hand: Heart 7, Pericardium 7, Lung 9, Small Intestine 4, Large Intestine 4 and Triple Warmer (Sanjiao) 4.

Source points of the foot: Liver 3, Spleen 3, Kidney 3, Gallbladder 40, Urinary Bladder 64, and Stomach 42

Since a strong relationship is said to exist between a source point and the organ for which it is named, source points are especially ideal places to test the validity of that aspect of TCM theory. [65] In one study investigating these relationships, researchers looked at whether or not the source point for the kidney, called K-3 (shown in Diagram 2-16), might influence kidney function in a measurable way. Applying electro- acupuncture to the equivalent point on laboratory rats, the rat kidneys were

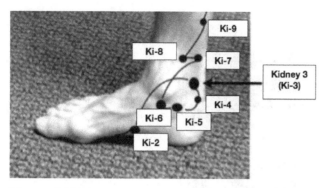

Diagram 2-16

Foot and Ankle Aspects of the Kidney Meridian

The arrow indicates the source point "Kidney 3" (Ki-3)

later excised and subjected to analysis. Researchers found that, when compared to a control group of rats which did not receive the acupuncture treatment, the treated rats showed a positive (threefold) increase in biological changes related to kidney function. Presumably in reaction to the K-3 source point treatment, kidney vitality appeared to improve in ways that supports life function and detoxifies the body. [66]

This observation leads us to believe that the location of source points plays a role in healthy organ function. Applied to humans, this observation suggests that they are situated near the wrists and ankles, either by design or in terms of evolution, in order to provide beneficial stress associated with regular turning and twisting movements at those locations.

Internal Energy Pathways and Body Design

Consider the following: first, that the source points are located near the wrists and ankles, and second, that some research supports the notion that source points have a relationship to the organ for which they are named. Taken together, the merging of these two attributes presents a novel way of thinking about the relationship between visceral organ function and stimulation of the body's myofascial meridians. This notion of "co-evolution" relates to the way we humans turn, stretch, and twist our bodies, and how these actions trigger subtle, but consistent, health influences that are reflected in deep responses within the body.

In other words, the location of source points near the wrists and ankles suggests that optimal organ function might be maintained through movement resulting from their intimate link to physical interaction with the natural environment.

Normal human motion, especially for those of us living in a more natural environment, involves daily twisting and turning. Often, these actions are accentuated through exaggerated wrist and ankle movement, thus the location of the source points at the ends of our limbs offers clues to their meaning. Furthermore, their location, and their actions at those locations, provide insight into the meaning of "internal energy" and "energy medicine."

By the sweat of the brow you will work

Genesis 3:19

This hints at the secret meaning of source acupoints. They may not always lay passively in ways characterized by Tiller, citing Helms, in "loose connective tissue." Turning and twisting movements generate *strain* to the local hand or wrist source point. In response, the localized stress initiates a piezoelectric charge along the meridian line. As a justification for why source points are situated where they are, it is interesting to consider that the body might be designed, or have evolved, to rely on stress to the source points and those subsequent micro bursts of piezoelectric / bio-electric energy.

Tying together the description of the meridians by Myers and Dorsher, who suggest that the myofascial meridian structures, like the body's matrix of connective tissues, transmit stress along a meridian, it seems more than a coincidence that source points are located at just the right places to provide that kind of stimulation.

Consider that the kidney source point transmits stress that originates near the ankles. Subsequently, that strain is then reflected through the entire kidney meridian and, presumably, to the organ itself. Likewise, stress to the heart source point in the wrist, for example, from climbing a tree or pushing oneself over a large boulder, transmits stress through the heart meridian and, theoretically, also to the heart organ. In these examples, stress to the respective source points initiates a piezoelectric charge that, according to TCM theory, provides a positive influence on the organ for which that source point is named.

The nature of these interactions between source points, meridians, and the body's response to them implies that to at least to some extent, visceral organ health may be dependent on healthful stress derived from *natural* movement. This speaks to the design of the body, which has evolved to be responsive to the variable challenges of twists and turns that occur continually through one's encounter with irregular terrain.

One's encounter with natural obstacles sometimes causes extreme changes to foot shape (Diagram 2-17). Foot shape change-adaptation initiates stress to source points. Subsequently, stress is transmitted differentially throughout the entire myofascial structure. Consider, for example, that in some cases, foot shape change from walking on uneven surfaces will trigger reactions far from the foot, such as in the shoulders and neck, and it appears as though this kind of stress comes with benefits.

It is proposed that a kind of *energetic nourishment* takes place through natural movement. A natural environment, with obstacles and challenges at every step, produces a kind of "massaging" of the foot, where numerous acupuncture points are stimulated.

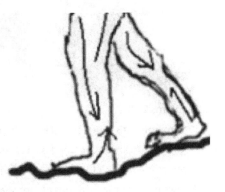

Diagram 2-17
Extreme Foot Shape Change in Response to Variable Terrain

Utilizing healthful stress along energetic meridian lines has provided new insights into both the benefits of exercise, and how one can improve their practice of energetic exercises such as *qigong* and *hatha* yoga. This might help explain why certain practices like these stimulate the body's energetic and immune system, while reducing or counteracting the impact of denatured lifestyles that most of us face in modern cities.

Source Point Stimulation to Enhance Athletic Performance

Exaggerated foot shape can induce stress along a given myofascial meridian, and in turn, this beneficial tension can influence the body's energy system. These proposals suggest another avenue of investigation: is it possible that a person's more conscious engagement with the foot's myofascial meridian source points could influence athletic performance?

In an attempt to study these relationships, our martial arts group began to experiment with how exaggerated movement might affect athletic performance. To our surprise, we found that exaggerated foot position exercises did improve "athletic connection," while also affecting other athletic markers, such as improved reaction time. Images demonstrating the principle applied to martial arts training are shown in Diagrams 2-18, and a brief video can be viewed via the link included in Box 2-19.

We found that when intentionally changing / exaggerating foot positions to activate and stimulate source points, the individual becomes increasingly able to consciously trigger the feeling of stressful tugging along the myofascial meridians. As a result, the sense of exaggerated foot position becomes easier to access in training. Although initially tested as a training method for athletes seeking to improve "connection" and power, regular practice of the technique translates into other activities, such as walking and running. **

** More discussion on body shape as it relates to the flow and balance of internal energy is included in Section XI.

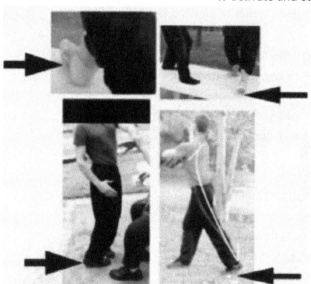

Diagrams 2-18

Experiment with Exaggerated Foot Shape

Note how the lower two images illustrate the improved connection through the athlete's body.

Arrows indicate the locations of foot shape exaggerations

Link to video: Working and Experimenting with Exaggerated Foot Shape

https://youtu.be/6YQnKruUQEA
or
https://chiarts.com/2-19

Box 2-19

Chapter 7

Variable Outcomes in TCM

*A*cupuncture and traditional medicine remain more art than science. Furthermore, skill in diagnosis, point selection, and application of other techniques vary widely among practitioners. Adding to the confusion is the fact that some studies using "sham" acupuncture have been shown to work as well as genuine acupuncture. [67] [68]

Ultimately, the practice of healing arts based on the traditional acupuncture meridians and acupuncture points, as well as acupressure, moxibustion, and massage, often rely on the intuition of the therapist, and as levels of intuitive ability vary, so do results.

Acupuncture and other TCM techniques, as well as other forms of bodywork, are not as effective when posture corrections are not included in the intervention. Consider a patient who suffers from chronic headaches. While in some cases it might be sufficient to use standard needle point prescriptions, such as gallbladder 20 (GB-20), urinary bladder 11 (UB-11) and large intestine 4 (LI-4), therapists who address the patient's posture, as shown in Diagram 2-19, will tend to obtain better long-term results. Photos 2-20 illustrate posture correction that might be included as part of a treatment protocol for chronic headaches and neck pain.

In terms of evaluating the efficacy of a TCM treatment, it is useful to include an additional note concerning the influence of a patient's belief in the outcome. Personality, along with factors such as expectation and psychological resistance, also play important roles in determining the outcome. In any therapy (including drug therapies), patient openness and expectation contribute to the success of the intervention. Furthermore, it is not uncommon for "energy workers" to encounter patients who would rather stay in pain than admit to benefiting from strange "alternative" methods like acupuncture or "energy work."

Thus, acupuncture and other TCM techniques applied the same way to two different individuals, and for the same presenting problem, do not always produce the same result. Acupuncture and TCM come with a world view, and it does matter whether or not the patient embraces a belief in "*qi* energy" and the efficacy of a technique such as needling. For some patients, openness to alternative approaches like *qigong* or acupuncture can pose a threat to their

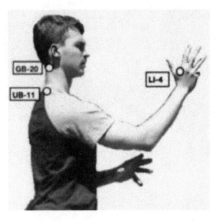

Diagram 2-19
Locations for Points GB-20, LI-4, UB-11 and LI-4

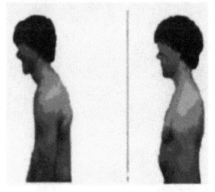

Photos 2-20
Comparison of Posture Habits

Posture habits contribute to the relative effectiveness of acupuncture and other therapies. These photos show the posture of a patient before and after correction.

Left: Habitual "head hanging forward."

Right: Upright and suspended posture correction.

pre-existing world view. In these cases, whether conscious or unconscious, a person with rigid perceptions of health and medicine can prove resistant to treatment.

Endnotes

1 Veith, Ilza (translator), *The Yellow emperor's classic of internal medicine: A new translation of the neijing suwen with commentary*, University of California Press, Oakland 1975 p.53.

2 As traditionally described, body fluids, or *jin ye*, are the body's nourishing and lubricating fluids. They include mucus, semen, tears, and sweat. The *jin ye* include two types, *jin* and *ye*. The *jin* are "lighter" and more "pure." They moisten and nourish the skin and muscles. In contrast, the *ye* fluids are denser and comprise the fluids in the internal organs, brain, and bones.

3 As cited in http://www.itmonline.org/5organs/heart.htm

4 Adapted from the Joseph Needham's translation of a portion of the *Tung Chung-Shu Chhun Chhiu Fan Lu Needham, Joseph, Science and civilization in China*, Vol. 2, Cambridge University Press, 1983. pp. 275-276.

5 As translated by Joseph Needham, *Science and civilization in China*, Vol. 5, p. 210.

6 Needham, Joseph, *Science and civilization in China*, Cambridge University Press, 1983 Vol. 2, p. 280.

7 Needham

8 Ni, Maoshing, *The yellow emperor's classic of medicine: A new translation of the neijing suwen with commentary*, p.4.

9 Needham, Joseph, *Science and civilization in China*, Cambridge University Press, 1983 Vol. 6, p. 75.

10 Also see references to Dr. Hans Selye's work on the relationship between stress and health in Section IX

11 Curran, James, "Huangdi neijing" *British Journal of Medicine*, 2008 Apr 5; 336(7647): 777.

12 Needham, Joseph, *Science and civilization in China*, Vol. 6 pp. 67-68.

13 For example, the famous physician Sun Simiao, in *Prescriptions worth a Thousand*, suggests a health regimen which includes burning of herbs at select points. He writes the following:

"After enjoying excellent health for ten days, one should employ moxibustion at a few points in order to drain out [noxious] wind and *chhi* [*qi*]. It is well, day by day, to harmonize the *qi*, adjust the circulation, massage oneself, and practice gymnastics. Do not take good health for granted. [Just as one] should not forget danger in time of peace, try to prevent the coming of disease beforehand."

As cited by Joseph Needham, *Science and civilization in China*, Vol. 6, p. 69.

14 Gwei-Djen Lu & Joseph Needham, *Celestial lancets: A history and rationale of acupuncture and moxibustion*, Cambridge University Press, 1980 p. xxi.

15 As Maciocia explains, "Overflow of *qi* runs into the extra meridians and irrigates the space between skin and muscles. The extraordinary vessels all derive their energy from the kidney and all contain the essence *(Jing)*... They circulate the essence around the body, thus contributing to integrating the circulation of nutritive *(Ying) Qi* with that of the essence. For this reason, the extraordinary vessels are the link between pre (early) heaven *qi* and post (later) heaven *qi*." (Maciocia, p. 820). Later Maciocia quotes Li Shi-zhen, who explains:

"The extraordinary vessels are the root of the Great Avenue of Pre-Heaven, the Governing, Directing and Penetrating vessels [du-ren-chong mai] are the source of creation. As Maciocia describes it, the Directing and Penetrating Vessels serve and important role in embryology and act as a 'genetic blueprint' along which the other energetic meridians are formed" (Maciocia, p. 821).

Maciocia, Giovanni, *The foundations of Chinese medicine: A comprehensive text for acupuncturists and herbalists*. Second Edition Churchhill Livingstone, 2005.

16 Ishida, Hidemi, "Body and mind," *Taoist meditation and longevity techniques*, Center for Chinese Studies, University of Michigan, 1989 p. 59.

17 Robert Becker, MD, *The body electric*, William Morrow & Company, Inc. New York, NY 1985.

18 Electrical correlates of acupuncture points. IEEE Transactions on Biomedical Engineering. 1975, p.22. (November): 533-535. As referenced in Oschman, p.69, Acupuncture meridians have been shown to be low resistance pathways for the flow of electricity. Reichmanis, et al. "Electrical correlates of acupuncture points." IEEE Transactions on Biomedical Engineering. 1975. 22 (November): 533-535.

19 Reichmanis, M, et al., "D.C. skin conductance variation and acupuncture loci," *The American journal of Chinese medicine*, Vol. 4, Issue 1, 1976.

20 Discussed in more detail later.

21 Omura, Y. "Connections found between each meridian (heart, stomach, triple burner, etc.) and organ representation area of corresponding internal organs in each side of the cerebral cortex; release of common neurotransmitters and hormones unique to each meridian and corresponding acupuncture point and internal organ after acupuncture, electrical stimulation, mechanical stimulation (including shiatsu), soft laser stimulation or QI Gong" Acupunct Electrother Res. 1989;14(2):155-86.More information on the Bi-digital "O" Ring test can be viewed at http://www.bdort.org/videos.html

22 For example, Yoshiaki Omura, MD, in his work using a variation of muscle testing called the Bi-Digital O Ring Test (BDORT) (also discussed in Sections III and IV), found that the standard location for an important acupuncture point called Stomach 36 (St-36) is incorrect. See "Anatomical relationship between traditional acupuncture point ST 36 and Omura's ST 36 (True ST 36) with their therapeutic effects: 1) inhibition of cancer cell division by markedly lowering cancer cell telomere while increasing normal cell telomere, 2) improving circulatory disturbances, with reduction of abnormal increase in high triglyceride, L-homocystein, CRP, or cardiac troponin I & T in blood by

the stimulation of Omura's ST 36—Part 1." *Journal of Acupuncture and Electrotherapy Research*, 2007;32(1-2):31-70.

23 Oschman, James, *Energy medicine; The scientific basis*, Elsevier Ltd, 2000 p.71.

24 The experiment involved two groups: the experimental group which were treated with shielded hands and the control group with non-shielded hands. Subjects in both groups received acupuncture at point ST.36, then tested for changes in the direct current potential between St.37 and St.39. Results showed that the shielded hands group responded to only one of the steps used in the experiment.

Lee, M.S., et al, "Is there any energy transfer during acupuncture?" *American Journal of Chinese Medicine* 2005;33(3):507-12.

25 Needham, Joseph, *Clerks and craftsmen in China and the West*. Cambridge: University Press, 1970, p. 289; also, Felix Mann, *Acupuncture*, New York: Random House, 11971, pp. 1-2. As cited by Davis, Devra Lee, *American Journal of Chinese Medicine*, Vo 3, No. 1, pp. 5-26, 1975.

26 Gori, L, "Ear acupuncture in European traditional medicine," *Evidence-Based Complementary and Alternative Medicine*. 2007 Sep:4 13-16

27 Authoring an article written for an on-line technology and science series, "Discovery Blog," Jennifer Viegas cites lead study author Maria Anna, whose article on the Ice Man was published in the Journal of Archaeological Science. She reports that the Ice Man's tattoos have a dark blue color, deriving from the imbedded soot." She adds, "There are groups of one, two, three, four and seven tattoo lines parallel to the longitudinal axis of the body, and so they're parallel to Chinese acupuncture meridians."

Researchers believe the cross-shaped tattoo on his knee, and another one on his left ankle, also lay over Chinese acupuncture "trigger points." Strengthening their argument is the fact that the soot-made markings are located on parts of the iceman's body not typical for tattoo displays, diminishing the notion that they served a more ornamental or aesthetic function.

Prior research showed that Oetzi [the name given to the Ice Man] did suffer from a variety of ailments that might have benefited from acupuncture. These included a bad back, degeneration of the hip, knee and ankle, and "severe abdominal disorders," primarily caused by whip worm, an intestinal parasite that can cause diarrhea.

Before the more recent studies on this mummy, historians believed the earliest acupuncture took place in China around 3,000 years ago. Since the iceman is much older, Pabst and her colleagues now think this therapeutic technique may have been independently discovered by many different prehistoric European and Asian cultures."

Pabst, M., "The tattoos of the Tyrolean Iceman: a light microscopical, ultrastructural and element analytical study," *J. archaeological science*, Vol 36, Issue 10, October 2009, pages 2335–2341. http://www.nbcnews.com/id/31965532/ns/technology_and_science-science/t/oetzi-icemans-tattoos-came-fireplace/#.UccbdlUldr0 By Jennifer Viegas updated 7/17/2009

28 McCann, Henry, DAOM, LAC, DIPL. OM, "Tung's acupuncture: An introduction to a classical lineage of acupuncture." *The Journal of Chinese Medicine*, Feb 2006.

29 Peacher, William G. MD, "Adverse reactions, contraindications and complications of acupuncture and moxibustion." *American Journal of Chinese Medicine*, Vol. 3, No. 1, pp. 35-46 1975.

30 Melzack R. and Wall, P.D., "On the nature of cutaneous sensory mechanism," *Brain*, 85: 331-356.

31 Davis, Devra Lee, "The history and sociology of the scientific study of acupuncture," *American journal of Chinese Medicine*, Vol. 3, no. 1 pp. 5-26 1975.

32 Lee, et al., "Endorphin release: A possible mechanism of acupuncture analgesia," *Comparative medicine, east and west*. Vol. Vi., No. 1. pp. 57-60, 1978.

33 Bressler, David and Kroening, Richard, "Three essential factors in effective acupuncture therapy," *American Journal of Chinese Medicine*, Vol. 4, No. 1, pp. 81-86. 1976.

34 Bressler, David and Kroening, Richard, "Three Essential Factors in Effective Acupuncture Therapy," *American Journal of Chinese Medicine*, Vol. 4, No. 1, pp. 81-86. 1976.

35 Holographic theories are discussed in Section III, primarily under the label of *wai san he, "Outer Three Relationships."*

36 Bressler, David, PhD and Kroening, Richard, MD, "Three essential factors in effective acupuncture therapy," *American Journal of Chinese Medicine*, Vol. 4, No. 1, pp. 81-86, 1976.

37 Bressler, p. 82.

38 Gerber, Richard, *Practical Guide to Vibrational Medicine*, William Morrow, 2000, p.26.

39 Gerber, pp. 263-264.

40 Ibid, p. 264.

41 Ibid., pp. 53-55.

42 Ibid., p.54.

43 Ibid., p.58.

44 William Tiller, William, *Science and human transformation, Subtle energies, intentionality and consciousness*. Pavior Publishing, Walnut Creek, 1997, p. 142.

45 Also known as an ion transporter, an ion pump moves ions across a plasma membrane. As described in Wikipedia, in the body, the primary ion pump / transporters are "enzymes that convert energy from various sources, including ATP, sunlight, and other redox reactions, to potential energy stored in an electrochemical gradient. This energy is then used by secondary transporters, including ion carriers and ion channels, to drive vital cellular processes, such as ATP synthesis."

Source: Wikipedia https://en.wikipedia.org/wiki/Ion_transporter

46 William, Tiller, *Science and human transformation, Subtle energies, intentionality and consciousness.* Pavior Publishing, Walnut Creek, 1997, p. 302

47 Eisenberg, David, MD, "Energy Fields, meridians, chi and device technology," *Energy medicine in China: Defining a research strategy. Noetic Sciences Review,* Spring 1990.

48 Tiller, William, citing J. Helms, *Acupuncture energetics: A clinical approach for physicians*, Medical Acupuncture Publishers, Berkley, CA 1995.

49 Tiller, William, *Science and human transformation: Subtle energies, intentionality and consciousness.* Pavior Publishing, Walnut Creek, 1997 pp. 118-119.

50 Tiller, p. 120.

51 Ibid., pp. 117--121.

52 Ibid., pp. 120-121.

53 Ibid., p. 93.

54 https://en.wikipedia.org/wiki/Fascia.

55 Myers, Thomas W. *Anatomy trains: Myofascial meridians for manual and movement therapists*, Elsevier, Ltd., 2009.

56 Dorsher, Peter, "Myofascial meridians as anatomical evidence of acupuncture channels," *Medical Acupuncture*, Vol. 21, No. 2, 2009, p. 2.

57 Dorsher

58 Ibid.

59 Ibid.

60 Langevin HM, YANDOW, JA "Relationship of acupuncture points and meridians to connective tissue planes," Anat Rec. 2002; 269:257-265 as cited in Dorsher's article, see the previous endnote.

61 Dorsher,

62 Ibid

63 Li Ding, *Acupuncture meridian and acupuncture points.* China Books & Periodicals, Inc., 1992

64 Holmes Keikobad, "Using Acupoint Heart 7: An anatomical approach." *Medical Acupuncture.* June 2009, 21(2): pp. 111-113.

65 Ding Li writes "Clinically, research has shown that pathological changes of the zangfu organs are often manifested at the twelve Yuan (source) points. For example, tenderness at a Yuan (source) point often indicates pathological changes of the associated meridian and the internally related organ." Li Ding, Acupuncture, meridian theory and acupuncture points," *China Books & Periodicals*, Inc.; Beijing: Foreign Languages Press, 1992

66 Investigators found a three-fold up-regulation in the kidney after the acupuncture. NAD-dependent isocitrate dehydrogenase* and quinone reductase, the proteins involved in energy metabolism, the reduction of endogenous quinones, chemoprotection, and electrophilic stress, were identified. The data indicated that acupuncture at the KI-3 of the kidney meridian was able to increase NAD-dependent isocitrate dehydrogenase and quinone reductase expression in the kidney, and supported the relationship between the kidney and KI3. Chun-Ri Li, et al, "Effects of acupuncture at taixi acupoint (KI3) on kidney proteome," *The American Journal of Chinese Medicine*, Vol. 39, No. 4, 687–692.

*One of two enzymes that catalyze the conversion of threo-ds-isocitrate, the product of the action of both aconitase and isocitrate lyase, to α-ketoglutarate (2-oxoglutarate) and CO2; one of the isozymes uses NAD+ (participating in the tricarboxylic acid cycle), whereas the other uses NADP+

67 Uğurlu F, et al, "The effects of acupuncture versus sham acupuncture in the treatment of fibromyalgia: a randomized controlled clinical trial." *Acta Reumatol Port.* 2017 Jan-Mar;42(1):32-37.

68 Lowe C, "Sham acupuncture is as efficacious as true acupuncture for the treatment of IBS: A randomized placebo-controlled trial." *Neurogastroenterol Motil.* 2017 Jul;29(7). doi: 10.1111/nmo.13040. Epub 2017 Mar 2.

Section III
(Mostly) Taoist Yoga & Qigong (Ch'i Kung)

The sages lived peacefully under heaven on earth, following the rhythms of the planet and the universe. They adapted to society without being swayed by cultural trends. They were free from emotional extremes and lived a balanced, contented existence. Their outward appearance, behavior, and thinking did not reflect the conflicting norms of society. The sages lived over one hundred years because they did not scatter and disperse their energies.

— The Yellow Emperor's Classic of Medicine[1]

III

(Mostly) Taoist Yoga & Qigong (Ch'i Kung)

Introduction to Section III

*T*his section looks for clues to the meaning of "internal energy" in the Chinese Taoist [2] and Tibetan *tantric* energetic yogas, with special attention directed to the practitioner's subjective experience during practice. Here we consider how a practitioner interacts with, and manages, sensations within the body that are often described as electrical, magnetic, or internal heat. The ability to generate, and then intentionally control, experiences like these separate the novice from the adept.

While the beginner's practice sometimes involves their awareness of what feels like an electromagnetic pulse in at the body's "energy centers," the advanced practitioner is distinguished by their masterful ability to trigger these sensations at specific targets in the body, such as along the spinal corridor, or the "energy fields," of the lower abdomen.

All sensations are not equal; many can be quite powerful, and some can be profound. With enough time spent engaged in the practice of energetic meditation, energetic yoga, or *qigong*, practitioners will begin to notice the appearance of a special class of perceptions within the body. Depending on the particular tradition, at very advanced levels these function as a kind of internal feedback, which can usher in the experience of bliss and joy associated with spiritual awakening.

For many practitioners, the presence of these sensations is evidence that one's physical experience is inseparable from transcendence, or the stuff of spirit. Over time, the practitioner learns that these sensations exist along a continuum, and that the distinction between the mundane and the spiritual is not all that firm. Eventually, it is discovered that the waters separating the physical from the etheric can be crossed by one who prepares the properly constructed yogic-energetic meditation vessel.

While the subjective experience can seem very real to the practitioner, the interpretation of these sensations incorporates theoretical constructs to explain the phenomena. In meditation, as well as the movement arts that developed on the Indian subcontinent, the practitioner's experience of subjective bodily feelings is equated with the presence and control over "energy" in and around the body, referred to as *prana, shakti,* or *kundalini*. By way of cross-cultural comparison, for practitioners in the Chinese meditative and healing arts, sensations of heat, pressure, or electrical-like tingling throughout the body, whether deliberately stimulated or passively perceived, are all identified in terms of internal *qi* or *nei qi*.

* Use of the term "yoga" follows suggestions by Charles Luk and others that it be used as an umbrella term which describes a variety of physically-based "energetic" health and advancement of consciousness regimens, particularly as applied to Chinese Taoist health and rejuvenation exercise.
See Charles Luk, Taoist Yoga [3]

Chapter 8

The Taoist Traditions

*T*wo millennia ago, some early Chinese Taoists — later characterized by John Blofeld as the first hippies [4] — abandoned mainstream society and moved to remote places, where they could commune with nature. They left the bustle of the cities and towns to seek the goal of many Taoists then, as now, which was to experience the nameless truth that reveals itself only through quiet and solitude. Immersed in the stillness away from humanity's caravan routes, the conditions were right to observe their thoughts, breath, and energy flow. From this pristine vantage point, they developed mind and body exercises to harmonize with the flow of nature and attune mind and body to the perennial wisdom of the primordial *Tao*; the nameless source beyond words.

The present chapter includes a general introduction to Taoist physical and mental yoga and is not intended to be a scholarly discussion of Taoism or Taoists. However, since this chapter and those that follow include an overview of practices that are generally labeled as "Taoist," such as Taoist meditation and Taoist *qigong*, it is necessary to include a few words on what I mean by the term *Taoist*.

At first glance, it would seem that defining terms like Taoist and Taoism would be a simple task, but there is more debate about the meaning of "Taoist" and "Taoism" than the casual reader of these subjects might suspect. Moreover, various sinologists continue to debate the meaning of these terms, further muddying the waters with each new distinction.

The religion, philosophy, and collection of practices that are generally labeled as Taoist trace themselves to the primary text of Taoism, the *Tao Te Ching* (道德經). A general meaning of the term Taoist is suggested by distinguished sinologist and historian, Nathan Sivin, who writes that for the common observer, the term Taoist denotes:

> Nothing more specific than a frame of mind-nature-loving, perhaps, or mystical in a naturalistic way, or unconventional––in discussions that are meant to be about a religion––an association of persons who hold a body of beliefs. [5]

However, as Professor Sivin continues, distinctive qualifiers of the meaning of "Taoist" and Taoism are elusive. Consider, for example, depending on use, that the term Taoist might in any given instance be sentimental, intellectual, social, or bibliographical.

Taoism is neither a unified religion nor a single philosophical stream, and some practices described as Taoist are not exclusively so. For example, individuals and practices labeled as "Taoist" might refer to those casually ascribed to the philosophy of Taoism. Furthermore, there were, and remain, not only Taoist shamans and priests, but other entirely different sets of practitioners that may be considered Taoist or have Taoist leanings, such as the inner and outer alchemists. Adding to the discussion, not only are there practitioners of Taoist magic and rituals, there is even a historical category of a type of Taoist mystic called "Far Roaming," who believed that through meditative trance, they could travel beyond the confines of their bodies and visit far and distant lands. Furthering the confusion toward a meaningful definition of Taoists and Taoism are the *fangshi* (方士), "master of the recipes," meaning shaman, who practiced arts like astrology and divination. [6]

However, the present work does not join in the academic arguments over what constitutes a Taoist or Taoism, nor does it pursue the variant definitions thereof. Designed for the casual reader, in the pages that follow, the disciplines and practices referred to as Taoist are those that are generally represented as such. Those are the traditions that, loosely or otherwise, trace their roots to the respective writings attributed to Lao Tzu [7] and Chuang Tzu in the sixth or fourth century BCE. However, it should be noted that, as Sivin points out, these are not be thought of as a single unified group emerging from a common line, but instead "a handful of authors scattered throughout history." In discussing such writings, Sivin explains how they:

> Meant one thing to their writers, another to their compilers, another to each reader, and quite another to moderns. None of these brings the same assumptions to them, and each finds different "original meanings" in them. [8]

"Inner" and "Outer" Alchemy as Referenced in the Present Work

At its most basic level, Taoist yoga is a collection of tools that the initiate applies toward the mastery of mind and body. As the writer on Taoist practices Hedemi Ishida explains, the traditional Taoist yogic-meditative view is that control over the body leads to control over the emotions, and that this ultimately leads to tranquility and "emptiness of mind." [9]

Restated, the aim of Taoist internal yoga is first to control the body, which in turn leads to control over the emotions, and ultimately "tranquility and emptiness." [10] Both active and passive Taoist yogas are considered in the present work, and later, the Taoist quietest-contemplative tradition will also be considered.

Taoist Inner Alchemy

The Chinese internal alchemy-yoga tradition is called *neidan*. As with the basics of TCM discussed in Section II, the Taoist *neidan* tradition is likewise concerned with three aspects of the body's energy system. They are the energetic elements of *jing, qi,* and *shen. Jing* is nutritive and reproductive essence. *Qi,* in context of the tripartite *jing, qi, shen* representation, refers to both the energy that moves through the channels and organs, but is also the energy of metabolism, respiration, mobility, and immunity. *Shen* refers to the most etheric and refined aspect of human energy, and aspects of human experience characterized as psyche, spirit, and emotions.

The earliest references to inner alchemy appear around the same time Buddhism was making its way into China. Although correlation does not prove causation, this may account for what some scholars see as the influence of Indian religion, particularly Buddhism, on the development of the Chinese internal, *neidan,* tradition. On this note, Isabelle Robinet, whose specialty is Shangqing Taoism and inner alchemy, suggests that the Taoist *neidan* traditions might have developed as a Chinese (national) and Taoist (philosophical) "reaction to Buddhism." [11]

Dating back to the second century, the oldest known book on Chinese inner alchemy is the *Cantong qi* (參同契). Although the date when the doctrine and systematized practice of *neidan* inner yoga emerged is debated, it is generally accepted to have developed as a recognized tradition from the eighth century, with two main branches emerging between the twelfth and thirteenth centuries. [12]

The Southern and Northern Schools comprise the two main branches of the *neidan* tradition. The Southern School focuses on first cultivating one's existence or *ming* (命), and then cultivating one's *xing* (性), with *Ming* referring to the physical body and *xing* to the mind. The Northern School, on the other hand, focuses first on one's cultivation of *xing.* The Taoists taught that such cultivation could be achieved through "clarity and quiescence" (*chingjing,* 清靜). [13]

According to Robinet, what ties the *neidan* authors together is the concern for training the mind as much as the body, and the tendency to synthesize various Taoist currents with Buddhist speculations and Confucian lines of thought, making references to the *Yijing (Book of Changes)* and incorporating alchemical practices. [14]

For the Taoist yogi, the goal was simple: return mind and body to their inherent pristine state. For a Taoist alchemist, the ideal state of *xiantian* (先天), or "primordial (also transliterated as "earlier") heaven," was a goal that could be realized by the expert practitioner, who refined mind and body energy and became sensitive to, and harmonious with, nature's rhythms. Although the practice of physical and mental yoga to maintain health predates the Taoists, they are most probably drawn from shamanic dances designed to influence the weather. [15] [16] For the purposes of health, longevity, and sometimes as a quest to attain immortality, the Taoists created passive and active yogas.

Their quest led to the development of physical and mental yogas (note, as detailed below, "mental yogas" are distinct from meditation), many of which are still in use today. Some of these yogas were, and are, active, while others were, and still are, practiced as passive exercise. Through the accounts of the early practitioners who documented their experiences in order to pass on the traditions to later generations, the Taoist yogis compiled an invaluable record that reveals essential secrets of the nature of internal energy, along with the myriad ways to master one's life force.

Active, or "movement," exercises of the Taoists — including stretching and breathing art forms — were designed to manage, enhance and balance internal energy within the body. However, as mentioned earlier, the range of practices embraced by the Taoists also included passive yogas or the holding of static postures, which, rather than utilizing physical exercise in order to stimulate and revitalize the body's energy, relied upon the power of focused awareness directed to locations within the body. In today's parlance, they unlocked the power of attention to consciously influence the nervous system.

Whether engaged in active or passive (moving or static) yoga, the first task for an initiate was to gain some awareness of his or her life force. In both active and passive examples, the practitioner's primary goal was to become sensitive to the flow and rhythm of internal *qi*, or *nei qi* (內氣), [17] within the body. Blofeld describes the Taoist yogi's pursuit as one to "discover whether life had meaning, if so what, and then live in frugal but happy accord with nature's rhythms."

Since the 1950s, both active and passive yoga have generally been categorized under the umbrella term *qigong* (氣功). However, over the course of millennia, they were known by other names. Other terms for Chinese health-energetic exercise include *nei gong* (內功), meaning "inner work," and *yang sheng* (養生), "nurturing life," exercise. Relatedly, *yang xing* (養形) pertains to the cultivation of the body, while exercises directed to the maintenance of mind and spirit are called *yang xin* (養心) and *yang shen* (養神).

When employed as a physical discipline, the practice of Taoist exercise and posture holding falls into the category of *dao yin* (導引), "pulling and stretching." Other terms that sometimes apply are *an mo* (按摩) and *xing qi* (行氣). *An mo* refers to massage and *xingqi* translates as "moving the *qi*." [18]

Although the term *qigong* dates back only to the 1950s, [19] references to *qigong*-like practices can be found as far back as the fourth century BCE. Note that there are currently hundreds of traditions/ schools/methods of *qigong* with various names, many of which trace their lineage to legendary or historical founding masters.

Active vs. Passive Forms of Taoist Yoga / *Qigong*

On those distinctions between "active" and "passive" subtypes of Taoist yoga, in general, "active forms" include aspects of the previously mentioned physical forms of *dao yin*. Translated as "twisting and pulling" (or alternatively, "guiding and pulling"), physical forms evolved into branches of self-healing gymnastics and contributed to the development of martial arts like *t'ai-chi ch'üan (taijiquan)*. Interestingly, there is some suggestion that these disciplines, and in particular those that teach that health could be influenced by means of posture and the holding of specific body positions, might have contributed to the development of western gymnastics. [20]

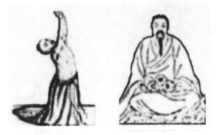

Images 3-1
Active and Passive Styles of Taoist Yoga
Left: *Dao yin* physical or active yoga
Right: *Nei guan* passive yoga and meditation [26]

In contrast to active yoga, this section also introduces some techniques that involve the practitioner learning to focus attention within the body, known as *neiguan* (內觀), or *neishi* (內視). Both are synonyms for "inner contemplation," and for the purposes of the present chapter, they are collectively referred to as *neiguan*, with *nei* meaning "inner" and *guan* holding several meanings. *Guan* can refer to a kind of watchtower, or a Taoist monastery or abbey, but, perhaps more fittingly, the term can also apply to breathing exercises inspired by the Buddhist practice of mindfulness meditation.

Many different techniques and practices can be classified as internal yogic *neiguan* practice. These include breathing exercises, visualization, self-massage of acupuncture points, and learning to place attention to subtle bodily cues, such as the pulse and heartbeat. Both active *dao yin* and passive *neiguan* methods are designed to "balance" the flow of *nei qi* internal energy, either willfully or through passive observation. Active forms accomplish this through movement and posture designed to align the body's internal energy systems, whereas passive forms access and moderate the body's energy systems through the powers of intentionality.

Becoming an Immortal: Compounding the Elixir

The inspiration for *neidan* inner yoga tradition sprang from the outer alchemists. The outer alchemical, or *waidan* (外丹), tradition can be traced to at least the third century CE. However, the notion of Taoist alchemy is often misunderstood in the West. Unlike European alchemy, which most often directed toward the transformation of base metals into gold, the Chinese proto-scientific alchemical practitioner, relying on carefully followed rituals, would construct his *danshi* (丹室) "laboratory," where he sought to compound the immortality elixir, or *dan* (丹). The alchemist believed that when digested, this elixir would allow him to attain physical and / or spiritual immortality, along with supernatural powers.

Through procedures conducted in their crude laboratories, the alchemists mixed and boiled compounds together with elements such as mercury, in order to attempt to extract *essence*. Later, they would subject the manufactured compounds to the influence of the sun and moon, which they believed would help formulate the primordial compound and ultimate secret elixir of life. They believed that ingestion of the *dan* would alter the course of their lives. It allowed a man to become an immortal. Thus, the *dan* elixir they sought was believed to reverse the normal course of mental and physical deterioration, and return the partaker-practitioner to the uncorrupted, prenatal state before being born, referred to as "primordial (or 'earlier') heaven."

The Inner Yogic Alchemist

In contrast to the outer alchemist, the inner alchemist, or *neidan* (內丹), practitioner sought to transform alchemical-energetic aspects within his or her own body. In Chinese alchemical terms, the transformation of elements necessary to produce this result still hinged upon successful creation of the *dan,* with the key difference being that for inner alchemists, the subtle mix of energetic forces that made up the elixir were naturally occurring, but lay dormant in the body until activated.

The Three *Dan Tian*
Henri Maspero (1883-1945) described the *dan tian* energy centers associated with the Taoist yogic practice as being located in three areas of the body: head, chest, and belly.

Box 3-2

Description of the *Dan Tian* - The Body's "Cinnabar Fields"
By Ko Hung (Ge Hong) 葛洪 (283-363)

The Tao ("the Ultimate One") has its names and demeanors. It is nine-tenths of an inch tall in man, and six-tenths of an inch in woman. It resides at two and four-tenths of inches below the navel in the lower dan tian, or

below the heart at jianggong 絳宮 and jinque 金闕, in the middle dan tian, or between the eye brow in the depths (of the skull): the location of the first

inch is named ming tang 明堂; the location of the second inch is named

tongfang 洞房; and the location of the third of the inch is named upper dan tian. These names and locations are crucial for Taoists; they have only have been transmitted orally to those who have taken the "blood-oaths" generation after generation.

Wang, Ming 王明. 1996. Clarification on the Inner Chapters of Baopu zi, Baopuzi neipian jiaoshi 保朴子內篇校釋 **

Box 3-3

** Adapted from the citation provided in http://www.literati-tradition.com/meditative_practice.html [21]

The Internal Tradition

Since the focus of the present chapter concerns Taoist inner alchemist traditions, it is useful to note that while inspiration and much of the terminology for Taoist inner yoga, or the inner *dan* (內丹) tradition, flows from the outer tradition, there is no historically clear or distinct line between the outer and inner schools. Prior to the Yuan dynasty, some alchemists simultaneously engaged in practices from both traditions, believing that each was essential to the other. [22]

It is probable that the toxicity of their alchemical formulas contributed to the decline of the "outer tradition," since highly poisonous elements, such as lead and mercury, were often included in the compounds they manufactured. It is of interest to note that the emperor Qin Shi Huang died from ingestion of an alchemical formula in the third century BCE, and more recently, the eighteenth-century emperor, Yong Zheng, is likewise said to have expired after he ingested an external alchemist's prescription. [23]

In contrast to the "outer" practice, the *neidan* yogic practitioner viewed the body as a microcosm, or model in miniature, of the larger universe, and, as a general statement, followed the doctrine that the "true laboratory was within." [24] In their quest to manufacture the "inner elixir," or *neidan*, their body and mind became cauldron and stove. In many examples, the inner alchemical Taoists adopted the language of external alchemists as metaphors in their yogic pursuits. As the term implies, the inner yogic Taoist focused not on the outer *dan*, but on the inner *dan*, which could be cultivated in the energy centers of the body, known as the *dan tian* (丹田), literally, the "cinnabar fields," or alternatively, the "elixir fields").

As traditionally described, the body has three *dan tian* energy centers: head, chest, and lower abdomen (Boxes 3-2 and 3-3, above). Of these energy centers, the *dan tian* of the lower abdomen was, and remains, especially important for inner alchemy, energetic meditation, *t'ai-chi ch'üan,* and other energy techniques.

The Body's Electromagnetic Energy Centers

This is a good place to reflect on the meaning of the *dan tian* centers as special locations, where the body's energetic fields can be awakened, actualized, and mentally and physically engaged.

The reason those energy centers of the body, such as those of the lower abdomen, became the focus of attention to the Taoist, among other energetic practitioners, was not arbitrary. These are special regions, known since ancient times to numerous cultures due to the special sensations that can be generated there. They are areas of the body that are known to become charged by, and responsive to, intent. In other words, focusing on these energy centers in the body can generate particularly strong emotional and other nervous system responses.

For the most part, the body's major energy centers lie along, or in line with, the spinal corridor. In the Taoist inner alchemical-yoga traditions, emphasis is placed on the *dan tian* centers, and in particular the *dan tian* of the lower abdomen. Thus, it may be appropriate at this point to devote a few words to considering *why* the lower abdomen energy center might be considered so important.

The importance of areas like the *dan tian* is obvious to most experienced meditators. When a person correctly aligns the body, releases all unnecessary tension, and focuses attention to the lower abdomen, they will experience obvious changes. Feelings that are produced in the area of the lower abdomen include warmth, and sometimes powerful electromagnetic (EM) sensations. However, before one is able to work with these sensations, the quiet practice of stillness meditation must first be engaged. There are three steps:

- First, attain correct vertical posture of the body
- Second, release all unnecessary tension
- Third, direct focused attention to specific areas within the body

The first requirement, achieving correct vertical orientation, is not trivial, and is often more challenging than one might suspect. Since more nuanced discussion of posture as it relates to "energy" is covered in Section XI, only a few points pertaining to sitting meditation are included here.

One example of how posture influences one's ability to become sensitive to, and engage with, the internal energy system pertains to sitting; specifically, how one sits in relation to the tailbone, as sitting with the tailbone tucked under inhibits the flow of "energy" in the body. The issue is more significant than is generally realized, which is why meditation teachers often check that students are lifting (suspending) from their pelvic floor muscles and not "sitting" on their tailbone. Likewise, if the head is not properly supported, the meditator will carry excess tension in the jaw. Some related observations on jaw tension are included in the Endnote. [25]

The second point concerns the requirement to release the body's excess tension. Again, this is not a minor point, since nearly all of us carry more tension than is necessary, and most of it is carried unconsciously. For example, many us hold tension in our shoulders, back, and neck. Until this unnecessary tension is released, one cannot fully experience the EM and magnetic-like sensations in the body that are associated with energetic meditation and energetic yoga.

After completing the first two requirements, one is able to attend to the third point. This concerns the art of placing one's awareness deep within the body. When these steps are successfully followed, the practitioner will begin to notice new sensations within the body. Among the more interesting of these are those that can be best described as electromagnetic vortices that move about within the body's core. These experiences can be very powerful, especially for the more practiced meditator, who will sometimes observe a synergistic effect that enhances the experience when the energy centers align. †

† More on this subject in Section V, and more advanced demonstrations of a practitioner applying electromagnetic-like vortexes for close combat are included in Section XII

Chapter 9

Neidan Inner Yoga

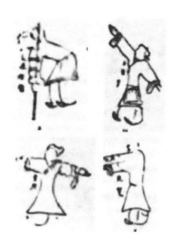

Figure 3-4

Examples of Ancient Yoga in China

Four sketches of Taoist yoga from a manuscript found in the second century, Mawangdui tomb: "Manual of Nourishing the Life-Force by Physical Exercise and Self-Massage." Next to the top left figure is written: "Using a pole to unite yin and yang." [35]

For the Taoist practitioner of inner yoga, the ultimate aim was to cultivate the *zhen dan* (真丹), or "true elixir of immortality." As conceived by the Taoists, for most individuals this remained an untapped resource throughout their entire lives, and to address this challenge, the inner yogic-alchemists sought to awaken and vitalize one's "true elixir." They believed the process would lead to the restoration of *zhenqi* (真氣), or "true *qi* energy." In this regard, the Taoist yogi's obsession with restoring the body's true *qi,* also known as primordial or *yuanqi* (元氣), relates to what might be thought of as a frequency of life energy named *xiantian,* or "primordial heaven" (先天). "Primordial heaven, "also referred to as "earlier" and "prenatal," can be thought of as a vibratory influence lost to the infant the moment that the umbilical cord is severed between mother and child. Thus, the principal aim of the Taoist energetic meditators was to return the body to the full and realized state that was present before birth, since birth represents separation from *source* and the beginning of the individual's decline.

In some ways, the ancient yogi's search can be compared to today's stem cell research as a way to restore youth and vitality. To achieve this goal, the yogic-meditator would engage in a transformative process whereby one's coarse (most dense and unrefined) aspect of *qi,* known as *jing* (精) energy, associated with semen, transmutes into a refined aspect of body "spiritual" energy named *shen* (神). Through *lianqi huashen* (錬氣化神), or "converting the *qi* into spirit," the Taoist yogic meditator, relying on his body's *huaji* (化技), or "mechanisms of change," sought to restore primal, natural energy, and thus return to the refined "prenatal" state of the *source.*

For the Taoist yogi, the *dan tian* energy center of the lower abdomen, also referred to as the "true cavity of *qi*" (真氣穴), was one of the most important bodily locations for refining and transmuting internal energy. Other areas involved in the transformation process included the solar plexus, the *huang ting* ("yellow hall") in the mid-torso; [27] and a point in the middle, posterior to the front of the forehead, known as the *ni wan.* In terms of the inner alchemical process, the Taoist yogi transmuted and transported unrefined *jing* from the abdomen to these locations where essence could be transformed. Lu Kuan Yu, in his introduction to the English translation of Chao Pi-ch'en's *The Secrets of Cultivation of Essential Nature and Eternal Life,* describes the process:

When the generative force moves to obey its worldly inclination, the purpose of regulating the breathing is to draw the force up to the lower [*dan tian*] cavity under the navel so as to hold it there and transmute it into an alchemical agent which is transformed into vitality in the solar plexus. [28]

As Lu explains, the microcosmic orbit meditation (covered in Section V) "produces and nurtures an immortal seed in the lower *dan tian* cavity under the navel, where it radiates, lighting up the heart. This light reveals the formation of the immortal seed, when all breathing appears to cease, and pulses seem to stop beating in a condition of complete serenity." [29] More than a thousand years ago, a Taoist practitioner described the training:

Therefore, those who seek to restore and nourish (their primary vitalities) all imitate it, saying that 'to return to the source' is the important thing about 'embryonic respiration'. Formerly it was always said that the Pool of *qi* (*qihai*, in the lower tantian) was the source of *qi*, but this is not so. If one does not know where it stops, there is no benefit from the 'returning.' The immortals of old always handed down (the true doctrine) by word of mouth, never committing it to writing, but I am anxious to reveal it to my like-minded brother –– therefore I say that the root and origin is right opposite the umbilicus, at the level of the nineteenth vertebra (counting from above), in the empty space (in front of) the spinal column, at the place where it approaches the bladder from below. It is called the Stalk of Life *(ming ti)*, or the Gate of Life *(ming men)*, or the Root of Life *(ming ken)*, or the Reservoir of Semen *(jing shi)* where men store their semen, and women their menstrual blood. This then is the origin of the qi of longevity and immortality...." [30]

Taoist Physical Yoga

Since ancient times, Taoists have believed that physical movement is essential to circulate the power of *qi* within the body. Old adages are still relied on to illustrate the relationship between movement and maintenance of one's health, such as, "running water does not stagnate," and "a moving door harbors no worm." [31] The Taoist beliefs that yogic movement and the holding of specific yogic postures could influence the practitioner's health were introduced to Western readership in the late 1700s, by the French Jesuit missionary to China, Cibot. His account of Taoist yoga records the missionary's favorable impression of these health-promoting yoga postures:

The various postures of the *Cong fu [gongfu]*, if correctly performed should cause a clearance of all those illnesses which arise from an embarrassed, retarded, or interrupted circulation. But consider, how many diseases are there which have a cause other than this? One may well ask whether, apart from fractures and wounds which injure the organization of the human frame, any such diseases exist. [32]

Taoist yoga was, and continues to be, practiced for many reasons. Designed to stimulate changes within the body's energy system through the application of specific physical postures, the goals of practice include spiritual enlightenment and general health maintenance, as well as providing supplementary training for martial artists. The efficacy of Taoist yoga continues to be investigated today, with more recent research looking at the therapeutic applications of Taoist yoga in clinical settings, and the potential benefits of the technique in controlling blood pressure and aiding rehabilitation. [33] Note, Taoist yoga as a spiritual practice will be covered in Section V.

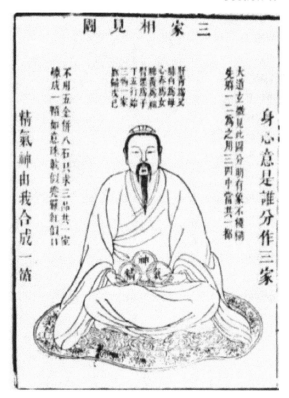

Figure 3-5

Seventeenth-Century Woodblock Print of Taoist Meditator

The three circles at the energetic practitioner's lower abdomen show the merging of the three aspects of "qi energy," *jing, qi,* and *shen*

Image from Joseph Needham, *Science and Civilization in China*

The Three Treasures: *Jing, Qi,* and *Shen*

Central to the beliefs adopted by the inner alchemists from the external school was the notion that production of the *dan* elixir required cauldron and stove. Adopted by the internal traditions, in those disciplines, the metaphor of the cauldron was applied to bodily locations where *qi* could be cultivated, nurtured, and transformed. Most important among these locations were the *dan tian* "cinnabar fields," and in particular the *dan tian* center of the lower abdomen.

The Taoists believed that by focusing attention to the *dan tian* — and directing specialized breathing and *dao yin* exercises to the area involving "twisting and pulling," in conjunction with other techniques — the three treasures of *jing, qi,* and *shen* could be compounded and transformed within the body. Note that the 1600 CE woodblock print in Figure 3-5 illustrates a practitioner with focus directed to the three aspects of *qi* in the lower abdomen. ‡

‡ Some reports of physical sensations associated with Taoist yoga focused on the *dan tian* were introduced earlier, and more theories on the meaning of these sensations are considered in Section V.

Diagram 3-6

The Three Treasures

The foundational formula holds that coarse energy transmutes into the *qi* of the channels, and then into *shen*, or refined "spiritual energy."

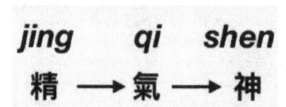

Jing, Qi, Shen

Early in their training, TCM students are taught that the body is made up of three densities of internal energy. This lesson, often given on the first day of traditional medicine class, provides the traditional formula that explains the relationships between the three aspects, or densities, of *nei qi* internal energy:

In this formula depicting the three aspects of "inner *qi*," *jing* is considered the densest representation of the life force, and *shen* the subtlest. Originally, the character for *jing* referred to pure, bleached rice; however, in the context of Taoist inner alchemy, *jing* became associated with bone marrow and semen (or, in female alchemy, menstrual blood [34]). As pertains to male practitioners, it is important to distinguish between *jing ye* (精液), or seminal fluid, and *jing qi* (精氣) as an energetic essence. This point will be returned to later on.

As an example of the earliest energetic-physiological principles that would eventually merge traditions of inner yoga, traditional medicine, and sexual alchemy, *jing* essence is said to be manufactured by, and thereafter stored in, the kidneys. *

> * The distinction between modern medicine description of kidneys as organs vs. the TCM / Taoist alchemist model was included in Section II.

Essence

Jing is a mixture of "prenatal / primordial" and "post-birth" elements. Also referred to as hereditary and acquired, in this scheme, the body's prenatal *jing energy* derives from *source* and is the *essence* inherited from one's parents, while the *jing* of later heaven is the energy derived from food, exercise, and breathing. In modern parlance, these can be thought of as: 1) a genetic influence — both strength and weaknesses — from one's parents, and 2) the degree of self-work (psychological self-examination, self-actualization, self-cultivation, and self-improvement), diet, and exercise discipline that a person maintains. Together, these co-influences determine one's health and longevity.

Chapter 10

The Meaning of Sensations:

Internal Yoga / *Qigong* as a Biofeedback System

*A*t this stage of our quest to learn more about the meaning of internal energy, three challenges must be addressed. The first has to do with how to interpret the sensations that are associated with, or described as, "internal energy." In the examples of the *qigong* and *t'ai-chi* masters, a particular class of sensation that the practitioner feels within the body are often referred to as *qi* energy. However, at this point we cannot say with true certainty whether or not something called *qi* energy exists. All we know for certain is that experienced practitioners identify sensations in their body, such as warmth or "electrically tingling," as the phenomenon of *qi* or internal energy.

Comparatively, in the case of the Tibetan *tantric* yogi, the experience of sensations within the adept's body is considered evidence of what is known in their culture as *lung-wind*, which, in many ways, can be compared with terms favored by the *t'ai-chi* and *qigong* practitioner. Similarly, in the example of *hatha* yoga, the experienced practitioner will name that same class of sensations occurring during practice as manifestations of *prana*. Thus, the first challenge is to ask whether or not these experiences are universal, and shared between traditions, or distinct phenomena unique to each.

The second challenge involves the question of whether or not something called "internal energy" exists as part of physical reality. Just because a practitioner might refer to sensations experienced during practice as *"qi,"* *"prana,"* or *"lung-wind,"* we cannot simply assume that something beyond the individual's subjective experience exists in a measurable way. At this juncture, all we can say with certainty is that experienced practitioners often encounter similar subjective sensations associated with the practice of yoga, *t'ai-chi*, *qigong,* and energetic meditation. This brings us to the third challenge.

Although subjective, which means limited in terms of the ability of others to agree that the phenomena we are discussing are "real," the kinds of sensations and personal experiences we are talking about still hold clues to the meaning of internal energy. Since they potentially encapsulate knowledge that will help us understand the nature of "internal energy," a closer look at these sensations is warranted.

Consider the way many energy practitioners describe their experience of feeling "energy" between their open-facing palms while engaged in *qigong* practice. In the same manner, reflect on the experience of warmth an advanced practitioner of Taoist or Tibetan energetic meditation describes as coursing through, or paralleling, the spine during their energetic practices. In order to explore the implications of these subjective sensations, both an approach to investigation and a new term are needed that will allow us to explore the interpretation of these experiences in and around the practitioner's body. At the same time, we need a working term that might remove the weight of the culture-laden assumptions that are embedded in terms like *qi, prana,* and *lung-wind.*

At this point in our investigation, it is useful to experiment with a few exercises for ourselves. Such a phenomenological approach will not only allow us to interpret sensations related to the practice of *qigong* and energetic meditation, but to do so without applying culturally specific terms such as *prana, mana,* or *qi.*

Through this experimental approach, we can gain insight into the meaning of subjective experiences described by some practitioners, such as the feeling of an "energy field" between one's open palms. This allows us to consider whether or not these kinds of experiences might actually be caused by a still-to-be-defined "energy," or if, as will be discussed later, they point toward an entirely different class of phenomena. Likewise, we, as amateur detective investigators, may discover that varying the practice by aligning the fingers in a certain way produces an increase or decrease in these kinds of sensations. This is another example of how one's experience while observing the phenomenon of sensations appearing within the body could further contribute toward the defining of what is meant by "internal energy."

Through one's experiences with "energetic" exercises such as those that follow, the investigation into these kinds of sensations is available to every practitioner with an open mind. In much the same way that one can learn to mentally attend to the slightest breeze passing over the cheek when wind hits the face from a specific compass point, one can become sensitive to feelings of "energy" surrounding the body. Although subjective, these provide important clues, since sensitivity of some sort or other to sensations perceived within the mind and body form the basis of *every* kind of *qigong,* Taoist, Indian, Tibetan, or any other form of energetic yoga and meditation. It's all about sensitivity, and in particular, the mind's ability to notice and consciously interact with these sensations as *signals.*

However, as just noted, this stated goal will be difficult to achieve, since the meaning of "internal energy" remains ambiguous. Thus, until more meaningful definitions of *qi, prana,* and similar terms become available, it would be useful to substitute them for another term that would allow us to investigate the meaning of these kinds of sensation. A useful term would be one that allows an interested person to experiment and practice with, as well as access the benefits of, energetic yoga / *qigong* without necessarily believing in — or, for the time being at least, even feeling the need to define — enigmatic and controversial terms like *qi* or "internal energy."

Thus, to meet this investigative requirement, the term signal is suggested. Although most often these sensations (feelings in the body) are identified with the presence of internal energy (feeling the *qi*), strength (is your *qi* strong or weak?), or the flow of internal energy through the body ("my *qi* is blocked!"), these descriptions are still subjective. Use of the term *signal* allows one to explore the experience without the need to define it in terms that are, at present, theoretical constructs. In utilizing this approach, *attention to sensations* in the form of *"signals"* can be interpreted and usefully developed as a personal biofeedback training system.

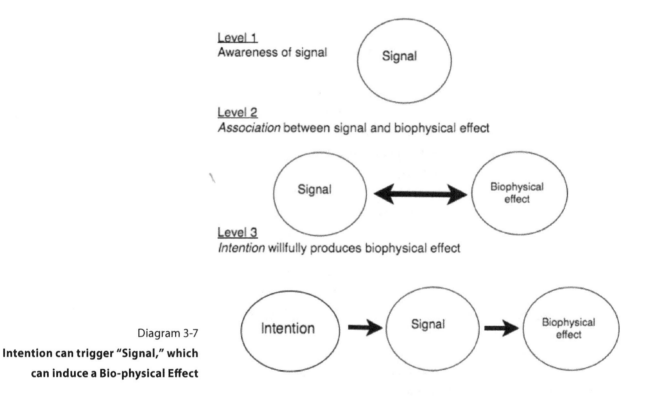

Diagram 3-7

Intention can trigger "Signal," which can induce a Bio-physical Effect

Signal as Biofeedback

For the remainder of this chapter, so-called "energetic practices," including *t'ai-chi, qigong,* and energetic meditation in all its forms, will be considered biofeedback practice. However, in the application of the biofeedback principles that follow, the kinds of biofeedback described here do not involve the use of a biofeedback monitor. Instead, this use of biofeedback involves one's ability to pay attention to subtle sensations within the body.

In each of the Asian traditions cited above, the practitioner learns to attend to subtle sensations within the body and to then trust and rely on them, before consciously reproducing them as biofeedback *signals* that can trigger physiological or more advanced "signal" changes. Examples include the increase in sensation or conscious direction of signal along supposed energetic pathways; the key point being that the power of attention directed toward biofeedback signals can be used to influence aspects of the normally unconscious nervous and, presumably, mind-body subtle energy systems.

Although traditional practitioners of Asian arts might, in their respective tradition, not think about their practice as a form of biofeedback, the principle of biofeedback applies to disciplines such as *qigong*, yoga, and energetic meditation in the way that they merge one's directed attention with subtle cues within the body.

Examples of how a cue can be observed and practiced within a biofeedback context is found in the way a particular cue can be used to induce warmth within the abdomen or along the spine. The biofeedback aspect applies when the practitioner attends to, and then willfully reproduces, the subtle cue within the body, and then adjusts their training (posture, breath, release of tension, attention, etc.) to access, *magnify*, or consciously direct the particular phenomenon they are emphasizing.

Sensations inform the practitioner that they are on the right track. Reproducibility and willful control over these kinds of sensations will, over time, lead the practitioner to mastery of that particular tradition.

To emphasize an earlier point, for the purposes of embracing these subjective experiences, at this stage it doesn't matter whether or not the perceived signals are actually something that might be called *qi, ki, prana,* or another variation of internal energy, or even if they are sensations that have nothing to do with *qi* or internal energy. What matters is that these repeatable biofeedback-based experiences provide valuable clues to the meaning of internal energy, regardless of how we define them.

Signal

While experiences of *signal* will vary between individuals, some aspects are shared among all participants. It should be noted that in the early stages of "energetic practices," such as in the examples that follow, it is not uncommon for a new practitioner to have some trouble learning to become aware of and work with *signal*. If this applies to you, be patient. Your ability to experience *signal* will improve with continued practice, open-mindedness, and patience.

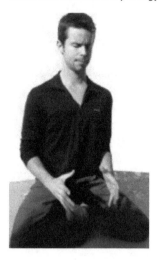

Photo 3-8

Sensing the Signal Between the Palms: Cross-Legged Posture

Note: Qi, *prana*, or "energy" sensing exercises, like those described here, are proposed to function through the body's embedded antenna receiving-transmission networks. As described here, these are proposed to allow one's *intention* to extend outward. Thus, it is STRONGLY RECOMMENDED that before engaging any type of "energy sensitivity" exercise, the practitioner first prepares themselves by prayer, or setting the intention, to interact with and be guided by a positive or benevolent source. This is believed to protect the individual during these kinds of practices. The antenna thesis is developed further in Section XII.

The best way to start is by adopting a relaxed, sitting, or kneeling position, as shown in Photo 3-8. Once ready to begin the practice, release all unnecessary tension, and when relaxed, place your open-facing palms near to each other, copying the hand orientation of the person shown in Photo 3-8. If you have previously attended a meditation, yoga, or t'ai-chi class, there is a good chance that you are already familiar with this exercise.

With practice, you will be able to observe *signal* not only between your open palms, but elsewhere in and around the body; ultimately, it will be felt wherever attention is directed. *Every* form of attention-directed internal / subtle energy training comprises three steps. The first involves the practitioner learning to perceive a sensation in the body associated with their goal. For example, if the goal of a particular exercise is to relieve back tension, the practitioner uses the "signal" to increase warmth to that area.

In contrast, if the practitioner's goal is to develop non-contact healing skills, such as the methods described in Section IV, they will work toward developing an ability to create a warm and tingling sensation in the lower abdomen, and then project that healing force onto the patient. As another example, if the practitioner's goal is to develop a light touch / minimal effort form of "internal power" for self-defense, the focus will be on channeling what feels like an electric current through the body. After considerable practice, the skilled practitioner is able to direct this representation of internal energy against an opponent. **

** Use of this application is covered in Sections VIII and XII.

Next, identify the body cues that accompany *signal* and will lead to success, such as relaxation of muscular tension in the area of the shoulders, or increased warmth in the lower abdomen. With regular practice, an unconscious link will form between the bio-physical *signal* and *intention*. In other words, through practice, *intention* becomes so closely identified with the signal and its bio-physical effect (e.g., relaxation of the shoulders) that placing attention to the target goal can immediately trigger the desired physiological response. This is an important step, whereby "energetic practice" begins to become a form of biofeedback training.

During this stage, the practitioner identifies subtle sensations in the body that will allow them to consciously interact with their perception of "energy." Subsequently, the practitioner begins to gain some degree of conscious control over certain aspects of the normally unconscious autonomic nervous system. An example of progress at this stage is the practitioner's ability to intentionally increase blood supply to the legs, which is indicated by increased warmth in the area. A link to a training video created by a practitioner working with *signal* is included in Box 3-9.

Magnetic Resonance

As in the example cited in Photo 3-8, a common report by practitioners engaging in regular practice with an open mind is the sense of magnetic resonance between their open hands. Sometimes, the sense of magnetic energy between the open palms can be very strong, perhaps even to the degree that it seems as though the two open palms cannot be pushed together. I have heard first-hand accounts by those who claim this was their experience, and for them, for a few moments or longer, it was impossible to join their palms together. In these kinds of examples, one's personal experience associated with *signal* can be especially intense. The notion that the body possesses magnetic fields, or at least what is perceived as magnetic fields, that can be engaged with and consciously manipulated is an important point. At this juncture, it is useful to include a few comments on the meaning of these sorts of sensations in and around the body.

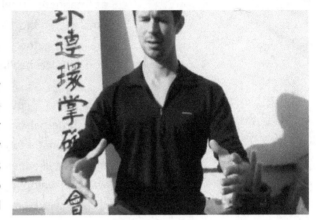

Working with Resonance
A video demonstrating this can be viewed at
https://www.youtube.com/watch?v=nH-dkUEd1ns
or
https://chiarts.com/3-9

Box 3-9

The Meaning of Magnetic-like Sensations

One of the more important clues that may help us reveal the meaning of "internal energy" has to do with the practitioner's experience of magnetic fields within the body, as it appears that all advanced practitioners of the "energetic traditions" experience the sense of magnetic centers or pulses within their bodies. Referring back to citations included in Chapter One, there is a long record of descriptions of a relationship between the experience of magnetism and "energy." One example noted there is that of nineteenth-century scientist von Reichenbach, who believed that a person could deliberately direct a magnetic field external to the body. Likewise, there was an entire class of scientists during the Renaissance who, referring to themselves as *magnetists,* focused their research toward the meaning of the mind-body "magnetic fields."

The theory that a strong magnetic field could be generated by an individual is expressed by Jan Baptista van Helmont, who postulated that the *vital effluence* radiated from every object in the universe, and it is not insignificant that he referred to this as his "great secret." Like van Helmont, many of the most well-known energetic healers through history attributed their gifts to an ability to become sensitive to their body's magnetic resonance fields. Consider the exploits of Valentine Greatlakes, also cited in Chapter One, who was documented for his ability to heal otherwise incurable maladies; it seems more than coincidental that he referred to his healing technique as "magnetic stroking." Later, we will address how the ability to consciously emit a large bio-electrical field is one of the criteria relied upon by modern era investigators researching the possibility that a person can mentally direct non-physical healing powers.

Two points summarize the preceding paragraphs. First, that no matter how "internal energy" will eventually come to be defined, mastery over the enigmatic force will be associated with the control over the kinds of magnetic-like feelings we've been talking about. Secondly, the most direct way of developing conscious control over that mysterious internal energy is through working with the "signal" as a biofeedback system.

Working with Biofeedback

A number of techniques can trigger experiences like those just described, including the feeling of magnetic fields or vortexes within the body, all of which involve the use of *signal*. For the practitioner, the experience of *signal* can be initiated through passive or active methods. In the classic Chinese yoga and meditation traditions, passive methods employ "listening," since they involve paying attention to cues within the body. This area of study falls under the category of *neiguan*.

Three requirements influence the individual's ability to work with *signal*: *inner calmness,* an open, positive and non-judgmental attitude; and the *intention* to perceive *signal*. The practitioner's condition of inner calmness promotes the synchrony of biological rhythms, which is an essential prerequisite for mastering one's internal energy.

With a few exceptions that will be addressed later, the experience of working with *signal* is usually safe and pleasurable. It is enjoyable to learn to observe the subtlest sensations within the body, and then discover how attention to these can consciously induce warmth, pressure and electric-like tingling. These are the same sensations that Taoist yogis, *neidan* alchemists, and other energetic meditators have relied upon for thousands of years, to inform them of the flow of *qi* in and around their bodies.

It is useful to consider systematic training that can increase one's ability to work with *signal*. Here is one example:

1. Acquire Signal

If you have ever attended a yoga, *t'ai-chi,* or *qigong* class, there is a good chance that you have already been introduced to this practice. The exercise illustrated in Photo 3-10 can be performed while lying down or while seated or kneeling.

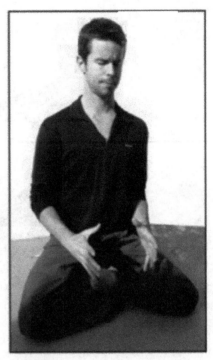

As illustrated in the photo, begin by holding your hands in a palm-open position, six to eight inches apart. If seated, sit with your back as straight as you can comfortably manage, since a hunched over posture tends to interfere with the ability to work with *signal.*

The initial goal is to learn to feel *signal* in the otherwise empty space between your two open palms, so simply relax and search for a sensation of "energy" in that area. This is a crucial step to take before learning to work with sensations that most practitioners identify as the control of subtle energy in and around the body.

Photo 3-10
Open Palm Signal Exercise
(Repeated from Photo 3-8 for the convenience of the reader)

More often than not, the sensation between the two open palms can be experienced as warmth / pressure, and with practice, most practitioners experience *signal* as an electrical-magnetic pulse. Once you reach this level, you'll learn to observe the feeling and then begin to understand how such a sensation can easily be identified (depending on the tradition) with terms such as *qi, ki, or prana.*

Although the experience of a particular sensation will vary between individuals, the sensation that you become aware of is the "feeling" you will identify as *signal.* Familiarity with your personal *signal* is useful for more advanced work, and with patience and regular practice, most people learn to feel pressure, or a slight electromagnetic sensation, between the hands akin to the repulse generated between two positively charged-sided magnets when they get near each another.

After a few moments, most individuals holding this position feel warmth or tingling between their hands. If you don't feel it at first, don't worry. Never try too hard to feel it, since over-trying can reduce your level of relaxation and thus block your ability to sense. When you do get it, observe the change that you feel in the empty space between your hands, and then feel free to play around with it. Just relax and imagine that your hands are "listening" to each other.

On overcoming difficulties, the following advice applies to one's work with any of the subtle cues described in this chapter, including the heartbeat of the heart-pulse method that will be presented later. If you are having difficulty acquiring the feeling of a particular cue, try imagining that you <u>are feeling it</u>. As a result, most individuals are eventually able to feel the particular cue associated with an exercise.

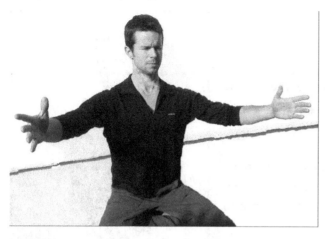

Photo 3-11
Working with *Signal*
In this example, the practitioner learns to maintain the *signal* and observe *resonance* while moving his hands farther apart.

Working with Resonance ("Resonance Training")

As shown in Photo 3-11, once you are able to perceive *signal* consistently between your open palms at will, you are ready to experiment with *signal* in new ways. Things are about to get interesting.

This extension of our *signal* experiment is based on the principle of "listening." It involves working in more nuanced ways with *signal* as a biofeedback technique, and the first step requires one to learn how to keep perceiving *signal* even as the hands move further apart.

Once you are able to feel *signal* in this scenario, try applying *signal* detection to your sitting, standing, and other postures. At this stage of practice, you will begin to notice how posture changes — even the smallest modifications — can influence *signal* strength in a yogic pose, or *qigong* technique.

This principle contributes to a concept that addresses the relationship between posture and one's ability to access maximum levels of efficiency and "energy," which will be addressed in Section XI.

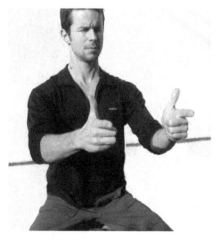

Photo 3-12
Concentrating Signal to the Fingertips ("Sword Fingers")

2. More *Signal* Work

After becoming confident in your ability to work with *signal* between your palms, begin exploring the meaning of sensations between your open palms in different ways. As suggested in Photo 3-11, start by slowly moving them further apart, and then bringing them back closer together.

While experimenting with this technique, be careful to maintain your awareness of *signal*. When you are able to sense the signal with your palms further apart, play with the concept of "breaking" and then reestablishing the "resonance response" by widening and narrowing the distance between your hands. The goal is to first be able to acquire, then purposefully turn off, and then reacquire your *signal*. Practice in a relaxed way and smile. Smiling relaxes jaw and facial tension, relieves stress, and promotes the flow of energy and blood.

3. Focus to Index Fingers ("Sword Fingers")

As illustrated in Photo 3-12, once you gain proficiency in working with *signal*, you can learn to concentrate the feeling of *signal* to different parts of the hand. Once you are ready, try to concentrate and focus the buzzy, electric-like, and (usually) increased warmth *signal* into your two index fingers.

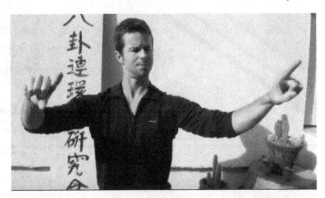

Success with this step means that you are gaining increased control over your ability to direct aspects of your blood and nervous system purposefully, and also gaining control over that enigmatic, yet to be defined *qi / ki / prana* internal energy.

Working with *Signal* and *Resonance* in Various Body Configurations

After becoming increasingly confident in your ability to sense and work with *signal* (buzzing, electrical-like, heat or pressure feeling), you are now ready to advance your use of *resonance* as a self-teaching tool.

At this stage, you are able to rely increasingly on signal to provide biofeedback, so that you can continue to make micro adjustments to your posture, *t'ai-chi*, yoga practice, and other endeavors based on paying attention to the *signal* feedback.

Intermediate Work with Signal and Resonance
A video demonstration of this technique can be viewed at:

> https://www.youtube.com/watch?v=vf8a6g1BtiU
> or
> https://chiarts.com/new-book-line-video-library/
> section-iii-box-3-13

Box 3-13

Working with **Signal** and **Resonance** in Various Body Configurations

Achieving Advanced *Athletic Connection and Alignment with "Resonance Training"
The top photo in the series shows broken (absence of) resonance. In the middle photo, the practitioner begins to feel and then "follow" the feeling of resonance. The lower photo shows the practitioner after achieving resonance between the two fingers.

"Athletic connection" is a new term, coined to describe the *ability to present effective and stable power* in context of a loose, wiry athletic state. It is not to be mistaken with strength of the kind found in muscle groups that are tense and resisting a force; the phenomenon presents in contact with a target.

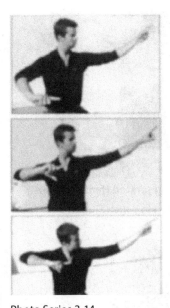

Photo Series 3-14

Breaking and Reestablishing Resonance

Begin by deliberately initiating the buzzy, electric-like sensation of *signal* in your index fingers. Then, play with the feeling of putting yourself slightly in and out of optimal position, while at the same time learning to observe which positions make you feel stronger, as well as those that make you feel weaker.

A link to a video demonstration of the exercise is included in Box 3-13, and three stills of a more advanced practitioner playing with these types of finger-concentrated resonance *signals* are shown in Photo Series 3-14.

In this practice, the goal is to establish "communication" between the two index fingers. You will know you have it when you feel increased heat, pressure, and a "buzzy" feeling in both fingers.

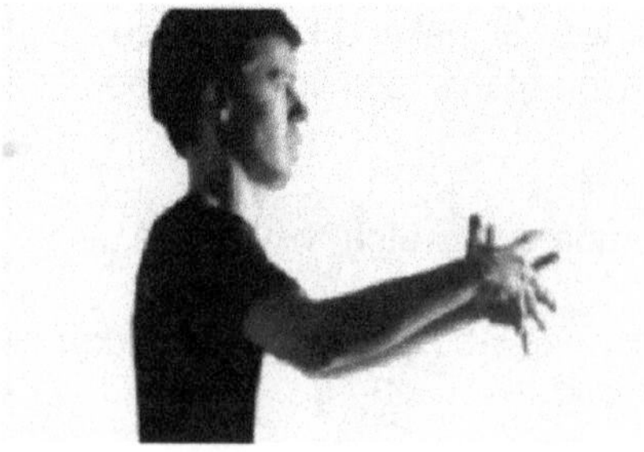

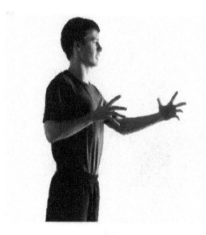

Photo 3-15

Standing and Movement Practice While Working with Signal

4. Intermediate Practice: Breaking and Reestablishing Finger Resonance †

Once you have enjoyed success in controlling the feeling of "energy" simultaneously in both fingers, you may wish to try a technique related to more advanced *qigong* / Taoist yoga training.

† The term "resonance" is used metaphorically, to explain the practitioner's experience of sensation. The term originated in the field of acoustics, and was adopted by researchers in electricity and magnetism. It is not common in neurology, except when talking about MRI's.

‡ It is useful to explain my equivocation in using the term "energy" vs. "feeling of energy." The reader may ask why I don't just make it easier by referring to the phenomenon simply as "energy?" The answer comes in two parts. First, no such "energy" has yet been accepted by conventional science. Second, Section XII includes an original thesis on the meaning of those sensations, how to interpret them, and their meaning in terms of a multi-dimensional definition of "internal energy." Thus, *sensations* like those described in this section might not be "energy," but instead those of a different nature.

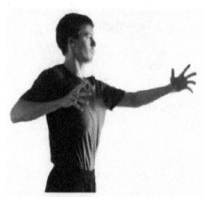

Photo 3-16

More Exaggerated Hand Position while Working with Signal

While making very subtle body adjustments, discover how you can reestablish the warmth, pressure, or electrical feeling you were working with earlier; experiment with the way a slightly relaxed and stretched elbow will increase *signal* strength. Stretching the small finger in just the right way can also create an improved sensation of energy flow throughout the entire body. Because it is based on biofeedback (self-detection) of signal rather than rote learning, this way of training is a quicker path to mastery. You are learning to align your body and become increasingly familiar with your attunement to your body's energy flow.

Photo 3-17

Increased Speed and Distance Between the Hands while Maintaining Attention to *Signal*

Referring back to the three images in Photo Series 3-14, note how they demonstrate progression in index finger-based resonance training. The upper photo in the series shows broken resonance, the middle photo shows the practitioner working with resonance, and the lower photo shows established resonance. The lesson here is that there are both more and less optimal physical alignments and postures.

To review, resonance training is based on the observation that, without our conscious awareness, we normally experience varying degrees of efficiency in how we move and hold our body. People are generally unaware that some poor postures create misalignment and produce a weakening effect on the body, or that learning to work with *resonance* can lead to discovering how slight posture corrections can allow one to feel better and more athletically integrated, and thus stronger.

A useful note for students of *qigong*, and internal energy arts like *t'ai-chi*, is that resonance practice helps you attune your internal energy system to its ideal balance. This form of resonance practice will deepen your understanding of yoga, *t'ai-chi*, and *qigong*. Study resonance by changing the distance and orientation of the index fingers in relation to each other. You can gauge your success by noting how quickly you can break and then reestablish resonance.

Through this approach, one will notice how the smallest movement can influence one's overall energy field. For example, note how a slight shift of the pelvic region might produce increased resonance, or, while guided by the feeling of resonance, observe how a slight inward turning of the knee while performing a posture or movement can influence its strength and integrity.

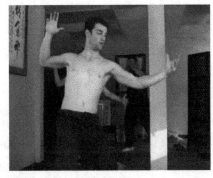

Photo 3-18

More Advanced Practice: Attending to Signal While in Motion

After gaining proficiency using *signal* as a biofeedback technique, try a more advanced practice that includes standing and movement. As demonstrated in Photo 3-15, begin by standing, and then tune into *signal* between the palms in the same way you did in the previous sitting practice. Once you have tuned into *signal* in the open space between the palms, begin to stretch and exaggerate your posture, as demonstrated by the practitioner in Photos 3-16 and 3-17. Gradually, while maintaining attention to *signal*, and also maintaining a tensional feeling in the palms and arms, begin moving one hand to the rear.

Perform this exercise in an isometric way, as if your rearward arm movement is resisting tension. Then, gradually increase the distance between the hands and move with increased speed, going as fast and as far as you are able to without losing the sensation of the *signal*. The distance between the hands gradually increases, as does the speed of movement. A link to a video showing a class practicing this exercise is included in Box 3-18.

More Advanced Studies of Signal: Movement
A video of students in a class practicing these exercises can be viewed at:

https://www.youtube.com/watch?v=TvTPffDs_Z4

or
https://chiarts.com/3-18

Box 3-18

Chapter 11

A Little More Advanced: The Outer Three Relationships

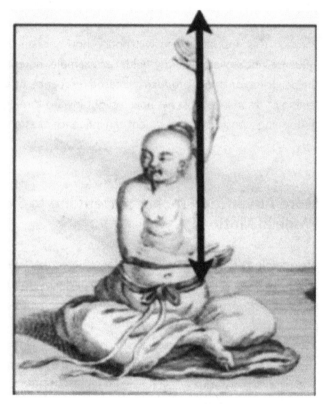

Figure 3-19

Wai San He — Is Energetic Alignment illustrated in an old Manuscript?
Drawings of a Taoist yogi from a 1779 French manuscript suggest that the practitioner was paying attention to the alignment of his wrists.

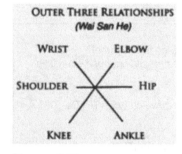

Diagram 3-20

外 三 合 **Wai San He**

"Outer Three Relationships"

The *wai san he* principles demonstrate how the elbow relates to the opposite knee, the wrist to the ankle, and the shoulder to the hip.

The *wai san he* (外三合), or "outer three relationships" (OTR), is one part of a pair of subdivisions of mind-body energetic principles known as the "six inner and outer relationships" (六內外合). More discussion of these relationships, with special attention to the other subdivision, *nei san he* (內 三 合), or "inner three relationships," will be covered later. The OTR is a system of energetic relationships within the body that is applied to traditional Chinese medicine, Chinese internal martial arts, and multiple forms of Taoist energetic yoga.

From the viewpoint of the OTR, the body is understood as a network of interconnected, or "holographic," relationships. As illustrated by the patterns featured in Diagrams 3-20 and 3-21, the OTR model demonstrates how some parts of the body have an energetic relationship with others. For example, as illustrated in the diagrams, when the right elbow is held just the right way in relation to the left knee, this "harmonizes," or creates a strengthening relationship with, the left knee. The OTR principle is common in energetic yoga and Chinese internal martial arts, providing an important diagnostic and intervention technique that also applies to some systems of traditional Chinese medicine. An example of this can be found in acupuncture, where, in some therapeutic interventions, a needle might be placed in the left elbow as a means of treating an issue in the right knee. Sometimes, however, the OTR principles apply to the same side of the body. Drawing 3-22 is borrowed from a paper on the subject, authored by Dr. Henry McCann, published in the *Journal of Chinese Medicine.* [36]

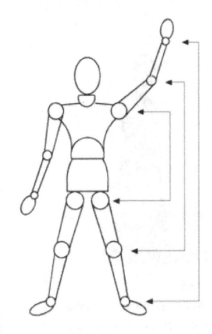

Figure 3-21
***Wai San He* "Outer Three Relationships"**
The Body's Energy Matrix

From Theory to Personal Experience

As demonstrated via the video link included in Box 3-18, because of its *signal-*feedback attributes, energetic practices such as Chinese yoga and *qigong* can be vehicles for exploring the body's energetic relationships. In the context of the OTR, this exploration converts the practice from theoretical to personal experience and practical application. In terms of the bio-mechanics that apply to the martial arts, one representation of OTR principles has to do with the way a strike is timed with the landing of the foot. In this context, when performed correctly, it represents the perfectly timed and coordinated hand and foot movement, where the execution of a step and a strike are synchronized. This OTR-based synchronization is in contrast to the more common way of foot / hand timing, where the foot sets slightly ahead of a hand strike. A video example that demonstrates both body mechanics and energetic body matrix principles can be viewed at the link in Box 3-23.

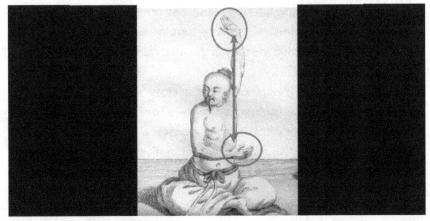

Diagram 3-22
The Outer Three or "Holographic" Relationships
This diagram is from a paper presented by Dr. Henry McCann,
Henry McCann, "A Practical Guide to Tung's Acupuncture," *Journal of Chinese Medicine.* [37]

Examples of *Wai San He* Outer Three Relationships
A video introducing *wai san he* "Outer Three Relationships" training for martial arts and body energy matrix study can be viewed at:

https://www.youtube.com/watch?v=_TFih-ke09gg
or
https://chiarts.com/3-23

Box 3-23

Exploring the Meaning of *Signal* and OTR Resonance

Using a variation of *signal* and *resonance* training, it is possible to test one's own OTR. In this case, OTR practice involves observing changes in the body brought about by making subtle adjustments to one's body position, i.e., pertaining to foot and hand orientation, and their relationship to each other. Consider that with each posture in an energetic practice, such as *t'ai-chi* or yoga, when the person is sensitive and open enough, he or she can become aware of how very slight changes to the body reveal the ideal position for a particular movement. This is due to the fact that when an aspect of the body deviates slightly from the optimal, it manifests as a weaker overall energy profile of a particular movement or posture. As an example, when the shoulder is not in optimal alignment with the hip, this will have a weakening influence on the energy system of the entire body.

Researching the OTR

Begin this exercise from either a sitting or standing posture. After reviewing the feeling of *signal* as presented in the earlier sections, hold your hand out in front of your body in the manner demonstrated by the practitioner in Photo 3-24. However, instead of searching for *signal* in the empty space between the hands, as was described in the earlier sections, now search for the feeling of *signal* between the wrist and the ankle on the opposite side of the body.

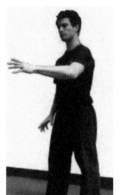

Photo 3-24

Working with Signal in the Outer Three Relationships

After assuming the approximate position where you feel your wrist might be in energetic resonance with the opposite ankle, experiment with this technique by moving your hand slightly, side-to-side at first, to break and then reestablish *signal* resonance. After a little practice, most individuals are able to find just the right positioning, where *signal* will simultaneously appear in both the wrist and opposite ankle. As previously described, when the relationship is optimal, most practitioners will feel pressure, increased warmth, or a buzzy, electric-like sensation simultaneously at the wrists and ankles.

With experience, one's awareness of these cross-body *signal* relationships will become stronger, and subsequently one's confidence in practicing the technique will improve. As with the earlier exercises, if you initially have trouble detecting *signal*, be patient, stay relaxed, and remain open-minded. If not at first, then eventually you will be successful in practicing the OTR *signal*.

Once you've gained confidence in your ability to detect and work with *signal* between the wrist and opposing ankle, experiment with slight changes that move the hand in and out of the optimal energetic relationship. Continue to experiment with your ability to detect and improve less optimal alignments in your yoga, *qigong*, or *t'ai-chi* by extending the practice to other body configurations. For example, experiment with the same wrist and ankle exercise on the opposite side of the body.

More Advanced *Wai San He* Matrix Work

Once you have achieved some success with the *wai san he* feedback sensation while sitting, start to experiment with experiencing the same sensations in other standing or moving exercises. The goal in this kind of practice is to feel the OTR sensations continually throughout your energetic practice.

Thoughts on *Wai San He* as the Body's Energetic Matrix

The Taoist yogis of ancient China had bodies identical to ours; they did not wake up one day and decide that some random stretch was essential to health. The sensations described in this section referring to the practice of *signal* are the same class of experiences as those observed and studied by those Taoist yogis long ago. However, one important difference between the ancient Taoist adept and most of us today is the amount of daily time they devoted to their practice. Through patient, quiet observation, they were able to observe how pressure to a specific location on the body could stimulate sensations like a flushing feeling, or tingling elsewhere in the body.

Through systematic observation of the subtlest bodily sensations, those skilled at paying attention to *signals* provided by their body were able to study their own hidden energetic connections. Part of their research led them to discover what we might today call the body's interconnected holographic matrix. This represents the way that different aspects of the body relate to one another, and how some parts maintain a holographic harmony with others. Among their various discoveries, a set of body relationships called *wai san he*, or the "three outer relationships," was an important contribution that no doubt furthered the development of the Chinese internal martial arts, such as *t'ai-chi ch'üan*.

Chapter 12

Dao yin Physical Yoga

As evidenced by the *Mawangdui* tomb drawings found on silk texts (Figure 3-25), the practice of Taoist self-healing exercise dates back at least to the first millennium of the current era, with other references suggesting that the practice is much older. For example, the fourth-century BCE Taoist philosopher, Chuang Tzu, made disparaging remarks about the practice of what he referred to as "bear-hanging" and "bird-stretching."

Figure 3-25

Outlines of Twenty-Eight Postures Found in the Second-Century BCE Mawangdui Tomb Scrolls

These images provide the earliest existing depictions of dao yin Taoist yoga / posture exercises. The characters next to the top-left image read, "Getting in touch with yin and yang with use of a long pole."

Source: Joseph Needham, Science and Civilization in China [45]

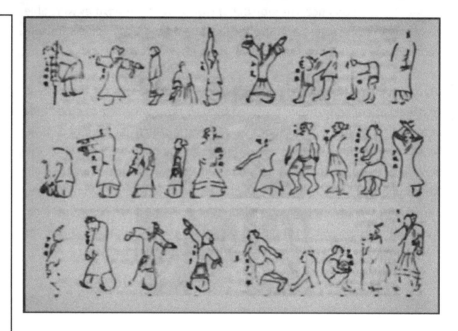

It is instructive to reflect on the description of Taoist yoga from other sources, such as the biography of third-century CE surgeon, Hua Tho, which includes a description of the practice:

> Wu Phu of Kuang-ling and Fan A of Pheng-cheng were both pupils of Hua Tho. Wu Phu followed exactly the arts of Hua so that his patients generally got well. Hua Tho taught him that the body should be exercised in every part but that this should not be over-done in any way. 'Exercise', he said, 'brings about good digestion (lit. causes the dispersal of the qi) of cereals... and a free flow of the blood. It is like a door-pivot never rotting. Therefore, the ancient sages engaged in *dao yin* exercises, (for example) by moving the head in the manner of a bear and looking back without turning the neck. By stretching at the waist and moving the different joints to left and right one can make it difficult

for people (to grow) old … It can be used to get rid of diseases, and it is beneficial for all stiffness of the joints or ankles. When the body feels ill, one should do one of the exercises. After perspiring, one will sense the body grow light, and the stomach will manifest hunger. Wu Phu followed this advice himself and attained an age greater than ninety, yet with excellent hearing, vision, and teeth.[38]

It is probable that the development of Chinese *dao yin*, or "physical yoga," was influenced from contact with other forms of yoga, particularly those of Indian origin. It is noteworthy that some scholars, such as Catherine Despeux, claim that this was the case and that *hatha* yogas, as practiced on the Indian subcontinent, were their source. [39] Taoist yoga can be subdivided into physical and mental practices. *Dao yin* "pulling and stretching" exercises are of the physical type. They are designed to invigorate and move internal energy through yogic stretches and the holding of specific postures.

Sometimes, *dao yin* exercises are performed along with self-massage, while other practices are performed in conjunction with breathing techniques. In contrast, mental *neiguan* yogas address the body's interior through focused, or passive, attention. However, these distinctions between physical and mental yogas are painted with a broad brush, since it is rare for Taoist yogas to be exclusively physical or attention-based. Physical approaches almost always include an intention component to move the *qi*, and forms of yoga that emphasize directed attention to the interior often include a physical component as well.

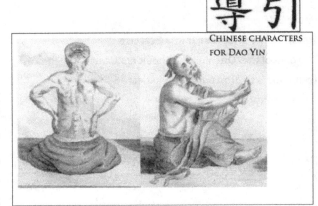

CHINESE CHARACTERS FOR DAO YIN

Three *Dao yin* Yogas

Including prescriptive routines and stand-alone exercises, there are many hundreds, if not thousands, of *dao yin* active yogas. As with the example of "Look at Moon," some of these are widely practiced, whereas others are seldom used. This chapter includes three *dao yin* stand-alone postures: "Opening the shoulder Joints," "Look at Moon," and "Awakening the Dragon." Opening the Shoulder Joints is a good example of a *dao yin* exercise that can be used for therapeutic applications to address neck and shoulder pain. Look at Moon represents the merging of traditional Chinese medicine with *qigong* and Taoist health practices, since it is designed to stimulate the channel on the back of the body that is associated with the outermost layer of defense against exogenous influences. The exercise is comparable with what can be thought of today as an immune enhancing function. Awakening the Dragon is a variation of the more widely practiced "Crouching Monkey" posture. It is included here as it represents the kind of *qigong* technique where one

Figures 3-26

Eighteenth-Century Etchings of Taoist Yoga

These images are from the first depictions of Taoist yoga appearing in Western print. These and similar drawings are from the French publication *Memories concernant L'Histoire, Les Sciences et Les Arts De Chinois*, published in 1779. It is interesting that the exercises shown in the image are still practiced today. In Figure 3-26: Left: a Taoist yogi massages his back to increase warmth and *qi* in the kidneys. Right: massaging acupuncture channel points on the webbing of the big toe to calm the liver.

side of the body creates the feeling of an electrical field that "communicates," or interacts / balances, with the opposite side of the body — in this example, wrist-to-wrist and knee-to-knee.

For all functional disorders affecting the torso, exercises are used that consist of maintaining a certain posture over a given span of time while the adept mentally guides the qi throughout the body.

Catherine Despeux [40]

Dao yin forms of physical yoga are most often performed in a static position, or through the repetition of sets of extremely slow movements. They are designed to balance energy, promote healing, and increase athletic performance. Their regular practice is said to "remove stagnation," clear energetic channels, and activate the body's bio-energetic reserves.

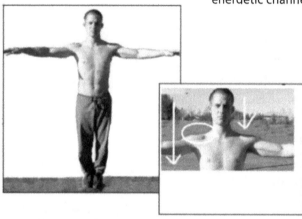

Those who practice circulation of qi may perfect their inner state, those who practice gymnastics [daoyin] may cure afflictions of the limbs

Catherine Despeux [41]

The "Opening the Shoulder Joints" (OSJ) exercise, shown in Photos 3-27, is a good example of Taoist yoga in that it combines stretching, breathing, and mental exercise. OSJ is useful as an adjunctive therapy for neck and shoulder pain. Correctly performed, within a few minutes of holding the arms outward in this way, a *traction* effect will be produced. This is an orthopedic technique for relieving pressure on the spine or bones, which can be traced back to ancient times. The practice of holding the technique helps the muscles of the shoulders and upper back release in order to accommodate the arm positions. As habitual tension in the shoulder complex starts to relax, OSJ tugs at the neck and shoulders.

Photo 3-27
Opening the Shoulder Joints Exercise
The goal of the "Opening the Shoulders Joints" technique is to drop out the shoulders and release tension

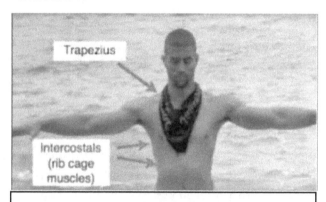

Opening the Shoulder Joints Training
A video showing the Opening the Shoulder Joints training can be viewed at the following link:

https://youtu.be/BqsNcrIi1RI
or
https://chiarts.com/3-28

Box 3-28

In the language of the body's channel and energetic system, OSJ promotes energetic balance at the juncture of six channels (three *yin* and three *yang*) as they pass from the torso to the arms. These are the *yin* energetic channels of the lung, pericardium, and heart; and the *yang* energetic channels of the large intestine, triple burner, and small intestine. The exercise is particularly valuable, since half of the major channels pass through these locations.

In surprising ways, exercises like the OSJ provide a training advantage in other endeavors. This point is illustrated by how one practitioner used the technique to enhance his *conga* drum playing. Sal, a senior instructor in our organization, used the OSJ as a warm-up technique before drumming practice, and he believes that the exercise helped him see a dramatic improvement in his overall performance. Sal shared the technique with his drum instructor, who became so impressed with his own increased power and control after practicing the technique that he now regularly employs the posture as a warm-up exercise for his students.

"Looking at the Moon"

As mentioned earlier, Looking at the Moon (LAM) is a perfect demonstration of the interrelationship between Taoist yoga and traditional Chinese medicine. Illustrated in Photos 3-29, the exercise creates gentle, continuous stress along the entire *taiyang* channel system, and is useful as a strength, rehabilitation and preventative technique. In traditional terms, the latter use is known as "repelling the exterior."

Repelling the Exterior

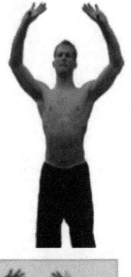

Credited to the famous Chinese physician Zhang Zhongjing (150 - 219 CE), Zhang's *exterior - interior* theory describes the body's channel system as a series of protective layers from the outside to the inside of the body. Consisting of the Urinary Bladder (UB) and Small Intestine (SI) channels, the *taiyang* channel system acts as the body's first defensive shield against the invasive influence of *exogenous* [42] or "pernicious" influences, such as cold, heat, dampness, etc.

Looking at the Moon is also a supplement for athletic training. When practiced regularly, the exercise creates an overall feeling of springiness, or *song,* * throughout the body. Furthermore, the practice engages the body's myofascial channel system, a subject introduced in Section II and addressed more in later sections. Benefits associated with the practice include tension release in the shoulders and back, and, for martial artists and Western-style boxers, an increase in "explosive" power.

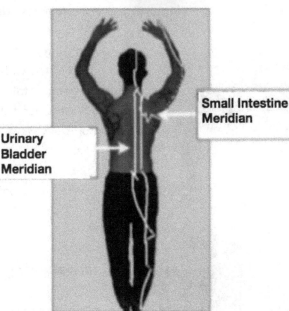

Small Intestine Meridian

Urinary Bladder Meridian

* Covered in Section XI

Practices

Holding your palms above your head in the manner shown in Diagrams 3-29, gently stretch into the exercise and work on developing the feeling of a springy-connectedness throughout the entire *taiyang* channel system. When correctly performed, a stretchy-tugging

Diagrams 3-29

"Looking at Moon" and the *Taiyang* Channels

The "Looking at the Moon" posture stimulates and balances both channels of the taiyang channel system. (Note, for illustration purposes, although running bilaterally along both sides of the spine, the channel, with two branches is shown on the right side only.)

feeling should be felt laterally (outside) from the feet to the small fingers of the hand. Ultimately, you will recognize this gentle tension as what is referred to as the *song-peng* continuum. ** The stretch should feel slightly challenging, but not painful. The goal of the exercise is to develop a feeling of stretching or tugging through the entire body, which can be compared to a person using athletic stretching / exercise bands.

**Defined in Section XI

When it comes to the effects of the exercise on the small intestine channel of the arms and hand, the exercise triggers a bit of healthful tension that starts deep in the shoulder complex and travels all the way to the outside corner of the small finger. When you feel a tug along the entire channel, hold onto that feeling and work with it.

Train to feel the sensation of elastic stretchiness through the entire *taiyang* system. Look for the feeling of gentle tension that originates in the location of the "funny bone" in the elbow. When you get it right, you will notice a stretchy-tug at that location, and once the exercise is complete, the gentle tension continues up the back of the arm and traverses behind the scapula (shoulder blade). From the shoulder blade, maintain a gentle but firm stretchy feeling to the hollow of the collarbone, and continue the stretch to the muscles on the side of the neck, over the cheek to the ear, and then to the corner of the eye. As with any gentle stretching practice, start with only a few minutes and gradually increase the length of time holding the posture. Intermediate to advanced practitioners may practice ten to twenty-five minutes a day, or every other day.

Looking at Moon (LAM) exercises the full range of tendons and ligaments associated with the elbows and wrists. When correctly performed, LAM promotes total body athletic connection* to such a degree that the practitioner is able to express an advanced level of integrated athletic force, or "body wave," which in the internal martial arts is known as the "Dragon Palm."

(A few more notes on Looking at the Moon are included in Endnote [43])

Awakening the Dragon

The Awakening the Dragon (ATD) exercise provides two benefits; one as an upper and lower body physical integration practice, the other energetic. As a physical practice, the exercise stretches and strengthens the muscles of the lower back, while its energetic aspects allow the student to influence and interact with internal energy cross-principles. In other words, the practice includes the feeling of magnetic energy traveling along one side of the body, which can influence and interact with the sense of magnetic energy on the opposite side.

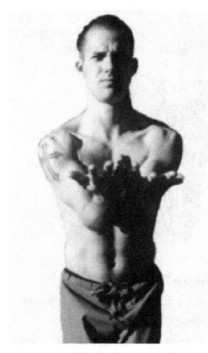

Photo 3-30
Awakening the Dragon

ATD is particularly useful in training the flexor iliopsoas muscles (Diagram 3-31) deep in the lower back / upper legs. In terms of traditional medicine, it activates important energetic centers and pathways associated with the kidneys and kidney energy.[44]

Awakening the Dragon develops whole body power and expression by strengthening the unique set of muscles that join the lower with the upper body. Some of the energetic attributes of the exercise are described later.

Start the practice by bringing your knees together. Then bend the knees forward while arching the back in order to assume a slight crouching position. Taking the posture shown in Photo 3-30, the goal is to find a crouch position that feels a bit uncomfortable. Your goal is to challenge the core muscles of the body, so unless you are already in condition and accomplished in disciplines like surfing or rock climbing, the muscles of the lower back and upper legs will be challenged.

Next, similar to the instructions that accompanied the LAM exercise, work to engage your entire body from the core psoas muscles to the fingers, paying particular attention to the small fingers on both hands. Continue this whole-body integrated stretch as you join your small fingers together in the manner shown in the photo, making slight adjustments as you search for the deep tug of the psoas that expresses all the way to the small fingers. If correct, "pull" from the exercise should be felt through the shoulders and lower back. Start with only a few minutes a day and then gradually increase the time holding the static posture for up to ten minutes at a time.

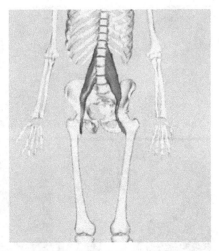

Figure 3-31

Iliopsoas Muscles

The iliopsoas is the combination of two muscles, the *Illiacus*, and the psoas major. The *Illiacus* originates on the pelvic crest and attaches to the femur. The psoas major begins on the lumbar vertebrae of the lower back and attaches to the large femur bone in the upper leg.

Awakening the Dragon as an Electro-Magnetic Resonance Practice

One of the reasons that the ATD posture is included in this chapter is because of the way the exercise can increase the practitioner's feeling of electromagnetic energy *(signal)* flow in and around the body. One variation that demonstrates the power of the exercise as a psychological calming technique involves learning to pressure / stimulate a point on the heart channel referred to as *shen men*, or "spirit gate."

Spirit Gate (Heart 7)

Notice the point between the two joined wrists shown in Photos 3-32. Acupuncturists refer to this point as Heart 7 (H-7); the therapeutic and energetic use of these body cross-connection points demonstrates a convergence between TCM and *dao yin*-style exercise.

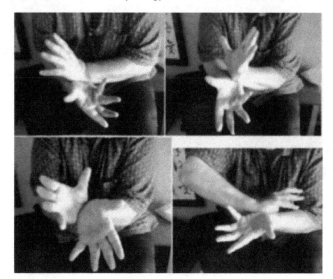

Photos 3-32

Hand Positions that Enhance Energy Conduction Through *Shen* Men, "Spirit Gate"

(Acupuncture Point "Heart 7")

The emotional balancing aspect of the exercise relies on both the application of sustained pressure between the medial aspects of the two wrists and directed intention to the point, with both being directed to the connecting *shen men* / "spirit gate" points. The practice relaxes the body and calms the emotions. A variation of the exercise involves pressing these two points together while changing hand shape, as shown in Photos 3-32, which triggers cross-body energetic balance through the heart channel.

Applying Cross-Body Energy Relationship Principles

It is good practice to exercise cross-body relationships. While holding the ATD posture, work with feeling cross-body "energy" sensations small finger-to-small finger, wrist-to-wrist, and, if you are flexible enough, inside elbow-to-inside elbow. Other cross-body locations not shown in the photo are knee-to-knee and ankle-to-ankle.

Relaxation does much more than relieve bodily tension. It interrupts the brain's release of stress–stimulating neurochemicals, and stress is the number one killer in America. Lowering stress reduces heart disease, high blood pressure, and pain.

Dr. Andrew Newberg, How God Changes your Brain [46]

Chapter 13

Neiguan: Inner Yoga of Directed Attention

The previous chapter introduced some of the benefits of *dao yin* physical yoga practice, describing how its benefits are derived from creating gentle stress along myofascial channels. ** By contrast, *neiguan* "inner yoga" exercises derive their benefits through mental practices, such as directed attention and visualization. In this category of exercise, beneficial influences are gained from the practitioner's attention to internal processes, such as the heartbeat and pulse, stimulating psychophysiological changes within the body.

> ** The use of "myofascial" as an attribute of "channels" will occasionally be used to stress / emphasize the physically real nature of the channel structure (as opposed to an imaginary energy line), as was described in Section II.

Inner yoga techniques can be general or specific. General techniques influence the energy fields † of the entire body and promote relaxation and a positive attitude, whereas other *neiguan* exercises are very specific, and can be used to address specific issues such as pain in specific areas of the body or increased circulation. Inner yoga can be further subdivided into active and passive types. Active inner yoga, through directed attention, targets specific areas, channels, or energy centers of the body. An example of passive inner yoga is found in the way a practitioner might learn to relax tense muscles throughout the entire body. By contrast, learning to detect and direct attention to the pulse at various locations throughout the body is an example of a more active type of mental yoga practice.

> † Although in one sense, the "energy fields" being discussed here refer to the as-yet-undefined qi of traditional Chinese medicine, these most probably also refer to the synergistic bio-fields of the body that are generated by the organs (most notably the heart), and the cumulative bio-electrcial fields on the cellular level.

Passive Yoga and the Heartbeat

A good example of passive Taoist yoga is in the way one can use awareness of the heartbeat as a relaxation, meditation, and self-healing technique. The notion of working with the pulse as a mind-body training is an ancient Taoist technique. As Ishida explains, observing the pulse is a form of working with the body's "protective and constructive energies:" [47]

> One can imagine the pulse as the waves of the various fluids flowing around the body. It is in these waves, sent out originally from the heart, that the spirit takes up its residence. [48]

Ishida adds: "Assuming that the pulse represents the basic wavelike nature of all the energies of the body, one may depict their relationship as follows: [see Diagram 3-33]"

In traditional terms, the notion of the arterial pulse being connected to "mind" that moves around the body is expressed in ancient Taoist and Confucian texts (Diagram 3-33). Consider that the *Huainanzi* states that "the mind moves around throughout the body [because of the pulse]," [49] which, as Ishida explains, forms the basic understanding that led to the formation of Taoist practices that emphasized first control over the body and then management of the emotions, which in turn leads to tranquility and emptiness of mind. [50]

Passive *neiguan* exercises, when utilized as a relaxation technique, usually begin in the most relaxed position possible. However, once proficiency is sufficient, many techniques can be adapted to walking, running, and even as a technique to improve athletic performance. The benefits of the exercise described below, known as "heart-pulse training," are often noticed immediately, especially the relaxation and calming effects.

An example of how the heartbeat and pulse can be used to reduce stress is illustrated by in the experience of a client who, following service as a Marine Corps officer, started a small business in Malibu, California. We met weekly at her office for training in meditation, martial arts, and *qigong*. During some of our sessions, she would describe her business challenges. She would often seem angry and upset about the day's mishaps, and on one day in particular she was distressed to the point that she was unable to concentrate on the planned lesson. Detailing the stressful events of the day, she provided a verbal list of things that had gone wrong, from office landlord issues to product containers that had failed to be delivered as promised. Instead of the planned lesson, I asked her to lie on the floor, face up, placing her hands over her chest, and instructed her to observe the heartbeat.

A minute or two later, she began to relax. She continued to practice placing attention on the heartbeat, and, seeing the relaxation of her tense facial and jaw muscles, I knew that she had calmed down. After a few minutes more, I asked her to once again review the day's events. This time, although the

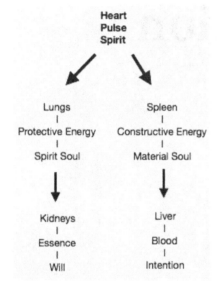

Diagram 3-33

Aspects of Mind and Pulse as Represented in Classic Traditional Chinese Medical Texts

Based on the depiction by Hidemi Ishida, "Body and Mind: The Chinese Perspective," Taoist Meditation and Longevity Techniques

information she conveyed was the same, her description of the day's events was new and improved. As she repeated the list of the day's calamities, her mood was lighter, and at times she seemed close to laughter.

Rather than feeling angry and frustrated, she now observed the day's events from a new perspective, viewing them as a sequence of humorous events. Although the same day's events remained part of her experience, the way she described them, and presumably her immune system's stress response, was significantly different. The principle is explained in the *Secret Teachings of the Red Monk,* which states:

> Find the place in your standing, walking or sitting. Then become aware of your heart pulse. Sense your pulse move through your entire body. Move with and follow the pulse. Learn to connect and at no time become disconnected from this. This is the master tool of the high arts.

—Secret Teachings of the Red Monk

Important: Never end pulse practice with attention focused at or near the head. Instead, always end by observing the pulse at the lower abdomen, hips, or feet.

Learning the Heart-Pulse Method

Step 1: Practice with the Heartbeat

Begin by lying completely flat, face up. Lying on a hard (but not cold) surface is better than a soft bed. If you can do it without much discomfort, lie with your head flat and without a pillow. Place your relaxed hands across your chest and release unnecessary tension.

Close your eyes, and become aware of your heartbeat. If you cannot feel it at first, be patient. Eventually, you will be able to feel your heartbeat fairly easily, anywhere and anytime that you choose. The effect of this simple exercise is *more powerful* than you will be aware of. It gives you conscious control to immediately influence and calm your nervous system.

Through your relaxed hands on your chest, become aware of the sensation of the heartbeat in your chest as detected through your hands. For most individuals, as they start to become aware of their heartbeat, they also notice an involuntary deepening of their breath. This is a good sign relating to *entrainment,* the attainment of synchrony between various body rhythms, which will be addressed in Section VII and again in later chapters.

Step 2: Distal Training

Next, attempt to detect the feeling of the pulse in another area of your body. The hips, abdomen, or anywhere in the pelvic area will provide a good pulse signal to work with. Identifying the secondary location is often challenging to begin with, but it is a *very important* part of the training. The technique requires you to notice and pay attention to an internal biofeedback *signal* (the pulse) anywhere in your body.

To help you find and intentionally engage the pulse, use your hands as a pulse-detection "instrument," placing them on your lower abdomen. While doing this, keep your hands very relaxed — think of them as sensitivity / detection instruments — and if you have trouble relaxing them while keeping them in place on your abdomen, try hooking your thumbs into a belt loop. The aim is to keep them as relaxed as possible while you learn to feel the pulse in the abdomen.

With your hands in position on the lower abdomen or pelvic area, search for the sensation of the pulse. As an example of how internally-directed focus can influence a specific area of the body, as well as *the entire nervous system*, during this step most individuals immediately notice relaxation in the area. Since this step leads to increased circulation, most individuals will feel improved warmth and blood circulation to their legs and feet. When you perceive increased flushing warmth in the lower body, relax and enjoy the sensation for a moment longer.

With practice, the act of intentionally attending to the pulse becomes easier. Search for the feeling of the pulse originating deep within the abdomen. Then, with your attention turned inward, search for the feeling of the beating pulse from the blood moving through the arterial vessels. Just as with Step 1, you might notice the occurrence of a sudden deep breath as tension releases; if this happens, just relax and observe. This is another good sign, as it means that you are gaining some conscious control over normally unconscious aspects of the nervous system.

Step 3: By Attention Only

Next, learn to trigger the same sensations that you are concentrating on, but without using your hands as a "signal detector." In this step, the goal is to consciously pay attention to the pulse in your body, using your attention to trigger, and become aware of, the feelings of warmth and flushing at various locations, while using internally-directed focus alone. This is a significant accomplishment, since it is a sign that you are gaining more conscious control over normally unconscious processes.

Next, begin by lying flat, face up, with your hands open, relaxed, palms facing upwards. When you are ready, place attention on the heartbeat in your chest. As in Step 1, some individuals might have difficulty with this at first, especially if they are tense or stressed. If you are feeling anxious or nervous, notice, as you attend to the heartbeat, how this produces a relaxation response. As you relax, observe how your breathing will sometimes deepen automatically.

Step 4: Targeted Attention

This step involves learning to attend to, and observe, your pulse in different areas of the body. With practice, it will become increasingly easy to observe to the pulse wherever and whenever you wish. Here is a typical sequence of attending to the pulse / relaxation training:

- Place attention to the heartbeat at the center of the chest.
- Then, observe the pulse at the lower abdomen.
- Back of the neck –- above the top thoracic vertebrae.
- Back to the center of the chest.
- Then back to the abdomen.

Then the pelvic area. When you complete this step successfully, you will be able to direct and influence the pulse in any area of the body you choose.

With practice, the yogic art of attending to the pulse can be undertaken while a person is sitting or standing. When perfected, the pulse as a *signal* can be attended to while one is moving, talking, or even as a background *signal* while one is participation in sports. Practice your "pulse training" while sitting or standing, working to develop the awareness of the pulse in your lower back, abdomen, or another area throughout your normal day.

† Section VII includes examples where the protocol is applied to mock combat practice.

Alternative Practice: Partner Work

An alternative way of practicing involves cooperating with a partner, who can help you through the various steps while you learn to relax and concentrate.

The partner will help you to monitor the pulse cues in your body. After you are successfully able to feel your heartbeat, place your hands by your side.

Begin by closing your eyes and relaxing. Then, your partner will assist you by lightly placing two fingers on the areas on your body, as indicated in the sequence listed in step 3.

Begin with your partner placing two fingers on the center of your chest. Attend to the pulse at the location where they are touching very lightly.

With your eyes closed, practice feeling the pulse at the exact position where your partner is lightly touching, for example, on the abdomen, hips, or legs. When you feel a sensation at each target, acknowledge this success with a slight nod of the head rather than speaking.

Ask your partner to review the sequence suggested in step 3 in a calm and patient manner. Your partner should move on to the next target in the sequence only after you have indicated that you feel the pulse at the particular target location.

Box 3-34

125

Heart-Pulse Method as Adjunctive Therapy

Due to its ability to induce health-enhancing and powerful mind-body states, the heart-pulse method is valuable either alone or in combination with other therapies. As will be described in a moment, in some cases, the passive therapy of the heart-pulse is one of the only non-pharmaceutical interventions available.

One example of the therapeutic value of the technique is in the way in which it helped a patient I worked with at the Natural Health Medical Center of Los Angeles, who I'll call Jana. A middle-aged woman of Middle Eastern descent, Jana had been diagnosed with chronic fatigue syndrome. She appeared depressed and exhausted and was so physically weak that she seemed to have difficulty sitting. Consequently, I asked her to continue the interview lying down on the exam table.

Jana explained that her daily life was ruled by constant physical pain and weakness, and for someone not familiar with chronic fatigue syndrome, it can be difficult to imagine the debilitating nature of this disease. Although I specialize in therapeutic exercise, breathing techniques, and meditation, I wondered what on earth I could offer someone in Jana's position.

I asked her to relax and breathe slowly, in order to give me time to think of something to try. It then occurred to me that because of its passive, gentle nature, the heart-pulse method would be one of the few exercises that she could perform. Following a similar protocol to what was described earlier, I began to teach her the technique, first asking her to place her hands over her chest and attend to the feeling of her heartbeat. Initially, she was so tense that she couldn't feel her heartbeat, so I asked her to *imagine* feeling her heartbeat.

After a minute or so of imagining the feeling of her beating heart, she began to be able to feel it for real. A moment or two later came the first hints that the stress was beginning to release its hold. A few moments after that, her breathing became less strained and her facial tension relaxed slightly. As she continued to work with attention to the pulse in her chest and abdomen, a little more tension was released, and then two tears rolled down her face. The simple act of attending to the subtle internal signal of the beating heart began to break her body's life and death-like grip of chronic tension.

Dr. Hoang, the center's director, agreed that the heart-pulse method seemed to help, and we continued the treatment for several weeks until her medical insurance coverage for the visits expired. However, a few weeks later, Dr. Hoang informed me of his surprise to learn that the large (and usually extremely conservative) HMO‡ that provided for Jana's care had approved additional therapy sessions with the unorthodox treatment. Jana's attending psychiatrist had written a special letter to the HMO's patient care supervisors, asking that the unusual therapy be continued.

‡ Health Maintenance Organization, in the U.S., an organization that
provides health insurance

Like Jana, many of us hold chronic tension in our bodies; the pattern of this kind of physical stress can be insidious and not easily recognized. Often, we are unaware of the negative health effects of this kind of chronic stress and tension. Jana's experience matches the results of hundreds of other students, clients, and patients I've taught this technique to over the past twenty years. Their stories provide strong anecdotal evidence of the potential benefits of the heart-pulse method as a useful intervention to mitigate mental and physical stress.

Final Comment on the Value of the Heart-Pulse Method

I continue to be amazed by the multifaceted helpfulness of the heart-pulse method. It provides one with the power to consciously influence the blood and nervous system in targeted areas within the body, and thus can be a helpful adjunctive therapy to address numerous conditions. I hope that the efficacy of the technique will one day be investigated through clinical trials. Over the last couple of weeks before adding this note, the method adjunctively helped one client minimize the length and severity of an upper respiratory lung infection after he directed his mental focus to the pulse in the upper chest. In that example, the technique provided not only the sensation of a strong pulse to the upper lung, but also increased warmth throughout the entire upper back, which he reported as being helpful. Another elderly person with poor circulation used the method to increase warmth to her legs, and I have used it to relieve muscle stiffness in my lower back and hip muscles. On another occasion, I employed it to help relieve congestion and "foggy head" by attending to the pulse at the soft palate of the upper mouth.

Although a technique like this should never be tried without a medical professional's instructions, nor relied on as an exclusive alternative to conventional medical care, my impression is that this technique, involving the art of attention to the pulse targeted at specific areas of the body, helps the body recover faster. An adjunctive self-therapy, it represents the power of the conscious mind to work in concert with the body's unconscious healing processes in order to speed recovery. Furthermore, it also allows the patient to play a role in their recovery from many infirmities that, like the self-treatment of bronchitis mentioned in the earlier paragraph, would otherwise involve remaining passive and waiting for the immune system and pharmacology to perform the job of healing. The potential of this technique is too important to be ignored.

Chapter 14

Neiguan Advanced Practices

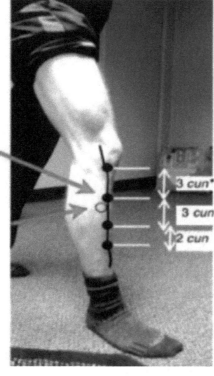

Traditional location of acupuncture point St-36 (Stomach 36)

Approximate location of OT-36 (Omura's True 36) about 1.5 cm from St-36

3 cun
3 cun
2 cun

Figure 3-35

Partial View of the Stomach Acupuncture Channel

(Originally presented in Section II, the image is presented again for the convenience of the reader.)

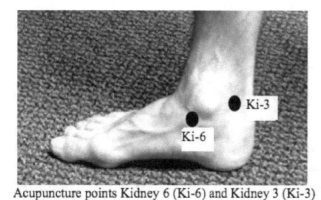

Ki-3

Ki-6

Acupuncture points Kidney 6 (Ki-6) and Kidney 3 (Ki-3)

Diagram 3-36

Two Acupuncture Points near the Ankle

*T*his chapter includes examples of more advanced *neiguan* techniques. The exercises described here demonstrate how one can consciously influence the body's energetic system through directed intention to its energy centers, channels, and acupuncture points. As will be covered shortly, research supports the notion that this kind of influence is indeed possible.

One of the most important aspects of advanced *neiguan* practices has to do with the ability to influence acupuncture points and channels. Significant to the present chapter is the notion that these kinds of "energetic practices" involving directed attention can immediately and directly influence the body's subtle energy system. In Taoist practice, the exercise is called "turning the vision and hearing inward" and "focusing the mind in the points." [51]

As an example, one study investigated whether it was possible for an individual to stimulate an acupuncture point through mental focus alone. In that study, researchers chose Stomach 36 (St-36); this acupuncture point, previously discussed in Section II, is located on the lateral side of the calf, three *cun* — "acupuncture inches" — below the knee.

Illustrated in Figure 3-35, and as previously covered in Section II, St-36 is a well-studied point, which, when stimulated through acupuncture, is known to increase white blood cell count. In one study, researchers wanted to ascertain if these same sorts of results could be initiated not through needles, but through mental focus alone. Studies showed that mental focus directed to the point could trigger an increase in white blood cell leukocytes when subjects imagined the achy feeling of stimulation to the point that Chinese acupuncturists refer to as *deqi*. [52] [53]

Neiguan Channel Activation

This chapter introduces two *neiguan* inner yoga exercises, both of which demonstrate the power of a person's focused attention to influence acupuncture points and channels. The first exercise focuses attention on kidney point 3 (Ki-3), located on the inside of the foot between the anklebone and the Achilles tendon (Diagram 3-36). The second uses directed attention targeted upon the kidney channel, which runs upward on the inside of the leg from the bottom of the foot, then to Ki-3 and thereafter ascends along the medial side of the leg to a point called Governing Vessel 1 (GV-1), located midway between the tip of the coccyx and the anus. As described in the traditional maps of the channel, at that point the channel enters the kidney organ and connects with the bladder, before ascending along the front side of the torso (the lower aspect of the kidney channel is shown in Diagram 3-37).

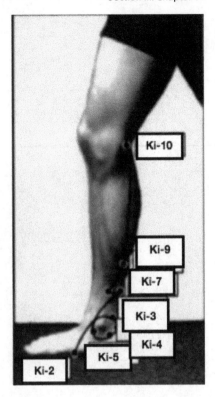

Diagram 3-37
Lower Medial Aspect of the Kidney Channel

In TCM parlance, both techniques promote "kidney function." As discussed in Section II, through the lens of traditional medicine, kidney function is much broader than what is described in Western physiology; an example of this is that in the traditional model, the kidneys are said to store "sexual essence." In the context of TCM, this aspect of energetic physiology pertains to not only sexual function, but also processes related to what, in modern physiology, would be concerned with hormonal balance. These are crucial to life extension and the optimal functioning of the body's immune system, which makes addressing "kidney function" important for stress management, since stress and anxiety deplete the kidney's *qi*. Thus, exercises that nurture "kidney function" can be thought of as a kind of antidote to the pernicious and depleting influences of stress that often accompany modern life.

Exercise 1: Activating Ki-3

This exercise is useful as a way of mentally stimulating points Ki-3 and Ki-6, shown in Photo 3-35. Activation of these points is known to calm psychological stress, and, when used regularly, the exercise promotes a deep, calm sleep. Begin by locating and massaging points Ki-3 and Ki-6; this will help you get in touch with the feeling of those points being stimulated and aid in your learning to stimulate the points mentally.

Step 1. Lie flat, face up, and completely relax. As with any mental yoga, it is also helpful to start by placing your hands over your chest and feeling the heartbeat. This helps you place your attention away from the outside events of the day and focus within. Paying attention to the heartbeat also helps you to tune in and harmonize your internal rhythms.

Step 2. Attune to sensations you feel in the area around the ankle, with particular attention to Ki-3. Your goal is to mentally create a dull, achy feeling at the acupuncture point. To enhance the function of the energy channel, imagine there is an energetic-magnetic connection that crosses between both legs at points Ki-3 and Ki-6. With practice, most people will feel a bilateral-interactive magnetic interchange between the two points and channels. When this happens, the sensation will be as if one leg is magnetically interacting with, and correcting imbalance in, the other. The successful result should feel similar to the sensation of buzzy electricity between the palms, which was part of the resonance training discussed earlier.

When you feel that warm, buzzy electrical sensation bilaterally in the ankles, or improved warmth along the kidney channel, intend to increase these sensations. Your ability to mentally interact with and increase sensations like these in your body is a sign that you are beginning to engage mentally and trigger positive changes in your acupuncture points and channels. Observe the buzzy feeling and experiment with increasing or decreasing the sensation. When this happens, you will begin to experience increased warmth in both ankles. With daily practice, most practitioners feel these kinds of responses after a week or two.

Exercise 2: Vibrating the Kidney Channel

After you experience some success with the warm, buzzy feeling associated with the activation of the Ki-3 point, you are ready to try "Vibrating the Kidney Channel."

Begin by lying relaxed and flat on your back. Next, mentally trigger the areas at or near acupuncture points Ki-3 and Ki-6 in the same manner as described in the previous exercise. Then, relax and mentally attend to the feeling of warmth moving up and around the inside of your legs; the path that this feeling takes should more or less approximate the lower aspect of the kidney channel as shown in Diagram 3-34.

With practice, most individuals report the sensation of magnetic buzzing traveling up the legs. This is an indication that they are accessing the healthful, restorative energy of the kidney channels, providing a kind of personal and no-cost restorative acupuncture treatment that you can use as often as you wish. The sensation that moves up the leg is reminiscent of what I felt when, as a child, I played with a 9-volt battery and stuck it on my tongue. With practice, the sensation within the channel becomes stronger. Once you feel sensations along the kidney channel and you practice the inner yoga for a week or so, you should be able to feel it easily.

As the practitioner notices a warm-tingling feeling traveling up the leg, they will gain an increased feeling of calm and relaxation. With continued practice over time, a strong pulse will be noticed in the lower back. This is a good sign.

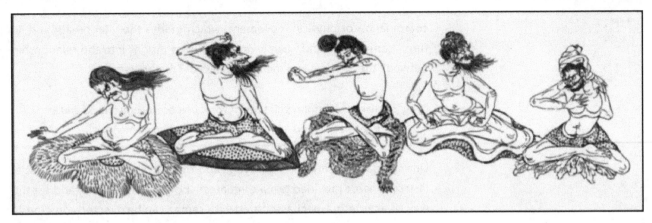

Image 3-38

Tibetan *Tantric* Yoga [54]

Chapter 15

Comparing Energetic Yoga Systems

*E*arlier, a challenge was presented concerning the meaning of "energy" in the context of energetic yoga. It is possible that by way of cross-cultural comparisons of energetic yoga systems as practiced in various traditions, we might reveal more clues to the meaning of "energy" in energetic yogas. In this light, it is useful to make a comparison between Taoist energetic yoga and a Tibetan *tantric* energetic yoga known as *trul khor.*

> In order to have a supple mind, you need a supple body. In order to have a supple body, you need a supple mind, so exert yourself in yogic practice.
>
> Khenpo Tsultrim Gyamtso [55]

Trul khor (ཙ་རྩལ་འཕྲུལ་འཁོར)

Sometimes translated as "magical movement instrument,"[56] *trul khor* is an introductory-level Tibetan Buddhist *tsa-lung* (ཙ་རླུང) "channels and energy" practice comprised of a series of 108 postures. Sketches of some *trul khor* postures, depicted on the walls of the Dalai Lama's summer temple at Lukhang, are shown in Image 3-38. *Trul khor* yoga is said to increase the practitioner's control over breath and internal energy; the practice involves coordination of physical movement, which guides the vital breath and, in turn, "carries the mind." Lama Yeshe provides insight into the relationship between the physical and mental aspects of Tibetan yoga.

> When you perform [this style of yogic practice] energy blocks and "negative thoughts are eliminated with each movement." [57]

One comparison between Taoist yoga and Tibetan *tantric* yoga is that special instructions are provided to male initiates in both traditions. They address the way an energetic aspect associated with semen can be directed consciously within the body's energy channels through these kinds of physical and mental yogas. This instruction will be addressed further in Section VI.

More on Energetics

The Tibetan *tantric* yogic practice of *tummo* (གཏུམ་མོ), or "inner heat," provides another clue to the meaning of conscious control over subtle energy within the body, as warmth within the body, and especially along the spine, is a derivative of practice. Although *tummo* is covered in more detail in Section V, and is only briefly introduced here, it is worth noting that from the viewpoint of the *tantric* tradition, the practice of *tummo* inner heat is said to activate the *vajra,* or "lightning bolt body." It is useful to mention that the devotee's ability to generate intense warmth along the spinal corridor is comparable to the experience of warmth along the spine that is sometimes reported in Taoist microcosmic orbit meditation, a subject also covered in Section V.

Since the Tibetan *tantric* practice of *tummo* interacts with, and engages, the practitioner's *lightning bolt,* vajra deha, or "diamond body," it is useful to consider that this refers to an energy field, or "subtle energy structure," that is said to underlie the person's physical body. [58] The subtle energy *vajra* body is made up of energetic flows, or "winds," along with a special form of *lung-wind* called *thigle.* In *tantric* practice, the energetic relationship between the "melting" of *thigle* through "inner heat" is an important part of the practice of *tummo..* ‡

> ‡*Tummo*, or the practice of "inner heat," in the context of energetic meditation is addressed in Section V, and in relation to the transmutation of sexual energy in Section VI.

Other aspects of the practice involve the practitioner learning to activate spiritual-etheric physiology within their body, which unites one's subtle energetic physiology. As explained by Lama Yeshe, inner heat produced through *tummo* meditation "melts" the *thigle* drops contained throughout the body's energetic channels. For the practitioner, this results in the experience of *bliss* and induction of advanced states of consciousness, which furthers the *tantric* practitioner's goal of attaining enlightenment.

The three aspects of what are considered to be body and mind energy-physiology in *tummo* practices are *tsa* (ཙ channels or nerves), *lung* (the body's "wind" energies) and *thigle* "drops." Although dispersed throughout the body's energy channels, *thigle* droplets primarily reside in either the top of the head or below the navel, and are either white or red in color.[59] [60]

As noted above, the practice of *tantric* yogic to master the flow of subtle energy in the body is called *tsa-lung*. Shenphen Dawa Rinpoche, son of HH Dudjom Rinpoche, provides a useful description of *tsa-lung*:

> My specialty is in the training of yoga. These are the teachings of the Buddha, and more particularly, these are the teachings of Guru Rinpoche. These relate to the three essences: essence of nerves, essence of wind, and essence of the seed - it's called *"thigley"* *[thigle]*. From the yoga point of view, the training is to learn how to bring purification to the wind, nerve, and essence. The heart of the teachings of the protectors and dakinis—their essence—is based on the practice of the yoga. This has been my training. It's a whole field of awareness. We are totally affected by that: we have so many nerve obscurations resulting from sicknesses, wind obscurations manifesting as mental disturbances, *thigle* obscurations arising as a degeneration of our cells, bringing negative emotions up. *"Tsa"* is nerve [channel], *"lung"* is wind, and *"thigle"* is seed. In the gross aspect, it is seed, in the subtle aspect it is the realization of the mind, which relates to clarity and luminosity. So, when we are talking about rainbow body, and the perfection of Dzogchen, perfection of Dzogchen comes with the perfection of *tsa-lung,* which will greatly enhance complete understanding of awareness. ... In *tsa-lung-thigle* we learn how to bring it *[karma]* out, so that it can be heated and purified by the wisdom heat.[61]

A further comparison that can be made between Taoist and Tibetan energetic yoga systems is how the balance of psychological factors influence the flow of energy in the body, and how these, in turn, influence one's physical health. The inter relationship between one's energy balance and physical health is expressed in a comment by Lama Thubten Zopa Rinpoche: "Once in Dharamsala, when I had *lung* or wind disease, Lama [Yeshe] told me [that] 'with achievement of *bliss* and voidness there is no *wind* disease. There is no place for tightness if you have *bliss* in your heart.'" [62]

Endnotes

1 Ni, Maoshing (translator), *Yellow emperor's classic of medicine, A new translation of the neijing suwen with commentary*, Shambhala, Boston 1995 p.4.

2 Consistent with comments in the opening pages of the present work, although for the most part Chinese characters are transliterated using the *pinyin* system of transliteration, there are a few exceptions where Chinese is Romanized in the Wade-Giles style. Examples of Wade-Giles transliteration in this chapter are Tao, Taoism, the *Tao Te Ching, t'ai-chi ch'üan* and its abbreviation, *t'ai-chi,* Lao Tzu, Chuang Tzu, Ko Hung, and Hua Tho.

3 See Lu K'uan Yu (Charles Luk) *Taoist yoga & immortality*, Samuel Weiser, Inc., York Beach, ME 1973

4 John Blofeld's description of the Taoists as the first hippies is too elegant to paraphrase, and is included here in its entirety:

As for Taoism being the progenitor of the first hippies, close on fifteen hundred years ago there flourished some widespread taoistically-minded communities known as the Light Conversationalists. Their prescription for discovering whether life had meaning, and if so what, was to live in frugal but happy accord with nature's rhythms, which generally involved fleeing from places where man-made laws imposed artificial limitations of people's spontaneity. They rather hoped to discover true understanding of life's meaning by seeking it in the stillness of their undisturbed minds; meanwhile, just in case life might offer nothing meaningful to understand, they enlivened their days with widely unconventional behavior and by conversing at deliberate fantastic levels for the fun of it.

Blofeld, John, *The secret and sublime: Taoist mysteries and magic*, Penguin Group 1973, p.14.

5 Sivin, N., "On the word 'taoist' as a source of perplexity. With special reference to the relations of science and religion in traditional China," *History of religions*, Vol. 17, No. 3/4, Current Perspectives in the Study of Chinese Religions (Feb. - May (1978), pp. 303-330.

6 Sivin, p. 305.

7 Virtually no sinologists believe that Lao Tzu (Laozi) was historical figure.

8 Ibid., pp. 303-330

9 Ishida Hidemi, "Body and mind: The Chinese perspective," Livia Kohn (Editor) *Taoist meditation and longevity techniques.* Center for Chinese Studies, University of Michigan, 1989 p. 55.

10 Hidemi, p. 55.

11 Robinet, Isabelle, "Original contributions of nei tan," *Taoist meditation and longevity techniques*, p. 299

12 "Religious Daoism," *Stanford encyclopedia of philosophy*, Aug 2016.

13 The practice of *chingjing* is described in the Tang Dynasty's (618-907 CE) *Classic of Clarity* 清靜經, which presents the principles in a in Buddhist-like framework.

14 Robinet, Isabelle, "Original contributions of *nei tan,*" *Taoist meditation and longevity techniques,* Livia Kohn (editor) p. 300.

15 Nathan Sivin, in his introduction to Joseph Needham's *Science and Civilization in China,* Volume 6 writes: "Physical and meditational techniques of self-cultivation, we now know, pre-dated the Taoist movements, were widely practiced by non-initiates, and were not in any sense peculiar to Taoist masters." Nathan Sivin (Editor), From the Introduction, Needham, Joseph, *Science and civilization in China,* Volume 6, Cambridge University Press, 1983, p. 11.

Later in the same text, Professor Needham speculates that Taoist health exercise regimens may have derived from the dances of ancient rain-bringing shamans. Needham writes, "but in any case, they were associated with the idea, as old in Chinese as in Greek medicine, that the circulatory system was liable to become obstructed, thus causing stasis (yü) and disease." Needham, p. 77.

16 Despuex, Catherine, "Gymnastics: the ancient traditions," *Taoist meditation and longevity techniques,* University of Michigan Center for Chinese Studies, 1989 p. 238.

17 As covered in Chapter One, the word / character *qi* has many uses in the Chinese language, and variations on the usage can refer to emotion, the weather, breathing and many other things. When preceded by the word *nei,* or "inner," the meaning refers to the "inner qi" of the body's channel and organ system. More detail is provided below.

18 Referring to the practice of circulating *qi,* Professor Needham writes, "There were two ways of making it circulate. Concentrating the will to direct it to a particular place, such as the brain, or the site of some local malady, was termed *hsing ch'i [xing qi].* Visualizing its flow in thought was 'inner vision' *(nei shi)…*"   Needham, Joseph, *Science and civilization in China,* Vol. 5, Cambridge University Press, 1983 p. 148

19 Voigt, John, "The man who invented qigong," *Qi: The journal of traditional eastern health and fitness*

20 Professor Needham writes, "There is considerable reason to believe that information about practices from Asia influenced the growth of calisthenics in modern Europe. This influence was marked from the eighteenth century onwards."

Needham, Joseph, *Science and civilization in China,* Vol. 6, Cambridge University Press, 1983 p. 7.

An additional comment on this subject by Professor Needham can be found in Volume 5, where he also makes a note of the apparent influence of Taoist *tao yin [dao yin]* exercise on the development of Western gymnastics. The suggestion is based on the work of Stockholm, Sweden based P.H. Ling. Ling, a former fencing teacher and pioneer of western gymnastic theories which included his approach to development of health maintenance exercise. See Needham, Joseph, *Science and civilization in China,* Vol. 5, Chemistry and Chemical Technology Spagyrical Discovery and Invention Physiological Alchemy Cambridge University Press, 1983, p. 173.

21 Wang, Ming 王明. 1996. *Clarification on the Inner Chapters of Baopu zi, Baopuzi neipian jiaoshi* 保朴子內篇校釋 Beijing: Zhonghua shuju. as cited by http://www.literati-tradition.com/meditative_practice.html

22 Needham, Joseph, *Science and civilization in China,* Vol. 5, Cambridge University Press, 1983 p. 35.

23 https://www.revolvy.com/topic/Chinese%20alchemical%20elixir%20poisoning

24 Needham, Joseph, *Science and civilization in China,* Cambridge University Press, 1983, p. 289.

25 In my experience working with clients over several decades, the unconscious persistence of jaw tension is a counter influence for the body's ability to relax on multiple levels. It seems that a one's inability to relax jaw tension may be related to those clients experiencing immune system issues. These observations are supported in the literature. As an example, the following is from a web article describing the relationship between jaw tension, the lymph system and fascial health:

> Excessive contractions in muscles can lead to tightness in all of the tissues, restricting the flow of lymph. A healthy lymph system supports a fluid membrane balance throughout the whole body; any condition of pathology can be traced back to a fluid-membrane imbalance. **Skin conditions such as acne, rash, cellulite and, in extreme cases, lymphedema can result from poor lymphatic drainage.**
>
> Lymph nodes are part of the lymphatic system — an important aspect of the immune system — responsible for the differentiation of 'self' from 'other', as well as what serves from that which doesn't. This network carries fluid, nutrients and waste material between the body tissues and the blood. Lymph nodes filter the fluid – trapping bacteria, viruses and foreign substances (anything deemed unsupportive to the organism) – and the lymphocytes (specialized white blood cells) destroy them. Stagnation or blockages in these nodes can mitigate the filtration process, therefore increasing the amount of toxins in the blood and lymph. An excess of toxins in these fluids can cause acne in skin that has increased levels of sebum and blockages in its pores.

"Why Jaw Tension Might Be To Blame For Your Breakouts," *The Chalkboard: A guide to living well.* http://thechalkboardmag.com/how-jaw-tension-causes-breakouts-acne-stress-and-skincare

Note: A discussion of jaw tension, as well as a specific technique to address the issue, is included in Section XI.

26 Images borrowed from Joseph Needham, Science and Civilization in China.

27 Note: Some scholars suggest that *huang ting,* literally the "yellow court," refers to the heart, and not the solar plexus.

28 Chao Pi-ch'en, originally titled *The secrets of cultivating essential nature and eternal life,* from the introduction to *Taoist yoga: Alchemy & immortality* by Lu Kuan Yu, Samuel Weiser, Inc. 1973.

29 Lu Kuan-Yu, *Alchemy and immortality*: Samuel Weiser, Inc., York Beach, Maine, 03910, 1973 p. xiii.

30 Anonymous, Tang or Sung dynasty (618-1126 CE) texts, *Thai his ken chih yao chueh* (Instructions on the essentials of understanding embryonic respiration). As translated and cited by Needham, Joseph, *Science and civilization China,* Vol 5, Cambridge University Press, 1983, pp. 186-187.

31 As Needham explains, "Already in the *Lü shih chhun chhiu* we can find the aphorism that 'Running water does not stagnate, nor does a door-pivot become worm-eaten, because they move.'" Needham, Joseph, *Science and civilization in China,* Cambridge University Press, 1983 Vol. 6, p. 77.

32 Cibot, *Memories concernant l'histoire, les sciences les arts de Chinois,* 1779, as translated into English by Professor Joseph Needham, *Science and civilization in China.*

33 The Official *Journal of Naturopathic Physicians* reported the following:

> Lee, et al., randomized 36 adults with hypertension to either a waiting list control or a *Qi gong* group that practiced two 30-minute Qi gong programs per week for 8 consecutive weeks. Systolic and diastolic blood pressure was significantly reduced in members of the Qi gong group after 8 weeks of exercise. Significant improvements in self-efficacy and other cognitive perceptual efficacy variables were also documented in the Qi gong group compared to controls.
>
> •Lee et al randomized 58 patients with hypertension to either a *Qi gong* group (N=29), or a control group (N=29). Systolic blood pressure and diastolic blood pressure decreased significantly in the Qi gong group, such that both became significantly lower after 10 weeks in the Qi gong than in the control group. Also, there was a significant reduction of norepinephrine, metanephrine, and epinephrine compared to baseline values in the Qi gong group. The ventilatory functions, forced vital capacity and forced expiratory volume per sec, were increased in the Qi gong group but not the control. The authors conclude that Qi gong may stabilize the sympathetic nervous system, is effective in modulating levels of urinary catecholamines and blood pressure positively, and improves ventilatory functions in mildly hypertensive middle-aged patients.

34 For male aspirants, the goal was to send the *jing* upwards to "nourish the brain." The corresponding practice for women was to "irrigate the brain with nectar." Joseph Needham, *Science and civilization in China,* Vol. 5, Cambridge University Press, 1983 p. 237. More details on the subject are provided in Sections V and VI.

35 *Thai-chhing tao yin yang shhg ching* (Manual of Nourishing the Life-Force by Physical Exercises and Self-Massage). From the *Mawangdui* tomb, as cited by Needham, Joseph, *Science and Civilization in China,* Cambridge University Press, 1983 Vol. 3, pp. 156-157.

36 McCann, Henry, "A practical guide to Tung's acupuncture," *Journal of Chinese medicine,* February 2006

37 McCann

38 From the *San Kuo Chih ("Romance of the three kingdoms")*, the biography of surgeon Hua Tho, as translated by Joseph Needham, *Science and civilization in China*, Vol. 5 pp. 160-161.

39 Despeux, Catherine, "Gymnastics: the ancient tradition," *Taoist meditation and longevity techniques*, University of Michigan Center for Chinese Studies, 1989, p. 231.

40 Despeux, p. 255.

41 Ibid.

42 As opposed to *endogenous* disease and how they are related to excess emotions, discussed in Section II

43 A new practitioner to the Looking at the Moon (LAM) exercise should start by practicing only a few minutes at a time, then gradually increase practice time. It is best to start with five to ten minutes. Later the exercise can be extended for up to forty-five minutes per session. The athletic power developed from Look at Moon derives from the exercise's effect from integrating power through the myofascial meridians of the arms, shoulders and back.

In practice, turn and open the palms upward to the terminal position **very gradually.** This will help develop the total body connection.

An additional value of the exercise is its ability to mitigate the effects of high impact athletic training on the body. This is so since overuse of dominant muscle groups disproportionally places stress on key joints, and LAM, because of its body integration properties, counters this exercise imbalance.

In practice of LAM, a common mistake at the beginning is to overuse the shoulders to achieve the posture. Instead, slow, patient practice allows your shoulders to naturally stretch and release tension throughout the entire back, and continue to maintain the gentle stress all the way down the legs. With time, the practitioner learns to de-emphasize over use of the elbows and shoulders and allow the back and leg muscles bear the weight of lifting the arms, which in turn opens the energetic channels of the shoulder blade and back.

As mentioned in the main text, work on opening and stimulating the energetic channels with minimal turning of the elbows and joints. Avoid overturning one joint to relieve stress on the muscles of the forearm. (For example, by overturning the wrists so that the upper shoulder and back muscles are not effectively incorporated into the exercise).

44 Here, referring to the broader energetic "organ" system of Chinese traditional medicine that was covered in Section II. In this example, taking its name from the "kidney" which, as covered earlier, encompasses a broader meaning beyond the organ and organ function described in modern physiology.

45 Needham, Joseph, *Science and civilization in China*, Vol. 5, *chemistry and chemical technology spagyrical discovery and invention physiological alchemy*, Cambridge University Press, 1983.

46 Newberg, Andrew MD, *How God changes your brain: Breakthrough findings from a leading neuroscientist.* Ballantine Books, NY 2010, p. 155.

47 Ishida, Hidemi, "Body and mind: The *Chinese perspective"* Taoist meditation and longevity techniques, Livia Kohn (Editor) *Taoist meditation and longevity techniques.* Center for Chinese Studies, University of Michigan, 1989 *p.* 56.

48 Ishida

49 In the traditional Taoist view, the mind is not located in a single place within the body, but moves around through various body locations. Hidemi Ishida describes the principle of the moving mind in the following way

> When the mind is fixated on one spot, it cannot pay attention to another. This means that the fluids of the constantly flowing body tend to concentrate in one place or another at any given time. Thus, "when energy fills everything, the mind is also present everywhere." This in turn means that every tiny and remote part of the body is filled with awareness, and the movements and actions of the body are coordinated to perfection.

> *Ishida, Hidemi,* "Body and mind: The Chinese perspective: Taoist Meditation and Longevity Techniques," Livia Kohn (Editor) *Taoist meditation and longevity techniques.* Center for Chinese Studies, University of Michigan, 1989 p. 56.

50 Ibid.

51 Wile, Douglas, *Art of the bedchamber: The Chinese sexual yoga classics including women's solo meditation texts*, State University of New York, 1992, p. 37.

52 It is common for an acupuncturist in a Chinese-speaking situation to ask the patient, *"Deqi le mei yuo?"* meaning, "Do you have the achy feeling of the *qi* stimulation?"

53 Subjects in the study were allowed to touch acupuncture point St-36 before beginning the mental stimulation process. Results of the study show that patients who had previously received acupuncture showed greater results than patients who had not.

O'Connor, J. and Bensky, D. "A summary of research concerning the effects of acupuncture." *American journal of Chinese medicine*, 3:377-394, 1975. As cited in Milovanovic, Miomir, et al., "Mental stimulation of acupuncture Point zusanli (St-36) for rise of leukocyte count: Psychopuncture." *Comparative medicine east and west*, Vol. VI. No. 4. pp. 307-311.

54 Illustrations by Sergio Verdeza based on photographs presented in Ian's Baker's, *The Dalai Lama's Secret Temple.*

55 Rose Taylor Goldfield, *Training the wisdom body,* from the forward by Khenpo Tsultrim Gyamtso. Shambhala Publications, 2013 Boston, MA. p. 4.

56 http://www.shambhala.com/snowlion_articles/spinning-the-magical-wheel/

57 Yeshe, Thubten, *The bliss of inner fire: Heart practice of the six yogas of naropa,* Simon and Schuster, 2005 p. 99.

58 As described in Tibetan Buddhism, the body exists simultaneously on three levels: the gross, subtle body and very subtle body. The gross consists of bones, muscles, organs and other physical structures. The subtle body—the vajra body—is comprised of the body' energetic systems, which includes the main channels in front of and paralleling the spine, the energy – winds and "drops" the energy system is activated through energetic meditation — as well as the "wheels" or *chakras* that branch off from the main energy channels (see Yeshe, p. 84-85). The mind moves through the subtle energy channels with the "winds." The subtlest energy field manifests after death.

59 Red being female, white is male, but every person has both.

60 Lama Yeshe, *The bliss of inner fire: Heart practice of the six yogas of naropa,* Simon and Schuster, p. 206.

61 An interview with Dudjom Tersar lineage holder Shenphen Dawa Rinpoche from the following website: http://www.tersar.org/continuity.html

62 Yeshe. p. xvi.

Section IV
Non-Contact
Energetic Healing

...by laying my hand upon the place, and by extending my fingers towards it. Thus, it is known to some of the learned that health may be implanted in the sick by certain gestures....

— *Hippocrates, Fifth Century BCE* [1]

IV

Non-Contact Energetic Healing

Introduction to Section IV

*C*ontroversy persists around whether something called "internal energy" might exist in our physical reality. However, that controversy pales in comparison to the dispute surrounding the question of whether or not a healer, relying on minimal or no contact with a patient, can transmit a healing force. * This is one aspect of the larger question of whether non-physical influence can interact with the material world in demonstrable ways.

The chapters in this section include an overview of a few select forms of non-contact healing. It should be noted that there are *many* forms of non-contact healing to be found in numerous traditions. Thus, the non-contact healing practices discussed here are not intended to represent a comprehensive overview of all forms of energetic healing. Chapter 16 includes an overview of various non-contact healing traditions that have been practiced around the world from ancient to modern times. In Chapter 17, we seek to uncover clues that shed light on the meaning of subtle, human-directed non-physical influence. In Chapter 18, our search focuses on non-contact healing known in China as *wai qi* (also written *waiqi),* or "emitted energy" practice. Chapter 19 includes a discussion of the dangers of non-contact energy healing. Chapter 20 includes an overview of research and design problems related to non-contact healing research in the West. Chapter 21 presents an alternative explanation for non-contact healing, and the end of this section includes an Afterword with recommendations for researchers of Chinese style non-contact healing.

---

* The energetic model discussed in this section describes healing that is "fixed in time and space" (as in, brain → intention → energy "fields" surrounding the body → influence on the patient). Note that there is an alternative model of healing which is not addressed in the present work, known as "non-local healing." A leading expert on the non-local theory, Larry Dossey, MD, believes that healing and conscious experience can take place beyond the local. According to Dossey: "The non-local model.... is not confined in space and time to the brain and body, although it may work through the brain and body and is not confined to the present moment." **

Box 4-1

** Additional discussion about non-local healing is provided in the Endnote [2]

As noted in Box 4-1, the present section looks at *local,* as opposed to *non-local,* healing. These forms of healing, when and if validated, would be those that will one day be describable, and accepted, in terms of accepted physical laws. Whether the effect of this kind of healing is due to the healer's ability to emit electromagnetic, infrared, "information," or another, yet to be discovered medium, these forms of healing, if validated, may one day be shown to be subject to the laws of cause and effect. As noted in Box 4-1, the forms of energetic healing considered in these pages do not address the *non-local* healing, such as that described by Larry Dossey, nor do they address the type of healing that might be affected by religious prayer or by holy persons. To reemphasize a point, this section is not so much a discussion of energy healing per se, but rather, another thread of our search for clues into the meaning of "internal energy" as a measurable and intentionally directed human influence.

Chapter 16

Energetic Healing: Ancient and Modern

*T*he belief that one person can heal another through the projection of a consciously directed energetic force is an ancient one. Dating back earlier than 1550 BCE, the *Ebers Papyrus* [3] describes a person who could transmit healing energy to the sick. Likewise, the belief in minimal or non-physical contact healing appears in many, if not all, traditional cultures. For example, a *curandera,* a shaman in Mexican and Mesoamerican cultures, practices a form of energy known as *limpia* — Spanish for "cleansing" — to treat a wide range of disorders.

One *curandera* describes their healing art, sometimes referred to as *curanderismo,* as an effective treatment for a diverse range of disorders, from eating problems, diabetes, and heart problems to chronic pain.[4] The *curandera* shaman relies on a variety of tools to help the patient. These include education on lifestyle, bodywork, and the use of energetic cleansing implements, including crystals, feathers, and branches, which are brushed over the patient to cleanse their energy field, a process called *limpia,* or "cleansing." [5]

The Essenes of the Old Testament practiced non-contact healing,[6] and from ancient times to the present, the Hawaiian people have maintained a long oral tradition that describes how an individual possessing sufficient personal power can heal others. In the Hawaiian culture, whether healer, chieftain, or other person of importance, *personal power* comes to the individual through their strong relationship with the spiritual force, *mana.*[7] In this culture, the traditional healer, a *ka'ike huna,* uses mental power to influence external phenomena. Thus, *mana* is a valuable asset in Hawaiian culture, and the *kahuna* enjoys great prestige. The earliest Greek healers practiced their art through touch in the Asklepian temples, and spiritual healing is still practiced in many Christian churches, having been associated with the "light" since early times. [8]

Richard Gerber, MD, who was cited in Section II due to the use of energetic healing in his medical practice, writes that some ancient kings were "purportedly successful in curing diseases," such as tuberculosis, through the laying of hands. Gerber describes energetic healing as involving "mentally directing a visualized stream of inhaled energy through [the healer's] hands and into the patient's body." [9] As Gerber explains, in some ancient cultures, the ability to heal was considered a spiritual gift, normally ascribed to the power of the king, or the gifts of a revered healer. That belief was later adopted by Christians and attributed to the power of Jesus.[10]

In more recent times, the first Western physician to proclaim the principle that "energy" could heal was the Swiss physician and alchemist Paracelsus. Paracelsus believed the human being to be primarily energetic, and that through an energetic exchange, one person could influence another without physical contact. According to Paracelsus, the human being was defined by an outer layer that was not of flesh, but a radiant "luminous sphere," which "could be made to act at a distance." [11]

Some early Western scientists strongly believed in the reality of an invisible healing "energy," and several dedicated a large portion of their life's work to attempting to prove the objective existence of subtle human "energy" and "energetic healing." Proponents of such causes included the highly-regarded scientist Carl von Reichenbach, discoverer of kerosene, paraffin, and creosote who, along with a handful of colleagues, believed that one day the proposal of an invisible healing force would be accepted as part of mainstream science. In his investigations, von Reichenbach drew on the reports of "sensitives" that could visually perceive the subtle energetic forces:

> You know that, whenever you touch a sensitive with your fingers, you exercise an effect upon him which he can feel and, when in darkness, see. But it is not even necessary to come into actual contact with him; the mere approach of your fingers produces effects that are considerable.[12]

Reichenbach describes the abilities of "sensitives" to visually perceive what, for most of us, remains an invisible force:

> [A normal person] can produce "very strong excitations" [of this force] at a distance of several inches; but by sensitives of a middling degree of sensitivity [they will be able to feel this energetic force] a foot off, or even at a distance of several feet. And in the case of high-sensitives the effect goes far beyond that – to the end of the room; in fact, I have had several cases in which the effect made itself clearly perceptible at the astonishing distance of twenty and thirty paces and more.

Franz Mesmer was, as previously mentioned, a physician and scientist who spent years studying the effects of magnetism and magnetic fields on the human body. However, he eventually came to believe that magnets were unnecessary, and that the magnetic healing influence could be transmitted directly from healer to patient. The process involved the healer first concentrating the life force in his hands and then transferring it to his patients.[13]

More clues as to the nature of energetic healing can be gleaned by comparing and contrasting the non-contact healing traditions of different cultures. In this vein, we might ask to what extent the healing force described by Mesmer might be related to the healing energies of the shamans in ancient cultures. A related question is whether the healing energy studied by Reichenbach might be the same force known to the Chinese *qigong* masters as *qi*. Regarding Mesmer's work, an interesting clue regarding the meaning of internal energy is found in his patients' sometimes strange reactions to his healing energy. For example, after receiving Mesmer's healing treatments, some patients experienced violent convulsions or episodes of uncontrollable laughter. [14]

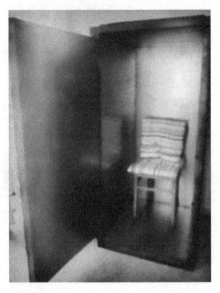

Photo 4-2

An Orgone Accumulator Based on William Reich's Design

Source: *Wikipedia Commons*

William Reich is the most notable early-twentieth century physician to apply energetic fields when treating his patients. Reich, a student of the famous Austrian physician and founder of psychiatry, Sigmund Freud, believed that a magnetic-energetic force he called *orgone* could treat both psychological and physical issues. After immigrating to the United States, Reich became noted for his attempt to trap and "bottle" what he believed to be the elusive genii of energetic health, through an invention he called an *orgone accumulator*. Orgone accumulators varied in size from about a that of a shoebox to a very large device (Photo 4-2), with the larger version being big enough to allow a patient to sit comfortably while undergoing treatment. However, his claims regarding the efficacy of orgone treatments, and especially his assertions of it being a cancer cure, put him at odds with the U.S. government. Because of his claims, he was convicted and imprisoned, where he died in 1957.

Another controversial topic at the time was was Reich's belief that a relationship existed between sexuality and energetic healing. No doubt his outspoken views on this matter were another reason why the U.S. government took exception to his ideas. As Reich saw it, blocked sexual energy was the root of most diseases suffered by both individuals and society at large.

> The temptation to deny the sexual etiology [underlying cause] of so many illnesses is far greater in the case of sex-economy † than it was in psycho-analysis. [15]

> † Reich explains the use of his term "sex-economy" in the following way:

>> "It was only with great effort that I succeeded in establishing the term 'sex-economy.' This concept is intended to cover a new scientific field: the investigation of biopsychic energy." [16]

According to Reich, not only "psychic illness" (psychological disease), but also behavioral problems he called "irrational actions" resulted from "disturbance of the natural ability to love."

The vital energies regulate themselves naturally, without compulsive duty or compulsive morality — both of which are sure signs of existing antisocial impulses. Antisocial actions are the expression of secondary drives. These drives are produced by the suppression of natural life, and they are at variance with natural sexuality. [17]

Chapter 17

Possible Scientific Explanations

This chapter looks at scientific studies and science-based theories that might provide insight into the meaning of "internal energy" in the context of "energetic healing." Subjects covered here include a brief overview of the various theories that purport to explain how patients receiving non-contact "energetic therapies" might receive benefit from the treatment. Evidence will be considered that is presumed to support the notion that this unconventional form of healing might be attributed to an unknown "energy." Other explanations will also be considered, such as to what extent expectation and belief might also play a role in this kind of therapy.

Diagram 4-3
Measurement of
Human Bio-fields
Composition of Seto's Bio-Magnetic Field Emission Measurement System From "Detection of Extraordinary Large Bio-magnetic Field Strength" [18]

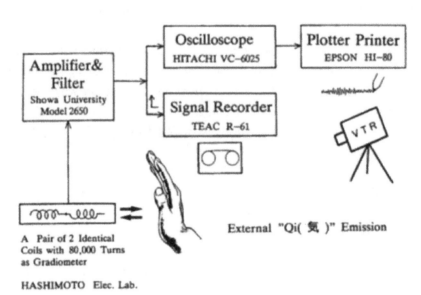

Externalizing (Emitting) Energy

An important question to consider when exploring the meaning of internal energy is whether or not it is possible for a person to emit a *measurable* healing force. In a study published in China in 1977, researchers claimed to have proven that such a force exists, and that it *was* measurable. Investigators referred to the energy they observed as "emitted *qi*," and claimed that they were able to measure electromagnetic (EM) energy emitted by a *qigong* master. Reporting their results, investigators described what they referred to as *qi* energy as being "much like infrared rays, EM waves, static electricity, magnetism, and the flow of tiny subatomic particles." [19]

In their attempt to develop models to explain how this kind of non-contact healing works, some Chinese researchers apply what they describe as the Taoist model of *qi* energy to explain non-contact healing. For example, Kunio Miura believes that Chinese *qi* masters take the energy they transmit from their own bio-energetic stock. Accordingly, in the scheme proposed by Miura, non-contact emission of *qi* energy in the Chinese Taoist model depletes the *qi* master's store of energy. Therefore, after depletion, the *qi* master must revitalize their own energies through solo *qigong* exercise. [20]

Similarly, Japanese scientists Akira Seto, PhD and Chikaaki Kusaka, MD conducted a fascinating study supporting the notion that a non-contact healer does emit an energetic field. In their study, Seto and Kusaka relied on measurements from an EM field detector (Diagram 4-3) to document whether or not known practitioners of energetic practices might be able to intentionally emit a measurable bio-magnetic field from the palms of their hands. [21] [22] Investigators were able to document how *some* exceptionally gifted healers were, in fact, able to emit an extremely large EM field. Whereas normal human fields do not exceed 10-6 gauss, researchers detected large EM fields on the order of 10-3 gauss in the cases of these noted healers. ‡

‡ "Gauss," named after physicist Carl Friedrich Gauss, is a unit of measurement.

$$10\text{-}3 = .001, \ 10\text{-}6 = .000001$$

As with similar studies, Seto and Kusaka's investigation provides important evidence that it is indeed possible for some individuals to willfully emit an incredibly strong EM field. In the Seto study, the documented emissions measured an increase that was more than 1000 times the normal human EM radiation. However, although researchers have reliably documented these kinds of extraordinary EM emissions, they have been unable to determine their source.[23]

In another study of the same kind, Shanghai University Professor Shen Han Chang measured the emitted EM radiation of *qigong* masters. In that study, Shen documented how healers radiated both infrared and EM radiation, with measurements showing that some *qigong* masters emitted infrared radiation in the 1 to 4.5 micron range. Additionally, it was noted that the participants' palm temperatures elevated 4 to 5 degrees centigrade over background ambient levels. [24] [25]

Similar studies produced similar results, such as one which looked at healers and *qigong* masters, who the researchers referred to as "energy projectors." Investigators in that study documented how some of these individuals were able to generate large voltage pulses,[26] and although most "energy emitting" studies involve Chinese style *wai qi* healers, some have looked at other styles of energetic healing and yielded similar results. For example, one published article by Stanford University's William Tiller evaluated research that measured bio-electrical fields generated by Therapeutic Touch

(TT) practitioners.[27] This was a follow-up study to one conducted by Green *et al*, where non-contact therapists were recorded as producing body-potential surges ranging from -4 V to -190 V. On average, these electrical pulses were 3 times larger than the psycho-physiologic galvanic skin-potential (GSP) changes typically associated with emotional responses, 5 times larger than electrocardiographic (EKG) voltages, and six times higher than electroencephalographic (EEG) voltages.[28] Commenting on those observations, Tiller believes that some humans are able to emit bursts of subtle energy from "various body chakras,"* explaining that this takes place through a "subtle energy / electrical conversion process involving the acupuncture meridian system." [29] This observation, along with related speculation on the meaning of subtle energy fields that surround the body, will be returned to in Section XII.

> * Discussed more in Section V, a *chakra* is described as the intersection point, or "vortex," between the "etheric body" and the physical body, where wavelengths of emotional and mental energy converge.

Many of us who work with mind-body energy systems, such as *qigong* and internal martial arts, have had personal experiences that, for us, demonstrate the reality of subtle human EM fields. I had one of those experiences when I discovered that certain postures could generate a field which disturbed the functioning of electronic equipment.

My senior students and I became aware of the problem when we discovered that a microphone placed on an advanced practitioner's body during videotaping would sometimes pick up random static. At times, the interference was so strong that the voice instructions in the videos became unintelligible at key moments.

Investigating the unexplained static, we discovered that the interference was not related to a particular physical movement, nor any inadvertent movement of the microphone. Instead, the disruptive static would appear when a more advanced practitioner, with a microphone on his body, performed martial arts or *qigong* sequences that involved the concentration or extension of internal energy. Although the problem persists to this day, and especially while teaching more internal energy-based lessons using video conferencing technology, the microphone / static problems in a studio setting were, for the most part, resolved by purchasing more expensive equipment. I'm sure that other teachers of energetic arts and yoga have had similar experiences.

Schumann Waves

As suggested by the studies just cited, it appears that at least some *qigong* masters can emit a measurable energetic field. This raises the question, what might it be about an emitted bio-electrical field that could produce healing? One possible explanation is that electrical fields emitted by a healer might attune the recipient to the earth's EM field. Proponents of such a theory suggest that a healer's ability to emit specific EM frequencies helps synchronize the patient's EM field in a special way. According to this model, the interaction with the healer initiates an ordering, or anti-entropic, influence on the patient.

This theory suggests that emitted EM energy synchronizes the patient with the earth's EM pulsation, understood as Schumann waves. Schumann waves are the micro pulsations of the earth's magnetic field, generated by electrical storms that charge the ionosphere. They can be measured at approximately 7.8 Hz at any given time, and the resulting EM field occurs not because of local weather events, but due to the charging of the Earth's overall ionosphere by electrical storms occurring across the planet. These electrical charges create a predictable EM pulse that can be detected anywhere in the world, and proponents of the theory believe that a person's synchronization with these fields represents a basic EM set point that determines their ability to heal. Accordingly, when reset by an energetic healer, a patient formerly "out of harmony" with the Earth's field is readjusted to the EM frequency; ergo, anti-entropic healing influence has taken place.

Section II included discussion of Robert Becker's investigation of acupuncture meridians. In review, Becker demonstrated that, since they conduct current, the meridians possess an "objective basis in reality." Commenting on the relationship between Schumann waves and the ability of energetic healers to tap into "healing energy" associated with the EM field of the earth, Becker wondered if there was something special about the brain function of gifted healers that allowed them to tune their EM fields to the Earth's, and thereby transmit a healing influence to others.

Investigating how energetic healers functioned while in a healing mode, Becker identified similarities in brainwave patterns of individuals considered gifted healers. These similarities led Becker to speculate that, since it is possible to train the brain to "change frequency" with specific types of meditation training, an otherwise normal individual can, like the energy healers he studied, also learn to attune to the micro-pulsation energy surrounding the planet. This could potentially explain how otherwise normal individuals might also learn to replicate and emit the "healing frequency." As Becker explains:

> All matter, living and nonliving, is ultimately an electromagnetic phe-
> nomenon. The material world, at least as far as physics has penetrated,
> is an atomic structure held together by electromagnetic forces. If some
> people can **detect** fields from other organisms, why shouldn't some

people be able to **affect** other beings by means of their linked fields? Since the cellular functions of our bodies are controlled by our own DC [direct current] fields, there's reason to believe that gifted healers generate supportive electromagnetic effects, which they convey to their patients or manipulate to change the sufferer's internal currents directly, without limiting themselves to the placebo of trust and hope. [30]

Often the exact internal mechanism, or "switch," that allows a healer to influence their patient remains unknown to the healer. In support of this point, Becker cites a study conducted in the former Soviet Union, which documented a Hungarian colonel named Estebany, who was discovered to have unusual healing abilities. It was observed that horses Estebany trained recovered faster when exhausted, and healed faster compared to horses handled by others. These observations led to a more formal study of Estebany and his unusual abilities, with researchers finding that he could also influence wounds on mice to heal faster. It was noteworthy that Estebany didn't have to touch the mice physically, but only put his hands over the cages to increase healing. [31]

Chapter 18

Wai Qi Chinese Style Non-Contact Healing

*T*oday, some Chinese hospitals allow non-contact healers to treat patients alongside conventional medical practitioners, and this chapter takes a closer look at that particular form of non-contact energetic healing. While known by various names, this type of healing is most commonly referred to as *waiqi liaofa* (外氣疗法), and abbreviated as *wai qi* (外氣), meaning "externalized *qi*." The practice of "externalizing *qi*" often falls under the very large umbrella term, *qigong* (氣功). It is also important to mention that some practitioners and researchers, because of the non-contact healing art's relationship to the Chinese shamanistic tradition called *zhuyou*, claim this style of non-contact healing as a branch of Chinese medicine. However, there are some problems with this claim that will be addressed later.

As its name implies, *wai qi* non-contact energy healing typically involves no physical contact between patient and healer. There have been many hundreds, if not thousands, of studies that have examined the efficacy of Chinese-style *wai qi* energetic healing in both Asia and the West. The practice of *wai qi* healing, like other forms of non-contact healing, is based on the notion that a healer can transmit an invisible healing energy, which transits the otherwise empty space between the practitioner's palms or fingers and the patient. Normally, the distance between the therapist's hand and the recipient of an "energy treatment" is between 2-5 ft.

While the veracity of claims that an unseen healing force can be transmitted is *almost* universally doubted by Western scientists, in the East, and especially in China, Taiwan, and Japan, a subset of researchers are studying the phenomenon of energetic healing more closely. Their observations offer important contributions to the discussion of "internal energy." For example, in one study conducted at China's Xiamen University, researchers found evidence of positive changes in blood chemistry associated with *wai qi* treatment. The assumption made by researchers to explain this result was that the energetic healer, or *qigong* master, was able to influence the patient's blood chemistry energetically.[32]

In similar studies, researchers found evidence suggesting that *wai qi* was helpful for the treatment of neurological disease and paralysis.[33] Results like this offer the possibility that there may an invisible *natural force* that can be directed by will, and channeled through the hands and fingers of a healer to their patient.

Positive and Negative Energy

Some researchers believe that a *qigong* master can project two different kinds of *qi* energy. The different forms are classified as *healing* and *disruptive*, or alternatively, as "positive" and "negative" *qi*. This theory suggests that these different kinds of subtle energy produce different results. *Positive qi* promotes healing and growth, while *negative qi* induces weakening or destructive responses.

Yoshiaki Omura, a physician and senior researcher in the field of *qigong*, is widely regarded as one of the foremost experts on the subject of positive and negative *qi* energy. Omura conducted numerous studies investigating the nature of *wai qi* energy, and also claims to have been able to uncover the inner secrets of healers performing this style of non-contact healing.

In one study, Omura wanted to find out if external *wai qi* energetic healing could improve drug uptake in specific organs. The study looked at how a *qigong* healer could improve the effectiveness of a drug by targeting specific viruses present in a patient's organs. Results of the study supported the hypothesis that *qigong* treatment could improve drug uptake to targeted organs, and these experimental results advance our discussion in two ways. First, it is an example of the varied ways that researchers study Chinese non-contact healing, and second, the study demonstrates how Omura distinguishes between positive and negative *qi*.

Distinguishing between positive (+) and negative (-) *qi*, Omura explains that positive *qi* can enhance "circulation and drug uptake in diseased areas where there was microcirculatory disturbance."[34] By contrast, negative *qi*, according to Omura, has "completely the opposite effect and therefore has not been used [in those studies], although there may be some as yet undiscovered applications." [35]

As an example of research that looked at negative *qi*, one study examined the ability of an energetic master in China, named Bao, to emit either positive or negative *qi* as he chose. Bao's ability was tested at the General Naval Hospital in Beijing, where researchers asked him to annihilate bacteria in a test tube. As described in the published study, Bao could indeed *selectively* cause the bacteria to either flourish or decline. Researchers believe that the results demonstrated the presence of both growth and inhibitory influence that could be modulated through human intention. For researchers, Bao's demonstration was an example of conscious control over so-called positive or negative internal energy. [36] [37]

In another study investigating a practitioner's ability to emit positive *qi*, investigators looked at the effects of non-contact energetic treatment *in vivo* (human subjects). The study, published in the *American Journal of Acupuncture*, investigated whether the effects of energetic treatment on free radicals in blood could be measured. The study showed that *wai qi* treatment could in fact decrease the concentration of free radicals, with results suggesting that an unknown influence — presumably the application of subtle bio-energy treatment — can trigger a wide range of positive responses in the human immune system.

More on Chinese *Wai Qi* Non-Contact Healing

The Chinese non-contact healing practice of *wai qi*, or "externalizing *qi*," deserves a section of its own for three reasons. The first reason is because of the healing method's increasing popularity as an alternative health treatment, both in China and the West. Second, is because many proponents of the practice claim it is a lost branch of traditional Chinese medicine (TCM), which should, again, be included along with acupuncture and herbal medicine. Lastly, the third reason is that there is an ever-increasing number of scientific studies investigating the efficacy of that style of non-contact healing.

As noted earlier, some studies investigating non-contact healing have documented an extremely large EM field that the healers appear to project from their hands while in a mental state conducive to treating patients. Energetic researcher and author James Oschman suggests that the heat radiated by *qigong* practitioners from the palms of their hands may increase cell growth. Oschman characterizes some of these "emissions" as being so strong that they could "be detected with a relatively simple magnetometer, indicating a robust effect that should be easy to study." [38]

Oschman believes that the ability to accelerate cell growth in this way is evidence that Chinese-style energetic healing promotes DNA and protein synthesis. Alternatively, when used as a treatment for diseases, such as bacteriological infections, the technique utilizes "negative" or "inhibiting *qi*," which restricts or slows the metabolizing of pathogens. [39]

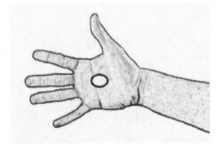

Figure 4- 4

The Lao Gong Point in the Center of the Palm

In acupuncture nomenclature, referred to as pericardium 8 (P-8), the point is indicated by the white circle in the middle of the palm.

Chinese Non-Contact Healers

Several thought-provoking studies have focused on physiological changes experienced by *wai qi* healers while they are in the *qi*-healing / *wai qi* state. These studies can be divided into two distinct areas: (1) the detection of external signals, and (2) physical changes to the healer's body while in the healing *wai qi* state. Investigation of external signals includes detection of infrared light, and EM emissions detected during healing sessions.

In one paper published in the Chinese publication *The Nature Journal,* Gu Hansen and Lin Housheng, of the Shanghai Institute of Nuclear Physics, looked at physical changes exhibited by *wai qi* healers. The measurements they observed compared energetic healers to non-practitioners, and researchers documented an unusual infrared radiation time spectrum that extended 1.2 cm from the *lao gong* (pericardium 8 / P-8) acupuncture point in the center of the hand (Figure 4-4) of the energetic healers. Investigators described the emitted infrared radiation in terms of an emission of "slow wave crests," which represented low-frequency amplitude modulation.

However, other possible explanations have been advanced to explain how healing might take place. One posits that a practitioner might be able to generate an "oscillating energy field," which, if true, suggests that healing might be explained in terms of a "healing vibration" emitted from that healer's hands. Oschman believes such a healing phenomenon is more likely a "blend of the fields generated by molecular, cellular tissue, and systemic oscillations within the body of the therapist." [40]

> Medical research is demonstrating that devices producing magnetic fields of particular frequencies can stimulate the healing of a variety of tissues. Therapists from various schools of energy medicine can project, from their hands, fields with similar frequencies and intensities. Research documenting that these different approaches are efficacious is mutually validating. Medical research and hands-on therapies are confirming each other. The common denominator is the pulsating geomagnetic field, which is called a biomagnetic field when it emanates from the hands of a therapist. [41]

As Oschman explains, bio-magnetic fields radiating from the hands of energy healers and certain martial artists, "show that practitioners can emit powerful pulsing bio-magnetic fields in the same frequency range that bio-medical researchers have identified for jump-starting healing of soft and hard tissue injury." [42]

Rats!

One way to investigate non-contact healing is to study the phenomenon outside of the influences of belief or faith in the healer. Thus, in some investigations, researchers study energetic healing on laboratory animals. One example of this kind of investigation took place in late 2000, with researchers looking at the effect of *wai qi* healing on "stressed out" laboratory rats. Scientists divided the rats into two groups, both of which were subjected to stress. One group received *wai qi* treatment from an energetic healer, while the other did not. Results showed that rats receiving energetic treatment maintained their weight (the measure demonstrating the effects of stress), whereas the rats in the control group lost weight. This suggests that an unknown influence, presumably the *wai qi* treatment, had a beneficial effect on the rat's autonomic nervous system. [43]

Cracking the Code: The Secret Inner World of the *Wai Qi* Healer

One challenge that has long limited researchers in their investigation of Chinese energetic healing is secrecy. Often, the Chinese healing tradition, like that of the martial arts, is rife with secrecy. In those circles, the specific technique used by a master of a particular school or tradition is often closely guarded. Thus, the oft-hidden nature of techniques prevents researchers from conducting a comprehensive examination of the phenomenon. For this reason, one study conducted by Omura to penetrate that veiled world is especially intriguing.

In an attempt to discover the inner thoughts and experiences of the *qi* master, Omura relied on a sophisticated variation of his patented muscle testing technique, called the Bi-Digital "O" Ring Test (BDORT). [44] Let us begin by considering what Omura observed regarding the effects of non-contact healing on the practitioner's body.

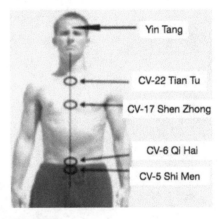

Figure 4-5

Physiological Changes During "Qigong State"

A Weakening Influence

Illustrated in Diagram 4-5, Omura reports that the practice of non-contact healing initiates significant changes at key acupuncture points. As shown in Figure 4-5, affected points were conception vessel 4 and 5 (CV-4 and CV-5), located below the umbilicus, along with several others. Significantly, during "outgoing *qi* therapy," those points experienced a weakening change to the practitioner's body during non-contact healing energy practice.

Relying on standard measurements that Omura developed for use with the BDORT protocol, results indicated a **weakening change** in these units from +4 in the pre-qigong state to between -3 and -4 during the *qigong* state at acupuncture points CV-5, CV-6, CV-17, CV-22, as well an "extra point" located between the eyebrows called *yin tang*. [45]

Omura's observations may suggest a "dark side" to energy work, since "lowering" or weakening of an individual's energy system from a positive to a negative, like that just described, is normally associated with pathology.

Relying on his sophisticated muscle testing technique as a way of glimpsing the normally veiled internal processes of the energetic healer, Omura used the

Omura evaluated the physiological state of *qigong* practitioners and patients during "Qi Gong State" using his variation of muscle testing called the Bi-Digital O-Ring Test (BDORT). According to Omura, both the qigong healer and patient experience marked changes during the qi gong experience at acupuncture points CV-5 *Shi Men* (stone gate), CV-6 *Qi Hai* (sea of qi), CV-17 *Shan Zhong* (chest center), CV-22 *Tian Tu* (celestial chimney), *Yin Tang* (seal hall), and *Bai Hui* (hundred gatherings, at the top of the head, not shown). [47]

BDORT technique first to identify, and then, along with fellow researchers, to replicate the secret techniques of the *qi* masters. After learning their secrets, Omura subsequently taught the procedure to other researchers, and even young children. The children that were taught the protocol were able to produce the same healing effects on patients as the accredited *wai qi* masters when, for example, attempting to lower blood pressure.[46] However, in the published study, Omura also details **health dangers to the practitioner** that are attributed to *wai qi* energetic practices. These, along with some of Omura's comments to me on the matter, are included in Chapter 19.

Chapter 19

Warning: Potential Self-Harm To Non-Contact Healers

Yoshiaki Omura, the developer of the "Bi-digital 'O' Ring Test" (BDORT), distinguished between two types of *qi* energy he calls positive and negative. Subsequently, the researchers experimented with applying the non-contact healing techniques to themselves and subjects. Significantly, they were able to duplicate the healing skills of the *wai qi* healers. However, it was troubling that when researchers themselves applied the non-contact healing protocol, they began to experience serious health issues, and subsequently abandoned the practice. It appears that practice of the *qi* master's secret method was damaging to the practitioner's stomach and gastrointestinal systems. These comments are from the published journal article:

> If the drug-uptake enhancement was still not sufficient for the drug to reach therapeutic levels in the diseased organ, direct application of (+) Qi Gong from the practitioner's hand often enhanced the drug uptake more significantly. **However, this direct method often results in the practitioner developing intestinal micro-hemorrhage within 24 hours which may or may not be noticed as mild intestinal discomfort with soft, slightly tarry stool.**[48] [emphasis added]

This suggests that *wai qi*-style non-contact healing may include an inherent danger, and, according to Omura, the observation potentially applies to all forms of non-contact healing. Could there be something about extending an invisible force, through what otherwise appears as empty space, which threatens the practitioner's health?

I learned of Omura's discovery of dangers to practitioners of non-contact healing during his presentation at the 2000 International Qigong Conference. However, because of the potential consequences for healers, he decided that he would not share what he learned about the secret techniques to presentation attendees.

However, Omura's discoveries about the secret world of the *qi* master were published in the *Acupuncture and Electro-Therapeutic Research Journal*. Thus, they are publicly available for anyone who takes the trouble to find them. In a few paragraphs, I will provide what Omura discovered in his investigation of *qi* masters, but I ask the reader's indulgence in carefully considering the following caveat.

Based on my personal experience of working with *wai qi* and other kinds of non-contact healers over many decades, I have observed the same kind of "danger to the practitioner" that Omura describes. As with the report made by Omura, the problematic areas I observed in non-contact practitioners often appeared to affect their stomach, intestines, and lower abdominal areas. In some cases, the damage presents in the form of chronic tension and dysfunction in the practitioner's lower back. Actually, I have never met a single non-contact healer who did not suffer from intestinal issues, lower back problems, or generalized weakness. Recently, a *reiki* healer asked me to help her understand the negative experiences she was having related to her practice. She said that she "felt terrible" after working with clients, and reported that it felt as though her "fingers were burning" when she practiced the therapy. My impression was that when she practiced, she was absorbing her patient's toxicity. It also appeared that she was storing that toxicity in her lower abdomen. Visually, my impression was that there was a large, dark mass in her lower abdomen. Upon hearing this, she immediately stopped offering the therapy.

I discussed the negative side-effects reported by *wai qi* non-contact healers, like those just described, with Omura after his presentation at the *qigong* conference, and our conversation touched on the danger to the energetic healer's stomach and abdominal region. I asked him if this was the general experience with healers, and he insisted that it was. According to Omura, every **non-contact healer, "100 percent," suffered from these kinds of health issues, "even if they denied experiencing these kinds of negative results."** Omura emphasized the point by stating that this was "true in every case," and even applied to famous Chinese masters he had studied, "even, if they did not want to admit to having such problems." Because of the possible danger to those who might try these techniques, I had mixed feelings about whether to include what Omura reports as the secret energy healer protocols in the present work. As mentioned earlier, although Omura's observations have been published in a peer-reviewed journal, he had declined to share them on a public forum.

In the end, my justification for including Omura's study is that the present work is intended as a survey of all research, discoveries, methods –– be it the good, the bad, or the ugly — in the realm of "energy" and "energy practices." Thus, the list of criteria provided in Omura's published study comes with something like the surgeon general's warning on a cigarette pack: "The practice could be (and probably is) dangerous to your health." It is the responsibility of readers and researchers considering this information to observe due caution.

Note: the information that follows is presented for research and discussion purposes only, and is not a recommendation for practice. Those interested in the practice of the *wai qi* healer are advised to seek guidance and counsel from a qualified master, and to not attempt the procedure without proper training.

Omura's Criteria for Attaining the *Wai Qi* Qigong State

(Information obtained from Omura's research of *wai qi* practitioners using the BDORT)

1. Concentrating the mind on the lower abdomen below the umbilicus (the *dan tian*).

2. Slowly breathing in deeply.

3. Constricting the sphincter muscle of the anus and pulling it up as high as possible.

4. Visualizing a large, shining sphere of light.

5. Visualizing the sphere of light covering the pathological part of the patient.

6. While simultaneously performing all of the above five steps, form the fingers and hand into a tubular shape and direct it at the patient's affected area.

The dangers described by Omura in relation to the practice of *wai qi* non-contact energy healing are consistent with my own observations. Non-contact energy transfer seems to affect practitioners, including some martial arts masters. Sadly, a dramatic example of gastrointestinal complications related to *wai qi* energy practice involves one of my own teachers. Before he passed away some years ago, the elderly and highly-accomplished master regularly visited our school in southern California.

At around 89 years of age, during what would be his penultimate visit, the master impressed us with his stamina; the youthful spring in his step belied his years. In fact, I have a clear memory of him, at one point during a break, spontaneously demonstrating a cartwheel! What a great example for us to aspire to! It showed us what we, too, might accomplish in our old age.

The master's vigor and supple youthfulness were an inspiration, and we were surprised to learn that he had even added something new to his instruction regimen. However, I believe that this new addition to his repertoire contributed to his sudden illness and ultimate decline not long thereafter. Out of the blue, at the end of one class being held in the parking lot behind our studio, the master told us that he wanted to project his healing *qi* energy to us. I had not previously seen him do anything like this during our 20-year master-disciple relationship, and to explain why I believe he had decided to project his *qi* to our group, some background information is helpful.

In the 1990s, in some parts of Asia, the phenomenon of mass *wai qi* energetic healing was all the rage, and a few *qi* masters were receiving a lot of media attention. In some cases, crowds filled auditoriums to attend and receive energy healing. Some of these gatherings had the feeling of an evangelist revival, characterized by overflowing emotions and sensationalism. A crowd of excited followers would wait anxiously for the master to take center stage, aim his open palms toward the attendees, and extend his healing *qi* power toward them.

Like spiritual mass healing services in other traditions, some of the faithful would join the master on stage. There, they described their sudden, miraculous recovery from whatever malady had afflicted them. At times, the afflicted would jump out of wheelchairs or throw aside crutches in response to the healing miracle. However, the highlight of the demonstration was always saved for the end, when the master extended his palms toward the audience and sent forth his energy. I believe that my teacher became aware of the popularity of some of these spectacles, and said to himself, "I, too, can do that."

At the end of that class, the master asked us to form a semi-circle around him. The ten-to-fifteen of us present formed the requested configuration, and, in physical proximity ranging from 5-10 ft away, he asked us to stand still and close our eyes (I didn't quite close mine, because I was too curious about what he was about to do). Then, imitating the stage performances of energy healers in Asia, he aimed his open hand at us and fluttered his fingers in our direction. Moving his hands back to send his *qi,* the movement began from his left, proceeded to the right, and then back again. The master's projection of *qi* was emitted so that everyone could experience a bit of it, and I suspected that this had recently become part of his regular routine with his students back home.

Over the course of the next year, the master's health went into a sharp decline. He began to experience serious gastrointestinal health issues, of which I never learned the official diagnosis. The worsening condition led to surgery and the complete removal of his stomach, and on his next, and unfortunately last, visit, he could barely walk, hardly resembling the previous year's cartwheeling marvel. Due to the removal of his stomach, the limited capacity of his digestive system required him to carry a thermos everywhere he went, from which he would take a small spoonful of nourishment every half-hour or so. He passed away not long after leaving us to return to his homeland.

I agree with Omura's view that the practice of *sending* or externalizing subtle energy comes with dire consequences. The practice of projecting non-contact energy to others may be very dangerous, and thus not something to be trifled with. As suggested by Omura's description of the weakening effects of *qi* projection, there seems to be some sort of connection between mastery over one's bio-energy systems and stress to the practitioner's lower abdomen.

It will be covered in the chapters that follow, especially those concerning the internal energy traditions of Tibet and China, how there also appears to be a relationship between the areas of the lower abdomen, internal energy, and advanced spiritual accomplishment. As with other energy practices, the area of the lower abdomen is often the locus of attention in energetic yoga and meditative traditions. As for the practice of "externalizing energy," there appears to be something especially stressful about the practice that might harm the practitioner's body. Perhaps, then, it is the case that most of us aren't designed with the necessary infrastructure to "play safely" with such a degree of "energy."

Speculation on *Why* Non-Contact Healing Might be Dangerous to Practitioners

In every form of energetic healing, whether acupuncture, energetic massage, or non-contact healing, a subtle and unspoken dialogue takes place between practitioner and patient. In acupuncture and massage, the exchange between therapist and patient operates through physical contact. However, regardless of whether or not physical contact takes place, effective treatment requires the therapist to "listen" and respond to the patient.

In each of those three therapeutic interventions, the practitioner adjusts the protocol in response to the unspoken exchange between therapist and patient. Conversely, in the case of non-contact healing, both the "dialogue" and treatment take place through "empty space," usually at a distance of a foot or more, between the therapist and patient.

Earlier chapters have presented examples of non-contact therapy in Chinese-style *wai qi*, and although no physical contact is made in this form of healing, the same kind of adjustments to the patient response are still required. Whatever it is that produces healing, ** whether a yet-to-be-named force, energy, or source of "information," it must transfer through the medium of "empty space" between the therapist's fingers or palm and the patient's body.

> ** When "local," as opposed to non-locally, per the definition of the type of healing that is addressed in this section, and described in Box 4-1

Diagram 4-6

Tiller's Schematic of Near (Reactive) and Distant (Radiated) Energy Fields

The illustration shows the radiated field pattern from an acupuncture point and meridian. Note that field demarcations A and B are the author's and not part of Tiller's original diagram.

(Diagram based on schematic from William A. Tiller's Science and Human Transformation)

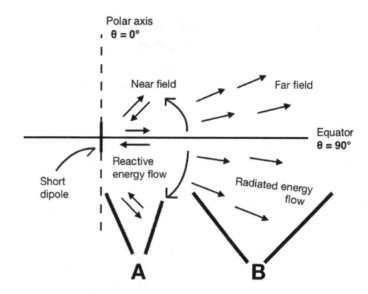

The Near and Distant Fields and Their Role in Healing

Section II included William Tiller's modeling of the human "energy field," citing the hypothesis that it functions akin to the fluctuating voltage radiation fields surrounding a simple dipole antenna. † At this juncture, it is useful to think about two aspects of Tiller's model, the first being the role of the close reactive vs distal fields in explaining the phenomenon of internal energy, while the second is the question of why the practice of non-contact healing appears to be harmful to the practitioner.

It is speculated that the near field, lying an inch or so around the body (represented by Demarcation A of Diagram 4-6), serves a protective function, and that the radiated "energy field" presented within this demarcation is quite different from the distal radiation field associated with Demarcation B. This is due to the bi-directional nature of the near field.

In the application of non-contact healing, such as *wai qi* therapy, even though physically separated from the patient, the therapist still must "feel" and adjust their technique based on their perceived response of the patient to the treatment. For example, if sensing the source of inflammation or deficiency in an organ or meridian system, the therapist adjusts to the patient's response. However, it may be significant that non-contact intervention usually does not take place within the hypothesized protective layer of the *auric*-reactive field, but instead from the (non-reactive) distal radiated field. This may be excessively taxing to the practitioner.

Nonetheless, because of the feedback requirement, in practice, the art of projecting healing intention outward, and then "listening" for feedback, must pass through not only ambient radio waves, but innumerable unknown entities in the "empty space" between practitioner and patient. Could it be that this kind of transfer and exchange exhausts the therapist?

† More nuanced discussion of these proposed radiation fields provides insight into the meaning of "internal energy," and is included in Section XII under "Speculation and Dimensional Stuff."

Chapter 20

Problems with Research and Experiment Design

*I*n recent years, a number of problems have been reported by investigators in the West attempting to replicate the results of *wai qi* energetic healers in China. In April 2005, Kevin W. Chen, PhD MPH, Associate Professor of Psychiatry at Robert Wood Johnson Medical School in New Jersey, reported information on a web *qi* research (energetic research) bulletin board following a discussion he had with a senior scientist in the field.

Posting on the online forum, Chen revealed that most funded studies in the US, including several major projects, had failed to achieve significant results in replication studies. In other words, studies on external energy treatment (EQT) — another name for *wai qi* non-contact healing — which had previously achieved significant results in Chinese studies, could not be replicated in controlled U.S. follow-ups. This was problematic, as it would make it difficult for researchers to receive grants to study external *qigong* in the near future.

Chen expressed his interest in discovering why the results in U.S studies differed from their Chinese counterparts, and summarized what Chinese researchers have learned in previous studies of EQT. Here are some of his main points:

1. Since *qigong* is a self-training or therapy process, most practitioners do not study [in a systematic way] external healing methods. Thus, it is not practical for all *qigong* practitioners to emit external healing for laboratory study purposes. Self-practice methods (internal training) should be promoted to "take full advantage of *qi gong* therapy as a self-empowerment method."

2. Results of external energetic healing studies in the U.S. suggest that not all *qi* energy "healers" can emit external *qi*. † Since some energetic healers, even known healers, can heal themselves or others, but fail to demonstrate this under laboratory conditions, researchers should not be surprised by their failure to replicate the findings from other investigational studies.

3. Even a qualified external *qi* healer with a good record in clinical studies may not be able to produce consistently positive results in *in-vitro* or *in-vivo*. To improve results, in some cases the energetic healer should be included in the experimental design.

4. External energetic healing is a "complicated technique or skill that is usually developed over a length of time. To achieve the effective emission of *qi* in a study, the practitioner needs practice and understanding of the sensors or methods used for measurement. They may also have some special requirements for the environment or control conditions, such as lack of extraneous sound and skeptical personnel. Therefore, it is important to have open communication with the *qigong* practitioner, and to allow them to practice and familiarize themselves with the setting before the studies commence." [49]

Chen also points out the importance of consciousness and *intent*, and how they are important variables to be considered in the methods and discussion aspects of clinical trials, despite not being fully understood *why*. It is also important to consider the patient's consciousness, mindset, and expectation as factors that could affect the trial outcome. Chen suggests that in documenting post-treatment results, the investigators limit questioning the patient about their pain. As he explains:

> The lesson we learned in this type of study is that when you ask the patients if they still feel the pain or symptom (or tumor), they will try very hard to locate the residual pain or symptom at the old location. Since the sick *qi* ‡ or the symptom may be recreated by his / her own consciousness, it is important not to dwell on the pain. Since external qigong therapy applies the intention and consciousness of the healer, it is also important to remember that everyone's consciousness has power and energy. When a patient thinks of the pain or symptom area for a long time, the sick *qi* or the symptom may be recreated by his / her own consciousness. [50]

Finally, Chen suggests that researchers need to observe the energetic healer's personality and emotional state, and determine how to make those factors a constant in the study. Given that the results of each study are directly related to the healer's subjective feeling and mood, the study should be conducted only when the healer is in a "good mood." Chen's posting underscores the role of subjective factors, such as consciousness, expectation, and intent in determining the success or failure of *wai qi* external energetic healing. He suggests that an expanded paradigm which includes these subjective factors would be valuable in understanding the phenomenon.

> † As suggested in the Afterword to this section, it may be presumptive for researchers to assume that measurement of extraordinarily large bio-electrical or infrared radiation is synonymous with *qi* internal energy. At this point, *qi* has not been clearly defined, and by making reductionist pronouncements like this, researchers are saying that

qi is simply an observed EM or infrared radiation phenomenon. An example is expressed through a statement such as, "this 'qi' is directed by a trained practitioner." It is the author's contention that when *qi / ki / prana,* or similarly named subtle energy phenomenon, is more fully understood, it will be established as something much greater than EM or other-field radiation. It is also important to keep in mind that claims of a "healing force" are extraordinary, since such statements assume the phenomenon is a yet undefined force of nature. More comments on this are included in the Afterword.

‡ Until an accepted definition is available, it is suggested that researchers be more cautious about the use of terms such as "sick *qi.*" Since, at the present time, a succinct definition of *qi* is lacking, it is not helpful to intermingle traditional concepts, e.g., "sick *qi,*" with scientifically accepted methods that are applied to investigations of the subject.

Lack of Consistent Definition of Internal Energy Training and Practices

As described by Chen, two of the reasons that non-contact energetic healing is so difficult to study under laboratory conditions have to do with the lack of definition and inconsistencies in *qi* training. There is no standardization of *qigong* training, and results are often dependent on the personality of the healer.[51] The systematic study of energetic healers is further complicated by the nature of healing traditions, and the tendency to combine them with mental, physical, spiritual, or religious aspects.

Expectancy Effects

The failure of U.S. researchers to replicate results of non-contact healer studies in China may partially be explained by the phenomenon researchers call *expectancy effects.* This research challenge can be imagined as represented by a two-sided coin.

On one side of the coin is the age-old problem faced by scientists, namely that researchers sometimes have an unconscious (and sometimes not so unconscious) bias in favor of data that supports the conclusion they are seeking. The other side of the coin is represented by individuals — patients, students, and experimental subjects — who unconsciously learn to report results and perform as expected, in order to please the authority figure of the teacher, investigator, or master. In this light, one probable reason for the inability of U.S. researchers to duplicate the results obtained by their counterparts in China may be due to the *expectancy effects* of patients in the Chinese studies. * In some cases, not only do the researchers expect a certain result from their investigation, but their patients do as well. Regardless of whether or not it is ever proven that something called *qi* exists, in Chinese culture, the patient's belief in the "power of *qi*" to heal will often be extremely strong, acting as testimony to the power of belief and the largely untapped potential of the mind.

*Additional discussion of "expectancy effects" as applied to martial arts is included in the Afterword to Section VIII.

Chapter 21

Information: A new Explanation for "Energy" Healing

One problem non-contact energy researchers face relates to the **amount** of energy that the technique would require in order to produce the desired healing effects. The problem applies to both *in vivo* studies (eg, blood radicals in patients) and *in vitro* effects (eg, the annihilation of bacteria in a Petri dish). Thus, it is imperative to consider other explanations that do not necessarily rely on a tremendous **quotient** of "energy." An alternative scenario involves replacing the notion of "energy" with the concept of *"information."* Here, we consider the *information theory* proposed by Kenneth Hintz.

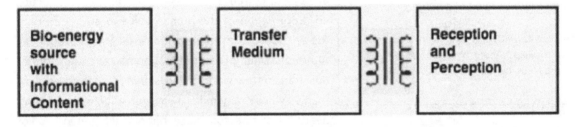

Diagram 4-7

Dr Kenneth Hintz's Block Diagram of Bio-energetic Components

Based on a Diagram from Hintz et al., "Bio-energy Definitions and Research Guidelines" [52]

Reduction of Entropy

Some aspects of energetic healing might be best explained not in terms of a practitioner's ability to project a quotient of "force" or energy, but in terms of the healer's ability to transmit anti-entropic information. The model suggests that rather than "energy," the practitioner transmits coded information which carries "instructions." In the context of energetic healing of any type, these instructions interact with the patient's subtle energy field (Diagram 4-7). Accordingly, information exchanged between healer and patient works because anti-entropic information instructs the patient's system to move from "relative disorder to one of less disorder." [53] [54]

As discussed at the beginning of this section, two types of phenomena fall under the umbrella of energetic healing: healing that appears to conform to known laws of physics, and forms of energetic healing that do not. Classifiable respectively as *local* and *non-local* (as presented in Box 4-1), the *information* model offers a new explanation for non-contact healing in the context of the principles of "local." In this light, *information theory* is presumed to act consistently with known laws of physics, such as bio-electricity. In contrast, long-distance healing, which falls into the category of non-local, does not appear to follow conventional laws.

Hintz's Proposed Model of two kinds of "Energy Healing"

Bio-energy that conforms to accepted definitions of "energy"

Detectable or measurable
by instruments or bio-markers

**Healing energy that
does not conform to
accepted notions of "energy"**

Includes healing at a distance,
which seems to defy spatial
and temporal rules of energy

* From Kenneth Hintz, PhD, et al. "Bio-energy definitions and research guidelines." Alternative Therapies in Health and Medicine. May/June 2003

Box 4-8

Hintz believes that energetic healing which conforms to known laws of bio-energetics will one day be shown to be "detectable and measurable by physical instruments or bio-markers" that conform to accepted definitions of "energy." He posits that these forms of healing will one day be shown to be "at least in part electrical, magnetic, or EM in nature." Hintz's two proposed forms of bio-energy are contrasted in Box 4-8.

Hintz's model of local, *information*-based healing can be understood as a kind of "bio-information" exchange between healer and patient that can be compared with telephone communication. In telephony, only a small amount of current is necessary to transmit the "encoded" information of the human voice to an appropriate "de-encoder" (the other person's telephone earpiece). Although, when presented to a human ear, the *information* transmitted via a coded signal is interpreted as a friend's voice many miles away, in reality, what is being heard is not an actual voice, but only a *representation* of the friend's speech. In other words, *information* creates a representation, but not the actual voice. The example provides a model for thinking about the way *information,* applied to healing, might be transmitted via a coded, anti-entropic signal that is then interpreted and responded to by the receiver's biological systems. To restate, according to Hintz's proposed model, the healing process takes place not through the transfer of an energetic force, but, as in telephony, through an extremely minute current, which is received and decoded at the terminal end (the "terminal sink" shown in Diagram 4-7).

Hintz defines a bio-energy *information* system as one comprised of the following aspects:

- a source that generates energy, and modulates it in some manner so that that it conveys information
- a coupling mechanism connecting the bio-energy source to a transfer medium

- a transfer medium through which the bio-energy flows
- a coupling mechanism connecting the transfer medium /bio-energy sink
- a terminal sink, which includes a mechanism for the perception of *information*

Hintz proposes that the healing benefit of *information* transferred between healer and patient works because of the way encoded *information* reduces *entropy*. In this context, entropy is the tendency for systems, including biological organisms, to deteriorate and break down.

According to Hintz's theory, an "energetic healer," when operating *intentionally*, [55] would be a person with an intuitive ability to consciously produce a harmonious signal, which then encodes and subsequently transfers the healing (anti-entropic) signal in the form of *information* to the recipient. In terms of healing, or in the case of "internal energy in the martial arts," the recipient's unconscious biological response to the *information* determines whether or not the anti-entropic encoding was successful.

Hintz's Bio-informational Model as an Explanation for the Effects of Energetic Healing

1. The practitioner must be able to attune to, and generate, a measurable bio-electrical field.

2. An ordering (or possibly disordering *) encoding becomes associated with the practitioner's bio-electrical field (when consciously initiated, this is most often due to *intention*—discussed below). In this model, the *information*-encoded bio-electrical field interacts with and influences the recipient

*The possibility of sending disordered or a weakening influence is suggested as possible explanation for some martial art abilities, as covered in Section VIII

Box 4-9

Conclusion to Section IV

*D*eciding how "non-contact healing" fits into the larger discussion of internal energy is challenging. While some evidence supports the hypothesis of an undefined non-contact healing force as a valid phenomenon, it is both interesting and frustrating that many important points that might lead to a more complete understanding of the phenomenon remain elusive.

Although much of the present section has focused on the Chinese phenomenon of non-contact healing, the practice exists in shamanistic forms across many cultures. As noted earlier, the Hawaiian shaman understands healing to manifest through the power of a *kahuna*, or person of power, who possesses sufficient *mana*. Likewise, in Mexican and Meso-American cultures, there is a belief that physical, emotional, and spiritual healing could be provided by the *curandera*, who conducts a *limpia*, or "cleansing."

Whether non-contact healing will eventually be explained in terms of a *force of nature* or as the result of an unidentified aspect of our shared psychology, the cross-cultural acceptance of "energetic healing" suggests that the notion is powerful. One day, its healing benefits may be described in terms of human directed "energy," or it might also be ascribed to a patient's belief in the healer. In either case, for many of us it is part of our nature to place faith in the idea that some among us have the power to heal the sick, not through drugs, herbs or surgery, but through psychic *intention*.

Is it possible that the belief that one person could heal another without contact may have surfaced at the same time as our ancestors painted their stories on cave walls?

Due to its shared practice among numerous ancient cultures, it appears that this little understood form of healing emerged as humans began to engage in more abstract thought. This suggests that faith in the existence of a healing energetic force may be tied to an evolutionary step related to the development of the higher brain. If so, the practice might be closely related to our ancestors' belief in the power of their intention to influence the physical world through will, magic, and ritual. The universality of non-contact healing across multiple ancient cultures indicates that we are hard-wired to accept the notion that healing is possible through mysterious forces beyond our comprehension. Its universal nature suggests that our brain can be set to *believe* and *expect* results from an energetic healer, like a shaman, *wai qi* practitioner, or spiritual healer.

Some of the most interesting evidence for the efficacy of non-contact healing and the objective existence of healing energy comes from physiological measurements of non-contact healers. Research investigating the bio-electrical characteristics of individuals referred to by researchers as "energy projectors" is especially intriguing. This field of investigation includes those studies of *qigong* masters who were documented as being able to emit measurable EM and infrared radiation. Other studies of energy projectors include measurements of the projector's ear lobes, which, during the energy projection process, indicate the presence of transient large voltage pulse.

Correlation vs. Causality

It is puzzling that in many studies, such as Seto and Kusaka's investigation of energetic healers, only a few members of selected groups were able to emit measurable EM fields. Thus, it remains unclear how such results affect the discussion of "internal energy." At this time, it may be too big a leap to equate the measured electric-magnetic pulses measured from the palms of some non-contact healers as "*qi*" internal energy. At best, results like these are correlational, but not causal. In other words, because electromagnetic bio-markers are present in *some* demonstrations of energy healing, it should not be assumed that EM energy *is* the manifestation of *qi*, or "healing energy." This point will be further explored in Section XII.

Signal

In Section III, it was suggested that, for practical purposes, instead of "energy," the term "signal" should be adopted. *Signal* provides a target goal without requiring a precise definition of "energy." Working with a concept like signal enables a practitioner to assume a particular psychological and physiological state, and then experiment with its effects on mind and body without the requirement to name the source of the experience.

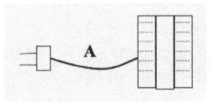

Diagram 4-10

Is it the Extension of "Energy" or Power Management Issues?

In this way, whether or not the *signal* being worked with really is *qi, ki,* or *prana* becomes less important. To reflect on the advantages of adopting this approach, it is useful to consider the metaphor of a heater or other electrical device, where a large amount of current is required for its operation. An investigator unfamiliar with the principles of EM current could potentially make the mistake of thinking the extraneous heat produced by a thin wire feeding the household electrical heater might be causal, and thus related to, or perhaps even synonymous with, the heat produced by the device.

Illustrated by A in Diagram 4-9, an overheated wire is not the force that empowers the heater. The overheated wire is the result of power management issues. In this example, a thicker cord providing less resistance would not be overly warm, and thus, the heater would not only produce less heat in wire A, but also be more efficient. In this example, it would be erroneous to associate heater function with an overheated electrical wire, as the two issues are independent of each other. In fact, if one were to place primary focus on the presence or lack of heat in the wire, the more important causal discussion of electron flow from plug to heating element might easily be missed.

Also, by placing too much attention on the artifact — in this case, designing a system to produce more heat in wire A — we know from the physics of resistance that we are in danger of destroying the whole system, and perhaps even causing a fire. This metaphor also suggests another explanation for the danger to *wai qi* healers, described by Omura and discussed in Chapter 19.

It is fascinating that in modern China, healing traditions rooted in shamanism have begun to merge with modern scientific inquiry. Today, *wai qi* non-contact energetic healing is beginning to be regarded as a legitimate branch of traditional medicine, and it is not uncommon to find practitioners of *wai qi* healing practicing in hospitals, and working in concert with acupuncturists and herbalists, to provide care alongside conventional Western-style medical professionals.

As the quest to establish *qi* as an objective *force of nature* continues, some researchers have taken a completely independent approach. This has led to suggestions that what is referred to as subtle, or internal, energy may in actuality be the "exchange of information" between healer and patient. This theme will be explored further in the sections that follow.

Afterword to Section IV

Comments and Suggestions for *Wai Qi* Researchers

This Afterword focuses on two main issues. First is the caveat that researchers be more careful when describing non-contact healing as an ancient form of traditional Chinese medicine. Second, that instead of thinking about *wai qi* as an ancient and lost branch of TCM, researchers be more open to the possibility that Chinese style non-contact healing might be better understood as an example of the healing power of the shaman, not the traditional doctor.

The notion that it might be possible for one person to heal another without making physical contact is fascinating, and, if proven true, speaks to the future evolution of the human potential; an exciting prospect indeed! However, it should again be noted that the majority of scientists do not accept the proposition that human intention and influence, whether in the form of *qi* or some other unidentified medium, acts as a *natural force*.

When broadly accepted, objective evidence supporting the idea that one person can influence another, not only through physical interaction, but through intention conveyed through the medium of empty space, will modify the science of physics.

This realization will establish *intention* as a verifiable force that can influence the physical world outside of one's own body. If one person can reliably demonstrate this, then, some day in the future, our descendants may find such ability commonplace.

Our descendants, inheriting our research and progress, would then reflect on us as representing a backwards era of undiscovered potential. They would regard us as those who had not yet realized the latent power hidden in our genetic blueprint.

The Chinese-style practice of non-contact healing still awaits comprehensive investigation. However, unless it is to forever be ascribed to faith or a fluke, it is essential that empirical investigation of the subject proceed with proper scientific protocol. Such protocol requires that the antecedents of any claim of tradition, special abilities, or unusual skills (e.g., the ability to heal without physical contact) be cited and fully explored. For example, if the following statement was made: "There was an physician named John Doe, who was able to heal patients with his thoughts," then one would expect numerous citations, whether *pro* or *con,* to support the existence and claims of John Doe, who was said to have healing abilities. In support of this point, these are exactly the types of reports that document the life of the American visionary and healer Edgar Casey, whose life spanned the late-nineteenth and early-twentieth centuries. In this case, many volumes exist on the subject of Casey and his work, and various related citations can be found that were made by news services and authors of the time.

Traditional Medicine or Shamanistic Practice?

Although *wai qi,* whether referred to as externalized *qi* or Chinese-style non-contact healing by another name, is frequently described in journal articles as "having roots deep in Chinese medicine," I find no credible evidence to support these claims.[56] However, it is noteworthy that the roots of some practices may refer to shamanism rather than traditional medicine. Consider, for example, that Chinese writer Bi Youngsheng refers to the roots of non-contact healing which he names "outgoing [qi] therapy" as being related to an ancient Chinese practice known as *zhuyou* (祝由) (also written *zhu you).* [57]

However, *zhuyou* is a shamanistic practice, and not a form of traditional Chinese medicine. In fairness, it is safe to say that the ancient roots of TCM can in fact be traced to shamanism, however, by the time of the Zhou dynasty,[58] Chinese medicine was already emerging as a distinct proto-scientific tradition. By that time, it had already begun to distance itself from the shaman.

Professor Philip S. Cho, in his doctoral thesis, describes the co-development between the *zhuyou* and the foundational beliefs that developed into traditional Chinese medical theory. Cho informs us that the ritual therapies associated with *zhuyou* were designed to "move and transform *qi* in the body," and that this is the central principle of Chinese medicine. However, other aspects of *zhuyou* distinguish it from traditional medicine, for example, the *zhuyou* relied on incantations to "expel hidden or occult pathogens that were minute and subtle as if ghosts." [59]

> A variety of manuals show how different healers interpreted the art. For example, Orthodox Unity priests at the Temple of Profound Mystery in 18 th century Suzhou rewrote the origin myth of *zhuyou* to make it a part of their tradition ....
>
> Critical of religious healing, scholar physicians in the region reinterpreted *zhuyou* as a secular therapy to treat emotional and spiritual disorders.

Rather than ghosts, the cause of disorder was flawed character, resulting in improper behavior or excessive harmful emotions.[60]

The role of the shaman as an explanation for non-contact healing will be returned to in a few paragraphs. However, pertaining to our discussion of the roots of TCM, it is important to distinguish between shamanism and the proto-scientific foundations of traditional medicine. Consider the following claim which appeared in an online text on Chinese non-contact healing, describing a technique known as "moving the *qi*," which is purported to be a non-contact form of Chinese medicine:

> For thousands of years, the Chinese have fashioned an art and a science of projecting vital life energy to heal illnesses. It was first called *Bù qì* (布氣) "Spreading the *Qi*." Now it is called "External Qi Healing Therapy" (*Wài qì liáofǎ* - 外气疗法). The basic technique has the practitioner emitting Qi [vital life energy] into the appropriate acupuncture points on the client's body. There are different methods, but most often the healer emits qi through the fingers and palms. There is no direct physical contact or touching and the client is fully clothed. [61]

There are other references to *buqi* — "spreading the *qi*." Kunio Miura writes that the practice was used in ancient China:

> To spread one's *qi* in order to heal a sick person one must first examine where, in his orbs, the problem is rooted. Then one takes one's *qi* through the mouth and places it into the patient's body. The patient faces the *qi* master, but before he receives the *qi* he should calm his mind and cleanse his thoughts. After the infusion, the patient should swallow the *qi*. Thereby demons and devil forces will be expelled; bad *qi* will be eradicated forever. [62]

According to Miura, *buqi* was practiced in the Song dynasty (960-1279 CE). In those references, its application involved physical contact to specific points on the patient's body. Like forms of *qigong* practiced today, the therapy generated warmth within the practitioner's body. One story cited by Miura is that of a Taoist nun, who treated patients by infusing *qi* through the mouth. It was reported that in one case, the practice resulted in the nun's embarrassment when the warmth experienced in her intestines caused her to become momentarily incontinent. [63]

Chinese terms are often difficult to translate into English, and sometimes change over time. Consider the use of the general term *qigong*. In the article, *The Man who invented 'Qigong,'* John Voigt informs us that in 1947, a Chinese clerk named Liu Guizhen developed a healing art based on focused attention and breathing. According to Voigt, in a search for a more palatable term than the originally proposed "spiritually healing," "psychological therapy" or "incantation therapy," the term "qigong" ("energy skill") became accepted as the new term for the therapeutic method in March 1949.[64] Subsequently, Liu began to teach and study *qigong* in hospital and research settings.

However, problems arise for modern day researchers when a practice like non-contact *qi* healing is credited to an un-cited, enigmatic, and "ancient source," since investigators are required to have a clear and precise understanding of a phenomenon, including antecedents, which they are examining. For example, consider the subtitle of one article published in *The Natural Medicine Journal* which states:

> Qi gong is one modality of traditional Chinese medicine (TCM) believed to be at least 4,000 years old. Written records referring to *Qi* and its effects are thought to be as old as 3,300 years (Shang dynasty oracle bones, Zhou dynasty inscriptions).[65]

As suggested by the subtitle, it is true that there are ancient traditions that can be called *qigong*, including *tuina* (推拿, also written *tui-na*), therapeutic manipulation, *daoyin* yoga, and from the early centuries of the first millennium, "energetic meditation." However, I have found no references to an ancient "external" *wai qi* practice in accepted scholarly texts. Thus, it may be premature to associate *Zhou* dynasty inscriptions with the practice of non-contact healing.

It is misleading to too hastily link the terms "external" and "internal" *qigong*. Furthermore, it may not be prudent to suggest, without supporting references, that non-contact energetic healing is part of the *ancient* practice of traditional Chinese medicine. As far as I can tell, there is no mention of a non-contact healing practice in the earliest Chinese medical text, the *Emperor's Classic of Medicine*. Furthermore, after conducting a search of Joseph Needham's *Science and Civilization in China*,[66] I found no mention of *wai qi* or non-contact healing. There is, however, the notable exception of the shaman tradition, which will be addressed in a few paragraphs.

Recently, I was referred to another contemporary source that reiterated the claim that non-contact healing practice was originally called "spreading the *qi*." Although I remained skeptical, this revelation did inspire me to re-read the relevant chapters in Wang and Wu's comprehensive 1936 *History of Chinese Medicine*, which informs us that:

> Only four branches of medicine were recognized in the Chou [Zhou] dynasty, the number had increased to seven during the Tang dynasty. These were diseases of adults, diseases of children, diseases of eye and ear mouth and teeth, cupping, massage, and exorcism.[67]

Wang and Wu inform us that during this period, "four kinds of doctors were differentiated: physicians, acupuncturists, masseurs, and exorcists. Special chairs were established with a *"Po Shih,"* or professor in charge, of each department." Furthermore, Wang and Wu provide the official repertory of the *New Tang [Dynasty] Annals,* which describes the organization of the Imperial Medical Bureau. The Tang Dynasty report is instructive on the organization of medical practice in ancient China, and is included in the Endnote.[68] Notably, there are no references to the practice of non-contact healing.

As with the search for historical sources in both the Needham collections and contributions to the literature by Wang and Wu, I came across similar information in examining the fourth-century *Pao Pu Tzu*. Although the author, Ko Hung, comments on every known health and longevity technique, from external alchemy to sexual alchemy and even wizardry, no mention is made of an art of healing without touch.

The unchallenged frequency of citations made in reference to this "ancient *qigong* practice" is troublesome, since evidence that the non-contact *qigong* technique was a branch of TCM remains sketchy at best. Consider another example from a published article:

> Basically, there are two categories of qigong: internal qigong and external qigong. Internal qigong or qigong exercise is self-directed and involves the use of movements, meditation, and control of breathing pattern, whereas external qigong or emitted qi, is usually performed by a trained practitioner using their hands to direct qi energy onto the patient for treatment. Their underlying mechanisms that provide potential benefits are different. [69]

I believe statements like these unintentionally act as a disservice to researchers investigating such an important phenomenon as *wai qi* non-contact healing. To both advance knowledge of the healing art and develop its credibility, it is important that we proceed with rigor and caution. Thus, suggestions of non-contact healing being traced back to ancient records on oracle bones may not only be inaccurate, but also unwise. Likewise, in the above quoted introduction to a published research paper, the author of the study takes for granted that there is such a thing as "external qigong or emitted *qi*," and that this "*qi*" is actually directed by a "trained practitioner."

I am not arguing for or against the possibility of non-contact healing as a real phenomenon, nor am I disputing the notion that this kind of healing might be accounted for by *qi* energy. My point is simply that it may not necessarily be an "ancient practice" with roots in Chinese medicine. Although, the practice might not be traceable to the foundations of TCM, it might instead be a newer practice. It is a leap for researchers to assume that "something," presumably *qi* energy, is transferred to the patient during a healing session, since other mechanisms might well explain the efficacy of non-contact healing. The "healing" may or may not have anything to do with "*qi* energy." It might be belief, it could be the work of angels, it could be the alignment of the planets, or perhaps some combination of all these. Thus, researchers (at least until *qi* is measurable and reliably defined), should not assume that "non-contact healing" is due to the practitioner's ability to emit an invisible and non-quantifiable force.

I do not mean the preceding statement to be dismissive of the highly educated, thoughtful, and well-meaning authors of the above cited articles. These are only a few examples from a long list of published papers on the subject, and my fear is that their claims may act as a red herring and mislead other researchers. Thus, it is a threat to serious investigation to assume non-contact healing with "qi" is an ancient and lost form of Chinese medicine.

Shamanistic Roots

In the 1950s, the first research into non-contact healing was introduced by the Chinese government, and since the 1970s, the phenomenon has been increasingly looked at by researchers throughout the world, especially in Mainland China. As cited earlier, some of these results are very promising. However, it is intriguing that the earliest record of something akin to non-contact healing may have its roots in shamanism.

One reason this distinction is important is that researchers, if examining non-contact healing as a technique of traditional medicine, *could mistakenly* consider the *wai qi* phenomenon as distinctly Chinese. Thus, it would be easy to overlook what the *wai qi* tradition might have in common with ancient the Hawaiian shaman or the prayers of a Christian mystic.

For example, if *wa qi* were uniquely Chinese, then it would be important to consider the *yin* and *yang,* as well as other aspects of a disease, within the context of TCM. However, if the roots of *wai qi* practice are shamanistic, this suggests that other factors universally found in shamanistic cultures, such as the relationship between the patient and shaman, belief and expectation of the parties involved, or social support from members of the group. Or, perhaps the cause that produces healing is really *qi* after all, and it is the case that skilled shamans in every tradition might really be able to emit some unknown force that the Chinese call *qi.*

In the Introduction to Volume Six of Joseph Needham's *Science and Civilization in China,* the editor, Christopher Cullen, describes several different kinds of sorcerers, or shamans. For example, there are the *fa-shi,* a term originally used to designate a Buddhist teacher. There is also a *wu,* or "medium." According to Cullen, there was some mixing of shamanistic tradition with other practices, which have since evolved to become known as *qigong,* or internal energy exercise.[70] Furthermore, Ko Hung, in 300 CE, describes the efficacy of Taoist breathing techniques when used in conjunction with charms and incantations. [71] Needham et al state:

> Probably before the beginning of the Shang kingdom, Chinese society
> had its 'medicine-men,' something like the shamans of the North Asian
> tribal peoples. [72]

Needham comments on the physicians of China becoming a respected, educated class in the following way:

> Considerable numbers of physicians were well educated in general literature, and with greater culture than their predecessors had possessed. Such men called themselves *ju i* ('Confucian physicians') as opposed to those they belittled as *yung i*, mediocre practitioners or quacks.[73]

Needham et al also describes another kind of physician, the forerunner of the wandering mendicant:

> Prominent among those so denigrated were the wandering medical peddlers frequently seen in late imperial China, jingling their special kind of bell on a staff and handing out herbal remedies for the smallest of fees.

Perhaps the true origin of the non-contact healing tradition was the shaman, who, mixing spiritual beliefs and magic, no doubt had a profound effect on at least some of his patients. Also beyond doubt is the assertion that their philosophy contributed to the foundation of traditional medicine.[74]

Impressive evidence suggests that non-contact healing is a phenomenon worthy of serious investigation, and thus it is important that researchers in China and elsewhere continue to investigate the efficacy and mechanism of the technique. I hope that such investigation continues, but I also wish for investigators to be more cautious when considering whether the active ingredient / causative agent is, in fact, *"qi."*

It is important for researchers to consider that non-contact healing may not be a Chinese phenomenon with "deep roots" in ancient Chinese medicine. It is also worth considering that the phenomenon may speak to the universal power of the shamans of all ancient cultures to heal the sick. If true, investigators of non-contact healing should look for the roots of the tradition not in ancient Chinese proto-science, but in the shared universal experience of the shaman across the globe.

When we take the investigation of non-contact healing beyond the limited confines of "traditional Chinese medicine," we begin to compare Chinese-style healers with other traditions that produce similar results. There are many of these rich traditions, including not only the Hawaiian kahunas and Christian mystics, like Brazil's John of God, but other intriguing traditions such as the Quakers and Shakers.[75]

Perhaps the most striking aspect of an "energetic healer," modern or otherwise, is the power of the healer to affect another person because of their charisma; the characteristics of such a person have been noted. A text translated by Arthur Waley, from a 500 BCE source, describes the shaman in the following way:

The shaman, is a person upon whom a Bright Spirit has descended, attracted to him because he is 'particularly vigorous and lively, staunch in adherence to principle, reverent and just; so wise that in all matters high and low he always takes the right-side, so saintly *(sheng)* that he spreads around him a radiance that reaches far and wide ....'[76]

Is this a description of a person who is so strong in his *nei qi* internal energy that it radiates outward to heal others? If so, could this be the secret to healing without touch?

Endnotes

1 As cited by Wayne Jonas and Jeffrey Wayne in *Essentials of complementary and alternative medicine,* Lippincott Williams & Wilkins, May 1999, p. 370.

2 Dossey describes the non-local as "infinite, and by inference immortal, eternal, omnipresent" and in an on-line interview says:

> "These are spiritual ideas. I have tried to fortify or justify the non-local model. The evidence is overwhelming that mind behaves in a non-local way. If one honors the data, then one must conclude that the local model is incomplete. It is a matter of being a good scientist. If you honor the data, what kind of model must you make of the mind in order to account for what is happening?

> The concept is used in contemporary physics. Physicists have already had to make their peace with non-locality. Nick Herbert wrote a book, Quantum Reality, for lay people. In non-mathematical terms, Dr. Herbert describes the world as essentially non-local. It may be hard to imagine, but physics experiments have clearly shown that non-locality is the characteristic of the world at the sub-atomic level. Bell's Theorem has proven it. Non-locality is at home in physics and since physics is the most accurate science we've ever had, we are justified in using the term to describe a similar state of being at the level of mind."

From interview with Larry Dossey, MD, http://www.share-international.org/archives/health-healing/hh_bwrecovering.htm.

3 The *Ebers Papyrus* are named after the German Egyptologist Georg Ebers, who purchased the papyrus scrolls at Luxor in the winter of 1873-1874. Believed to be copied from older manuscripts, they are considered among the oldest and most important medical papyri of ancient Egypt.

4 Avila, Elena, *Woman who glows in the dark: A curandera reveals traditional Aztec secrets of physical and spiritual health,* Penguin Putnam, New York, 2000, p. 41.

5 Avila, p.84.

6 The Essenes were a Jewish sect that inhabited some areas of Judea from 116 BCE to 140 CE during the Hasomoneasn *(Hashmona'im)* dynasty. During this period, one of their groups lived in Qumran, where the Dead Sea Scrolls were discovered, and some scholars believe the Essenes may have authored the scrolls. They lived a communal life and many practiced celibacy.

7 In Pan Pacific culture, it is believed that an entity's "life" is derived from its *mana* or spiritual component.

8 Is "light" another term for "energy?" It is of interest that early Christians in their baptism ceremony referred to in their initiation practice as "light" and some of these traditions included the gift of a lighted candle to the newly initiated to symbolize their newfound inner light. Note, other references to "light" are described later in the context of *wai qi* energetic healing.

9 Gerber, Richard, *Vibrational medicine,* Bear & Co., Rochester, VT, 2001, pp. 264-265

10 Gerber, p. 263

11 The Academy of Parapsychology and Medicine 1992, as cited by Trish Dunning (Editor) *Complementary therapies and management of diabetes and vascular medicine,* John Wiley and Sons, Ltd, 2006 p. 181

12 F.D. O'Byrne, Translator and author of the Introduction, *Reichenbach's letters on Od and magnetism: Published for the first time in English, with extracts from his own works, so as to make a complete presentation of the Odic Theory.* London, 1952 p.39

13 Gerber, Richard, *Vibrational medicine,* Bear & Co., Rochester, VT, 2001, p. 265

14 Swann, Ingo, *Psychic Sexuality: The bio-psychic "anatomy" of sexual energies* Panta Rei/Crossroads Press, 1998/2014 Psychic *sexuality,* Panta Rei, [Crossroads Press digital edition] Retrieved from Amazon.com Kindle Reader locations 1032-1055

15 Reich, William *Function of the Orgasm,* Translated from the German by Vincent R. Carfagno, Farrar, Farrar Straus and Giroux, New York, 1973, p. 5 Original manuscript, *Die Entdeckung des Orgons, Erster Teil: Die Function des Orgasmus,* Copyright © 1968 by Mary Boyd Higgins as Trustee of the Wilhelm Reich Infant Trust Fund

16 Reich, p. 5

17 Ibid. pp. 6-7

18 Seto, et al., "Detection of Extraordinary Large Bio-magnetic Field Strength" *Journal of Acupuncture and Electro-Therapy Research,* Vo. 17, pp. 75-94

19 Miura, Kunio, "The revival of qi," *Taoist meditation and longevity techniques,* edited by Kohn, Livia, Center for Chinese Studies, University of Michigan, 1989

20 Miura, p. 343

21 Seto, A., et al. 1992 "Detection of extraordinary large biomagnetic field strength from the human hand." *Acupuncture and Electro-Therapeutics Research International Journal 17:75-94.* As referenced by Oschman, p. 79.

22 Investigators in the Seto and Kusaka study used a specially arranged magnetic field detection system consisting of a pair of two identical coils with 80,000 turns and a high sensitivity amplifier. Each of the coils were rolled in opposite direction, actuating what investigators referred to as a gradiometer. It is noteworthy that this phenomenon is not common to all energetic healers. The cited study examined 37 "healers," and found that of these only three exhibited the described large bio-field effect. This point will be addressed again in Section XII. Seto, A, et al, "Detection of extraordinary large bio-magnetic field strength from human hand during external qi emission. *Acupuncture and Electro-Therapeutics Research Int.,* Vol. 17, 1992 pp.

23 In the study of thirty-seven individuals classified as energetic heal-ers, only three were able to generate a measurable electromagnetic frequency. The frequency of electro-magnetism in these individuals was measured to be between 4 and 10 Hz. Some select comments presented by Seto et al in the published report:

"We encountered the following interesting phenomenon. The sub-ject …. was able to send out *qi* energy from her palm, which was ob-served clearly as strong bio-magnetic field emission. … [The results] indicated that the human extraordinary large bio-magnetic field strength is never derived from the internal body current alone. ….

… we cannot find the internal body current which corresponds to ex-tremely large current in order of 10mA. The large human bio-mag-netic field emission in this experiment is not only exceeding unusual but also astonishingly special in every respect. The origin of the hu-man extraordinary large bio-magnetic field remains still uncertain. ….

It is necessary to specify a true origin of the bio--magnetic field emit-ted fro the palm of unusual individual. The human body usually can-not secure the current source of strength which is necessary for gen-eration of the extra-ordinary large bio-magnetic field in the order of mGauss. Therefore, another energy source which is equivalent to the large current flow, must exist by all means, as an origin of the human extraordinary large bio-magnetic field.

In order to resolve a contradiction of a quantitative issue, we assume the existence of a parameter such as another energy source in the human body.

Qi is not magnetic field but "deep force" behind our observable dimen-sion rather than existing physical quantity such as magnetic field. [Em-phasis added]."

From discussion and conclusion, Seto, et al, "Detection of Extraor-dinary Large Bio-Magnetic Field Strength from Human Hand during External Qi Emission," *Acupuncture and Electro-Therapeutics Research, Int. Journal*, Vol. 17. pp. 75-94, 1992

24 In a paper published in the Chinese publication *The Nature Journal* Gu, Hansen and Lin Housheng of the Shanghai Institute of Nuclear physics reported an unusual infrared radiation time spectrum 1.2 centimeters from the Lao gong acupuncture point in the center of the hand of advanced *qi gong* practitioners compared to non-prac-titioners. The infrared radiation of the advanced practitioners in the study had a group of what the researchers described as slow wave crests, which they referred to as low-frequency amplitude modula-tion. See Gu Hansen, Lin Lousheng, (1978), "Preliminary Experimental Results of the Investigation on the Materialistic Basis of 'Therapy of Qi Mobilization' in Qi gong. Ziran Zachi (*The nature Journal*/ Chinese) 1:12

25 As cited by William Tiller in *Science and human transformation: Sub-tle energies, intentionality, and consciousness*, p.15

26 In this case, electric pulse generation by the *qi gong* masters was measured by an electrode attached to the ear lobe. Researchers found that instead of the usual 10-15 millivolt baseline with ~ 1 milli-volt ripple, in energy projectors, ear lobe voltage often plunged -30 to -300 volts and then recovered to baseline in ~ 0.5 to 10 seconds.

This astoundingly large voltage pulse was 10^5 times normal! In the time span of a single 30-minute healing session that took place inside a special environment, one healer manifested 15 of these anomalous-ly large voltage bursts (each greater than 30 volts) with each main burst being composed of 5-6 sub-pulses convolved in one burst "en-velopes."

As cited by Professor William Tiller in *Science and human transforma-tion: Subtle energies, intentionality and consciousness*, pp. 14-15

27 Therapeutic Touch (T.T.) is an "energy healing" system developed by Dora Kunz and Dolores Krieger in the 1970s.

28 From the Abstract:

A simple electric dipole model, in the static limit, was used to analyze simultaneous voltage recordings from the ear of an experienced non-contact therapeutic touch specialist and from four surrounding cop-per walls during a 30-minute therapy session wherein 15 ear voltage surges were recorded, ranging between -20 V and -80 V from baseline with time durations from approximately 0.5 to 12.5 s. In 13 of these 15 voltage surges, the origin of the dipole was located in the abdominal region and the dipole length extended from the ear to the feet with the ear always negative. In the other 2 cases a second dipole may also form in the head.

29 Tiller, William, *Some science adventures with real magic*, Pavior, p. 139

30 Becker, Robert, *The body electric: Electromagnetism and the founda-tion of life*, William Morrow & Co, 1985 p. 269

31 Becker, pp. 26-27

32 *Medical applications of qigong and emitted qi on humans, animals, cell cultures, and plants: review of selected scientific research. American Journal of Acupuncture* Vol. 19, No. 4, p. 199

33 Ibid.

34 Omura, Y., Application of intensified (+) Qi Gong energy, (-) elec-trical field, (S) magnetic field, electrical pulses (1-2 pulses/sec), strong Shiatsu massage or acupuncture on the accurate organ represen-tation areas of the hands to improve circulation and enhance drug uptake in pathological organs: clinical applications with special em-phasis on the " Chlamydia-(Lyme)-uric acid syndrome" and "Chlamyd-ia-(cytomegalovirus)-uric acid syndrome". *Acupuncture and Electro-therapy Research* 1995 Jan-Mar;20(1):21-72

35 Omura, Y., Application of intensified (+) Qi Gong energy, (-) elec-trical field, (S) magnetic field, electrical pulses (1-2 pulses/sec), strong Shiatsu massage or acupuncture on the accurate organ represen-tation areas of the hands to improve circulation and enhance drug uptake in pathological organs: clinical applications with special em-phasis on the "Chlamydia-(Lyme)-uric acid syndrome" and "Chlamyd-ia-(cytomegalovirus)-uric acid syndrome". *Acupuncture and Electro-therapy Research* 1995 Jan-Mar;20(1):21-72.

36 Xin Yan, et al. 1999 Mat Res Innovat (1999) 2:349-359

37 In studies conducted by researcher Feng and colleagues, a *qi* master named Bao held bacteria-laden test tubes in her palm for one minute. In one study between 44%-89.8% of *E. coli* and 66.7%-98% of *Shigella* were dead after being subjected to a *qi* emission with "termination" intention. In another experiment, E. Coli increased between 2.4-6.9 times when *qi* energetic treatment was matched with "growth" intention.

Feng, Lida, et al., *Proceedings of the First Annual Meeting of the Beijing Qigong Scientific Research Society,* Beijing, China, 1981.

38 Oschman, James, *Energetic medicine: The scientific basis,* Churchill Livingstone, 2000, p. 102.

39 Oschman, p 82.

40 A magnetic field is created by an electric field in motion. For example, an electric field can be created by putting an oscillating (alternating) electric current through a conductor such as metal. See Oschman, *Energy Medicine,* p.156

41 Oschman., p. xiv.

42 Oschman, James, *Energy medicine: The scientific basis* Churchill Livingstone, 2000.

43 ITOH Tomoko, SHEN Zaiwen ITOH[2] Yasuhiro, TAMURA Akira and ASAYAMA Masami, "The Effects of Wai Qi on Rats under Stress Based on Urinary Excretion Measurements of Catecholamines, *Journal of International Society of Life Information Science, Vol.*18, No.2, September 2000 [Proceedings of The Tenth Symposium of Life Information Science]

44 Developed by Dr. Omura, the bi-digital O Ring Test is an adaptation of Applied Kinesiology (AK) muscle testing where a third party acts as a "testing instrument," thus separating the researcher from the person or object being tested. The "bi digital O Ring test involves using this method while the "testing instrument" subject closes the thumb upon the index finger. Subsequently, testing of the strength or weakness of the closed thumb and finger "O Ring" is presumed to indicate truth (stronger) or falsehood / stress (weaker). Omura, using this "test" as a way of collecting data in a number of areas, including detecting of errors in traditional acupuncture charts, location of cancer and virus concentrations within diseased organs, and, apropos to the present chapter, revelation of otherwise secret interior processes of *qigong* energetic healers.

45 Omura

46 Omura

47 In the study, Omura taught the technique to four children who had little or no knowledge of *qi gong* or traditional Chinese medicine. The four children ranged in age from eight to eleven. Of these, one was able to attain the *wai qi qigong* state in less than half a day, one after less than two days. The other two children were inconsistent in being able to reproduce the state.

Omura, Y., et al, "Unique changes found on the *qigong* master's and patient's body during the non-contact *qigong* treatment; their relationships to certain meridians and acupuncture points and the re-creation of therapeutic Qi Gong states by children & adults." *Acupuncture and Electrotherapy Research* 1989;14(1):61-89.

48 Omura, Y, Beckman, S.L, "Application of intensified (+) Qi Gong energy, (-) electrical field, (S) magnetic field, electrical pulses (1-2 pulses/sec), strong Shiatsu massage or acupuncture on the accurate organ representation areas of the hands to improve circulation and enhance drug uptake in pathological organs: clinical applications with special emphasis on the 'Chlamydia-(Lyme)-uric acid syndrome' and 'Chlamydia-(cytomegalovirus)-uric acid syndrome.'" *Journal of Acupuncture and Electrotherapy Research*, 1995 Jan-Mar;20(1):21-72.

49 From Dr. Chen's notes to an online *qigong* research forum

50 From Dr. Chen's notes to an online *qigong* research forum

51 "An evidence-based review of qi gong by the national standard research collaboration" *Natural Medicine Journal*, 5-1-2010

52 Hintz, Kenneth, et al, "Bio-energy definitions and research guidelines," *Alternative therapies in health and medicine.* May/June 2003, 9, 3. p. A13

53 Hintz

54 Insight into the relationship between energy and entropy in thermodynamics is provided by William Tiller, PhD, who in *Science and Human Transformation* discusses the meaning of information. There, Dr Tiller writes that "Over the past 50 years we have begun to realize that information gained in a particular event or process is negative entropy and that although in the course of evolution, the potential of the physical universe continually decreases, the content of information continually increases.

The informational content spoken of here can be in two forms. It can be in the form of physical order or organization of a physical structure or organization of the internal structure of an entity or it can be in the form of knowledge (a different kind of organization) . . .."

See William Tiller, William, *Science and human transformation: subtle energy, intention and consciousness*, pp. 175-176.

55 However, as suggested in the earlier story involving Colonel Estebany, some healers are not consciously aware of their ability to emit healing "energy" or "information."

56 I often wondered how it was possible for researchers to make, what seems to be, such an obvious and potentially serious, research error. It is conceivable that in the case of some well-meaning non-Chinese researchers with a background in experimental science, while in the process of investigating the non-contact healing phenomenon, approached their Chinese speaking colleagues and asked questions such as, "how does this kind of *qi* - energy research fit in with Chinese tradition?" The answer could easily be one not based on review of scientific journals, or previously relied upon research protocols, but based on Chinese cultural lore that the native speakers grew up with. The offered answer could have easily been taken at face value, "there

are two kinds of *qigong*, 'internal' (inner development) and 'external' (referring here, to the external expression of *qi*-energy, 外氣功). In this context, some authors refer to the "sending" of *qi*-energy across empty space as *fafang* or *fafang waiqi*.

57 Per the Chinese website, *Baidu*, referring to prayer, "the art of *zhuyou* makes use of talismans, spells, prohibitions, and sacrifices to cure illness." https://baike.baidu.com/item/%E7%A5%9D%E7%94%B1%E6%9C%AF/7681732

58 Western Zhou dates from the eleventh century BCE to 771 CE.

59 Cho, Philip S., "Ritual and the occult in Chinese medicine and religious healing: The development of zhuyou exorcism," (January 1, 2005). *Dissertations available from ProQuest*. Paper AAI3197659. http://repository.upenn.edu/dissertations/AAI3197659.

60 Cho.

61 Tianjun Liu, Xiao Mei Qiang, *Chinese medical qigong* (Google eBook), Singing Dragon, May 28, 2013, p.291.

62 As cited by Miura, Kunio, "The revival of qi," *Taoist meditation and longevity techniques*, p.344.

63 Miura, p. 344.

64 Voigt, John, "The man who invented 'qigong'" *Qi: Journal of Traditional Eastern Health and Fitness*, Autumn 2013.

65 NMJ Contributors, "An evidence-based review of qigong by the National Standard Research Collaboration," *National Medicine Journal*, May 2010, Vol. 2, Issue 5.

66 Of three of the highly-regarded tomes (Volumes 2, 5, and 6)

67 Wang and Wu, *History of Chinese medicine, Being a chronicle of medical happenings in China from ancient times to the present*, National Quarantine Service, Shang Hai, China, 1936.

68 In the Department of Medicine were one professor of medicine of the 8th grade, A class, and one assistant of the 9th grade, B class. The students were taught the subjects of internal medicine, ulcers and swellings, children's diseases, ear, eye, mouth and teeth affections, and cupping. In the Department of Acupuncture were one Professor of Medicine of 8th grade, B class, one assistant of 9th grade B class, and ten acupuncturists also of 9th grade, B class. The students were taught the signs of the pulse and the special 'points' for puncture. The Department of Massage had one Professor of Massage and four masseurs, all of 9th grade, B class. They gave lessons in physical exercise, and treated cases of fractures, injuries and wounds. The Department of Exorcism was in the charge of the Professor of Exorcism, an official of the 9th grade, B class who taught people how to chant incantations, drive away pestilential influences and fasting.

Wang and Wu, p.75

69 Source purposely emitted.

70 Cullen, Christopher, from the forward to Joseph Needham, et al.,

Science and civilization in China, Vol 6. p. 11,

71 Cullen., p. 11.

72 Ibid. pp 40-41.

73 Ibid.

74 Needham writes: "There can be no doubt that Taoist philosophy and religion took its origin from a kind of alliance between these ancient magicians and those Chinese philosophers who, in ancient times, believed that the study of Nature was more important for man than the administration of human society," Needham, Vol. 6, p. 58.

75 Bradford Keeney describes a link between the spiritual ecstasy between the Shaker tradition and their ability to heal. As Bradford explains, the relationship between shaking and healing has been known throughout the world, yet the value of trembling, vibrating, quaking, and shaking as a medicine for the body, mind, and soul had been all but lost in recent time, particularly among the more literate and technologically developed cultures."   (Keeney, p. 2).

Citing the work of Peter Levine who, according to Keeney, found that animals in the wild rarely get traumatized. After a near death attack, the animal goes "somewhere and tremble, shake, pant, take deep breaths, and exhibit rapid eye movements. Free from the language-making of a cerebral cortex, they don't get engaged in language-based therapy and treatment. Wild animals simply allow their reptilian brains to trigger shaking medicine." (Keeney, pp. 31-32).

The origin story of the Shaker healing tradition is fascinating. According to the tradition, in the early-nineteenth century, a man named John Slocum had died. While a group of friends waited with the body for the casket to arrive, to their shock and amazement he suddenly returned from the dead, bringing with him a new form of "shaking medicine." Reminiscent of the experience of tummo "inner heat" which we will discuss in Section V, Slocum reported sensations of heat flowing through his body.

Keeney, Bradford, *Shaking medicine: The healing power*, Destiny Books, VT. 2007.

76 Waley, Arthur, *The nine songs*, p. 10, Forgotten books, 2014.

Section V
Energetic Meditation

Now that we have some idea of the mind's nature and how it works, we must bring it under control and master it. In order to do this, it is said that we must keep our body perfectly still. Moreover, if the body is straight, the subtle channels will be straight. If the subtle channels are straight, the wind-energy will be unobstructed. And if the wind energy is unobstructed, the mind will rest in its natural, unaltered flow.

— *Dudjom Rinpoche*

V

Energetic Meditation

Introduction to Section V

Energetic Traditions in Meditation

*I*n some spiritual traditions, it is believed that a person who masters the flow of energy within the body can attain not only enlightened spiritual insight, but also awaken supernatural powers. The chapters in this section look to those traditions for more clues that might reveal the meaning of "internal energy."

The previous three sections focused on the meaning of internal energy in the disciplines devoted to healing one's self and others. Section II considered healing in the context of traditional Chinese medicine, Section III looked at the mental and physical techniques of Taoist energetic yoga, and Section IV focused on the controversial question of whether it might be possible to heal without physical contact. The present section examines how practitioners within select energetic meditation traditions learn to master the flow of subtle energy in and around their bodies. It will also examine how it might be possible for one to gain the kind of control over the flow of internal energy within the body that leads to expanded consciousness.

Consider, for example, the belief shared among the energetic meditation traditions that life functions along a continuum which ranges from the physical, to the etheric, to the spiritual. Accordingly, those traditions rely on various mechanisms within the body to convert physical energy into spiritual energy.

That conversion of the physical to the spiritual takes place along a set of structures. Some of these, such as the spine, are physical, whereas others, such as the energetic centers along the central axis of the body, known as *chakras* in Sanskrit, are etheric. Founded on the principle that the mind is inseparable from the body,[1] this belief underlies the energetic yoga traditions covered in this section.

Since there is no clear demarcation between the mind and body,[2] the influence is bi-directional. Mind influences body; body influences mind. Thus, as suggested in the quote from Dudjom Rinpoche which introduces this section, postures that facilitate the flow of energy also influence the mind and spirt, and in the same manner, a person's thoughts also influence their physical body.

For the Tibetan *tantric* Buddhists, the most advanced level of spiritual attainment is enlightenment. For the ancient Taoist[3] *neidan* (內丹) practitioner, mastery of the currents that make up the mind-body energy system leads to immortality. In another Taoist meditation tradition, the ultimate expression of spiritual understanding is to attain the state of *ho Tao* (合道), mystical union, or "harmony with the *Tao*."

As for those super-normal abilities, the power appears in different forms. Sometimes, the awakened psychic power that comes from mastering one's internal energy is the ability to read another person's thoughts. At other times, power presents as control over the elements; for example, the ability to put out fires, not by any physical means, but through the power of intention.

Tibetan *tantric* practitioners refer to internal energy as *lung* (རླུང), or *"wind."* The highly regarded Tibetan lama, Gyalwa Yangpönga (1213-1258), taught that when *lung* combines with breath control, special powers are awakened. In addition to the all-important "emergence of the mind's natural state," other powers that can awaken include "heightened states of awareness, mystical experiences, clairvoyance, and blissful physical sensations." [4]

The literature detailing these internal energy traditions is extensive. Much of it is ancient and all of it is highly nuanced, thus it is impossible for the present work to consider more than a small fraction of the available literature and concepts. The Eastern disciplines that are considered in this section represent only a sampling of the energetic meditative traditions. Please note that while the focus of a significant amount of the material that follows is a brief overview of Taoist and Tibetan *tantric* practices, these are only two of the many Asian meditation traditions.

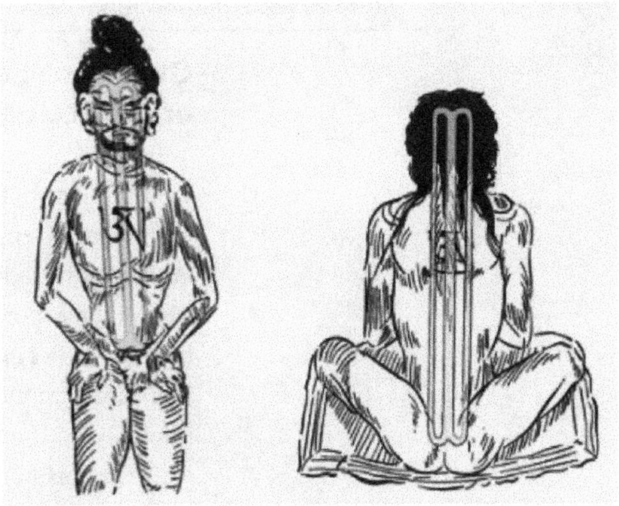

Figures 5-1

Tibetan Yogis and the Main Energy Channels of the Upper Body

The *Sushumna* is shown in the center with the *Ida* and *Pingala*, respectively, to the left and right side of the spine.

Illustrations by Sergio Verdeza, based on Ian Baker's photographs presented in *The Dalai Lama's Secret Temple.*

The Taoist types of meditation covered in this section include *neidan* meditation, which is an aspect of the *neidan* inner yoga covered in Section III, and *Shouyi*, or "guarding the One," which traces its roots to the beginnings of Taoism. An overview of Taoist mystical practice is also presented. We begin with a general summary of energetic meditations.

Box 5-2

Tantra and Tantric Practices
The terms *tantric* and *tantra* are derived from the Sanskrit word meaning "woven." Buddhist *tantric* practice refers to several disciplines including prayer, visualization, and physical yoga. These direct the practitioner toward the development of progressive realization, which culminates in the achievement of Buddhahood—the state believed by Tantric Buddhists to be endowed with the ultimate potential to benefit living beings. *Tantra*, as traditionally described, is considered a transformative path where human energies, rather than being stifled, ignored, or used for selfish purposes, are focused toward achieving advanced spiritual understanding.

The practice of *tummo* described in the present chapter is one form of *tantric* practice. There are two distinct lineages of *tummo*: the lineage stemming from the *Dzogchen* path, and the *Mahamudra* tradition. Dzogchen's path of *tummo* is one aspect of *tsa-lung* ("channels" and "wind") training, while the Mahamudra tradition of tummo is one of the Six Yogas of Naropa.

Ian Baker, who writes extensively on the art and culture of Tibet and the Himalayas, offers the classic definition of *tantra* as the "secret path that allows us to penetrate the veils of obscured vision." *Tantra*, called *gyu* in Tibetan, "refers to the unbroken continuity of enlightened energy that permeates all aspects of existence and connects all sentient beings."

(See Ian Baker, *The Dalai Lama's Secret Temple*, pp. 50- 51)

Overview: Comparison of Subtle Energy Structures and Practices

Common to both the Taoist and Tibetan *tantric* energetic meditative traditions is the belief that the flow of life energy can be consciously directed. In the Taoist traditions, mastery of one's internal energy has as its goal the transmutation of coarse energy at the lower *dan tian* energy field. In that tradition, one's *qi* is transformed into spiritual energy as it travels upward. In the Tibetan *tantric* tradition, management of one's subtle energy is focused primarily on the melting of a form of energy referred to as *thigle* * (ཐིག་ལེ), which comes in red and white "drops" and resides primarily in the central channel.[5][6] When practicing, the yogi-meditator focuses attention and breath on the secret center below the navel [7] and, while relying on breath control, "fans the flames of the red drops that reside there." [8] In response, this action melts the white *thigle* drops that reside primarily at the crown *chakra* (energy vortex) at the top of the head. According to Lama Yangpönga, this causes "the descent of melted *thigle* white drops and their union with the red." As Yangpönga explains it, the union of white and red destroys the "mind's discursiveness and brings about the natural state, innate wisdom." [9]

* Pronounced theeg-lay

Other differences between the Tibetan *tantric* and Taoist *neidan* traditions are noteworthy, and these include the goals of practice. For the *tantric* practitioner of the Tibetan tradition, the quest is enlightenment. By contrast, the Taoist alchemist and energetic meditation practitioner sought union with the Tao, *ho Tao,* and the "coming together of energy." Professor Livia Kohn emphasizes this point with a quotation from the *Chuang Tzu:*

> The human life is a coming-together of energy. If it comes together, there is life. If it scatters, there is death. [10]

As introduced in Section III, in the Tibetan system, the internal energy *lung* (རླུང་) is said to flow through the *tsa* (རྩ) channels. This is one aspect of *tantric* physiology which describes the energetic, or *vajra,* body as consisting of many subtle layers made up of energetic channels, *lung,* and vital essences.[11]

When the practitioner attains sufficient control over the flow of internal energy within the body through the yogic-meditative practice of *tsa lung thigle,* an energetic interaction may be initiated between the *lung-wind* and the *chakras.* The principle *chakra* energy vortexes are located along the spinal corridor. These function as energetic valves that connect the etheric with the physical body, and function as an interface between an individual's emotional experience and the etheric world.

It is worth noting the emphasis of the central channel running along the axis of the spinal corridor in Tibetan *tantric* tradition. According to Yangpönga, the central channel is not the spinal cord, but instead runs parallel to the spine. Its function is to connect the crown *chakra* at the top of the head with the sexual centers. [12] Yangpönga describes the central channel in the following terms:

> The upper end of the central channel penetrates the Brahma aperture at the crown of the head [crown chakra], while the lower end enters the secret center below the navel [secret chakra]. [13]

Here, referring to subtle energy within the channels as "air," Lama Shenphen Dawa Rinpoche describes the process of energetic meditation in these words:

> Once you have brought in the wisdom air, next visualize the central channel. This is very important. The central channel is the basis of our memory and reflects the three *kayas.*[14]

As described by Lamas Yeshe and Zopa Rinpoche, the three *kayas* are the Dharmakaya (truth body), sambhogakava (enjoyment body), and nirmanakaya (emanation body).[15]

In contrast, the Taoist *neidan* meditator is concerned with the transmutation of coarse *jing* (精) into refined *shen* (神), or spiritual energy. Compared with the goals of the *tantric* practitioner, the Taoist meditator does not seek enlightenment, as such, but instead perfection of body and mind leading to the status of *zhen ren* (真人), or "true person." Accordingly, this kind of perfection could, depending on the Taoist tradition, lead one either to mystical union with the Tao or physical immortality; the latter being the state which Joseph Needham describes as "a youthful body in a kind of earthly paradise." [16]

Chapter 22

Esoteric Energy Traditions in the West

*T*he oldest descriptions of an energy physiology which describes how semen can be consciously directed from the genitals to the brain are found not in China, India or Tibet, but in ancient Greece. However, there is some evidence to suggest that the doctrine might have even earlier origins.

The hint of a more ancient source of the belief comes from the Middle East, where evidence of the teaching that seminal energy could be converted into mental energy survives in the form of a stone vase dating back to 2050 BCE. The vase features imagery of a snake moving from the base of the spine to the brain, which is the same metaphor used in Eastern traditions to represent the migration of energy upward along the spine. [17]

However, the oldest textual evidence of the belief that semen retention contributes to mental function can be traced to Greece and Sicily. Even before the time of Plato, the Greek philosopher, Diogenes of Apollonia (425 BCE), taught an "energy-physiology" that, in various key ways, can be compared to the *tantric* traditions of India and later Tibet.

Another fascinating similarity between the ancient Greek energetic traditions and those originating on the Indian subcontinent is the description of the two primary energy channels that run parallel to the spine. For example, akin to the way energy channels are depicted in *tantric* imagery (Figures 5-1), ancient Greeks described the energetic channels along the spine as "two veins pre-eminent in magnitude [extending] through the belly along the backbone, one to right, one to left; either one to the leg on its own side, and upwards to the head, past the collar-bones, through the throat." [18]

To explain the similarities between ancient Western doctrines and those of India, Professor Thomas McEvilley suggests that the notion of sexual energy migrating from the genitals to the brain might have originated with the Greeks, and thereafter diffused to the Indian subcontinent. Much like the belief found in Asian energetic traditions, the Greeks also taught that long life was associated with the conservation of semen. An example is found in the way Aristotle described how spinal fluid was related to sperm,[19] while another useful comparison lies in how the Greeks, like the ancient Chinese, believed that a man's conservation of semen contributed to a long lifespan. [20]

The Greek belief in the Timaeus can be traced to a period before Plato — and the trail leads primarily to the Sicilian and South Italian schools of medicine, which were connected with the Pythagorean and Orphic communities in the same area. These schools taught that semen comes from the brain and is of one substance with the spinal marrow, by way of which it travels to the genital organ through the spinal channel that Indians call sushumna and Greeks called "the holy tube." [21]

The pre-Socratic writer Heraclitus (535 – 475 BCE) also taught that the *aion,* or "lifespan," was related to retention of seminal fluid. McEvilley writes that Heraclitus, "taught the [doctrine of] retention of semen and a qualified sexual abstinence." [22] McEvilley proposes two hypotheses as explanations for why similar themes are found in both Eastern and Western traditions. The first is the possible diffusion of pre-Socratic lore from India to Greece between the sixth and fifth centuries BCE, while a second theory suggests that the concept of spinal fluid being related to semen is a more universal notion, originating in proto Indo-European times.

However, the belief that conservation of semen provides mental and physical advantages is not only an ancient one, as the same instruction is often found today in the guidance provided by coaches to athletes. For example, athletic trainers and bodybuilders sometimes instruct male athletes to minimize ejaculation, especially in the run-up to a competition, because of the positive benefits that they believe limiting emission has on the body. Bodybuilding champion Bill Pearl describes the energy associated with sex drive and athleticism as "an amount of energy that cannot be measured," and he believes this represents a particular type of "energy" beyond the influence of testosterone. As Pearl explains, it is responsible for the "'backbone and grit,' which cannot be estimated until being put to the test." [23]

Pearl believes that this yet-to-be-understood energy source is one of the chief factors responsible for superior athletic performance, and that the body's response to the chemical processes triggered by it is responsible for the greater wealth of energy reserves that are created by the internal secretions of the sex glands. "The quantity of this secretion cannot be measured," he says, "nor its quality estimated." In describing the relationship between optimal performance and the secretions of the sex glands, he writes:

> The physical type of individual in itself will not be sufficient to judge a man in this respect. The man himself will be totally unaware of the superior or inferior quality of this secretion as well, as the energy and stamina that it creates, until he is put to the test.
>
> So, it is also with the man who is endeavoring to develop muscle bulk and specific muscle power. He may have no knowledge of the deficiency or inferiority of internal sex secretion until he fails to develop his muscles and improve his strength by systems of exercise that should, by all the rules of exercise bring about marked improvement. Additionally, after failing he may not know why he failed, for there are few who can tell

him. It may be that all he will be required to do, in order to make his body more responsive to his efforts, will be to conserve or increase his sexual energy. (Emphasis added)

Could it be true that there is a yet-to-be-identified substance in the body that, in males, is closely associated with semen and testosterone, and that can enhance brain performance? Cross-cultural similarities concerning the doctrine suggest that there may well be.

Alternate Hypotheses

There are at least three other possible explanations for why similarities might have developed in the doctrines of diffused cultures. The first concerns how individuals, while in a relaxed state, can consciously induce blood supply to the nerves and areas of the body through the practice of directed attention. [24] In practice, focused attention, directed deep within the body's core, would stimulate changes in blood flow. The results would be to produce feelings of pressure, warmth, and other sensations, such as the feeling of an electrical current moving through the body. Long ago, a practitioner sitting in deep meditation might have noticed that directed attention could stimulate these kinds of changes deep within their interior. The adept would then observe that the inwardly directed, highly-focused attention could produce these kinds of perceptible changes in their practice.

Although the adept's perceived changes would eventually be explained by modern science as conscious influence over hormonal levels and blood supply, the explanation offered by the ancient practitioner would be quite different. In the case of the latter, the observed altered state might very well be explained in terms of mystical or spiritual language.

Another possible explanation is the ability of very experienced meditators to perceive extremely subtle body rhythms. For example, one of these very subtle rhythms might easily be the practitioner's sensitivity to minute bodily responses that correspond to the ebb and flow of the spinal fluid on its journey from the ventricles of the brain to the sacrum.

In this light, it is useful to consider the subtle movements the body makes in response to spinal fluid ebb and flow, as documented by John Upledger, DO (1932 -2012), who, based on his observations, developed the CranioSacral Therapy (CST) system. The impetus leading Upledger to his therapeutic system can be traced to a discovery he made one day while assisting with spinal surgery. During the procedure, Upledger was tasked with immobilizing the patient's spinal cord. However, to his frustration, he found that he was unable to hold the spinal cord completely still, as it repeatedly slipped out of his hand. He observed that the outermost layer of a three-tiered system encasing the patient's spinal column had a rhythmic, or pulsatile, movement of its own that was distinct from pulse or breath, and he subsequently became fascinated by the discovery. This led to him investigating the mysterious "wave" further, ultimately resulting in the creation of a new system of bodywork.[25] His research informed the discussion of the possibility of a yet-to-be-fully explored bio-mechanical system of the body, which could well explain what some practitioners of energetic meditation perceive as a link between the sacrum and the cranium.

Over the course of his investigations, Upledger documented how the entire nervous system is linked by the rhythmic movement of the cerebral spinal fluid, from the brain to the tailbone, and ultimately, the entire body. As suggested by Upledger's theory, the ebb and flow movement initiates extremely subtle movement-responses that are reflected throughout the body. Therapists trained in Upledger's CST learn to perceive these extremely subtle rhythms in a patient's body with their palms and fingers.

In my own practice, I have developed ways of utilizing the CST rhythm described by Upledger's system to train athletes, meditators, and pain patients. The techniques are based on learning to observe this rhythm in one's own body, and, in my experience, these rhythms function as what might be considered a physical waveform that can be sensed and worked with in interesting ways. It is conceivable that this same flow, or rather, the body's responses to the cerebral spinal fluid ebb and flow, had also been noticed by ancient meditators in their deep meditation. If so, this supports the notion of a sensory link between the cranium and the nerves of the pelvic floor, such as that described by Upledger, may well have been perceived and consciously manipulated by yogic practitioners in order to produce what adepts would have described as a psycho-sexual connection.

Based on these observations, it is conceivable that energetic meditators, including the Taoists and *tantric* practitioners, might have, like the ancient Greeks, perceived these "energetic" rhythmic relationships between the sacrum and the brain. This idea is supported by Upledger's clinical work in therapeutically balancing the ebb and flow relationship between the sacrum and cranial base, which can improve one's ability to concentrate and has been used in treating attention deficit disorders.[26]

A third possibility that might explain similarities in ancient cultural beliefs is that a yet-to-be-discovered subtle physiology connects the sacrum and sexual centers with the brain. It is conceivable that when a person becomes aware of, and then accesses, this subtle physiology, that it triggers a radically profound change in the individual. In that case, well-practiced meditators across different traditions may have become aware of that same underlying physiology that connects the body in this way. For example, this awareness might also explain the observations such as those provided by *tantric* mystics, who claim that the physical body exists on a backdrop of an energetic body or blueprint. The Tibetan masters refer to this blueprint as the *vajra,* "lightning bolt," or "diamond" body.[27]

नाडी

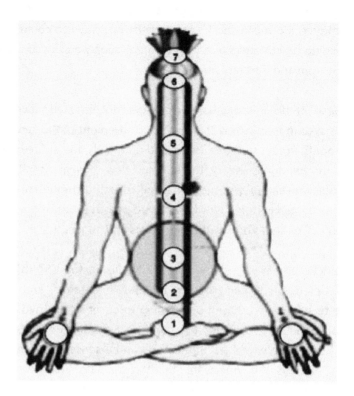

Figure 5-3

The *Chakra* (Circled Areas) and the *Nadi* (Connecting Tubes)

Source: Wikipedia Commons

Chapter 23

Chakras

*N*ewcomers to the practice of energetic meditation often encounter challenges to the way that they think about the mind and body. Among those challenges are descriptions of structures that are not part of known anatomy, most notably the psychic-energy structures lying along the body's central axis, known as *chakras*.

Chakras, literally "wheels," are locations where "energy" accumulates and energetic vortexes form. In Sanskrit, the *Ida* (इडा) and *Pingala* (पङ्गिल) are energetic lines that run parallel to the spine, crossing at key locations. *Chakras* form where these lines intertwine at intersection points along the central channel. The seven major *chakras* of the Hindu system are illustrated in Figure 5-3. In the Tibetan *tantric* system, they are referred to as *khor lo nga,* or "the five wheels," which, as the name suggests, refers to five *chakras.* These, too, are said to represent the etheric blueprint that underlies the physical body.

Although *chakras* are primarily considered an Eastern concept, they are also found in some esoteric Western mystical practices. The Cypriot Greek mystic, Daskalos, claimed that the *chakras* allowed him to receive communications from Jesus's disciple John the Evangelist. Sharing his experience, Daskalos explains that "the vibrations of the saint's presence are so intense that [his] material brain has a hard time channeling his teachings." [28] He described the *chakras* as "sacred discs" that act as psycho-noetic centers, conveying a type of etheric information, that also functions to transmit a *cosmic vitality* that makes healing possible. [29]

Regarding their capacity to imbue an energetic physiology, the *chakras* manage the interface between the body's "power" and emotional systems. They operate at key glandular locations, are closely tied to the body's nerve plexuses, and anchor emotions to the physical body. Functioning as "energy vortexes," they are gateways that allow an individual to interact with, and integrate, multiple levels of consciousness with one's emotional life. Proponents of these ideas believe that the mundane physical world represents only a small fraction of total reality. Thus, learning to activate *chakras* enables us to experience a broader spectrum of being.

The *chakras* engage, integrate, and represent the individual through physical and spiritual dimensions. In terms of a person's optimal functioning, a *chakra* can be either relatively closed or open, meaning less or more functional. *Chakra* functionality is expressed through the way one meets life's challenges and determines the ability to love or feel compassion. To this end, the *chakras* function as an extension of our sensory apparatus and allow us to live a more multi-dimensional life.

In the Hindu *chakra* system, the seven major *chakras* are located at the bottom of the spine, the genitals, the solar plexus, the heart, the throat, the third eye, and the crown. In this scheme, the *chakra* at the base of the tailbone represents grounding and survival; the second *chakra,* in the sexual centers, represents not only sexual love and intimacy, but also creativity; the third *chakra,* located at the solar plexus, represents the ability to imbue and express power; the fourth is the heart center, and responds to the expression of love; the fifth is in the throat, and represents one's ability to communicate; the sixth is in the forehead, and represents extrasensory visualization; the seventh, located at the top of the head, represents connection with the divine.

In the Tibetan *tantric* system, the five *chakras* are: the perineum, navel, heart, throat, and head. In addition, there are thirty-two main energetic channels that branch from the *chakras.* [30]

For a Tibetan Buddhist engaged in *tantric* practice, *chakra* work is an important aspect of secret training, and is reserved for advanced practitioners. As described in some Tibetan Buddhist sources, an adept working on the "completion stage" (*dzogrim*, རྫོགས་རིམ།), also known as the *perfection stage*, learns to access the *chakras* to bring the body's "winds," or subtle energy, into the central channel. Ultimately, the adept attains the union of *bliss* and *emptiness*, and through this process, becomes a *Buddha*.

Chakras in Western Mysticism

Several key individuals, and one major organization, are credited with popularizing the Indian teachings on *chakras* in the West. Especially influential were HP "Madam" Blavatsky, founder of the Theosophical Society (1831–1891); Charles W Leadbeater (1852-1934), who published *The Chakras* in 1927; and the Austrian mystic-philosopher Rudolf Steiner (1861-1925), who was noted for his writings and lectures on the topic.

The Western organization most prominent in its advocacy of subtle energy bodies and the introduction of *chakra* energy centers was the Theosophical Society. Formed in 1875, the society promoted beliefs from Hindu, Buddhist, and other Asian traditions.

Steiner focused on how one could develop what we would today refer to as psychic ability. At the dawn of the twentieth century, he became noted for his work describing the ability to perceive normally invisible realms and subtle energy associated with the body. Through lectures and writings, Steiner promoted the belief that individuals could increase their psychic capacity through a process of *super-sensibility*, or becoming aware of one's subtle energy fields. He taught that activation of the body's *chakra* system was key to developing super-sensibility skills, as the *chakras* function to open a specific range of emotional and mental "energy." In explaining how each *chakra* operates on a separate bandwidth which, in turn, activates an aspect of dimensional space, Steiner states:

> It must be clearly understood that the perception of each single organ of soul or spirit bears a different character. The twelve and sixteen-pet-alled lotus flowers [chakras] transmit quite different perceptions.[31]

Referring to the *chakras* as "organs of supersensible perception," Steiner posits that they function as spherical, multi-dimensional "organ" structures that are activated through an energizing process, with their actions being triggered through silence and "sustained active attention."[32] The process elicits a kind of spiritual initiation, resulting in awakened psychic energy from the "organs of supersensible perception." Of the various *chakras*, Steiner believes the heart, in the center of the chest, to be the most important. He describes the opening of the heart *chakra* as:

> A new center, located in the approximate area of the physical heart,
> becomes conscious. ... A great variety of movements and currents run
> from it to the various parts of the human body. The most important of
> these currents go to the lotus flowers, permeating them and their indi-
> vidual petals, and then pour out like rays into eternal space. [33]

According to Steiner, through this kind of attention the *chakras* eventually
become "warm, luminous, mobile, and of variegated color." At this point,
they begin to revolve within the subtle energy structures of the body, and
a new level of multi-dimensional perception awakens for the individual.
Working with the *chakras* in this way awakens clairvoyance and develops
supersensibility in the practitioner.

The *Chakras* and New Age Thought

Instruction that includes awareness and activation of the body's *chakra*
system is often included as part of "New Age" teaching and lectures. Teacher
and medical intuitive, Carolyn Myss, believes that the seven *chakras*
represent an individual's archetypal maturation through seven distinct
stages. As Myss explains, every thought and experience over a lifetime is
filtered through the *chakras,* with each acting as a kind of "database" which
records each life event. According to Myss, through the interaction of the
chakras and subtle energy fields, "your emotional experience becomes
your biology." [34] Different *chakras* become dominant at different times in a
person's life, and the dominant *chakra* operating at a given time determines
the individual's stage of evolution, with progression dependent upon the
mastery of a level of personal and spiritual power.

Myss's scheme of *chakra*-based lessons follow the description provided in
the earlier cited Hindu scenario, however, there are several additional points
worth mentioning. According to Myss, the second *chakra* also relates to
personal power in human relationships; the third, located at the solar plexus,
relates to ego and personality; the sixth, located at the third-eye in the
middle of the forehead, relates to intuition and insight. According to Myss,
the *chakra* at the top of the head, "pushes us to know and let go of untruths"
[35] and represents ascendency or union with the divine.[36]

Scientific Discussion of the *Chakras*

William Tiller, *professor emeritus* of Materials Science and Engineering at
Stanford University, whose works have been cited earlier, suggests that
chakras function to "emit bursts of subtle energy." [37] Tiller believes that
the *chakras* are involved in the body's conversion of subtle into electrical
energy through a process known as *transduction,* [38] and that they, along
with the acupuncture meridian system, operate as "*qi / prana* pumps." He

posits that when matched with "focused intention, they can raise the local EM [electromagnetic] gauge symmetry of their surrounding space and are thereby are able to "produce healings of great variety." [39] This is one portion of a complex proposal that may explain how observed phenomenon, such as electrical and electrical-like fields, joins with a proposed parallel subtle energy system that surrounds the body. **

**These ideas are explored in Section XII.

Chapter 24

Tibetan Tantric "Inner Heat" Meditation

A few terms pertaining to internal energy in the Tibetan *tantric* tradition:

Translated Tibetan	Tibetan Script	English Translation	Sanskrit
tsa	རྩ	Tube or Pipe "Energy Channels"	*Nadi*
lung	རླུང་	Wind / Subtle Energy	*Prana*
thigle	ཐིག་ལེ	Droplets "Essence"	*Bindu*
tummo	གཏུམ་མོ	Inner Heat	

Nadi

Nadi is the ancient *Sanskrit* term for the body's network of subtle energy pathways. Of these, the three primary *nadi* shown in Figure 5-1 are called the *Sushumna* (सुषुम्णा), which travels along the spine, and the *Ida* (इडा) and *Pingala* (पिङ्गल), both of which run parallel along the left and right sides of the spine.

Originating on the Indian subcontinent, the belief in these energetic pathways has long been part of Hindu *tantric* practice. An early description of the *nadi* system appears in the *Chandogya Upanishad*, where the body's subtle *nadi* system is compared with the arteries of the heart:

> A hundred and one, are the arteries of the heart. One of them leads up
> to the crown of the head. Going upward through that, one becomes
> immortal.[40]

Nadi pathways link the physical to the energetic and emotional bodies and are extremely reactive to thought and emotions. Negative emotions, especially anger, harm the *nadi*, and, when persistent, can lead to disease or illness due to negative emotions obstructing energy flow in the body.

In the Tibetan *tantric* tradition, the equivalent of the *nadi* are the *tsa-channels*. Like the Hindu *nadi*, they are important for both spiritual practice and traditional Tibetan healing, since they govern the healthful flow of *lung* subtle energy.

Tummo (Inner Heat)

Tummo (གཏུམ་མོ), or "inner heat," is an advanced Tibetan *tantric* practice that produces demonstrable effects within the physical body. *Tummo* is an energetic-meditative discipline through which devotees attempt to develop conscious control over their flow of subtle energy, *lung*, within the *tsa* energetic channels.

Tummo translates as "fierce woman," and the term is related to a female deity. The practice requires the adept to learn to consciously generate and control bodily heat, utilizing the warmth for both practical and spiritual benefits. Its potency increases along with the practitioner's ability to consciously control the flow of *lung* within the body, with the intention of directing it toward the ultimate goal of profound spiritual insight.

The "inner heat" of *tummo* is not metaphorical, but rather the manifestation of real, measurable warmth. At advanced levels, the degree of *tummo* heat generated by a practitioner is remarkable. When mastered, the adept gains control over body temperature to such an extent that they can sit barely clothed while exposed to extreme cold and snowy conditions.

Control over *tummo* heat also relates to the management of sexual desire and energy. This particularly applies to the flow of internal energy in the central channel that, when mastered, triggers a profound ecstatic experience.

Stories of inner heat meditation first reached the West via reports about Tibetan Buddhist monks and yogis in the Himalayas. There, living high in the snowy mountains, they were observed as requiring little or no clothing to keep warm.[41] In some *tummo* traditions, through a practice called *tummo rekyan*, the practitioner is tested for advanced accomplishment by demonstrating their ability to dry multiple wet sheets placed against their naked body.[42]

Like Taoist energetic practices, *tummo* involves focusing attention on the energy center in the lower abdomen, which in Tibetan *tantra* is referred to as the "secret *chakra*." In addition, the practice also requires specific postures, breath control, and visualization of the chakras.[43] The goal is to manipulate the form of *lung* referred to as *thigle.*

Thigle is the Tibetan translation of the Sanskrit term *bodhicitta.* For male practitioners, it is closely associated with semen. However, the term, as with the Chinese *jing,* is much broader, and applies to both male and female initiates. Yangpönga explains:

> *Bodhicitta [thigle]* is a factor of both body and mind. In terms of the body,.... *thigle* is the vital essence that nourishes both the coarse and subtle organic components of the body; it is also the male and female generative fluids. In terms of the mind, bodhicitta is the support to the mind itself, and its subtle aspect is inseparable from the mind's essence." [44]

As introduced earlier, in this form of *tantric* practice, breath control fans the flames of the "red" *thigle* drops at the lower abdomen center. This, in turn, melts the "white" *thigle* drops that reside primarily at the crown of the head, and the subsequent melting allows the red and white drops to merge. As Yangpönga explains, the process brings about a natural state of innate wisdom, and the experience of a special state known as *bliss:*

> This bliss is found within the temple of one's own body when the white vital essence at the head *chakra* is melted by the practices of inner heat or union with a consort. When the vital essence melts, it descends through the *chakras,* giving rise to bliss of different degrees, the last of which is known as the innate bliss. In this experience there is no subject-object dichotomy and no pleasure tainted by ordinary attachment. Although innate bliss is the very nature of ordinary consciousness, it remains hidden unless discovered through those powerful experiences. [45]

The possibility that a person might be able to consciously generate special abilities, like the incredible warmth associated with *tummo,* is intriguing. For this reason, the phenomenon can easily become the focus of attention for Westerners. However, it is important to keep in mind that, for practitioners, demonstrations of *siddhi,* or "psychic powers," are considered trivial. Those training in *tummo* are taught not to be distracted by early successes, but to concentrate on the attainment of more advanced states of consciousness. Lama Thubten Yeshe, a respected authority on the subject, teaches that *tummo* is designed to bring the "airs" [wind / *lung*] into the central channel, in order to help the practitioner awaken to "clear light."

Eliminating Obstacles

According to Tibetan *tantric* theory, *tummo* awakens when a practitioner is sufficiently advanced to have gained control over the body's internal energy. At this point, a fire stirs within the practitioner, which, although usually metaphorical, can also sometimes manifest as physical warmth that is intense enough to be unpleasant.

Beyond physical warmth, *tummo* is considered a psychic fire that burns negative "trash" accumulated by the ego. Guilt, fear, and judgment are examples of the extra and burdensome trash that "burns" in its blaze. Lama Yeshe explains, "We do not have bamboo, pine, or olive trees to burn as our inner fuel, but we do have plenty of ego garbage and superstitions." [46]

Because of the intense nature of the practice, inner heat meditation is considered a faster path to enlightenment. As with other *tantric* practices, *tummo* is believed by proponents to lead to the ultimate state of liberation, or Buddhahood, in the shortest time possible. [47]

Due to its intensity, *tummo* also comes with a cautionary note relating to incorrect or premature practice, warning that if the "winds" within the body are made to move incorrectly, it can result in serious illness. Thus, it should be emphasized that the practitioner undertakes advanced energetic practices like *tummo* only under the proper guidance of a bona fide teacher. Yeshe explains:

> The winds gather where the mind focuses, and sometimes the wind moves the wrong way and produces physical and emotional pain. To avoid this, sufficient practice of "empty-body" meditation, "vase" breathing and other preliminary exercises should be mastered first. [See Box 5-5] [48]

Box 5-5

Tibetan *Tummo* "Inner Heat" Preliminary Practices

Empty Body Meditation:
This is a preparatory practice, used before one can "see" the body's interior. Through the practice, the initiate learns to view his or her entire body as completely empty and transparent. This training is said to assist with the next level, which is the ability to observe and interact personally with the *vajra* (energetic) body.
(see Lama Yeshe, pp. 103-104)

Vase Breathing:
"Vase Breathing" is a specific breathing technique. It is a preparatory exercise before one can begin *tummo*. This technique includes "dispelling of impure airs," "milking the air *[lung]* from the two side channels into the central channel," imagery, and controlled tightening of the pelvic diaphragm.

Bliss

Bliss has a special meaning in the Tibetan *tantric* tradition that is closely tied to the experience of "clear light." *Bliss* and *clear light* are terms for the practitioner's experience, which result from optimal management of the flow of energy within the body. For the practitioner, these experiences are profound and result from the conversion of sexual energy into spiritual energy. The process is related to the *tantric* practitioner's ability to transform the sensation normally associated with orgasm. Lama Yeshe describes the relationship between *bliss,* advanced consciousness, and sexual orgasm as follows:

> The yogi or yogini is simply saying, "I am not satisfied with the pleasure I already have. I want more. That is why I am practicing inner fire." [49]

Expanding on themes introduced earlier, the experience of *bliss* is often described in terms of pleasurable magnetic-like feelings throughout the body. Yeshe explains:

> The magnetic pleasure will automatically be activated, *thigle* will flow, and you will experience bliss not just in your channels and chakras but throughout your entire body. [50]

Thigle (ཐིག་ལེ)

At the heart of *tummo* is the practitioner's ability to gain yogic control over *thigle* † in the channels. Thus, we again encounter the relationship between internal energy, *thigle,* bliss, and the meaning of orgasm in the *tantric* Buddhist tradition.

In this context, *thigle* refers to the energy of sexual orgasm and sexual-like ecstasy leading to enlightenment; this aspect of *thigle* manifests from control over internal energy in the central channel that travels along the spine. The experience is "orgasmic," but also different from normal sexual orgasm. As Lama Yeshe explains, normal orgasm does not arise from the central channel, but from the *thigle* — an aspect of *lung* energy — touching the outside of the central channel that runs next to the spine. In contrast, *bliss* is related to advanced consciousness and control over the internal *winds [lung],* which in turn results in control over *thigle* in the central channel, a crucial aspect of advanced training.

> † Note that in the cited text, Lama Yeshe translates *thigle* "for convenience," as *kundalini,* explaining the term is more universal. However, when treated with a more nuanced comparison, characteristics of *thigle* are distinct from *kundalini* (this point is addressed in Section VI). Thus, to spare the reader confusion, when quoting Lama Yeshe, his use of the term *kundalini* is replaced with the Tibetan, *thigle* (see Yeshe, p. 84).

The experience of *bliss* is an important aspect of *tantric* yoga practice, and thus deserves special attention. The goal of *tantra* is neither to reject nor deny pleasure, and from this point of view, pleasure is a tool that helps transform and advance an individual's consciousness. As Yeshe explains, the practice involves never "forgetting to unify the father aspect of bliss with the mother aspect of non-duality." [51] However, the experience requires a commitment to practice, where the practitioner's deep concentration "unifies [pleasure] with the wisdom that realizes emptiness." [52] The practice of bliss eventually gives rise to "great blissful wisdom," which in turn leads to enlightenment. [53]

Tantric Energetic Physiology

At this juncture, it is useful to take a closer look at the relationship between *lung* and *thigle*. As introduced earlier, *lung* is translated as "wind" or "energy," while *thigle* has several meanings and translations. The Tibetan word *thigle* derives from the Sanskrit word *bindu* (बिन्दु), meaning "dot" or "point." However, the term has other meanings. For example, it is used to describe the "spheres of rainbow light" that manifest around advanced meditators when they attain a particularly deep meditative trance state.[54] For practitioners of Tibetan *tantric* meditation, *thigle* has the additional meaning of an aspect of *lung* energy thought of as a "droplet," or "essence," which circulates in the energetic channels.

In this context, *thigle* exists throughout the *vajra* body blueprint, and, as introduced earlier, they are either red or white in color. Most red *thigle* reside in the lower body, in the energy center between the navel and sexual organs, which, as was also introduced earlier, in males is referred to as the "secret chakra." In contrast, most white *thigle* reside at the top of the head in the crown *chakra*. However, *thigle* are not limited to these two locations, and can be found within the more-than-a-thousand subtle energetic channels that run throughout the body. [55]

> Working with both white and red leads to health and spiritual wisdom
> — Gyalwa Yangpönga [56]

In some ways, *thigle* is comparable to the aspect of energy known in Taoist practices as *jing* (Chapter 25). In both Tibetan and Taoist traditions, *thigle / jing* are forms of internal energy associated with semen, with a key difference being that in the Tibetan tradition, females also possess *thigle*. Comparing *thigle* with *lung*, Tibetan tantric scholar and lama Namkhai Norbu Rinpoche explains, "They are not two separate things. The one is the essence of the other." According to Norbu, "When the *prana* [*lung* energy] is brought into the central channel, its essential nature — *thigle* — is activated and enters the channels," at which point the "dualistic mind is overcome, and realization achieved." [57]

Another notable comparison between Taoist and Tibetan *tantric* traditions is that male disciples are taught to avoid the loss of semen. As Yangpönga explains, in *tantra*, retention of semen is of vital importance: [58]

> Loss of semen implies not only the exit of vital essence from the body,
> but also the loss of recognition of the bliss that is the nature of the mind. [59]

More on Bliss

As mentioned earlier, in *tummo* practice, the adept achieves the state of bliss by setting fire to accumulated "negative energy." The practice "burns up 'dissatisfied' energy, bringing the practitioner total physical and psychological satisfaction." [60] Yeshe explains how to manage the experience of *extreme bliss*:

> As soon as we experience any bliss, we should put effort into generating the wisdom of non-duality. Bliss should be digested and transformed into wisdom, otherwise the experience becomes one of ordinary pleasure. [In this scheme] bliss becomes wisdom; wisdom becomes bliss. [61]

For a more experienced practitioner, the experience of *bliss* brings increased sensitivity, especially to one's own body:

> Your body is organic, and you need to learn to listen to its rhythms until you feel that each cell in your nervous system is talking to you. When you develop such sensitive awareness of your body, it's almost as though you can tell it what to do. Instead of clomping around heavily, your whole body feels light and blissful, as if you are walking on air. It is liberating. Simply touching yourself will produce bliss. We have that resource. Instead of being a source of pain, your entire body can become a source of bliss. You reach a point where your body and mind cooperate so perfectly that you feel body is mind and mind is body. There is an incredible sense of unity. [62]

For *tantric* initiates, the greatest hurdle is to convert the pursuit of pleasure into a force that can be used for the attainment of advanced consciousness. All *tantric* practices (and this is what makes them potentially dangerous if a person is not properly prepared and tutored by a qualified master) involve what is called "transformation of poisons," which Yeshe describes in the following way:

> What for others is bondage, for practitioners of tantra, is liberation... The tantric principle is based on recognition of the "mind's primal purity." [63]

The oft-cited image that illustrates the *tantric* doctrine of *transforming poisons* is that of the peacock; the bird that is unharmed by the ingestion of poisonous plants, and instead transforms them into spectacularly beautiful plumage.

But how does *tummo* relate to other schools of energetic meditation? A closer look at the "energetic physiology" of *tummo* provides insight. *Tummo* "inner fire" practice is one of the Six Yogas (meaning spiritual practices) of Naropa. These are the mind-body-energy forms of yoga revealed by the eleventh century Buddhist scholar, Pandit Naropa (1016-1100). The other forms of his yogas are Illusory Body, Dream, Clear Light, Intermediate State, and the Transference of Consciousness. ‡

‡ More discussion of *tummo* and *thigle*, in the context of *tantric* sexual practice, is included in Section VI.

Special Powers: *Siddhi*

Earlier, it was mentioned that *tantric* practice is sometimes accompanied by the sudden appearance of special powers, referred to in Sanskrit as *siddhi*. Examples of *siddhi* include the ability to read another person's thoughts and, according to some sources, even being able to gain control over the elements, like fire or the weather. There are various other examples of *siddhi*, such as one found in the Buddhist *tantric* tradition, which states that the yogi Yangpönga used *siddhi* powers to protect the local population from Mongol attack.[64]

One story of *siddhis* possessing the power to control the elements concerns a lama named Tsongkhapa (1357–1419). Once, as fire threatened to engulf his Lhasa temple, Tsongkhapa entered an advanced state of meditation and directed the flames to extinguish themselves, and his intervention is credited with saving the temple.[65]

Often, stories about *siddhi* powers contain a hint of playfulness. For example, Zhanag Dzogpa Tenzin Namgyal shares this story about the *siddhi* power of the Karmapa: *

> Once when the Karmapa visited the Phayul Monastery, residence of a famous *siddha* (*siddha* is the Sanskrit term for a master of *siddhi* powers), he lifted the *siddha's* sword, tied the metal blade into a knot, and then upon handing it back to his host said, "You see, I am a *siddha* too." [66]
>
> * * The Karmapa lineage is the first tulku (སྤྲུལ་སྐུ) lineage in Tibet. Predating the Dalai Lamas, a *tulku* in this context is a reincarnated master, who is a custodian of teachings, practices, and empowerments.

In practice, because *tummo* emphasizes the practitioner's attention to sensations within the body, it can interrupt the over-intellectualization that might inhibit spiritual progress. Commenting on the value of experience over intellectual debate, Yeshe states, "It is extremely important to let go in meditation such as inner fire. Intellectual cleverness does not work; it will only cause you to miss incredibly valuable experiences." [67]

As a final note on *tummo* practice, it is useful to think about the practice as representing a class of meditative disciplines that emphasize experiential over intellectual knowledge, and to view it more as mysticism than metaphysics. Thus, it is not a theological exercise in defining the nature of the divine, but rather an experience of the divine within the body of the practitioner.

Chapter 25

Taoist Energetic Meditation

The introduction to Section III included a note of caution regarding the terms "Taoist" and "Taoist practices." As mentioned there, such terms are frequently misapplied because they are ambiguous and multivalent, and the same semantic problems and cautionary notes apply to the present discussion of "Taoist" energetic meditation. This chapter has been written for the casual reader, and thus does not seek to join the academic discussion of what constitutes a "Taoist" or "Taoism."

The present chapter presents an overview of three Taoist meditation traditions: *Shouyi,* or "Guarding the One," a tradition with roots in the earliest beginnings of Taoism, and two types of Taoist *neidan* practices. However, before that discussion, it may be useful to consider the question of mysticism in early forms of Taoism.

The Quietest Tradition and the Taoist Mystic

The quietest tradition is often associated with what is sometimes referred to as Taoist mysticism. Influences that contributed to a Taoist mystical theology include those attributed to Lao Tzu, Chuang Tzu, Lieh Tzu, and Wen Tzu, who, when grouped together, Professor Harold Roth explains:

> …formed a Taoist school of philosophy devoted to cosmology and mysticism that advocated, among other things, the acceptance of death as just one more change in the eternal cosmic process.[68]

Early Taoism contains three components: a characteristic cosmological view, a political philosophy, and the practice of inner cultivation. The first of these components describes the Tao as the "unifying power in the cosmos." The second component comprises the body of political principles offered to address the social chaos at the time of its founding. The final component pertains to the origins of the Taoist mystical tradition and the practice of *inner cultivation,* which, as explained by Roth, involves:

> The attainment of the Tao through a process of emptying out the usual contents of the conscious mind until a profound experience of tranquility is attained.[69]

213

The point is emphasized in the earliest Taoist mystical text, the *Nei Yeh*, which stresses self-discipline to waken and nurture one's full potential. As the *Nei Yeh* explains, without self-discipline, the individual will fail to attain physical, psychological, and spiritual fulfillment. Roth emphasizes again, as elucidated in the *Nei Yeh*, that only through self-discipline can one attain, "health, vitality, psychological clarity, a sense of well-being, a profound tranquility, and, ultimately, direct experience of the Way and an integration of this experience into one's daily life." [70] Roth cites the modern-day commentator, Chao Shou-cheng, to reinforce the point:

> Inward training means inner achievement. It refers to the practice, by which one cultivates and nourishes the inner mind and preserves vital essence and vital energy. [71]

Roth's observations are echoed by John Blofeld's description of the power of disciplined inner focus, which is capable of:

> Directing consciousness in upon itself; within the mind, where shrouded by the mists that hover in deep valleys, lies a treasure discoverable only by direct intuition. [72]

Quiet Sitting

A Taoist, seeking mystical union with the *Way*, begins by simply sitting and being quiet. Thus, meditation is appropriately termed *jingzuo* (静坐), or "quiet sitting." Another term adopted by early Taoists to describe their practice was *zheng* (正), which in normal usage means "correct" or "straight." However, as illustrated in Box 5-3, for early Taoists, the Chinese character took on a special significance, since it could also be used to represent their cross-legged style of sitting meditation practice.

正

The Chinese character *zheng* normally meaning "straight" or "correct" has a special meaning in early Taoist meditation

Box 5-6
The Chinese Character for *Zheng*

To a Taoist meditator, the character *zheng* represents the practitioner, who sits in a balanced, cross-legged style. This posture, characterized by a "square pattern" (suggested by the *zheng* character's construction), the Taoist meditator is then able to invigorate the flow of internal energy throughout the body:

When your body is not aligned (正, *zheng*)

The inner power will not come.

When you are not tranquil within,

Your mind will not be well ordered.

Align your body, assist the inner power.

Then it will gradually come on its own.

Tao Yeh, Chapter 11, [73]

The Chinese character for *Te* (also Romanized as *De*) refers to a type of "primordial power" or "potential"

Box 5-7

Te: **Power through Alignment with the Tao**

Therefore, this vital energy

cannot be halted by force

yet can be secured by inner power [*Te*, 德]

cannot be summoned by speech,

yet can be welcomed by awareness

Reverently hold onto it and do not lose it

This is called developing inner power [*Te*, 德]

When inner power develops, and wisdom emerges,

The myriad things will, to the last one, be grasped. [74]

The *Tao Te Ching* (道德經) serves as the foundational text of Taoism. It is a cryptic collection of social, political, and energetic-yogic teachings that are believed by its followers to represent the *Tao* or "path" that goes "beyond words." For Taoists, it represents a timeless philosophy of natural truths. The text's title is translated into English as *The Classic of the Way and its Power* (alternatively, *The Classic of the Way and its Virtue*).[75] As mentioned earlier, this text is traditionally attributed to Lao Tzu, who is said to have authored it around 500 BCE.

For many Taoists, the middle character of the title, *Te* (德), pronounced as well as Romanized as *De*, has an especially important meaning. The term is often translated through a moralistic Confucian lens as "virtue," however, RL Wing suggests that when translated this way, *virtue* fails to capture the original Taoist meaning of *te.* This point is especially important for Taoist energetic practitioners, for whom the "power" translation suggests a kind of merging with the primordial force derived from the spiritual wellspring of the Tao. Thus, some writers on the topic consider a more profound and meaningful translation to be *power* or *potency*. As used here, *te* is the potency that germinates a sprouting plant, enabling it to come to fruition. As Wing explains, this view explores:

> A remarkable power that is latent in every individual. This power, which Lao Tzu calls *te,* emerges when one is aware of and aligned with the forces in nature *(Tao)*.[76]

In this context, when applied to humans, *te* can be thought of as a subtle universal source energy or "vibration" that one can "resonate with," and which quietly empowers a charismatic and influential person. Wing describes these kinds of powerful individuals as those endowed with the essence of the *Tao,* who:

> Never show their strength, yet others listen to them because they seem to know. They radiate knowledge, but this is an intuitive knowing that comes from direct understanding and experience of the ways of nature. They are compassionate and generous, because they instinctively realize that power continues to flow through them only when they pass it on. Like electricity, the more energy, inspiration and information they conduct, the more they receive. [77]

Taoist Concentrative Meditation

Shouyi 守 一, or "Guarding the One," is a philosophical term that can be used to inspire meditation, and which refers to the notion of keeping the mind under control. As an ancient theme in Taoist literature, the practice of guarding the One dates back to before the Han dynasty (206 BCE-220 CE) and can be traced to the Lao Tzu and Chuang Tzu traditions, sometimes referred to as philosophical Taoism.[78]

The *One* refers to what Taoists traditionally call the *xiantian,* or primordial state, which can be realized through concentrative meditation. As Livia Kohn explains, "*One* refers to four aspects of philosophical Taoism, a primordial state before creation, the principle through which creation takes place, the creative primordial force that sustains life, and the basic characteristic of 'all there is.'" [79]

However, guarding the One contains more than the essence of Taoist philosophy, as it also includes the earliest references to Taoist immortality practices. The relationship between guarding the One and the attainment of immortality is expressed thusly in the classic text *Guangchengzi:* "I hold on to the One, abide in its harmony, and therefore I have kept myself alive for 1200 years. And never has my body suffered any decay." [80]

Applied as a Taoist concentrative method — "stop your thoughts and guard the One" — [81] it refers to the adept who turns their attention inward and visualizes the inner light within the body. Through the practice of inwardly directed attention and visualizing inner light, the practitioner learns to "relax in serenity and attain cosmic consciousness." [82] Thus, the practice of guarding the One contains the essence of Taoist energetic practices, and leads to strengthening the *dan tian* energy center in the lower abdomen. [83]

Mysticism and Inner Alchemy

If you were traveling in the mountains of pre-communist China, you never knew whom you might encounter. British writer John Blofeld traveled through those mountains at that time and kept a record of his journeys as he went. On one of his travels, he encountered a person he identified as a Taoist recluse. The recluse's description of his meditative practice informs this discussion of Taoist immortality and spiritual practice, based on the following three aspects of his Taoist practice that he shared with Blofeld:

> To attain tranquility, so that "in the stillness of our hearts, we may apprehend the Tao within, and around us. This involves controlling one's passions and vanquishing excessive desires."

> To nourish vitality and prolong lives, to gain more time to refine spirit.

> Compound the *[dan]* golden pill. To compound the pill, one first learns to keep lustful thoughts in check, since sexual release is not helpful toward the goal. [84]

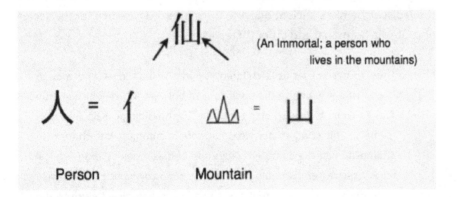

(An Immortal; a person who lives in the mountains)

Person   Mountain

Taoist *Neidan* Energetic Meditation

Diagram 5-8
Etymology of the Chinese Character for *Xian* or Immortal
(Also Romanized as *Hsien*)

The Taoist Inner Alchemist

For most Taoist inner alchemists, the goal was to attain immortality. To this end, the practitioner combined elements of heaven and earth, symbolized by the dragon and tiger, within his own body. There were two principle ways to accomplish this. Some sought to attain immortality through solo practice, while others pursued dual practice, or sexual alchemy. ** The second century CE text, *Instruction on the Regeneration of the Primary Vitalities,* describes the process involved in *neidan* alchemical transformation:

> There are two *qi*. One is yang and represented by the dragon and the element wood and by secretions. The other, *yin*, represented by the tiger, the element metal and by essences. When these two *qi* are brought into conjunction and made to react with transformation, then what results, is called the outer *wai tan [waidan]...*

> But, through conserving and harmonizing, working alchemical transformations within the viscera, exhaling the old and breathing in the new, and then transmitting upwards to the brain, and then showering downwards to the *dan tian* region of vital heat, restoring and transforming in endless cycles, passing through the heart and there collecting the five *qi* of the viscera, this is called the *neidan*. [85]

> ** Paired practice and sexual alchemy are covered in Section VI.

Through the rituals of *neidan* practices, the adept sought to reverse the otherwise natural tendency toward decline, aiming to restore youth and rejuvenate the body. Several methods were employed to achieve these goals, including visualization and breathing arts. Joseph Needham compares the Taoist alchemist's ancient quest to the modern-day search for the secret of youth via hormonal and other therapies:

> Thus 'to become as little children' was the neidan ideal, and though one must not minimize the undertone of holy innocence which all true Taoists would have wished to recapture, the physiological alchemists of medieval China had, in our view, far more in common with those who attempt to halt the aging of tissues and bodies today by bio-chemical means [such as] endocrinological treatments and hygienic exercises than with those who think in terms of a purely psychological 'return to the womb'. [86]

Through a process called *lienqi huashen* (錬氣化神), or "converting the *qi* into spirit," the Taoist yogic meditator, relying on *huaji* (化機), or "mechanisms of change," hoped to restore primal, natural energy, and return to the uncorrupted "earlier," or "primordial heaven" (先天) state. The hoped-for result was to reverse the aging process and attain immortality.

Merging the Three Treasures

Section III also discussed the importance of the *san pao,* or "three treasures" of Taoist inner alchemy traditions, *jing, qi,* and *shen.* Known as the three primordial energies, *san yuan* (三元), or three true energies, *san jen qi* (三真氣), the core of Taoist energetic practice involves the conversion of coarse *jing* into refined *shen.*

Conversion of *Jing* Essence

Section III also considered the methods that the inner alchemist might have employed when working with mind and body energy. Those techniques included visualization, prescriptive breathing practices, disciplined diet, absorbing the energy of the moon *(fu yue,* 服月) and the practice of sexual arts. For males engaged in Taoist practice, aspirants focused on "transforming the *qi* to nourish the brain," [87] while the equivalent practice for female initiates was known as "irrigating the brain with nectar." [88]

These are examples of alchemy practices that converted coarse *jing* into rarified *shen.* As with the Tibetan *tantric* traditions, an important part of the practice was to avoid depletion of sexual essence. For males, this meant eliminating, or at least minimizing, depletion of sexual essence. In contrast, for a female practitioner, loss of essential energy occurs through menses and childbirth. However, one's essential energy could be depleted in other ways. For example, one's energetic essence could be reduced by overthinking, worrying, sweating profusely, spitting, and the consumption of the "five grains" (meaning all grains, and referred to as the "five poisons"). Abstention from grains is called *bigu* (避穀). Ancient texts provide more insight into the practices of the *neidan* practitioner. One middle-late-twelfth century text describes their experience:

> The theory of the *neidan* in practices directed toward the attainment of immortality is nothing more than the mutual conjunction of the heart and the kidneys.

> Circulation of the *jing* seminal essence and *qi,* preservation of the *shen*-spiritual essence, the retention of *qi* and exhaling the old and breathing in the new. [89]

The text details the meditative practice of the inner alchemist as one involving the "mutual conjunction of the heart and kidney." This is an important clue, as it tells us about the kind of sensations the *neidan* meditators experienced during practice. The text describes how when one aligns and "activates" the body in specific ways, a special kind of arrangement can trigger some very interesting mind and body experiences.

Similar to the descriptions of *chakra* work, this set of instructions describes how one experiences a certain type of sensation when the body's energy centers align in just the right way. As described in the twelfth-century text just cited, when the body's energy centers are physically aligned and attended to, this can sometimes produce powerful emotional and (what we today understand as) electromagnetic field effects. For example, as suggested by the Taoist text, the sense of energetic vibrations within the body can be triggered through the merging of intention and specific physical postures.

In terms of posture, the text describes an alignment between the energy centers of the upper chest, associated with the heart and thymus when these energy centers physically align with the lower torso energy center associated with the kidneys. However, the practice of this energetic and physical alignment is more challenging than most of us realize. As will be covered in Section XI, unless otherwise corrected, the body tends to fall to the path of least effort, or slump. This happens because it takes less effort to allow the head to hang forward, out of optimal alignment, than to engage consciously in the active lifting of the head and chest. *Slumping* is not the alignment described in the Taoist text. Improper alignment of this kind not only inhibits the flow of energy through the "three passes," or *san guan*, but also serves as one of the more reliable markers of aging. Examples are seen in a forward collapsed head and neck, as well as the upper-back forward hunch colloquially referred to as a "widow's hump." In contrast, proper vertical alignment encourages activation of the meridians.

The Three Passes

The three passes, or *san guan*, are bottlenecks where the *qi* life force can easily get stuck on its upward journey along the spine from the tailbone to the head. The lowest bottleneck is the *wei lü* at the tailbone, the middle is in the upper-back, and the highest is at the base of the neck, at the occiput. Douglas Wile, in commenting on these bottlenecks, writes that, "the literature of inner alchemy is replete with special techniques — posture, breath, visualization, and sphincter contraction — for enabling the *qi* to rise against the current through these successively narrower 'three passes.'" [90]

This is a good place to address the meaning of *wei lü*. The term can refer either to the anatomical tailbone (wěilú gǔ; 尾閭骨) or an "energy center," and, depending on context, it can be structural (referring to a bone) or functional (referring to a chakra, or energy center). When talking about posture, it's fine to think of it anatomically, but when talking about the three passes, for example, it definitely refers to an energy center. Most general dictionaries only give wěilúgu, referring to the anatomical "tailbone," or coccyx, but specialized *qigong* and Taoist dictionaries give long discussion of the wěilú as an energy center, with much citing of chapter and verse from the inner elixir literature.

However, posture alone is not sufficient to activate the energetic relationship between the upper and lower body. Classical texts and modern commentaries alike speak to both the necessity and the potentiating influence of the power of consciously directed intention to induce changes in the mind-body.

As was discussed earlier, there exists the curious fact that directing attention toward specific parts of the body can influence the sense of magnetic pulse in the body, and those kinds of magnetic and magnetic-like sensations can intensify when mental and physical alignments are established between various body-energy centers.

For example, if one sits upright, releases all unnecessary tension, and then focuses attention on the lower abdomen, with patience and an open mind, most people will notice an increase in warmth in the area. Through sustained practice, one is even able to observe the pulse at specific locations throughout the body. As was covered in Section III, an easy self-test that demonstrates the power of intention to influence the body involves the placement of attention on specific areas of the body. First, relax all unnecessary tension, and then direct attention to the pulse at a specific location within the body, such as the perineum, genitals, or lower abdomen. With regular practice, a practitioner will observe how the combination of relaxation and attention can bring increased warmth and blood supply to the targeted areas. No doubt, this kind of practice, and the resulting sensations, captured the interest of the early *neidan* alchemists.

Microcosmic Orbit

One of the most well-known "Taoist" practices is the "microcosmic orbit." Also called orbital meditation, this form of energetic meditation is characterized by the practitioner's ability to initiate and control sensations. These are the sensations identified as the flow of energy along the body's front and rear meridians, known respectively as *ren* (任, conception) and *du* (督, governing).

It is likely that orbital meditation is a relatively recent practice, as references to the front and rear channels are not found in the meditation literature until the Sung (970-1279 CE) and Yuan (1271-1368 CE) dynasties.[91] By contrast, the principle that internal energy circulates within the body is much older. Since *qi* and blood are said to be coupled, the belief that energy circulates through the body is related to the observations by Chinese physicians regarding blood circulation.

The practice of orbital meditation involves the practitioner focusing attention on the *du* and *ren* channels (see Figure 5-9). This requires the practitioner to direct sensations, believed to be *qi* internal energy, through the body's front and rear central axes meridians. While performing these techniques, the practitioner will experience a host of sensations, including feelings of pressure and electrical-like signals along those channels, which might appear

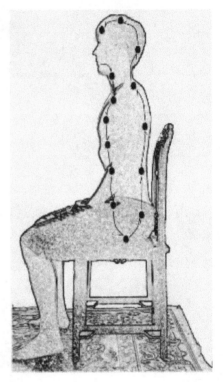

Figure 5-9

The Two Main Channels of Microcosmic, or "Orbital," Meditation

Originating near the genitals, in the scheme depicted in the drawing, internal energy first moves up the back through the du channel to the crown of the head. After completing a connection from the soft palate to the tongue on the inside of the mouth, it travels along the ren channel through the front center of the body.

with or without the presence of warmth. This migration of sensations along the *du* and *ren* channels informs the practitioner that *qi* is being directed through the principle channels along the frontal and posterior medial aspects of the body.

Although meditation practices like orbital meditation are traditionally associated with the Taoist alchemist's search for immortality, in modern times, aspects of this training have often adopted a more contemporary outlook. Nowadays, terms that are used to describe the purpose of practice, such as the "search for immortality," are often replaced with the "quest for longevity," and at times, energetic meditation is referred to as "longevity meditation." Chris Jarmey, a teacher and writer on the topic, describes the practice in the following way:

> The purpose of longevity meditation is to add more *Qi* to "elixir fields" [the body's energetic storehouses, the "*dan tians*"], so that you can have a virtually unlimited resource of energy for the purpose of extending your life as the most vibrant person possible in order to achieve your highest goals. [92]

However, as is the case with both Chinese medicine and martial arts, there is not one single approach to orbital meditation, but instead many variants. Thus, for the student of energetic meditation, it is useful to reflect on how various writers describe the practice. Taoist author Chao Pi-ch'en describes the training:

> When starting the exercise, inhalation and exhalation should succeed each other to stop all external disturbances so that spirit and vitality can unite. The practitioner will feel warmth below the navel, and this feeling may later last for the whole day. He will then notice that positive vitality first rises from the base of the spine; it will in time, as his practice continues, go up the backbone, and if his determination is firm, will pierce through the occipital region to reach the top of his head. So, if he has been taught the secret of alchemy, he can drive his positive vitality through the three gates (in the channel of control) at once. [93]

More insight into the practice is offered by Dr. Stephen Chang, whose description of the flow of energy up the spine follows the same basic scheme as Chao's, but with a few additional details:

> While locking sphincter, breath into *tan t'ien [dan tian]* energy center of lower abdomen, which activates sexual glands, energy begins to move upward along the back, as energy travels upward, it moves through the seven houses (glands) in succession, each time making a wheel like rotation around the gland it encounters on its upward migration through the body -- all this brought about by gradually training the breath to complete this on the inhale. [94]

Why Practice?

Proponents of orbital meditation believe the exercise restores youth and promotes longevity, and contemporary practitioners often describe the goals of the exercise in terms of empowerment and mind-body transformation. As Chang explains, an adept uses the microcosmic orbit to prepare "himself for this final transformation which occurs in a state beyond time and space, in which man realizes his true natural place in the universe." [95] This requires the practitioner to first attain an altered mental state, which prepares the individual for spiritual union with the primordial source.

As Chang explains, the practice converts the body's coarse *jing* sexual energy into *qi*, which "awakens life and health." This view of orbital meditation sees the process as transformative because of the effect of the exercise on the body's glandular system. In this view, the glands may be considered transformers, to be thought of as electrical generators that operate in the context of the body's storehouses of energy. [96] Chang describes orbital meditation as a yogic practice that utilizes the *ren* and *du* / front and back channels to trigger beneficial energetic changes along the medial aspect of the body. In turn, the process promotes anti-aging and empowering influences on the "seven glands," referring to the sexual glands (prostate and testes in the male, and ovaries, uterus, vagina, and breasts in females), plus adrenals, pancreas, thymus, thyroid, pituitary, and pineal gland. Chang points out that the conception and governing channels that run vertically along the front and back of the torso are the only two meridians where the direction of internal energy can be consciously changed. [97] Chang describes the rewards of practice:

> If impatience can be overcome, the rewards are indescribable. The spiritual eye of the practitioner is fully awakened, and he or she is raised to the level of the Hsien [Immortal] [See Box 5-8], or wise and immortal person. The Hsien is one who knows the secrets of the universe by being in complete union with the Tao, or God, exists perpetually, and has the power of the universe at his or her disposal. Is this not the true desire which lies in the hearts of all men? [98]

Chang's view of the hormonal glands as an "electrical system" is shared by some Western coaches and bodybuilders. For example, bodybuilding champion Bill Pearl refers to the hormones and secretions of the endocrine glands as "'spark plugs,' that provide stimulus and drive for the body as well as the mind." [99]

Microcosmic Orbit Details

The first steps of orbital meditation involve learning to pay attention to, and then control, sensations in the body that are associated with the movement and transmutation of internal energy.

It is noteworthy that, as with the practice of *tummo,* sensations within the body that the practitioner identifies as "energy" will "activate" and "move" along the spinal corridor with exceptional warmth or intensity. At times, these sorts of experiences can be unsettling, especially when they present as heat along the spine. Furthermore, with or without the presence of warmth, intense emotional experiences may accompany the practice, and it is not unusual for the practitioner to occasionally experience the feeling of being overwhelmed. However, unsettling experiences disappear when, according to the traditional Chinese alchemical-meditational model, the individual attains contact with *xiantian,* or "primordial heaven."

In rarer examples, the practitioner's experience presents as an extraordinary degree of objective bodily warmth. This raises the question as to whether this class of experience may be the same as *tummo* in the Tibetan *tantric* tradition. An excerpt from Jiang Weiqiao's 1914 book on energetic practice is relevant:

> All of a sudden, there was this intense rumbling movement in the cinnabar field *[dan tian]* in my lower abdomen. I had been sitting in quiet meditation as usual, but this was something I really couldn't control. I was shaken back and forth helplessly. Then an incredibly hot energy began to rise at the bottom of my spine, climbed up further and further until it reached the very top of my head. [100]

The practice of orbital meditation relies on the individual placing attention on the anterior and posterior acupuncture channels that lie along the medial aspect of the torso. In this regard, the normal flow of energy is upward along the spine from the perineum to the center of the brain. A continuation of the normal pattern is represented by the downward flow of energy over the front of the torso.

In the first stages of training, the practitioner directs sensations from the bottom of the spine up the *du* channel, and over the vertex to the energy center between the eyes called the "original cavity of the spirit." Next, the practitioner recirculates the energy down the front of the body, thus completing the cycle known as the "fire path."

Fire Path and Water Path

"Fire" and "water" paths refer to the directional flow of internal energy over the channels along the body's central axis. Lu Kuan-yu explains that the "fire path" triggers a rise of "generative" and "vital forces" along the *du* channel, and that the conscious direction of vital energy upward along the spine is known as the "ascent of positive fire." The subsequent movement of energy down the front of the body is referred to as "descent of negative fire." [101] In contrast, the conscious reversing of the aforementioned coarse, going downward along the spine and upward along the front channel, is known as the "water path."

Orbital meditation incorporates the movement of energy through what are traditionally referred to as the "four gates." Originally written for male adepts, those gates are located at the base of the penis, top of the head, the *dan tian* energy center in the lower abdomen, and *ming men* point in the lumbus. Lu also describes the base of the penis as the connection point for what he refers to as eight psychic channels. By the "eight psychic channels," he is probably referring to what is now known in TCM as the "eight extra meridians," which, according to current acupuncture charts, do not all pass directly through the region. However, since acupuncture charts have only recently been standardized, it is not surprising that there would be varying opinions on the track of meridian lines, especially in the case of the more esoteric "extra meridians," or "eight psychic channels." †

> † Some discussion on how descriptions of energy lines, acupuncture points, and meridians differ between traditions, and especially over time, were included in Section II.

Preparing for Practice

According to Taoist adept Chao Pi-ch'en, whose nineteenth century text was translated by Lu, one prepares for advanced energetic meditation by circulating breath [meaning *qi*] in the "eight psychic channels." According to Chao, failure to prepare correctly will lead to impurities remaining in the body, under which conditions the alchemical "Agent" [*dan* /elixir] cannot be created. [102] It is instructive to note some of the unusual sensations Chao experienced during his meditation practice, such as the perception of brightly colored lights and a feeling of disembodiment. ‡

> ‡ Chapter 26 includes notes on dangerous "energy practices," includ-
> ing possible psychological dangers.

As with other Taoist-alchemical practices, the goal of microcosmic orbit meditation is to draw energy into the lower *dan tian* below the navel, transmute it, and then direct it to the solar plexus, in a process referred to as "merging of forces in the 'yellow hall'" of the solar plexus.

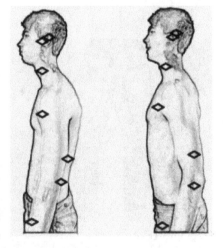

Diagrams 5-10

More Optimal Alignment of the Glands

Can posture and intention merge to influence "energy" and gland function? The left image illustrates less optimal alignment of glandular system. The right, more optimal alignment. The diamonds on each diagram indicate the "seven glands" described by Chang; those are, from top to bottom, the pineal, pituitary, thyroid, thymus, pancreas, adrenals, and sexual glands.

The Glandular System, Alignment, and Energetic Practice

There is an anti-aging and empowering exercise that can only briefly be introduced here. Inspiration for the practice derives from orbital meditation and related energy practices that regard the glandular system as "spark plugs," and are based Chang's principle of, "the glands as transformers." The practice is a good example of how posture and proper support of the body can merge with intentionality to trigger a synergistic effect that can supercharge the body's subtle energy system.

There are physical and intentional components to the practice. The physical part involves optimal alignment of the glands through posture, and activation of specific acupuncture meridians as myofascial piezoelectric structures. Directed intention activates the non-physical aspects.

The exercise is based on the principle that when the glands are more optimally aligned, a synergistic effect is produced that allows the mind-body system to function more ideally. Diagrams 5-10 are examples of less optimally aligned glandular systems.

When, in meditation or other quiet practice, the body is properly aligned, and attention is then focused on the glands along the body's center axis, the practice "charges" and transforms the exercise into a yogic practice. Correctly performed, the exercise produces a palpable influence on gland functioning. The resulting sensation is pleasant; it is that of a buzzy electric current running through the center of the body. For new practitioners, the exercise is best studied while in a sitting posture, however, the technique can also be practiced while standing.

To initiate the practice, assume a posture that triggers the tensional structures that run next to the spine. These fascial-tensional elements based on the myofascial lines described by Peter Dorsher, MD, *[103] are illustrated in Diagram 5-11. Next, while supporting as much of your frame as possible through myofascial tension support, relax all other unnecessary tension. This is a critical step, since release of excess tension is the precursor that allows the power of intention to interact with the glands. Next, intention is directed to the more optimally aligned glandular system.

*Myofascial meridians as fascial-tensional structures were introduced in Section II

For new practitioners, learning to suspend the body through consciously activated tension along the myofascial bands that parallel the spine can be challenging. This is quite different from the "normal" support of the body, which, through aging, relies increasingly on fulcrums. **

When you support the body through more reliance on myofascial-tensional lines, the muscles and myofascial elements next to the spine complain in

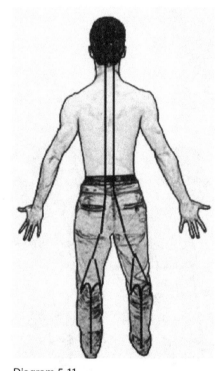

Diagram 5-11

Myofascial Meridian

Myer's "superficial back line." The myofascial lines, as anatomical representations of acupuncture meridian lines were described in Section II.

Diagram based on image in Peter Dorsher, MD, "Myofascial Meridians as Anatomical Evidence of Acupuncture Channels" [104]

response to you asking them to more actively support the body's weight. The goal is first to identify, and then over time prefer, the more engaged bouncy-stretchy meridian support of the body. Naturally, this results from regular practice.

** Soft tissue vs. fulcrum support of the body is covered in more detail in Section XI

The final step is to direct the influence of attention toward the glandular body centers. Although the effect of this alignment has not been scientifically studied, the impression is that the combination of posture and attention combine to activate health benefits in the endocrine glands.

When correctly performed, over time, the practitioner will experience certain changes. These observations include the perception of increased warmth in the area of the thymus in the center of the chest. With continued practice, one will also notice other sensations that are suggestive of hormonal and anti-aging benefits, such as increased confidence, improved mood, and a healthful flush of blood to the face.

Chapter 26

Warnings and Possible Dangers

$\mathcal{M}$editation is almost always beneficial. Recent studies by Harvard researchers show that, for regular practitioners, meditation decreases the amygdala's "fight or flight" stress response, and, significantly, the healthful benefits have been shown to extend to other aspects of the practitioner's life and promote emotional regulation.[105] Other research confirming the value of meditation includes a study conducted by UCLA's Department of Neurology, which showed that the brains of long-time meditation practitioners resist aging, and that meditators have "younger brains." According to the study:

> On average, the brains of long-term meditators were 7.5 years younger at age 50 than the brains of non-meditators, and an additional 1 month and 22 days younger for every year after 50. [106]

Further demonstrating the benefits of meditation, other research has documented how meditation could positively influence the immune system. In one particular study, scientists measured the body's natural killer cells and other immune system activity before and after forty minutes of meditation. Participants were divided into two groups: one group practiced an energetic meditation technique, the other did not. The study results demonstrated that the *qigong* meditation group showed a significant increase in natural killer cells, along with other immune system enhancements. [107]

Energetic meditation techniques develop calmness and promote self-healing. However, in the case of more intensive practices, some techniques can potentially be physically and emotionally challenging. Thus, more intense forms of energetic meditation should always be undertaken under the watchful guidance of a qualified teacher.

This chapter describes three categories of possible dangers that the practitioner should be aware of: 1) Potential nervous system and hormonal issues that may be associated with some more intense types of practice. 2) Dangers associated with "forcing" energy. 3) Dangers associated with seeking power.

Possible Danger 1: Nervous System and Hormonal Issues

The first category of potential danger concerns the stress of some types of practices on the hormonal and nervous systems. Thus, it is recommended that caution should be exercised in more intensive styles of meditation. Chang explains that some practices are potentially harmful when the individual "overloads" the body's energetic system. In one example, he describes stress to the diaphragm during the practice of "Immortal Breathing":

> Immortal breathing brings into the body very powerful levels of energy, and if the body is not sufficiently strong to handle it, nerves and glands may "burn out" from an overload of energy. [108]

Because of the broad use of the term, certain types of *qigong* practices are also considered forms of meditation. In China, there is a recognized psychiatric disorder related to those more intensive practices called "qigong deviation syndrome" (QDS). The condition tends to manifest in individuals with underlying psychiatric disorders. Some details from a published study on the disorder, including a case study of one individual, are included in Endnote. [109] †

> † Related discussions on the sometimes negative psychological side-effects of "energy practice" will be presented in Section VI, in the section covering *kundalini*.

In terms of psychological disturbances resulting from some forms of more intensive energetic practice, a report by one Western teacher of Eastern mind-arts (who wishes to remain anonymous) is included here. A master-level martial artist and healer, he shares his personal experiences relating to an especially intensive energetic practice:

> By the end of the week, I began to show symptoms of what is called "ultra-deviation" or Zeng Wang Xiang Gong... I began to experience green hallucinations and had an experience where it felt like my skeletal structure entered the back of my neck. I also began to have some strange thoughts or voices come through my head ... I believed I was going crazy... As the symptoms progressed and we [students in the class] began to panic, and we were told [by the teacher] "do not tell anyone about what is happening." During this stage, I would often wake up during the night vibrating like an enormous cell phone. There were many strange mental effects including voices and visual hallucinations. [110]

Due to the possibility of psychological stress that some practices can produce, anyone with a history of psychological or psychiatric disorders should be especially cautious before beginning any intensive *qigong* practice. As a rule, be sure to seek qualified psychological guidance before engaging in an intensive energy practice.

Possible Danger 2: Directing Physical Force Within the Body

Regardless of the discipline, a good rule of thumb is that practice should proceed in a gradual and relaxed manner. However, even greater caution applies to practices that involve the focused direction of physical pressures within the body.

This warning applies to *daoyin*, along with practices from other traditions where the devotee, through stretching, intensive breathing, diaphragm control, and bodily contortion manipulates the sense of pressure within the body. The warning applies to those examples where inordinate amounts of physical force are self-directed toward the heart or upper chest, as any excessive physical pressure to these areas can be extremely dangerous. These examples pertain to systems that incorporate the use of "forceful" pressure to the body as a means of manipulating internal energy. Since these can be potentially injurious to the practitioner, they will not be described here in more detail.

Possible Danger 3: Seeking Power

One of the most frequent warnings in the world's yogic and spiritual traditions has to do with the quest for power. An example of the kind of power that is ascribed to the practice of energetic meditation is the story of Lama Tsongkhapa. In that example, Tsongkhapa was said to have the psychic ability to control fire. According to reports, he once directed his intention to extinguish flames that threatened to destroy his monastery, [111] There are many other examples of a yogi or advanced meditator's expression of power.

However, regardless of whatever "powers" might appear, the best advice is that a practitioner not only ignore their appearance, but not seek it in the first place. The quest to attain power is universally considered a dangerous trap. The best rule to follow is to keep in mind that whatever power or enlightenment may come, it will come of its own, if at all, and the practitioner should remain unattached.

Chapter 27

Energetic Meditation: Alternative Views

*C*omparisons can be made between various meditation traditions, some of which provide more clues as to the meaning of "internal energy." As noted earlier, although there are important differences between the Tibetan *tantric* and the Taoist energetic meditation systems, there are also important similarities. It advances our discussion of the subject to consider whether these similarities might lead us to a better understanding of the *life force*.

This chapter focuses on three topics: the first concerns the effects of energetic practices on optimal physiology and mind-body functioning, referencing traditions such as Tibetan *tantric* and Taoist meditation practices. The second considers an area at the top of the head that, in the Taoist and TCM traditions, is called *bai hui*. A final point that is briefly addressed concerns the practitioner's experiences of "energy" along the "central channel," which is associated with the energy center of the lower abdomen.

Entrainment → Internal Coherence → Amplified Peace

The first topic takes a closer look at shared characteristics between Tibetan *tantric* and Taoist meditation practices. It concerns the psychophysiological effect of "energetic" practices on the practitioner, and, more specifically, it looks at the power of attention in terms of influencing one's psychophysiology.

Covered in more detail later, attention to one's biological oscillator, or rhythm, while one is in a relaxed state tends to induce a synchronizing, or harmonizing, influence with other bodily rhythms. This results in a physiologically measurable state called *entrainment*.

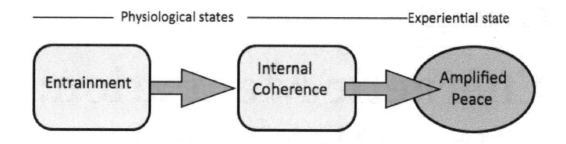

Diagram 5-12

Entrainment, Internal Coherence, and *Amplified Peace*

While in the entrainment mode, a practitioner can intentionally shift into the *internal coherence mode*, which can lead to the experiential state of *amplified peace.*

The ability to consciously induce *entrainment* ‡ has important implications for meditators. This is because the *entrainment* mode allows the experienced practitioner to intentionally shift into a deeper state of *internal coherence.*

> ‡ Having to do with the synchronization of biological rhythms. *Entrainment* is defined and discussed in more detail in Sections VII and IX.

While in the *internal coherence* mode, the subject's heart activity achieves a more stable pattern, which is associated with increased parasympathetic (non-stress and mind-body healing) activity.[112] * This is the aspect of the nervous system that induces relaxation and allows the body to engage in self-repair.

As documented by Tiller, and as illustrated in Diagram 5-12, subjects engaged in the *internal coherence* mode can enter a special experiential state, which Tiller refers to as *amplified peace.*

> * Section IX, Chapter 47, includes a graph of the internal coherence compared with other psychophysiological modes

Two kinds of observations regarding that experiential state warrant our attention. The first has to do with how subjects in experimental studies describe their experience as the sensation of "an inner electrical equilibrium." This observation pertains to the practitioner's report of their experience of a balance of electrical sensations throughout their body. Is it possible that their reports are of the same class of sensations reported by Taoist and Tibetan *tantric* practitioners since ancient times, describing the flow of "energy" through the body during meditation?

The next observation pertains to the transpersonal aspect of amplified peace. Research suggests that the experience aids the individual in achieving profound insight while engaged in the state, while Tiller describes how individuals report their experience as one where **"deeper than normal state of peace and centeredness is felt."** More discussion of the *internal coherence* mode is presented in Section X.

The "hundred gatherings," or *baihui* point

The second topic considers an energy center at the top of the head. The area is an important location in both the Tibetan *tantric* and Taoist energy systems, as well as other energetic traditions. In traditional Chinese medicine, the point, at the top of the head is referred to as "hundred gatherings," or *baihui* (百會), * and in modern acupuncture is referred to as Du-20.

The location and nature of this point provides yet another clue regarding the mystery of "energy" in meditation traditions. The full potential of this point is realized by experienced meditators when they consciously focus on it during practice.

> * Acupuncture point Du-20 is located on the top of the head, at the midpoint of the anterior hairline. It is the midpoint of the line connecting the apexes of the two ears.

For disciples of *tantric* meditation, the area is the focal point of secret practices concerning the melting of the "white" *thigle* drops. When an experienced meditator sits in a calm and inwardly focused state, and then directs attention to this point, it can induce a peaceful, total-body energetic experience.

However, the area is also important for other applications. For example, in TCM, the surface point at the top of the head is the acupuncture point used to treat vertigo and dizziness. However, treatment protocols describing the point suggest that the locus is not only used to calm the *shen* mental-emotional system, but also to stimulate the interconnectivity of the entire system from the top of the skull to the perineum. Demonstrating the potency of this acupuncture point, it is used to treat prolapse of the rectum and uterus. Presented for research and discussion purposes, the technique that follows is a more advanced energetic meditation technique, where the location plays a central role.

DISCLAIMER/ WARNING: The following is a more advanced meditation technique. It is included here for research and discussion purposes only. It should NOT be practiced without proper guidance from a qualified instructor of energetic meditation.

As discussed earlier, directed attention to a specific location within the body can sometimes induce a change to not only the specific point and immediate area, but sometimes the entire system from the top of the head to the perineum. What follows is a description of the experiences that a well-trained meditator will sometimes observe while focusing on acupuncture point *baihui* / Du-20.

While focusing inward attention on the point inside the skull, the experienced meditator will often notice a remarkable range of calming sensations. For example, when relaxed and focused, attention will sometimes produce a sudden release of chest tension, along with deepening and relaxation of breathing. This is an indication that the consciously directed attention is affecting the entire system.

The Universal Nature of Experience

Reports like these suggest the universal nature of experiences shared between various energetic meditation traditions. As in the example just cited, focus directed to the area can generate responses that are felt throughout the body. This commonality of experience suggests cross-cultural evidence for the location being a significant area.

One must wonder if sensations of flushing and relaxation, spanning from the genitals to the cranium, might be of the same class of sensations reported by Aristotle and Heraclitus. It appears that they also believed a fluid-connectedness to exist, which unites the highest with the lowest aspects of the physical body.

The implications for these kinds of cross-culture shared experiences seem too coincidental to be ignored. As McEvilley suggests, the knowledge of the energetic relationship between brain and lower torso may have spread between cultures of the ancient world. However, this may not have only been due to the sharing of lore, but perhaps because of the practitioner's universal experience with the power of directed attention.

> Touching below the navel when inner heat is activated causes you to feel pleasure in your entire nervous system, especially your crown chakra. The bliss of inner heat begins at the secret *chakra* [base of the penis] . . .[113]

As a final note to close this chapter, another clue as to the universal nature of these kinds of experiences is revealed in the way some points along the body's central axis can have a profound effect on the entire system. Here, reference is made to key locations where subtle energy is said to concentrate, and once again we see correspondence between the Taoist and *tantric* systems. Consider, for example, the importance placed on the lower abdomen energy center that the Taoists refer to as the *dan tian,* ** which also corresponds to an important energy center in the Tibetan *tantric* tradition. In terms of *tantric* practice, the importance of this energy center is emphasized through advice that the Dalai Lama once gave to Lama Yeshe: "Pressing a little just below the navel helps to increase bliss and inner heat."

** Depicted in Section III, Figure 3-5

Conclusion to Section V

*I*t cannot be said with certainty that *buddhahood*, immortality, or "mystical union with the Tao," exist in an objective way. Likewise, at this point, it is impossible to say whether a form of yet-to-be-identified "energy" exists that can be manipulated either through *tantric,* Taoist *neidan,* or other practices. However, what can be stated with certainty is that an experienced practitioner, while maintaining a peaceful and calm state, can positively influence his or her nervous and hormonal systems, brain wave patterns, and body rhythms.

This observation suggests that similar neurophysiological profiles may be shared between not only the highly accomplished *tantric* and Taoist masters, but also the accomplished meditator of every tradition. The regular practice of meditation leads to predictable psychophysiological benefits, while enhancing both physical and mental health. It triggers the body's production of anti-stress hormones, and increases pleasure–enhancing, mood-regulating neurotransmitters, like dopamine and serotonin.[114]

> Whenever concentration, bliss, and clarity are strong, you do not need to use these technical meditations. At those times, you simply let go and contemplate. When you reach the point where you can naturally and effortlessly hold the winds in strong vase meditation at the navel chakra, the airs will automatically produce blazing inner fire in the central channel.
>
> — Lama Yeshe [115]

Is "Energy" more Important than Technique?

As a practitioner reaches advanced levels of energetic skill, use of a specific technique becomes increasingly less important. At the most sophisticated stages, the adept's experience of inner peace suggests a profound common ground. When the discipline comes to fruition, the adept can enter the stage of experience Yeshe refers to as "clean-clear penetrative wisdom." [116]

Endnotes

1 Yangpönga, Gyalwa, *Secret map of the body: Visions of the human energy structure, Guarisco, Elio,* (translator) Shang Shung Foundation, 2015 p. 31.

2 Yangpönga, p. 31.

3 As described in the opening pages, in general, Chinese characters are transliterated using the *pinyin* system. However, there are exceptions where Wade-Giles transliteration of Chinese is relied on. Examples of Wade-Giles usage in the present section include *Tao* instead of Dao, and for consistency of style, *ho Tao* for "union with the Tao" is used instead of *he Dao.* Other examples of Wade-Giles transliteration in this chapter includes *Tao Te Ching,* and *Te.*

4 Yangpönga, Gyalwa, *Secret map of the body: Visions of the human energy structure, Guarisco, Elio,* (translator) Shang Shung Foundation, 2015, p. 63.

5 Yeshe, Thubten, *The bliss of inner fire: Heart practice of the six yogas of naropa,* Simon and Schuster, 2005, p. 145.

6 At this juncture, it is useful to comment on the varied meaning and definitions of *thigle.*

As applied to Tibetan *tantric* meditation and yoga, *thigle* is a "seminal drop" which carries "essence." In this context, the term most often refers to a male's sexual essence. However, there are other meanings. *Thigle* can also refer to the spheres of light that appear to the initiate during practice. *Thigle* also refers to the two principal essences of the body that are worked with in *gsang snags* secret mantra practice known as *thigle kar dmar.*

7 Yangpönga, Gyalwa, Secret map of the body: Visions of the human energy structure, Guarisco, Elio, (translator) Shang Shung Foundation, 2015 p. 55.

8 Yangpönga, p.91.

9 Ibid.

10 Chuang Tzu (Zhuangzi) as cited by Kohn, Livia, "Taoist insight meditation," *Taoist meditation and longevity techniques,* University of Michigan Center for Chinese Studies, 1989 p. 196.

11 Chuang Tzu, p. 39.

12 Yangpönga, Gyalwa, *Secret map of the body: Visions of the human energy structure,* Guarisco, Elio, (translator), Shang Shung Foundation, 2015., p. 46, 51, 55.

13 Yangpönga, p. 55.

14 An interview with Dudjom Tersar lineage holder, Shenphen Dawa Rinpoche, from the website: http://www.tersar.org/continuity.html

15 https://www.lamayeshe.com/glossary/term/dharmakaya-skt-tib-ch%C3%B6-ku-eng-truth-body

16 Needham, Joseph, *Science and civilization in China,* Vol. 2, Cambridge University Press, 1983, p. 141.

17 McEvilley, C., *The shape of ancient thought: Comparative studies in Greek and Indian philosophies,* Allworth Press, New York, 2002, p. 27.

18 As cited by McEvilley, p. 211.

19 McEvilley, C., *The shape of ancient thought: Comparative studies in Greek and Indian philosophies,* Allworth Press, New York, 2002, p. 211.

20 McEvilley, p. 210.

21 Ibid.

22 Ibid

23 Pearl, Bill, *Keys to the inner universe: World's best built man,* Typecraft, Inc Pasadena 1979, pp. 28-29.

24 Rossi, Ernest, *The psychobiology of mind-body healing: New concepts of therapeutic hypnosis* (Revised Edition) W.W. Norton, 1993.

25 Perhaps the most difficult to observe and work bodily rhythm has to do with the ebb and flow of the cerebral spinal fluid on its back and forth journey from the ventricles of the brain to the sacrum. Although the cerebral spinal fluid rhythm is too subtle to work with directly, it is possible for a person to consciously interact with the rhythm by learning to observe the body's subtle responses to it. Examples include the body's response to the rhythm (as described by Upledger) as the slight inward to outer and back again shifting of the clavicle in a movement that is separate from breath, and the subtle outward and inward flaring of the pelvic girdle. A few more examples of working with this rhythm to enhance athletic training are included in Section VII.

See John Upledger, D.O., *Your inner physician and you,* North Atlantic Books, Berkley, 1997 p. 12.

26 Upledger, John, D.O., *Your inner physician and you,* North Atlantic Books, Berkley, 1997.

27 Elio Guarisco, commentator on the works of the tantric yogi Yangpönga, describes the *vajra* body as "a mandala* that acts as the basis for the divine path, whose subtle aspects are the male and female deities." Guarisco, Elio, (translator), Yangpönga, Gyalwa, *Secret map of the body: Visions of the human energy structure,* Shang Shung Foundation, 2015 p. 30.

* A geometric figure representing the universe in Hindu and Buddhist symbolism

28 Markides, Kyriacos C. *The magus of Strovolos: The extraordinary world of a spiritual healer* Penguin Books, London, 1985 p. 9.

29 Markides., Kindle location 204.

30 Yangpönga, Gyalwa, *Secret map of the body: Visions of the human energy structure, Guarisco, Elio,* (translator) Shang Shun Foundation, 2015 p. 88.

31 Steiner, Rudolf, *Knowledge of higher worlds,* Rudolph Steiner Press, p. 146.

32 Steiner, p. 68.

33 Ibid., p. 146.

34 Myss, Caroline, *Anatomy of the spirit,* Crown/Random House, New York 1996, p. 68.

35 Myss, p. 87.

36 Ibid., pp. 29, 87, 129.

37 Tiller, William, *Some science adventures with real magic,* Pavior, 2005 p. 23.

38 Transduction is the process of converting of energy from one form to another and is covered in more detail in Section XII.

39 Tiller, William, *Some science adventures with real magic,* Pavior, 2005 p. 23.

40 From the *Chandogya Upanishad,* as quoted by McEvilley, See McEvilley, C., *The shape of ancient thought: Comparative studies in Greek and Indian philosophies,* Allworth Press, New York, 2002 p. 206.

41 There are a few demonstrations of *tummo* practice that can be viewed on the internet. One can be accessed via the link: https://www.youtube.com/watch?v=GiJvD2BPOhA

42 The number of frozen wet shawls that an adept is expected to dry as a demonstration of mastery varies from lineage to lineage.

43 Yangpönga, Gyalwa, *Secret map of the body: Visions of the human energy structure,* Guarisco, Elio, (translator and editor) Shang Shun Foundation, 2015 p. 91.

44 Yangpönga, Gyalwa, Gyalwa, *Secret map of the body: Visions of the human energy structure,* Guarisco, Elio, (translator) Shang Shun Foundation, 2015, pp. 59-60.

45 Yangpönga, p.96.

46 Ibid., p. 144.

47 Ibid., p. 4.

48 Ibid., p. 119.

49 Lama Yeshe, *The bliss of inner fire: Heart practice of the six yogas of Naropa,* Wisdom Publications, Sommerville, MA 1998 p. 83.

50 Yeshe p. 144.

51 Ibid., p. 182. The following definition of non-duality as provided in *The Bliss of Inner Fire: Heart practice of the Six yogas of Naropa:* "Emptiness, non-existence; fundamental nature and totality. Non-duality is the absolute nature of the self and all phenomenon; ultimately, everything is empty of existing dualistically, inherently, truly, or from its own side."

52 Ibid., p. 21.

53 Ibid.

54 Thondup, Tulku *Incarnation: The history and mysticism of the tulku tradition of Tibet,* Shambala Publications, 2011.

55 Lama Yeshe, *The bliss of inner fire: Heart practice of the six yogas of Naropa,* Wisdom publications, Sommerville, MA 1998 p. 83.

56 Yangpönga, Gyalwa, *Secret map of the body: Visions of the human energy structure,* Guarisco, Elio, (translator/editor) Shang Shun Foundation, 2015, p. 91.

57 Norbu, Chögyal Namkhai, *The Crystal and the way of light: Sutra, tantra, and dzogchen,* Shambhala, Snow Lion Publications, 2000, p. 124

58 Yangpönga, Gyalwa, *Secret map of the body: Visions of the human energy structure,* Guarisco, Elio, (translator and editor) Shang Shun Foundation, 2015 p. 92.

59 Ibid., p. 92.

60 Lama Yeshe, *The bliss of inner fire: Heart practice of the six yogas of naropa,* wisdom publications, Sommerville, MA 1998 p. 133.

61 Yeshe, p. 146.

62 Ibid., p. 86.

63 Ibid., p. 51.

64 Yangpönga, Gyalwa, *Secret map of the body: Visions of the human energy structure,* Guarisco, Elio, (translator) Shang Shun Foundation, 2015, p. 21.

65 Yangpönga, 158.

66 http://www.rinpoche.com/stories/krmpamiracles.htm

67 Lama Yeshe, *The bliss of inner fire: Heart practice of the six yogas of naropa,* wisdom publications, Sommerville, MA 1998 p. 155.

68 Roth, Harold, *Original Tao: Inward training (Nei-Yeh) and the foundations of mysticism,* Columbia University Press, 1999 p. 4.

69 Roth., p. 6.

70 Ibid., p. 11.

71 Chao Shou-cheng, as cited by Roth in *Original Tao.* See Roth, Harold, *Original tao: Inward training (Nei-yeh) and the foundations of mysti-*

cism, Columbia University Press, 1999, p. 12.

72 Blofeld, John, *The secret and sublime: Taoist mysteries and magic,* Dutton, 1973 p. 181.

73 Tao Yeh, Chapter 11, as translated by Harold Roth, Roth, Harold, *Original tao: Inward training (Nei-Yeh) and the foundations of mysticism,* Columbia University Press, 1999 p. 66.

74 Roth p. 14.

75 Following Wing's suggestion that *te,* the middle character of the *Tao Te Ching* be translated as "power" instead of "virtue," which, as introduced earlier, is a later Confucian influence. According to Wing, *Te* speaks to potentiality of the Tao, a central theme of Taoist practice. See also, Waley, Arthur, *The way and its power: Lao Tzu's Tao Te Ching,* Grove Press, 1958.

76 Wing, R.L., *The tao of power: Lao Tzu's classic guide to leadership, influence, and excellence,* Doubleday, NY 1986 pp. 12-13.

77 Wing

78 Kohn, Livia, "Guarding the one: Concentrative meditation in Taoism," *Taoist meditation and longevity techniques,* Center for Chinese Studies, The University of Michigan, p. 125.

79 Kohn, Livia, "Guarding the one," *Taoist Meditation and longevity techniques,* Michigan University Press, p. 127.

80 As cited by Livia Kohn, , See Kohn, Livia, "Guarding the one," *Taoist meditation and longevity techniques,* Michigan University Press, 1989, p. 129.

81 As cited by Livia Kohn, See Kohn, Livia, "Guarding the one," *Taoist meditation and longevity techniques,* Michigan University Press, 1989, p. 150.

82 Kohn, Livia, "Guarding the one," *Taoist Meditation and longevity techniques,* Michigan University Press, 1989, p. 133.

83 Kohn, pp. 135, 155.

84 Blofeld, John *The secret and sublime: Taoist mysteries and magic,* Dutton, 1973 p. 127.

85 *Hsiu Chen Pi* or *"Esoteric Instruction on the regeneration of the primary vitalities"* as translated by Joseph Needham, *Science and civilization in China,* Cambridge University Press, 1983, pp. 35-37.

86 Adapted from the translation by Joseph Needham, in *Science and civilization in China.* See Needham, Joseph, *Science and civilization in China,* Vol. 6, Cambridge University Press, 1983, p. 26.

87 炼精化气、炼气化神

88 Needham, Joseph, *Science and civilization in China,* Vol. 5, p. 237.

89 Adapted from Joseph Needham's translation Passage from *Chih*

Kua' Chi ("Pointing the Way Home to Life Eternal"), part of a collection of Taoist treatises called the *Tao Tsang (Daozang)* 道藏 Joseph Needham, Science *and civilization in China* Vol. 5, pp. 34-35.

90 Wile, Douglas, *The art of the bedchamber: The Chinese sexual yoga classics including women's solo meditation texts,* State University of New York, 1992, p. 38.

91 Wile, Douglas, *The art of the bedchamber: The Chinese sexual yoga classics including women's solo meditation texts,* State University of New York, 1992, .p. 41.

92 "Daoist Meditations," *Tai chi and alternative health,* issue 38 p. 24.

93 Chao Pi-ch'en, *The secrets of cultivating essential nature and eternal life,* As translated by Kuan Lu Yu, Taoist *yoga alchemy and immortality,* Samuel Weiser, York Beach, ME, 1973, p. 87

94 Chang, Stephen T., *The complete system of self-healing internal exercises,* Tao Publishing, San Francisco, 1986, p. 202.

95 Chang, p. 171.

96 Ibid., p. 199.

97 Ibid.

98 Ibid., p. 201.

99 Pearl, Bill, *Keys to the inner universe: World's best built man,* Typecraft Inc., Pasadena, p. 32

100 Weiqiao, Jiang, *Quiet sitting with master Yinshi,* as cited by Miura, Kunio, "The revival of qi," *Taoist Meditation and longevity techniques.* p. 333.

101 Lu Kuan Yu, Taoist *yoga alchemy and immortality,* Samuel Weiser, York Beach, ME, 1973, p. 35

102 Lu, p. 26.

103 Ibid.

104 Dorsher, Peter, "Myofascial meridians as anatomical evidence of acupuncture channels," Vol. 21, No. 2, 2009, p. 4.

105 https://news.harvard.edu/gazette/story/2012/11/meditations-positive-residual-effects/

106 http://www.phoenixisrisen.co.uk/?p=15911

107 Before and after a 40-minute meditation, the levels of (NK) cell activity and Interleukin (IL)-2 in venous blood were simultaneously measured to study changes. The study found that the levels of NK cell activity and IL-2 showed a significant increase when compared to the findings achieved from a study conducted on a group of subjects who had no experience in *qigong* meditation. HIGUCHI, Yuzo, KOTANI, Yasunori·HIGUCHI, Hironobu,·MINEGISHI Yukiko, TANAKA Yukio· Chang YU Yong· and Shinichiro MOMOSE "Immune Changes during

Cosmic Orbit Meditation of Qigong," *Journal of international society of life information science,* Vol.18, No.2, September 2000 [Procedures of the Tenth Symposium of Life Information Science] .

159.

115 Yeshe, p. 147.

108 Chang, Stephen T., *The complete system of self-healing internal exercises,* Tao Publishing, San Francisco, 1986, p. 200.

116 Yeshe.

109 In Western diagnostic systems, QDS syndromes are often labeled "Culture Bound Phenomenon." Psychological effects associated with the disorder include motor phenomena, perceptual changes and the patient's report of a sense of chilliness, skin itching, numbness, soreness and feeling bloated. From "Appendix III: Crackdown on falun gong," *Dangerous minds: political psychiatry in China today and its origins in the Mao Era.* Published by Human Rights Watch and Geneva Initiative on Psychiatry. August 2002. The following is one of the case studies included with the report.

CASE STUDY

Mr. A is a 22-year-old unmarried worker. He began to [teach] himself Qigong from books the "Wu Qin Xi" (exercise mimicking the gestures of five animals) on November 26, 1984 for the treatment of lumbago. Ten days later, he suddenly had "special senesthesiopathy" with "Qi" flowing adversely in the head and abdomen. When "Qi" flowed into his head, he felt fullness of head and chest distress. When showing [demonstrating] a Qigong gesture, he suffered agony and anxiety, and even attempted to commit suicide. Two hours later he was sent to Shanghai Institute of Qigong for help. Guided by a Qigong master he recovered. The next day he became delirious and claimed that he could hear the voice of evil spirits; he prayed to Buddha for help but only lost his self-control. During the intervals between the attacks, the patient was normal. But he could not work normally due to insomnia and difficulty in coping with Qigong deviation.

On January 15, 1985, the patient got upset because he was prevented by his family from doing Qigong exercise. He felt so hopeless that he attempted to commit suicide by bumping his head into a car. He was then sent to a hospital for psychiatric treatment. There were no abnormal findings in his physical and laboratory check-up. There was no history of psychosis in his family either. He was treated in a timely fashion by ECT. Two days later, his father took him back home. Now he is followed up by a Qigong master and is so far in good health state.

110 Personal e-mail correspondence with the author. Name purposefully emitted.

111 Lama Yeshe, *The bliss of inner fire: Heart practice of the six yogas of Naropa*

Wisdom Publications, Sommerville, MA 1998 p. 158.

112 Tiller, William A, et al., "Cardiac coherence: A new, noninvasive measure of autonomic nervous system order" *Alternative Therapies,* Vol. 2, No. 1, January 1996.

113 Yeshe, *The bliss of inner fire: Heart practice of the six yogas of Naropa,* Wisdom Publications, Sommerville, MA 1998, p. 145.

114 Newberg, Andrew MD, How *God changes your brain: Breakthrough findings from a leading neuroscientist.* Ballantine Books, NY, 2010, p.

Introduction to Sections VI and VII

*P*revious sections have focused on relatively mainstream discussions of the meaning of internal energy for healing and meditation practices. Supporting points for those discussions have relied on documentation taken from reliable sources that could be used, depending on one's viewpoint, to argue either for or against the theory that "internal energy," such as *qi* or *prana*, might or might not exist in a form akin to electromagnetism, as a yet-to-be-recognized *natural force*. However, when discussing the transmutation of sexual energy and the meaning of *qi* in martial arts, such as in the case of *t'ai-chi chüan*, the reliability of sources is sometimes questionable.

In the case of *t'ai-chi*, and Chinese martial arts literature in general, sources sometimes mix historical facts with myth; the origins of *t'ai-chi*, for example, are often traced to an enigmatic alchemist-monk. As will be addressed in Section VII, this claim is dubious, and mostly not regarded as credible by scholars. Likewise, many proposed *t'ai-chi* lineages also lack scholarly support. Consider the origin story of the Yang Lu-chan style, where some traditions hold that Yang learned his art by spying on Ch'en family practitioners, while other sources claim that the art can be traced to the discovery of a lost manual found in the back of a salt shop.

Are these origin stories important? Does it matter whether or not Grandfather Yang learned his *t'ai-chi* surreptitiously while observing martial arts practice in the Ch'en village, or if these are factual accounts or fairytales? For many, it may not. However, for some aficionados of the art, it is important to know if the discipline they practice was handed down by a master in a cloud-topped monastery many centuries ago. For them, it not only informs the discussion, but also affects their own skill development to consider that the genesis of their art was more recent. They care that the art might have developed from the collaboration of a group of individuals, who through trial and error developed their physical practice, along with the cultivation of a particular body-mind state. For the serious internal martial art practitioner, this is a crucial issue.

Myth Perceived as Fact

As in the example just cited, sometimes the origin of *t'ai-chi* is credited to a man named Zhang Sanfeng (Chang San-fang), but historical evidence does not support such an assertion. Martial arts historian Prof. Douglas Wile writes that Zhang was first suggested as the originator of *t'ai-chi* in the middle 1800s.[1][2]

The Zhang myth is a good place to begin our discussion on how tales can, over time, take on the aura of fact. According to one common *t'ai-chi* creation story, Zhang is said to have developed a fighting style based on his observations of, or his dreams about, a fight between a bird of prey and a snake. However, historians have been unable to ascertain if Zhang, supposedly an alchemist who lived, depending on the source, in either the twelfth, thirteenth, or fourteenth century, ever actually existed. In contrast, although historical evidence supports the notion that some *t'ai-chi* postures may be traceable to the Ch'en family village about three hundred years ago, [3][4] other evidence suggests that the practice developed more recently. [5]

In much the same way that a magical character named Zhang is said to have been the originator of *t'ai-chi*, the legend of the *Wudang (Wu Tang)* monastery being the birthplace of internal martial arts also captures the imagination. The source of this legend is no doubt the fertile imaginations of the writers of Chinese books, such as Huang Zongxi in 1669, followed by the filmmakers and comic book publishers of the twentieth century. These sources elucidate the mountain monastery as the place where, for hundreds of years, monks trained in a style of "soft" martial arts, as a kind of *yin-yang* counterpoint to the "hard" combat skills of the famed Shaolin monastery.

Fables masquerading as facts are found in other areas, and the water becomes murkier still when one discusses the possibility of "secret arts" said to derive from the supposed merging of Buddhist and Taoist "internal energy" practices. Although there might have been some exchange between Taoists and Buddhists, especially in the early years of the first millennium when Buddhism entered China, there is no evidence that Buddhist monks and Taoist recluses exchanged information regarding their respective fighting systems. Nevertheless, some authors claim this was the case.

Unlike the Shaolin monastery, which was destroyed for the final time in 1928 due to its political and paramilitary activities, pre-Communist Chinese authorities had no reason to fear peaceful monks engaged in non-political practices. Thus, if secret (non-political) doctrines ever existed that represented a blend of Taoist and Buddhist practice, they would still be in use today. Moreover, with *few* exceptions, Buddhists from India entering China were not concerned with the development of internal power, and certainly a monk's goal would never be to attain the physical immortality sought by Taoist *neidan* alchemists.

Although it is possible that some variants of Indian or Tibetan *tantric tummo* "inner heat" meditation made their way into China, in general, the notion of "secretive" energetic training among Buddhist monks is not factually based. Nevertheless, claims of "secret traditions" can be found in popular stories relating to the martial arts in both the East and the West. In some cases, books, seminars, and online presentations from this genre are represented as "secrets of ancient Buddhist and Taoist arts," and their promotional material is designed to appeal to those seeking both "power" and, in the case of *tantric* yogic sexual practices, great sex. This may well be a salesperson's dream pitch, offering potential customers amazing power and an improved sex life for the price of a book or a seminar.

Caveats noted, in most cases, Asian fables are harmless; the serious student need only differentiate between popular beliefs and more academically supported information. Unfortunately, though, the proliferation of myth as historical fact is easily found in the work of some writers — often those translating texts published in Taiwan — who describe "secret" internal arts taught in "the ancient days of the *kung fu* art." One must consider whether this kind of merging of myth and tradition is helpful, or whether its prevalence in Asian martial arts comic books and films is a disservice to the reader.

Ultimately, the answer depends on who is reading the material and why. In the case of a teenager or young adult finding inspiration from a romantic story, myth merged with quasi-history can be inspirational. However, as a teacher of the internal tradition, I encourage those wishing to replicate the all-but-lost skills of a past generation to seek a deeper understanding and investigate the authentic roots of their practice. When they, like their predecessors in the martial arts, discover the essence of their practice, they will then be able to pass on this knowledge to future generations. Without such effort directed toward uncovering the authentic sources of their disciplines, the energetic arts will continue to wither, and fewer transmitters of deeper knowledge will be around in the future.

For a serious adult practitioner investigating the step-by-step evolution of the "soft" and "energetic" martial arts, larger-than-life stories of those arts born in a mountain-top monastery a thousand or more years ago are not helpful. Instead, for the mature seeker, it is more useful to ask questions about the evolutionary conditions that might have contributed to the art's initial development. For example, the term *neijiaquan* appears as early as Huang Pai-chia's (Huang Baijia) seventeenth-century *Neijia Quanfa* ("Boxing methods of the Internal School"). However, it did not become a common classifier of martial arts styles until the nineteenth century, [6] and for practical purposes, not until Sun Lu-tang's use of the term to characterize a category of martial arts based on "soft" power, in books published in the 1920s.

But, are these points important? Again, it depends on who wants to know and why. In the case of the serious student striving to *advance* optimal use of body and mind, and investigate what is purported to be the amazing skill of a past master, they must look into the question of whether something significant might have been discovered in the martial arts circles of China's northern plain in the late-nineteenth century. In the pages that follow, it will be argued that at that unique time and place, a new approach to what can be called integrated body-mind training sprang forth in a *systemized way*, that ultimately led to the art we know today as *t'ai-chi ch'üan*.

The authentic master of the future will be one who seeks to replicate the sublime skills described by pioneers of the art. It is their job to unearth clues that may reveal the essence of the art that, at present, lays buried deep within the enshrined tombs of past generations. We have the same mental powers and physiological aspects as those past masters, and so, if they were really able to perform amazing feats against opponents, so can we!

Clues to the realization of our body-mind potential reside in the instruction manuals and ancestral knowledge passed down from generation to generation. In order to place these clues within the correct context, consideration must be given not only to the written words of past masters, but also to their appearance in terms of social, political, and cultural factors. From these, we can discover a few things about past masters and how they trained, but we must also reflect on whether or not there could really be a secret *x factor* that led them to the pinnacle of skill.

Based on my experience of nearly five decades of study in both the West and East, the remarkable skills associated with nineteenth and twentieth-century *t'ai-chi* and other related arts are, even in Asia, largely all but lost. It is the sincere student's task to rediscover how past masters might have studied and trained, and then apply these insights to their own practice today. Following this scheme, the replication of great skills should not be so difficult, but it is important to ground these, not upon a shaky foundation of lore, but through a closer and unbiased look at more relevant historical evidence.

The Problem of Secrecy

Another challenge is how to evaluate claims from controversial texts, something which is particularly problematic when background information is unavailable. Consider a text cited in Section VI on topics concerning the transmutation of sexual energy. As a source, the section includes a text by an author who chose to avoid criticism and public scrutiny by keeping his identity secret, but despite the veracity of many aspects of his report being suspect, the information was nevertheless included because of the paucity of information on the subject — here I am referring to claims of a present-day female sex cult.

In the example just cited, the unknown author describes his encounters with the "White Tigresses," as he claims to have been allowed to associate with this secretive cult in Taiwan. Using the pseudonym Hsi Lai (literally, "Coming from the West"), the writer claims to have been privy to the inner sanctum of the cult, detailing, among other claims, the patroness's secrets that were employed to train young women in sexual arts. Hsi Lai further professes to have been granted access to otherwise closely held information, and to have been permitted to review handwritten copies of ancient texts related to the practice.

Such claims are extraordinary, but even though his writing is impossible to verify, I nonetheless cite Hsi Lai since any information on exotic Taoist female sexual cult practice is nearly impossible to come by (and besides, the material is fun to read). Even if only partly true, information like this could be of value to those interested in the subject of internal energy, especially in terms of female practices.

I do not want to be too critical of writers like Hsi Lai, who keep their sources or identities secret, as there are times where I've had to do the same. For example, in Section VIII, which discusses internal energy in martial arts, as per an agreement with one source, the identity of a scientist who proposes a hypothesis to explain the bio-mechanics of internal energy in martial arts is withheld, owing to his past role as a researcher in classified government projects. This creates a challenge for the reader. With source information kept secret, how is it possible to discern truth from falsehood? In examples like these, the reader must decide for themselves how to judge the veracity of the claims.

Dating Chinese Texts

Another problem arising from the intertwining of lore with fact concerns the dating of Chinese texts. Often, relevant texts are attributed to antiquity, or predated hundreds or even thousands of years earlier, in order to heighten their prestige and authority. Thus, the problem of dating material applies not only to determining the authenticity of a relatively recent text, but older ones as well. In some cases, texts determined to be between one and two hundred years old may be represented as being a thousand years of age or older.

To illustrate how the dating of "ancient" manuscripts applies to our discussion of internal energy, consider one of the most important texts of traditional Chinese medicine, the *Huangdi Neijing,* or *Yellow Emperor's Classic of Medicine.* Introduced in Section II, the *Neijing* presents a useful example of confusion over dating. Attributed to the Yellow (or "first") Emperor, the *Classic* is often said to have been written about five thousand years ago. In contrast, Joseph Needham dates the text to around 100 BCE, [7] while Wong and Wu, in their 1936 classic, *History of Chinese Medicine,* suggest that it was most probably written at the end of the Chou dynasty (249 CE). [8] However, in the introduction to Ilza Veith's well-known English language translation of the *Classic,* he informs us that the opening part of the text, under a different title, is first mentioned in the annals of the Han Dynasty (206 BCE – 25 CE). Furthermore, Veith contends that the earliest mention of the second part, the *Su Wen,* came in the second century CE.[9]

In examples like the *Emperor's Classic,* authority is sometimes ascribed to a text due to the Chinese reverence for antiquity, but is knowledge of the actual date important? If we were to trust that an ancient source of knowledge was truly available five thousand years ago, it would mean that the ancients did, as some traditionalists claim, have access to a perennial wisdom. If true, we would then be led to revere the knowledge of the wizened sages of a bygone era. However, if the foundational text of Chinese medicine was really an amalgam of medical knowledge compiled over the previous five or six centuries,[10] this would promote the idea of trial and error as a natural part of an evolving knowledge base.

If the knowledge is the product of trial and error over subsequent generations, this would inform the student that their own progress is part of an evolving process rather than something absolute, and acceptance of such a belief could encourage practitioners to deepen their own research. In this way, each has the opportunity to contribute to the encyclopedia of a continuing knowledge database. Such a position presents the revered text not as a mystical source originating thousands of years before the present era, but as a compendium of later Han and Chin dynasties, representing the best understanding of the practice of medicine at the time.

From my point of view, the *Nei Ching* is best understood as the product of an historical lineage of documents and ideas. This approach is especially relevant to the discussion of the meaning of *nei qi,* or "inner *qi,*" of traditional Chinese medicine. For example, it is useful to consider when and why "internal energy" was first believed to be separate from "breath." [11]

It is hoped that these comments and suggestions will be helpful to readers in their pursuit of understanding internal energy in the contexts of sexuality and the martial arts.

Endnotes

1 On the Zhang Sanfeng (Chang San-fang) myth, according to Professor Wile, "The name Zhang Sanfeng does not appear in the Ch'en family or Wu/Li/Hao family manuscripts and thus is a product of the last days of the Ch'ing or early Republican period," Wile, Douglas, *Tai-chi's ancestors*, Sweet Ch'i Press, 1999, p. 49.

It is useful to consider that Zhang is often cited by internal martial arts teachers, and especially *t'ai-chi ch'üan* teachers, as the founder of a style of martial arts at the Wudang (Wu Tang) Monastery in Hebei province. In this regard, author and publisher Michael Demarco cites noted sinologist Anna Seidel, who states, "His biographies and legends lack even the faintest allusion to his being a boxing master . . . We know next to nothing about Zhang Sanfeng's historical existence and his thought." (As cited by Michael DeMarco in "The Origin and Evolution of Taijiquan," *Journal of Asian Martial Arts*, Vol. 1, No. 1, 1992, Seidel, Anna, *"A Taoist Immortal of the Ming Dynasty," Self and society in Ming thought*, W. T. Barry, editor, New York: Columbia University Press, 1970, pp. 483-531.

2 The martial arts scholar Gu Liuxin detailed Tang Hao's investigation of the Wudang myth in the Study of Shaolin and Wudang, where he writes: "In 1920, he [Tang] used lots of historical material to prove that Bodhidharma and Zhang Sanfeng knew nothing about marital arts, and that at the theory that Shaolin martial arts started from the Indian monk Bodhidharma and that taijiquan was invented by Zhang San-feng was incorrect." As cited by Brian Kennedy in *Chinese Martial Arts Training Manuals: An historical survey*, North Atlantic Books, 2005, Berkeley, CA, 2005, p. 48.

Kennedy goes on to say, "While it is true that the Wudang Mountains were home to a great number of Taoist temples, it is equally true that none of the three Wudang martial arts were invented there or owe much of their development to that area." Kennedy, p. 84.

3 Wile, Douglas, *Lost t'ai-chi classics from the late Ch'ing dynasty*, State University of New York, 1996, p. 16.

4 DeMarco, Michael, *"The origin and evolution of taijiquan," Journal of asian martial arts*, Vol. 1, No. 1, 1992.

5 Due to the paucity of evidence supporting the claim of the Ch'ens as the founders of *t'ai-chi*, the fact that *t'ai-chi* classics were written in the early twentieth century and transmitted through the Yang family, as well as other seminal contributions to the art by the Yangs, Professor Wile hints that the Yang family, not the Ch'ens, may be the originators of t'ai-chi ch'üan as we know it today. Wile, p. 33. More discussion on this point is included in Section VII.

6 However, there is mention of an "internal" martial art, and some literature describing the notion that *qi* energy could optimize the warrior's potential in combat. These references date to at least the mid 1600s. Of particular note is Huang Tsung-hsi's philosophical discussion regarding cultivation of *qi* energy (*Tai-Chi Ancestors*, p.41), the concept of coordinating the entire body (*Ancestors*, p. 43) and description of an "internal art" being counter to the brute force of Shaolin

(*Ancestors*, p. 47). Huang writes: "Now there is another school that is called 'internal' which overcomes movement with stillness. Thus, we distinguish Shaolin as 'external.'" As translated and quoted by Douglas Wile in *Tai Ch'i Ancestors*, p. 51. More on Huang in Section VII.

Adding to the discussion of disciplines purported to merge "internal energy," or "*qi* cultivation," with ancient Chinese yoga and martial arts in the mid-eighteenth century, Chang Naizhou (苌乃周) created a style that intertwined martial art with meditation, and which Professor Wile describes as "all but extinct." (*Ancestors*, p. 71). Chang's art emphasized *qi* development (*Ancestors*, p. 76), *qi* circulation (*Ancestors*, p. 77) — insisting that stagnation can be removed by movement (*Ancestors*, p. 77) — and emphasized the importance of focusing the body's qi on a single point. (*Ancestors*, p. 78). More on Chang in Sections VII and VIII.

7 Needham, Joseph, et al., *Science and civilization in China*, Vol. 6, p. 47.

8 Wang and Wu, *The history of Chinese medicine*. Originally published by the National Quarantine Service of Shanghai, 1936. Reprinted by Southern Materials Center, Inc, Taipei, 1977, p.7.

9 Veith, Liza, (translator) *The yellow emperor's classic of internal medicine*, University of California Press, Berkeley, 1949 p. 8-9.

10 According to Needham et al, "No one disputes that [the Neijing is the] systematized clinical experience and the physio-pathological theory of the physicians of the preceding five or six centuries."

Needham et al., *Science and civilization in China*, Vol. 6, p. 47.

11 It is helpful to note that Ko Hung, the most highly regarded alchemist in the fourth century CE, has not yet made the distinction that *nei qi* is a bio-energetic force separate from breath.

Section VI
The Transmutation of Sexual Energy

Huang Di asked, "If a wise one who follows the Tao at over one hundred years of age, can he or she still retain the ability to procreate?

Qi Bo answered, "Yes, it is possible. If one knows how to live a correct way of life, conserve one's energy, and follow the Tao, yes, it is possible. One could pro-create at the age of one hundred years."

— *Yellow Emperor's Classic of Medicine* [1]

Section VI

The Transmutation of Sexual Energy

Introduction to Section VI

The Transmutation of Sexual Energy

*T*his section looks for clues to the meaning of internal energy in those beliefs and practices, wherein the life force is understood to exist on a continuum that interacts with, and transforms, the individual. Here, we consider whether sexual energy could indeed act as a mutable force that can invigorate every aspect of life and well-being, from sexual expression to the attainment of advanced consciousness.

Can sexual energy be consciously converted within the body? Can a person's ability to manipulate "sexual energy" lead to enlightenment? Any discussion of human-directed subtle energy would be incomplete without considering the bio-energetic systems, such as those of Tibet, India, and China, that describe sexual energy as a transmutable force linked to spiritual wisdom and advanced consciousness.

Our search to uncover the secrets of the life force focuses on sexual energy within three distinct traditions:

1) Chinese Taoist [2] sexual yoga.

2) Indian yogic *kundalini*.

3) Tibetan Buddhist *tantric* practice.

In each of these, there is a special meaning to sexual energy beyond procreation or pleasure. Significantly, in each of the traditions, key perspectives on this subject are shared with the others.

The subjects introduced here are extremely broad. Each of the traditions considered has, over the course of more than two thousand years, produced an enormous volume of material regarding sexual energy, its transmutation, and its management. Thus, the present work can merely scratch the surface. It will consider only the most basic of concepts within these disciplines that relate to the role of sexual energy as it pertains to the life force, as well as its relationship to the advancement of consciousness.

For the Taoist inner alchemist learning to transmute his or her sexual energy, the goal is to obtain long life, or perhaps even physical immortality. Meanwhile, as introduced in Section V, the practitioner of Tibetan *tantra* pursues mastery over an aspect of internal energy known as *thigle* (ཐིག་ལེ) *, which awakens an advanced level of insight. This awakening allows the lama or yogi to more quickly attain realization of the *nature of mind*, which itself leads toward buddhahood.

> * An aspect of *tsa lung thigle* (རྩ་རླུང་ཐིག་ལེ) as a practice, and as was introduced in Section V

In the case of the practitioner of *kundalini* yoga, the prize is to stimulate and awaken dormant energy at the bottom of the spine. According to this tradition, the process allows the initiate to connect with *Brahman,* the Universal Principle and Ultimate Reality in the universe. In some cases, the individual's contact with divinity becomes so great that they become a *siddha,* or person of great power and wisdom.

Chapter 28

Sexual Energy in Western Traditions

*B*efore discussing the spiritual-sexual aspects of the Taoist, *tantric,* and *kundalini* traditions, it is useful to once again note how a concept that is often thought of as uniquely Asian — here meaning a relationship between sexual energy, access to enlightened thought, and spiritual knowledge — is also found in Western sources. Examples of the relationship between sexual energy and spiritual ecstasy are found in the earliest Christian traditions; consider the first organized Christian sect, the Moravians, who believed that true communion between God and man could only occur when sexual desire was combined with prayer. [3]

In Christianity, and in particular Catholicism, the notion that sexual energy can be transmuted is expressed through the concept of sublimation. Examples of sublimated sexual energy being said to have initiated mystical experiences are found in the legends of Catherine of Sienna and Padre Pio, St. Francis of Assisi, and many others. Then there are the creative sublimates, like Hildegard of Bingham and the Florentine Monk Fra Angelico, who went into ecstasy painting scenes from the life of Jesus.

As in the sublimation of creative energy through calligraphy, painting, music or meditation, these Christian examples are all said to be expressions of the transformative power of spirit. Here, creative sublimation is said to be the product of years of purification exercises, prayer, chants, celibacy, solitude, fasting, and silence. In the Christian tradition of strategies, these practices are designed to generate spiritual energy in preparation for illumination and, in the Eastern orthodox tradition, union, or *theosis*, with the divine.

Another example of Christian belief merging with what might be called a kind of sexual alchemy is found in the mysticism of the Swedish scientist, philosopher, and spiritual leader Emanuel Swedenborg (1688-1772). Teaching that erotic love binds the physical to the spiritual nature, Swedenborg believed that each act of intercourse on Earth produced a guardian angel in Heaven, [4] and, according to scholar Marsha Schuchard, more radical members of the Swedenborgian sect struggled to publish the founder's more explicit writings on Cabalistic marriage and erotic trance.[5] It is of interest that Swedenborg instructed his followers in techniques reminiscent of Taoist and *tantric* teachings on the body's energy channels, with an example being his description of a type of "respiration of the loins," which connected the genital area to the soles of the feet. [6]

Similarly, a close associate of Swedenborg, the highly-regarded poet and artist William Blake (1757-1827), also believed that sexual ecstasy brought one into union with "the Creator." Blake, along with several of his fellow artists, pursued, often practically, the notion that ultimate empathy with Christ's suffering could be realized through sex. Like some Taoists and *tantric* practitioners, their process emphasized the retention of seminal fluid during intercourse, a theme also present in various Eastern traditions.

As previously discussed, the instruction that a male should avoid, or at least minimize, ejaculation during sexual intercourse as a spiritual or psycho-energetic practice is found in several Eastern traditions. These traditions hold that due to a perceived energetic connection between the genitals and the brain, seminal retention nourishes the higher centers. This practice, too, was not without its Western adherents, as demonstrated by Blake, who also sought to maintain an erection for as long as possible, in order to use the charged sexual energy to initiate mystical visions. According to Schuchard, the practice put tremendous pressure on Blake's wife, who "enabled her husband to achieve the prolonged erection necessary in order to induce the mystical visions." [7]

As part of his psycho-sexual discipline, Blake practiced control over the cremaster muscle, thus impeding the flow of semen through the seminal vessels and maintaining an erection without emission. He, like many other psycho-sexual practitioners, believed that the technique allowed the essential fluid to be fed back to the brain, and that only then would it be possible for prayer and desire to merge as a unified force.

Another parallel between Eastern and Western psycho-sexual practices can be found in Swedenborg's description of the way sexual energy is said to travel through "energy channels" to initiate visionary experiences. As part of the body's physio-sexual energy system, Swedenborg taught that internal energy pathways were essential to the process, and that accordingly, "the great toe communicates with the genitals." This belief was expressed in Blake's self-portrait *William*, which depicts the artist's body as being flung backward, with a flaming star descending toward his left foot.

It is interesting to compare Blake's view of the energy channels to that held in traditional Chinese medicine (TCM). Like Blake's conception of the flow of energy, the TCM view of the liver meridian likewise connects the great toe and the testicles (see Figure 6-1, and Endnote [8] for a description of the liver meridian pathway). Is this a coincidence? On one level, a person unfamiliar with the meridian system might ask what the liver meridian (in this example, the channel between the testicle and the great toe) has to do with sex. The answer arises from two further questions: could there be pathways in the body that trigger and convert the flow of sexual energy, and, as Blake and the Taoist *neidan* alchemists believed, could these pathways be important clues to the meaning of internal energy?

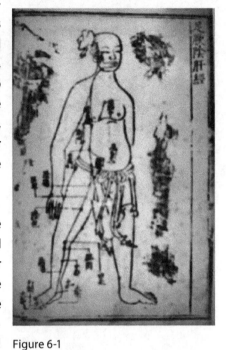

Figure 6-1

Woodcut Illustration from 1537

The liver channel of foot jueyin originates at the acu-point dadun ("big mound") and terminates at acu-point qimen ("portal of qi energy") of the lower abdomen

Source: Welcome Library, London

It is conceivable that individuals in different times and locations might have perceived these same energy flows within the body. From a cross-cultural perspective, it is interesting that some Westerners practicing their own version of sexual alchemy would have perceived the pathway of the liver meridian as described in traditional Chinese medicine, especially considering the shared observation of the channel's connection to the testicles.

For Swedenborg and Blake, their goal was to sublimate sexual energy into visionary energy. Through physical practices, they merged visualization with breathing exercises and worked to develop willpower directed toward erection without ejaculation, or at least postponing ejaculation for as long as possible. They believed that this allowed them to commune with the divine and the angels, and in this way, their practice was a kind of sexual alchemy that merged Cabalistic teachings with orgasmic trance.

Sexual Energy and Psychic Ability

In at least some examples, might there exist evidence of a relationship between sexual energy, a person's spiritual development, and psychic ability? If so, this could be considered yet another clue to the meaning of internal energy.

The suggestion that a relationship could exist between the experience of "energy," a person's ability to generate strong electromagnetic fields, and the experience of sexual energy can be deduced through various reports, such as those concerning Franz Mesmer's *animated magnetism*. Descriptions of Mesmer's work, already introduced in previous chapters, include reports by both men and women who experienced sexual arousal in response to his energetic-magnetic "healing fields." Others reported lethargy, after which the "cures" would become apparent. However, according to patient reports, sometimes their reactions to Mesmer's energetic-magnetic healing would trigger even more bizarre reactions. In some extreme cases, patients experienced ecstatic catharsis, which was apparently so stimulating that some female patients experienced "involuntary auto-orgasm," while males experienced "auto-ejaculatory release." [9]

Other clues suggesting a relationship between sexual and psychic energy are found in the notes of the nineteenth-century spiritualists. As introduced in Chapter One, the diaries kept by *séance* attendees describe bizarre, sometimes unsettling, experiences related to the presence of strong sexual energy during the sittings. [10]

In the mid-1800s, the noted German scientist Carl von Reichenbach, also introduced in Chapter One, proposed that the charisma of a highly influential person was tied to their "sexual energy." Reichenbach tried in vain to convince his colleagues that this was evidence of life energy as a natural force, conducting research into what he believed was a bio-energetic force he named *odic*, or *Od*. As part of his research protocol, Reichenbach relied on the accounts of *sensitives* — individuals with the ability to perceive "energy" visually, who we would today refer to as psychics — and their descriptions of energetic patterns around living things.

For Reichenbach, evidence of the *odic force* was found in the energy field surrounding a person, similar to what we refer to today as an *aura.* According to the *sensitives* he studied, Reichenbach documented not only the particulars of the aura, but also the various ways in which the *odic force* manifested. For example, he recorded the appearance of "energy" surrounding living things, as well as the energy patterns that were emitted from various body parts, including the fingertips, mouth, hands, forehead, feet, and especially the sexual centers.

Some sensitives engaged in Reichenbach's research reported that the emitted energy they observed around people in darkened rooms appeared as rays, beams, or undulating lights. [11] Reichenbach observed that in many instances, strong sexual energy accompanied the presence of psychic phenomenon. Ingo Swann describes Reichenbach's investigation of psychic forces reported during *séances*:

> One of the situations Reichenbach occasionally had to deal with involved erotic manifestations in the presence of "strong odic force." Such manifestations brought "disturbing" physical effects to some of his sensitives, some of his witnesses to the experiments, and apparently, sometimes to himself.

> Indeed, it seemed not uncommon that others besides the sensitives who felt "odic electricity" became "disturbingly aroused," and some of his sensitives fell into "temporary convulsions" and "were depleted" afterward. Some also lost weight.

> Some male and female sensitives could tell whether males were horny by special features of their odic energies and magnetic auras. However, the nature of the special features was either left undescribed [sic] or has been bleeped.

> Reichenbach's records, however, indicate in delicate terms that some female sensitives refused to work within the proximity of a horny male because of the "disturbing nature of their odic energies." Male sensitives were apparently not bothered with active female odic energies and seemed to enjoy their presence. [12]

A central question surrounding the meaning of *énergie vital,* is whether or not the energetic forces, like those studied by Reichenbach and Mesmer, might be in the same category as *qi, ki,* or *prana.* In this regard, it is useful to once again consider the observations of Sir William Crookes. Like Reichenbach, Crookes also attempted to prove that subtle energy was a natural force, and likewise believed a strong relationship existed between an individual with "strong energy" and sexual energy.

After studying the phenomenon, Crookes submitted his paper on the subject on 15 June 1871. Although regarded as one of England's top scientists, because his report affirmed the existence of the psychic force, the paper was highly controversial and never published. Crookes's report included his firsthand experience with this unnamed energy, wherein he described "tremulous pulsations in the vicinity of the loins." On Crookes's experience of sexual energy during *séances*, Swann writes:

> During the *séances*, many strange phenomena sometimes occurred which were not generally discussed or put officially into print. Sometimes, female mediums or sitters achieved spontaneous orgasm, which left them "exhausted." If male, they suffered erections of the male appendage, and sometimes spontaneously ejaculated in their undergear or trousers.

> Thereby, the concept of "tremulous pulsations of psychic force" took on new, if unofficial, potency--such as "force," that can rattle not only boards hooked up to strain gauges, but also erotically stimulate, to the point of achieving sexualizing ecstasy, the autonomic nervous systems of bio-bodies as well.

> Many reported being "disturbed," a Victorian code word for what we today would call horny and / or sexually aroused. [13]

Chapter 29

Alchemy and Sexual Yoga—Sexuality, Advanced Consciousness States, and Internal Energy

Modern physiology explains sexual arousal in terms of stimulation of specific areas of the brain, hormones, and the nervous system, and although the ancient Indian, Chinese, and Tibetan energetic physicians were ignorant of the physiology of the brain and nervous system in the modern sense, they nonetheless intuited the way mental activities might be related to the flow of the body's subtle energy.

The yogis of India, China, and Tibet observed and cataloged every subtle influence that might affect mind and body. The most accomplished yogic masters combined intuition with experience of what they perceived, either correctly or incorrectly, to be the flow of energy within their bodies, in order to forge powerful conceptual tools that could be used in their investigation of human potential.

Not unlike the way dietary guidelines might be used to enhance one's health and well-being, or how the use of a newly discovered herb might aid in healing a wound, sexual practices directed toward accessing one's hidden power and latent knowledge was likewise considered an important field of investigation. If certain forms of yogic stretching could relieve tension in the chest, then the infinite mysteries associated with sexual energy and intercourse could also provide valuable clues to aid the practitioner in other ways. For example, during periods when the Taoist inner alchemists were free to explore how sexual expression might serve as a gateway to shifts in consciousness, they were able to explore the meaning of those amazing electrical-magnetic-like feelings of sexual energy beyond procreation or pleasure.

Since the act of sexual intercourse has presumably not changed appreciably over human history, the experience of the ancient yogi-alchemist is still available today. It is easy to note the experience of an altered state of awareness, and the physiological changes that accompany sexual relations. The consuming feelings of love and attraction are powerful, and no doubt stimulate magnetic, or quasi-magnetic, forces within mind and body.

Whether observed by a monk in solo practice, or a yogi or yogini engaged in partner practice, it is also relevant to consider how the stimulation of sexual energy might induce an altered state, where breathing, focus, and awareness become modified.

Moreover, many of the more experienced practitioners might characterize their encounters with these interior forces as mystical, replete with attributes that would be characterized as aspatial and atemporal.

Likewise, during lovemaking, physical movement gives rise to elevated heart rate and changes in blood chemistry that combine to create altered states of consciousness; these contribute to, and reinforce, the altered state. For sexual energy explorers, these become roadmaps that lead them to pursue sexual yoga as a method of gaining insight into a broader spectrum of reality beyond the realm of the mundane experience.

Shared Aspects Between Traditions

Important conceptual commonalities exist between the *tantric* practitioners of Tibet and India, and the sexual yogic-alchemists of China. This observation applies to the power of sexual energy in particular, and especially to the relationship between sexual energy and the attainment of advanced body-mind states.

Each of these traditions holds that mastery of one's sexual energy could be converted into a potent physiological and spiritual force. For the Chinese sexual alchemists, the attainment of advanced abilities and full human potential required the transmutation of semen — or in the case of female adepts, a sexual essence — into a more rarefied and subtle form. As noted previously, in Taoist alchemy, this essence is known as *jing* (精, also Romanized *ching*), and thus it is important to reemphasize the distinction in Taoist sexual alchemy between *jing ye* (semen) and *jing qi* (sexual essence).

For the male adept engaged in the Taoist sexual transmutation arts, ** there were three main objectives:

1) Non-emission of semen during intercourse, or *coitus reservatus* (including *"retrograde ejaculation,"* or *injaculation*). [14]

2) Absorption of female sexual essence.

3) The achievement of transcendent states through the cultivation of sexual energy. [15]

Holding as they do similar beliefs, and as discussed earlier, Tibetan *tantric* practitioners refer to the sexual-energetic force as *thigle*. Other aspects shared between the Taoist and Tibetan traditions include instructions that the devotee focus mental attention to the lower regions of the body, particularly the genitals, perineum, and tailbone.

** Solo disciplines were discussed in Section V.

Of the traditions just cited, each holds that transmutation and / or masterful control of sexual energy opens a doorway to the attainment of full human potential. The many shared principles between the management of sexual energy and the attainment of advanced consciousness suggests that the relationship between sexual energy and advanced consciousness cannot be ignored.

In both traditions, a shared characteristic is the practitioner's conscious control over sensations. Another is the belief that this kind of conscious control leads the practitioner to control, and subsequently transmutation, of internal energy. In this light, it is useful to consider whether there might be neurological, biochemical, or other physiological explanations for what advanced practitioners of these traditions describe as enhanced mental and spiritual abilities.

This section also includes speculation on the meaning of the "transmutation of sexual energy" in terms of Western bio-medical physiology. Important here is whether "sexual energy" can really be willfully manipulated, converted, refined, or transmuted. Furthermore, we will assess the possible interpretations of those experiences classified as transmutation, but first it is necessary to define what is meant by "sexual energy."

The Sexual Energy Continuum

When used colloquially, nearly everyone has a sense of the meaning of "sexual energy," and yet the term remains both powerful and ambiguous. On the one hand, sexual energy might describe uncontrolled lustful desire, while on the other, the term could also describe electrical-like warmth or pleasurable feelings in the area of the genitals associated with blood flow. It is important to note that blood flow to the genitals and stimulation of the sacral nerve route, along with the presence of sexual-like sensations, can occur completely independent of sexual ideation. Thus, before one can consider the meaning of the "transmutation of sexual energy," the term "sexual energy" must first be defined.

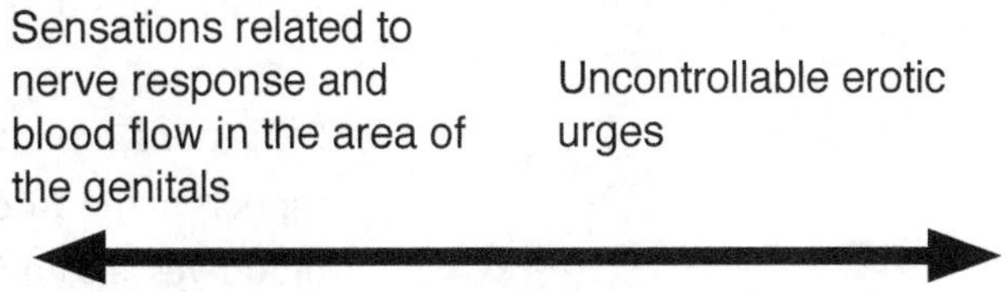

Sensations related to nerve response and blood flow in the area of the genitals

Uncontrollable erotic urges

← →

Diagram 6-6

The Range of Experience that can be Interpreted as "Sexual Energy"

Consider the possibility that the sensations and emotions that one identifies as "sexual energy" might refer to more than just the drive to have sexual intercourse. With this consideration in mind, there is a range of other experiences that can also be referred to in this way, some of which may explain age-old associations between the "transmutation of sexual energy" and the attainment of advanced consciousness. Pertinent to the discussion is whether it might be possible that "sexual energy" exists as a continuum of "energy" that incorporates a wide range of meanings and sensations. This way of looking at the meaning of sexual energy could begin to explain the interpretation of it in the context of psychic and spiritual-meditative traditions.

As suggested by the continuum depicted in Diagram 6-6, while one end of it represents experiences that might include "electric-like" energy sensations in the body's sexual centers — completely unrelated to sexual thoughts or desires — the other represents the experience of full-blown lustful desire.

When viewed as a range of sensations, thoughts, and emotions that form the continuum, the model provides a useful lens through which to think about the meaning of "sexual energy" beyond pleasure and procreation. Several traditions describe the idea that sexual energy can be transmuted into psychic or spiritual energy, including *kundalini, tantric,* and Taoist sexual alchemy; and a similar line of thought links sexual energy to the mystical traditions of some Christian sects, such as the Moravians and Swedenborgians. In various Eastern traditions, the meaning of sexual energy is viewed beyond lust or stimulation, and in some cases, it is even considered essential to the full human experience of the divine. This expanded view of sexual energy describes experiences and sensations relevant to a fully functioning nervous system; one that enlivens the entire system from the brain to the sacrum and genitals.

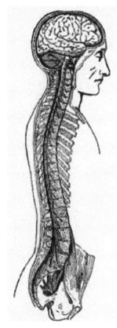

Diagram 6-7

The Human Nervous System from the Brain to the Genitals[21]

Physiologically, sexual desire is the culmination of multiple neural mechanisms, each controlled by different areas of the brain, that are activated at different times during the sexual experience. [16] When expressed through the euphoric and pleasurable sensation of sex, these signals primarily involve the limbic system. Also known as the paleomammalian brain, the limbic set is very close to the brain's base, and it is evolutionarily one of its oldest parts.

Sensations identified as sexual arousal are triggered by parasympathetic aspects of the autonomic nervous system, associated with vasodilation of the blood vessels and innervation to the genitalia. Human sexuality is defined by this parasympathetic response, along with other physiological markers such as increased heart rate. In the sexual response, there is simultaneously deactivation in the area of the brain relating to various external stimuli, particularly fear.

The possibility that a person might be able to gain some degree of conscious control over aspects of their nervous system provides new insight into the intersection of sexuality and mystical experience. It is conceivable that a highly advanced meditator or yogi could engage his or her mental focus to effect some degree of conscious control over the nervous system, and that part of this process would involve learning to consciously trigger sexual-like sensations.

It appears that, in at least some examples of highly-practiced yogis, the initiated force is so great that it could link mystical experience to the nerves of the lower body. Thus, this kind of nervous system control would include innervation and willfully induced blood flow to the sexual centers and areas of the perineum, tailbone, and pelvic floor muscles. As an example, consider the account of the energetic healer-nun that was cited in Section IV. Apparently, her healing power was connected to her ability to generate warmth in the area of her intestines. As detailed there, for her, the experience was so palpable that the experience of warmth in the lower abdomen caused her to lose bladder control.

Sexual Energy and Mystical Experience

It has been scientifically established that a person can consciously alter heart rate, [17] and there are other physiological measures that have also been documented as being malleable and responsive to conscious control, including blood pressure and several other aspects of neurophysiology. It is not inconceivable that, in a similar fashion, a disciplined practitioner might also learn to harness the power of highly focused attention to modify other psycho-physiological functions. There is no reason why a person with some degree of control over their nervous system might not also be able to consciously induce neurological responses that fall within the continuüm of "sexual energy."

Consider, for example, how some Taoist sexual-energetic texts describe aural and visual hallucinations associated with the practice. Other reported experiences include the practitioner's ability to intentionally cease breathing, and even eliminate the detection of their pulse during sexual alchemical-transmutation practices. [18] The trained practitioner's ability to gain this degree of conscious control over some aspects of their physiology could begin to explain at least some of the reports of ecstasy and altered body-mind states associated with practices related to the internal control over "sexual energy."

The notion that it is possible to awaken and work with one's nervous system in deeper ways than what is normally understood lends credence to the assertion that, through arduous and disciplined practice, practitioners might have learned how to harness these kinds of sensations within their bodies. It also supports the point that examples can be found in different geographical areas and in different time periods. Thus, it is not unreasonable to consider that some practiced individuals might have discovered how to manipulate their sexual energy in ways that could enhance or modify their normal sensory perception.

If an adept discovered that their focused attention could produce a new kind of experience, this discovery would have been explored further. This provides a new lens through which to view the meaning of sexual-like feelings, such as ecstasy, and the relationship between these and advanced spiritual practice. For meditators sitting in deep trances in caves, focusing their attention inward, the appearance of sensations such as these would have grabbed their attention.

Sensations associated with sexual energy, especially for a celibate practitioner, would certainly have caught their attention. Not having the distraction of outside stimuli, early monks, meditators, and alchemists looked to their own interiors for stimulation, as well as guidance on how to proceed. For Taoist solo practitioners, the "awakening of *yang*," where the male adept experienced erection during meditation, was considered an especially good sign. [19]

Awareness of sensations within the body guided the yogis in their practice. If, during the course of this kind of inner exploration, the yogi gained increased control over aspects of the nervous system associated with the reproductive system, changes in those centers, whether correctly or incorrectly understood, could easily be viewed as the "transmutation" of sexual energy.

It is conceivable that, in their deep meditative disciplines, practitioners accessed aspects of the brain and nervous system in ways that they might have identified as the transmutation of sexual energy. By extension, this kind of highly focused mental attention could, because of its effect on the body, have transformed into a kind of parasympathetic nervous system switch. When the switch was activated, it could easily have initiated profound experiences for the practitioner due to the sensory changes along the entire brain, right down to the genital spinal system corridor (see Diagram 6-7).

In this light, some practitioners, for example *tantric* and inner alchemy initiates, might have begun to associate an advanced level of nervous system control with sensations that they perceived as manipulation of and willful control over "sexual energy." The association between practiced nervous system control, along with what they perceived to be new levels of awareness and insight, could easily have become associated with the transmutation of sexual energy.

It should be noted that this model does not address the veracity of whether the practitioner might actually convert *jing* semen into a *shen* spiritual force, or control what is identified as *thigle* sexual energy in the *tsa* channels; nor even if the awakening of a dormant force such as *kundalini* is actually possible. However, this view does offer a psycho-physiological explanation for what is perceived by practitioners as the manipulation of sexual-energetic forces. Could this be part of the explanation for what the adepts of the past identified as the transmutation of sexual energy?

Consider, once again, the religious-mystical ecstatic experiences reported by Swedenborg, who was drawn to Cabalistic marriage because of his associations with Moravian and Jewish mystics in London. In his *Journal of Dreams,* Swedenborg explains how he sublimated his sexual energy to augment his personal mystical vision. His self-disciplined approach to sublimating his sexual energy involved achieving an erection by applying muscle control to the cremaster muscle, along with other sexual areas, while practicing breathing techniques. For mystics like Swedenborg, the result sometimes produced a sexually-charged transformative and ecstatic vision that replaced ejaculation. This was a profound experience, which Swedenborg believed would ultimately elevate him into the world of angels and spirits.

Another possibility that may explain the drive by some adepts to transmute their sexual energy involves the relationship between sexual energy, advanced consciousness, and a special type of energetic or *siddhi* power. † This point refers to the possibility of a brain-nervous system connection that was described by researchers such as Reichenbach, Mesmer, and others, as introduced in Chapter One.

It is conceivable that other yet-to-be-described relationships exist between nerve centers of the lower torso and brain neurology; the field of neurophysiology is relatively new, and discoveries relating to physiology continue to be revealed. As will be discussed at length in Section XI, consider the recent discovery of brain and lymph detoxification structures, which scientists have referred to as groundbreaking. According to one researcher, the new discovery fills a "major gap in understanding of the human body." [20] It is probable that the future will hold other discoveries about the brain and nervous system, and could these include newfound connections between the brain and sexual centers? If so, the sexual-spiritual ecstasy of the mystic who seeks to transmute sexual energy may yet be shown to have a physiological basis.

† Siddhis and siddhas are covered in Section XII

Chapter 30

Taoist Sexual Alchemy

Within silk books from the Western Han dynasty (206 BCE – 9 CE) *Mawangdui* (馬王堆) tombs, and among other sources, there exists a fascinating example of an at-least-two-thousand-year-old piece of literature, and the material includes some of the oldest surviving texts on Taoist sexual alchemy. Consistent with the explanation for how I use terms like "Taoist" and "Taoism" that appears early in Section III, it should be noted that although commonly referred to as Taoist sexual practice, the material describing solo and paired practice does not always delineate methods practiced exclusively by Taoists. That caveat noted, this chapter concerns disciplines and traditions that are generally referred to as "Taoist sexual-energy practices."

Taoist Alchemy and Medical Theory

The essential elements of Taoist alchemy and traditional medical theory have been presented earlier and need not be revisited in detail. However, since some aspects of alchemy and traditional medicine are shared with "Taoist" sexology, it is useful to review a few points.

Note that not only the lore, but also the "rules" of both solo and paired practice presented here are not universally agreed upon between the various traditions. From ancient times, treatises governing Taoist sexology were never monolithic. In Taoist subjects — and this is especially so in the cases of esoteric subjects such as Taoist sexology — although there is a consensus on a few main points, it is useful to keep in mind that there has never been *one* single prevailing "Taoist" view. Examples of differing points of view are reflected quite early in the literature. Consider the alchemist Ko Hung's discussion of the topic from the fourth century:

> Interlocutor: I have been taught that he who can fully carry out the correct sexual procedures can travel alone and summon gods and genii. Further, he can shift disaster from himself and absolve his misdeeds; turn misfortune into good; rise high in office; double his profits if in business. Is it true?

Ko: This is all deceptive, exaggerated talk found in the writings of mediums and shamans; it derives from the enlargements and colorings of dilettantes. It utterly belies the facts. Some of it is the work of base liars creating meaningless claims to deceive the masses. Their concealed purpose is to seek service from others; to gather about themselves pupils solely with a view to obtaining advantages for themselves in their own time.

The best of the sexual recipes can cure the lesser illnesses, and those of a lower quality can prevent us from becoming empty, but that is all. There are very natural limits to what such recipes can accomplish. How could they ever be expected to confer the ability to summon gods and genii and to dispel misfortune or bring good?

It is inadmissible that man should sit and bring illness and anxieties upon himself by not engaging in sexual intercourse. But then again, if he wishes to indulge his lusts and cannot moderate his dispersals, he hacks away at his very life. Those knowing how to prepare the sexual recipes can check ejaculation, thereby repairing the brain; revert their sperm . . . and [by conducting breathing exercises] they can thus cause a man, even in old age, to have excellent complexion, and terminate the full number of his allotted years. [22]

Clearly, Ko did not have a high regard for many of the Taoist sexologists of his time, and especially those who claimed special powers could be attained through practice of the exotic sexual yogas. However, as we will see shortly, some had other views, especially regarding the belief that sexual alchemy could lead the devotee to immortality.

Introduction to *Neidan* Sexual Alchemy

As covered previously, for the Taoist *neidan* alchemist, there were two main points of focus: the transmutation of *jing* essence into *shen* spirit and gaining mastery over the psycho-somatic mechanisms of body and mind that could initiate a transcendental state called *shen ming* (神明).

In paired sexual practice, the sexual yogi engaged in what Professor Douglas Wile refers to as a kind of "battle of the sexes;" [23] the goal of the male adept being to preserve his *essence* and use it for transformational purposes. [24] [25] The principle is expressed in the classic, *Essentials of the Jade Chamber*, which states: "To be aroused and not ejaculate is called 'returning the *jing*.'" [26]

Mostly written by and for the male initiate, the fundamental rule that applied to dual practice was that the male must not lose his semen during intercourse, and then, without emission, absorb the female's captured *jing* energy. A challenge like this was considered particularly arduous, since it required the practitioner to simultaneously stimulate and limit his expression of sexual energy. [27] The practitioner's belief was that the successful technique would aid the initiate toward the goals of long life, health, and immortality. Wile explains:

> Nothing seemed more logical to the Taoists than the pursuit of immortality by the attainment of higher and higher states of health, "reversing the aging process and reverting to youth." [28]

In contrast to the male's goal of limiting loss of sexual essence in the "battle of the sexes," the aim of the female initiate was to draw it out from the male and capture it. This theme is represented in a surviving fragment of a lost Chinese text, *Secret Instructions of the Jade Bedchamber* (玉房秘訣), which describes how the goddess Queen Mother of the West attained her immortal state:

> It is not only that *yang* can be cultivated but *yin* too. The Queen Mother of the West, for example, attained the Way by cultivating her yin energy. As soon as she copulated with a male, the male would immediately suffer illness, whereas her visage would become radiant and lush—even without make-up. She often ate curds and plucked her five-stringed lute. By this means, she harmonized her heart and stabilized her intentions, so that she had no other desire. It is also said: 'The Spirit Mother has no husband; she enjoys copulating with young boys. For this reason, [her methods] must not be taught to the world. For why would only the Queen Mother act like this? [29]

Thus, the male or female adept who most effectively guards their sexual essence could "recapture both the function and appearance of adolescence." [30] For the male adept, this meant that loss of semen was detrimental to his health, especially if he ejaculated too early, and should therefore be avoided. [31] In adulthood, the male's loss of sexual essence should be limited; a point emphasized in the P'eng Tzu classic:

> When *ching* [*jing*/ semen] is emitted, the whole body feels weary. One suffers buzzing in the ears and drowsiness in the eye; the throat is parched and the joints heavy. Although there is brief pleasure, in the end, there is discomfort. If, however, one engages in sex without emission, then the strength of our [*qi*] will be more than sufficient and our bodies at ease. One's hearing will be acute and vision clear. Although exercising self-control and calming the passion, love actually increases, and one remains un-satiated. How can this be considered un-pleasurable? [32]

The highest secrets regarding transmutation are closely guarded. However, a few basic points about how an adept would engage in Taoist sexual practice are known. One is an instruction for a male to practice sexual yoga with a woman he is not attracted to, in order to develop self-control. [33] Another is to keep emotional distance from women, so that they might be used as "fuel." [34] The equivalent female response to this strategy will be covered shortly.

Secrets

The highest secrets were never written down; they were verbally transmitted from master to initiate. Figure 6-8 shows a page from an inner alchemist's manual, which includes coded symbols as placeholders. They indicated points where guarded information was to be orally transmitted from master to initiate. As will be addressed later, knowledge of the sexual arts was mostly kept hidden from women. Wile remarks:

> The secret of the jade chamber warns those who would cultivate their *yang* must not allow women to steal glimpses of their art. [35]

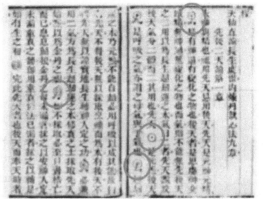

A page from the ancient Taoist alchemical text, *Nei Chin Tan*. The text includes the non Chinese symbols, which are markers indicating where the novice would be instructed in the their secret meaning by an initiate.

Jing-Qi-Shen

An overview of Taoist alchemy and notions relating to the conversion of *jing* (精) into *shen* (神) was offered in Sections III and V. Thus, only a brief review of a few main points is presented here. At the center of Taoist inner alchemy is the theory that advanced consciousness emerges from the conversion of the "dense" sexual substance, *jing*, into a refined spiritual essence, *shen*.

Together, the three "densities" of subtle *nei qi* energy form the *san pao*, or "three treasures" (三寶). These are the *jing, qi*, and *shen* that form the tripartite bio-energetic continuum. For the Taoist alchemist, the three treasures represent the possibility of progressive transformation through increasingly rarified stages, from the most physical to the most etheric elements of consciousness and spirit.

Ancient Taoist *neidan* masters believed that the relationship between the three treasures explained how the energies of body, mind, and spirit transmuted as a cooperative and intimately linked bio-energetic system. The Taoist adage that characterizes the nature of the three treasures and their preservation is: *Speaking little conserves the qi; ejaculating little preserves the jing; worrying little preserves the shen.* [36]

Joining meditation and medical theory with sexual yoga, in the context of the *jing-qi-shen* model, sexual alchemists perceived the physical form of the human body as the densest expression of life energy. The logical extension of this view is that at the opposite end of the energetic spectrum existed the subtlest, ethereal, and refined energy of *shen*, or spirit. In this context, the inner alchemist, through sexual yoga and other practices, sought to manipulate, unify, and transmute the denser aspects of the body's energy into the rarified form of *shen*. This process could manufacture the *dan* (丹) elixir within his / her body and mind, and thereby allow for the attainment of immortality. Ko Hung describes the retention of semen as part of a system that could awaken special powers.

Figure 6-8

Coded Symbols in a Taoist Alchemical Text

Taoist internal alchemy manual containing coded symbols, which served as placeholders to be interpreted by a master alchemist at points during instruction where the meaning would be communicated to an initiated disciple.

Source: Joseph Needham, *Science and Civilization in China*

> If you wish to seek divinity or genie-hood, you need only to acquire the
> quintessence, which consists in treasuring your sperm, circulating your
> breaths, and taking one crucial medicine. [37]

However, the energetic principles that describe life as a combination of bio-energetic *jing, qi,* and *shen* extend beyond Taoist sexual alchemy. They serve as foundational teachings that apply to a wide range of "Taoist" practices. The application of *jing, qi,* and *shen* principles ranges from physical and mental yoga (for example, the *dao yin* and *nei guan* yoga covered in Section III) to Taoist-based martial arts, including *t'ai-chi* and *baguazhang* (八卦掌), to acupuncture and traditional medicine.

Representations of the *jing-qi-shen* formula are reflected in the traditional doctor's diagnoses of a deficient or full kidney *jing* essence. They are evidenced today by the Taoist meditation and *t'ai-chi* instructions that advise practitioners to hold their tongues to the roof of their mouths, and in breath training, where it is standard practice to engage the diaphragm muscles to breathe deeply in order to initiate an internal massage that can awaken the *dan tian* energy of the lower abdomen.

Jing Essence

Although modern Chinese dictionaries define *jing* as semen, the archaic, alchemical, and yogic use of the word is much broader. Keeping in mind the distinction between *jing ye* (精液), or substance, and *jing qi* (精氣), an energetic essence, in alchemical usage, the term refers to both male and female sexual essence.

Jing essence plays a central role in Taoist yoga and meditation traditions, and especially so in Taoist sexual practice. In spite of its centrality in Taoist yogic arts and traditional medicine, a clear and concise definition of *jing* is not easily rendered. My Taiwan acupuncture teacher explained *jing* as a real physical substance closely related to semen, but again, not strictly so, since females also possess this enigmatic substance. Furthermore, as suggested by my teacher and other sources, the meaning of *jing* might actually be related to spinal fluid. However, it is interesting that, notwithstanding the discovery of a biological element synonymous with what the Chinese call *jing,* some writers describe *jing* in terms of an emotional or biological "urge." One writer on the subject, who uses the pseudonym Hsi Lai, offers the following definition of *jing,*

> [*Jing* is] the very primal urge people have to reproduce themselves, the behav-
> ior we apply in expressing our sexual desire, the substances contained within
> the sexual fluids—the regenerative force—all are *jing* or sexual energy. [38]

It is interesting to note that Hsi Lai's definition of orgasm includes not only sexual energy produced by the body, but also what he describes as a "substantive psychological force." [39]

As discussed in Section V, *jing* essence is divided into "acquired" and "inherited" attributes. In both cases, *jing* is considered an important part of life energy, which can be either strong or deficient. Where *jing* is strong, illness is easily conquered. However, when weak, the condition becomes more serious. While the physiological aspect of *jing* is stored in the kidneys and represents the body's reserve of sexual essence, it is expressed through such markers as clear eyesight, alertness, and intelligence.

Pertaining to males, there is a consensus in the Taoist and TCM literature that *jing* essence is depleted through excessive sexual release, and that lack of restraint is especially damaging to the kidneys. Aside from loss of ambition, [40] the pattern is predictive of a number of health issues, especially problems with the lower back and knees. In this light, one Taoist text on the subject advises that frequent sex with occasional ejaculation is superior to occasional sex with habitual ejaculation.[41]

Frequency of Sexual Intercourse and Loss of Jing

Both acquiring *jing* and minimizing its loss have long been considered important concerns. In the view of Taoist sexual cultivation, for males, the path to "eternal spring" was to seek the "spring-like youth" of young women. [42] The sexual classic *Ling Shu* says, "Nothing is more important for the *qi* of the man than the *jing* of the penis." [43] Thus, if a man experiences first sexual emission too early, this harms the *jing qi*. The medical classic *Su Wen* details the frequency of sexual release for a male: three times a month in spring, twice in summer, once in autumn, and none in winter. [44] By contrast, for females, *jing* essence is not depleted during intercourse, but through menses, and especially childbearing.[45]

Studies on the Effects of Ejaculation in Modern Scientific Literature

In one German study, researchers examined the effect of a three-week period of sexual abstinence on testosterone and testosterone-related factors, with both blood serum and cardiovascular parameters being monitored continuously during the period. The procedure was conducted for each participant twice, before and during the period of abstinence. The study showed that, for all male participants, higher testosterone concentrations were observed following the period of abstinence. [46]

Dual Cultivation and Solo Practice

Taoist sexology can be divided into two main categories: solo practice and paired, or dual, practice. Initiates of both traditions are concerned with transmutation of sexual energy, and it should also be noted that among Taoist practices, there was also a "pure practices" school, where physical-sexual interaction was totally rejected. As a replacement for physical intercourse, the adept performed a mystical marriage within his own body, where male and female elements were unified. [47]

The underlying principle of paired practice is that energy can be transferred from one person to another. [48] The Taoist practice of absorbing sexual energy is known as *caibu* (採補), and in this scheme, the skilled male master of sexual arts mixes his vital energy with the female's during sexual intercourse before later reabsorbing the vitalized essence. Note, the majority opinion is that this function is completed by non-emission. However, a minority opinion follows the notion of *injaculation*, which involves semen being reabsorbed back into the body without being emitted externally. In either case, the sexual prescription is for *jing qi* essence to be converted into *shen*, or "spiritual" *qi*, within the male adept's body. Upon reabsorption, the adept may experience a flood of energy throughout his body, which the *Mawangdui* texts refer to as *shen feng* (神風), or "divine wind." [49] The classic *Essentials of the Jade Chamber* states, "To be aroused and not ejaculate is called 'returning the *jing*.'" [50]

Since the ability of the male to reabsorb the converted *qi* essence was considered essential to long life and health, paired sexual practice, especially with young women, was prized as a precious medicine. It is one of the reasons why Chinese emperors kept many young concubines. [51]

Solo and Paired Practice

Also, and as introduced above, some types of sexual energy transmutation training were undertaken as solo practice. In those practices, the practitioner, while in deep meditation, would attempt to transform energetic forces within body and mind through visualization and focus. In Taoist paired practice, the use of special mental and physical techniques during intercourse allowed the couple's sexual fluids to mix. Then, through secret sexual arts, the properly trained male yogi combined these elements to create an enhanced *yang* and *yin* mixture, which was then reabsorbed back into his body. John Blofeld describes *dual cultivation* in the following way:

> It is true that those initiated into the yoga of dual cultivation, for which a sexual partner is required, find in it a fruitful aid to progress. Besides having the strength of will to stop short of emission, they know how to cause the *ching* [*jing*], now blended with the yogic partner's essence, to return and pass upwards, whereupon they experience great bliss. For them, "life blazes." However, the technique of returning the *ching*

is very difficult to master and quite impossible without an experienced teacher. [52]

However, dual practice was also dangerous, and few individuals possessed the necessary discipline that it required. Blofeld offers comments from a Taoist text, which introduces the challenges of dual cultivation:

> Only men of rare talent are suited to take on the dangerous yoga of dual cultivation. Men of lesser talent end by exhausting their stock of *jing* and *qi*, thereby impairing their health and being compelled to abandon forever the sacred task of creating an immortal body. In the end, they become mere libertines, effete and doomed to final extinction—such is what they chose to call cultivation of the Way! It would be laughable if one did not feel saddened by their loss. [53]

The Taoist inner alchemist sought to create *dan* elixir within the metaphorical laboratory of the lower abdomen. The alchemist, Ko Hung, discusses the process from the viewpoint of Taoist sexual arts:

> On the methods of correct intercourse, at least ten authors have written. Some claim they know how to replenish losses, cure illness, gather more *yin* or increase the *yang*, or increase the years and procure longevity. The essential here lies solely in reverting the sperm to repair the brain. God's Men [54] [*xian / hsien,* or "immortal"] have transmitted this method orally without any writing. [55]

But, instead of avoiding sexual relations to conserve essence, Ko's advice to aspirants is to practice moderation:

> Though one were to take all the famous medicines, without the knowledge of this essential it would be impossible to attain Fullness of Life. Man may not, however, give up sexual intercourse entirely, for otherwise he would contract melancholia through inactivity and die prematurely through the many illnesses resulting from depression and celibacy. On the other hand, overindulgence diminishes one's life, and it is only by harmonizing the two extremes that damage will be avoided. Unless the oral directions are available [to be passed from master to disciple] not one man in ten thousand will not fail to kill himself by attempting to undertake this [dual cultivation] art. [56]

It is of interest that Cheng Man-ching (1902-1975), a highly-regarded *t'ai-chi* master who helped popularize the art in the United States in the 1960s, like many teachers of the internal tradition, from Ko Hung to innumerable masters since, warned his students about the dangers of excessive sexual release. Cheng's advice to his students is included in Wolfe Lowenthal's *There are No Secrets:*

> It is necessary for a man to conserve the *ching [jing]*, the element in the semen that gathers in the *tan t'ien [dan tian]*. Ejaculation depletes the

jing. For a 16-year-old man, it takes the *jing* seven days to replenish itself after ejaculation. For a man of 24, it takes two weeks to replenish itself; for a man of 32, it takes three weeks; and for a man of 40 it takes 30 days. Once you reach 50, you should hold onto your *jing* for life. You have the potential of having 120 years of life. Depleting your *jing* is like taking money out of your bank account: you lose days of your life every time. [57]

Important Points

The foundation of Taoist bio-energetics is the *jing* of the *jing-qi-shen* formula, which is divided into two parts: acquired and inherited. Acquired, also called "postnatal" *jing,* is comprised of energy derived from daily life processes, such as the ingestion of food and exercise. Under normal conditions, acquired aspects of life-energy, when depleted, can be restored from correct diet and proper exercise. On the other hand, prenatal *jing,* once lost, is impossible to restore. In modern medical terms, postnatal *jing* is replenished through proper diet and care of the human frame. Its life essence is expressed in such bio-chemical processes as the manufacture of glucose, ATP, ‡ and basic metabolism. Prenatal *jing,* by contrast, refers to the vitality inherited through one's DNA blueprint. Thus, prenatal *jing* is inherited from one's parents at the time of conception. In Taoist alchemical terms, prenatal *jing* is the quotient representing a person's inherited constitution that allows them to recover from a long illness. The notion of innate *jing* energy is expressed in the observation that some people are inherently strong and resilient, while others are weaker.

‡ATP: Adenosine triphosphate is a complex chemical that is involved in many life processes.

As a self-healing reserve and an indicator of innate athletic ability, the available resource of inherited prenatal internal energy varies between individuals. Some people naturally possess more *jing* essence than others. This explains why some individuals can suffer a tremendous amount of abuse to their body through drug use, poor diet, and lack of exercise for many years, and then, in a relatively short time, achieve complete recovery. This is in contrast to others, who, while suffering only minimal self-abuse, can easily fall prey to disease and experience prolonged periods of ill-health. In many ways, DNA markers of inherited strength or weakness fit the model that Chinese inner alchemists in pre-modern times intuited to be a factor in human biology.

The notion that *jing* depletion can be detrimental to one's health cannot yet be supported through known bio-chemistry or bio-physics. However, as described in Chinese Taoist yogic and traditional medical theory, while complete depletion of acquired and inherited *jing* energy is associated with untimely death, partial depletion though excessive seminal release is predictive of weakness, bodily discomfort, and premature aging.

Sometimes called "enlightenment training," modern-day instructions in techniques to enhance or restore *jing* essence are still offered in the literature. For example, some writers on the topic, such as Yang Jwing-ming and Stephen Chang, believe that kidney *jing* can be nourished through self-massage and stretching exercises directed to the male organ. Both authors write that this category of solo practice can stimulate hormone production.
58

Inner Alchemy and the True *Dan Tian*

As noted earlier, the meaning of the Chinese character *dan* (丹) relates to the alchemist's formulae. In the tradition of the outer, or *waidan*, alchemist, the prepared laboratory compound, if consumed, would result in immortality. In contrast, *neidan* inner alchemists adopted the term as a metaphor for the development of the true *dan* within their own bodies through sexual yoga and other practices.

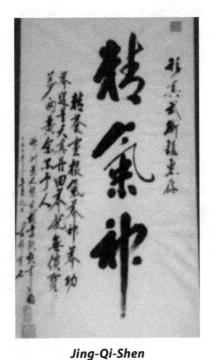

Photo 6-4
Jing-Qi-Shen Scroll by Master Liang Kequan
Scroll brushed by the author's late kung fu "uncle," with a translation that contains the directive to seek the *jen dan tian* (真丹田), or "true dan tian," worth many measures of gold.

Jing-Qi-Shen
. . . Ancient pearl of great value
Develop and search for the true *dan tian* ...
worth many measures of gold ....
Signed, "Liang Kequan, the writings of an old man"

Through yogic practice, meditation, and sexual alchemy, the search for the mysterious *dan* elixir as a source of youth and power has been an important quest for Chinese yogis and martial artists for generations. As an example of this ancient quest that continues to the present day, the scroll in Photo 6-4, brushed by Master Liang Kequan, contains instructions for searching for the precious *true dan tian*.

Taoist Sexual Yoga

Since the twelfth century, two distinct schools of *neidan* Taoism have emerged. Blofeld describes these as the Northern School, based at the White Cloud monastery outside of Beijing, which emphasized health and diet and eschewed Taoist sexual yoga; and the Southern School, developed in the Zhang monastery in Jiangxi province, which emphasized exotic magical practices and sexual alchemy. [59]

In the context of Taoist sexology, yogis of the Zhang monastery held that while the normal course of the union of *yin* and *yang* brings about procreation, the potential derived from the merging of these forces is considerable. This otherwise natural course can be interrupted, as the male aspirant, while being careful not to ejaculate, can mix and reabsorb the newly combined fluid. Through secret techniques performed during intercourse, *yin* and *yang* fluids merge to create a new compound, which is then reabsorbed into the aspirant's lower abdominal region to form a metaphorical "immortal fetus."

Modern writers on the subject sometimes describe Taoist sexology as a health and recreational regimen, with little or no reference to the notion of an "immortal fetus." Consider the view expressed by Dr. Stephen Chang, traditional physician and author on the subject:

> Taoism was the first philosophy to take human sexuality into full account, to present it in such a way that people could use it to transform themselves. [60]

Chang's statement describes Taoist sexual practices in modern terms, which, like their ancient counterparts, look beyond pleasure and reproduction. As Chang explains, benefits derived from Taoist sexual practice include enjoyment of sexual foreplay, sexual expression without the depletion of one's energy, the strengthening of sexual organs, and the use of sexual energy to heal ailments and strengthen the love bond. [61]

Female Taoist Practice

The descriptions of Taoist practices intended for female initiates also promises the return to a youthful spring. For the female practitioner, the goal was to shrink her breasts and limit or eliminate menses. In China, texts describing techniques developed for Buddhist nuns refer to the elimination of menses as "slaying the red dragon." [62] One technique, designed to eliminate menses gradually, includes meditation on points *qi hai* and *guan yuan* in the lower abdomen, *hui yin* at the perineum and cervix, *yong quan* at the ball of the foot, *yin tang* between the eyebrows, and *shan zhong* at the midline of the sternum.[63]

As with the instructions intended for male initiates, female practitioners too must calm their passions, but at the same time activate their internal energy in order to "overcome the natural stasis of *yin* and release the *yang* principle." According to the doctrine, this stimulates the *qi* to transform from "red" into "white phoenix marrow." [64] Because of deficiency and "cold," sex was forbidden during the women's "three periods:" menses, pregnancy and postpartum. [65]

As introduced above, it was due to these conflicting goals and methods of male and female sexual alchemists that set up the competition for *jing* essence. Where for the male, the semen withheld during sexual intercourse was the raw material of transmutation, for the female aspirant, the goal was to obtain male essence without giving up her *yin* fluid. This "differential alchemy," dating back more than a thousand years, most likely contributed to the Chinese folk belief in "fox spirits."

Fox Spirits

Fox spirits, or *huli jing* (狐狸精), are supernatural entities who, in Chinese folklore, were believed to disguise themselves as beautiful women in order to drain the *jing* sexual essence of unsuspecting young men. Akin to leprechauns in Irish folklore, fox spirits are regarded as mischievous fairies, said to be the source of various kinds of trouble that affect human beings. In *The Secret and Sublime: Taoist Mysteries and Magic,* Blofeld tells of the "fox towers," the dwelling places of the fox spirits, that he observed while traversing Buddhist and Taoist pilgrim routes of pre-Communist China. He devotes several pages to one particularly dangerous type of fox-spirit.

According to Chinese folklore, a *huli jing* poses as a young maiden. In this role, the fox spirit masters the art of sexual attraction to lure the unsuspecting male. Blofeld records the following advice offered by someone who believed that making a disparaging remark to a fox spirit had cost his brother's life: "If you ever chance to encounter a fox acquainted with human speech, I implore you to guard your tongue; your very life will depend upon your skill in exercising self-restraint." [66] Blofeld ends the section on *huli jing* with the following comment:

> Those tales of demons and fox-spirits, however far-fetched they may seem, will illustrate the atmosphere prevailing in many a Taoist monastery. The recluses and their followers accepted the reality of the spirits much as we Westerners accept the menace of the millions of invisible germs filling the earth's atmosphere. [67]

Bizarre, but is it True?

More recently, an author using the pseudonym "Hsi Lai" provided an intriguing account of a secret female Taoist sexual practice. Describing himself as a practicing Taoist with a background in "Chinese language, healing arts, and philosophy with notable teachers," Hsi Lai claims to have been allowed access to the inner sanctum of a cult of "White Tigress" female Taoist adepts, in order to document the techniques, methods, and history of a secret female clan located in Taipei, Taiwan.

In documenting the cult, Lai claims to have been able to examine secret handwritten copies of ancient texts that were written for female aspirants. The material, some of which is suspect, is nonetheless intriguing, and thus worthy of consideration.

According to Hsi Lai, while the goal of male aspirants is to cultivate and practice the retention of semen during intercourse, the role of the White Tigress is, through any means necessary, to acquire the male *jing* essence. As he explains, the White Tigresses, instead of allowing their sexual energy to be taken by men, specialized in depleting the *jing* essence of unsuspecting males (mainly through oral sex), in order to maintain youthfulness and beauty.[68]

Not to be confused with prostitutes, Hsi Lai explains, the members of the White Tigresses comprise a secret society headed by a female master "White Tigress." Within the sect, Taoist principles are taught through instruction in what he calls "all three interpretations" of Taoist practice, which include "first, undergoing sexual regeneration, then sexual alchemy, then spiritual alchemy—blending and developing all three over a nine-year period." [69]

Like many Taoist sects, the cult claims to originate with the mythical Yellow Emperor, who is supposed to have lived around 2,500 BCE. As the story goes, the Taoist legacy of sexology is traced to three female initiatresses, who instructed the legendary Yellow Emperor in the "arts of the bedchamber." According to the belief, the Emperor absorbed the sexual energy of 1,200 young female consorts, all without releasing his sperm. Accordingly, the procedure is said to have allowed him to become an immortal. [70]

Other aspects of female sexology training described by Hsi Lai include female adepts learning to curb menstruation in order to minimize loss of *jing-essence*. As Hsi Lai explains, a female at or near graduation enters a level called "Hunts for Prey," a state where she has gained enough "psychic power" to attract whatever she desires to satisfy her. In Hsi Lai's words, "like a hungry tiger, her senses become increasingly sharp." [71] As a final note, he describes the activation and depletion of *jing* energy in ways consistent with other Taoist teachings. For example, the development of *jing* begins at puberty, which triggers sexual development due to the production of testosterone in males and estrogen and progesterone in females.

Chapter 31

Kundalini and Super Consciousness

A beam of light will fill your head
And you'll remember what's been said
By all the good men this world's ever known.

"Melancholy Man", The Moody Blues [72]

Consider the possibility that a powerful force sits dormant and coiled at the base of the spine. Unless awakened, this aspect of internal energy remains passive. However, if and when it is roused, it initiates a wave of tremendous energy that pulses through the body, experienced as a highly charged and concentrated flow of energy from the tailbone to the top of the head. In its awakened form, its primary function is to initiate super genius. This scenario describes *kundalini* (कुण्डलिनी), potentially the single most powerful, and at the same time dangerous, form of internal energy. The awakened form of *kundalini* is not child's play.

To the experiencer, awakened *kundalini* manifests as a two-edged sword. While one side of the sword initiates genius and psychic powers, the other, due to its unwieldy nature, can inflict immense psychological and physical suffering. In some cases, the power unleashed from awakened *kundalini* can be so tremendous that it can even threaten to destroy its host.

This scenario introduces the *kundalini* subset of internal energy. According to some who have encountered this form of internal energy, it is described as simultaneously powerful and yet, whether by design or evolution, difficult to access. However, when awakened, it can become the gateway to the miraculous.

As described by proponents, awakened *kundalini* travels up the spine into a yet-to-be-mapped place in the brain, referred to as the *Brahma randbra*, which is described as the brain center that activates super genius. In contrast to the Taoist bio-energetics discussed earlier, *kundalini* awakening initiates a normally dormant force which can be so strong that, at times, the experiencer loses control over their volition. When this happens, the powerful *kundalini* force "takes on a life of its own."

Brief Introduction to *Kundalini*

The earliest references to *kundalini* date to the *Upanishads* (ninth century BCE – third century BCE). [73] Sitting like a coiled snake at the base of the tailbone, because of the connection between *kundalini* and hypersexuality, it is considered in the present section covering the transmutation of sexual energy.

Note that the views expressed in this chapter are of the minority opinion. The focus here is placed on the *kundalini* phenomenon as a potent form of mind-body internal energy. There is a larger body of work which describes the practices of *kundalini* yoga — as with other forms of Hindu-based yoga — as the path to worship of God or seeking union with the divine.

Gene Keiffer, a scientist who spent years investigating the phenomenon, believes *kundalini* is essential to human evolution. In his view, *kundalini* functions as the biological foundation of creativity and advanced thought, and thus the source of "spiritual inspiration [present] from the beginning of time." For Keiffer, *kundalini* represents the missing link to explaining the sudden advancement of human achievement throughout history, and "the golden thread that runs through the world's sacred writings." [74]

Some comparisons can be made between *kundalini,* the sexual energy-consciousness systems of China, and the *tantric* systems of Tibet. The obvious commonality is the activation and transmutation of sexual energy. In all three traditions, the process begins at the lowest energy centers of the body's core.

Gopi Krishna

Gopi Krishna came to the attention of the West after the publication of *The Biological Basis of Religion and Genius* (1972). In his descriptions of his personal encounters with *kundalini,* Krishna explains how his "*kundalini* activation" began in 1937. One day, while in seated meditation, he became aware of a strange sensation of movement in the area of his tailbone. As he continued to meditate, the sensations grew increasingly stronger, and, as the sensations continued to intensify, they became unsettling. Next, the strange feelings transformed into the sensation of something powerful traveling upward along his spine, until the movement of energy became so powerful that his entire body shook. The experience became overwhelming, and he felt that he was losing control over these sensations and that "something was giving way."

At that point, the sensations were no longer only at the tailbone and in his spine; he noticed some strange sensations appearing at the top of his head. At the very top of his crown, Krishna felt that a "new aperture had opened." These strange experiences were linked to the movement of *kundalini* energy rising in his spinal cord. [75]

The sensations continued over the following days and weeks, but with some differences, as along with the sensations came a sense of increased awareness and knowledge. Suddenly and unexpectedly, he knew a great deal about subjects he had never studied. For Krishna, this was evidence that he was not experiencing some kind of "normal" psychiatric episode, but rather that he had undergone something new and important. The knowledge he suddenly acquired included fluency in languages never studied. Krishna, a man with little formal education, began to write poetry in German, a language he had never studied. Here is one of his poems:

Ein Schöner Vogel immer singt
In Meinem Herz mit leisem Ton …
Und wenn vergist der Nachtwind auf
Die grünen Gräser seine Traänen, …
Dann der Vogel wacht [76]

[A beautiful bird always sings
in my heart with a soft voice
And when the night wind sheds
its tears on the green grass,
Then the bird is watching.]

Krishna was at a loss as he attempted to make sense of his new experiences. Then, occasionally and gradually, an entirely new sensation began to come over him. He would call the new experience *extreme bliss*. However, *bliss* came with a price. The experience of *bliss* alternated with the sense of internal terror, as he began to experience full-blown *kundalini* awakening. Fortunately, for most people, most of the time, the force remains dormant:

> Leaving out the extreme cases, which end in madness, this generalization applies to all men in whom Kundalini is more or less active, comprising mystics, mediums, men of genius, and those of an exceptionally high intellectual or artistic development only a shade removed from genius. In the case of those in whom the awakening occurs all at once as a result of yoga or other spiritual practices, the sudden impact of powerful vital currents on the brain and other organs is often attended with grave risk and strange mental conditions, varying from moment to moment, exhibiting in the beginning the abnormal peculiarities of a medium, mystic, genius, and madman all rolled into one. [77]

Due to its influence on the *Brahma randbra*, Krishna came to understand how full *kundalini* activation, along with its volatile power, possessed the capacity to bring forth either a great saint or a lunatic [78] (or perhaps, a lunatic who is a great saint?). The activation of the brain center totally drained his body's reserves, and its effects had a particularly powerful influence on the body's store of sexual energy. The awakened *Brahma randbra* fed off the body's sexual energy, and its appetite became insatiable. [79] The awakening initiated a host of heightened nervous system responses:

> With the awakening of *kundalini*, an amazing activity commences in the whole nervous system, from the crown of the head to the toes... the nerves whose normal existence are never felt by normal consciousness, are now forced by some invisible power to a new type of activity, which either immediately or gradually becomes perceptible to the subject.

> Through all their innumerable endings, they begin to extract a nectar like substance from the surrounding tissues, which, traveling in two distinct forms, one as radiation, one as subtle essence, streams in to the spinal cord . . . radiation, appearing as a luminous cloud in the head, streams into the brain. [80]

An Evolutionary Force

Krishna came to understand *kundalini* as an evolutionary force, and the underlying "blueprint stamped on the brain." [81] As Krishna explains, the "blueprint" contains sets of normally dormant internal codes that initiate a type of evolutionary advancement related to high creativity, the advancement of consciousness, and spiritual growth that he describes as the "evolutionary force in humankind." In his words:

> From my own experience, extending to a quarter of a century, I am irresistibly led to the conclusion that the human organism is evolving in the direction indicated by mystics and prophets and by men of genius. By the action of this mechanism, located at the base of the spine, depending for its activity mainly on the energy supplied by the reproductive organs. .... as the means to develop spirituality, super normal faculties and psychic powers, the mechanism has been known and manipulated from very ancient times. [82]

Kundalini's Sexual Appetite

According to Krishna, *kundalini* activates an insatiable sexual appetite because the awakened *Brahma randbra* brain center feeds off sexual energy. The process provokes what he describes as a "potential life and death struggle:"

> Once awakened, without the flow of energy from the reproductive organs to the brain that the process demands, the results would be insanity or death. [83]

Kundalini and Advanced Consciousness

Might there really be an aspect of brain biology that, as Krishna tells us, feeds from, and is responsive to, sexual energy? Could it be true that both sexual energy and the pleasure that accompanies it could somehow be related to super genius? The nature of these relationships between sexual energy and advanced consciousness seems to parallel the descriptions provided by some of the mystic-philosophers discussed earlier, such as Swedenborg and Blake.

Regarding the proposal that it might be possible for a person to suddenly gain access to knowledge never studied, this is supported by reports of people who have undergone a near-death experience (NDE). For example, psychiatrist David Hawkins, in recounting his own NDE, reports that the event initiated him into "advanced levels of understanding." In some ways, after his NDE — and this is remarkably similar to Krishna's experience – Hawkins, too, was suddenly able to access "formerly hidden levels of information," which in his case concerned the nature of consciousness and personality. Hawkins also describes the experience of pleasurable energy coursing through the spine:

> A sweet, delicious band of energy started to flow continuously up the spine and into the brain, where it created an intense sensation of continuous pleasure. Everything in life happened by synchronicity, evolving in perfect harmony, and the miraculous was commonplace. [84]

Hawkins's experience brought about a radical change in the way he saw the world:

> Everything and everyone in the world was luminous and exquisitely beautiful. All living things became radiant and expressed this radiance in stillness and splendor. It was apparent that all of mankind is actually motivated by inner love, but has simply become unaware... [85]

Sidebar/

Whether or not the experience had anything to do with *kundalini* activation I cannot say. However, for me, it serves as evidence for some type of latent power residing in the tailbone. The experience took place several years ago while I was presenting a series of seminars in South Korea.

One day, after the end of a long morning of training, we took a break and returned to our hotel for a brief rest. When I got to my bed, I laid down, exhausted and looking forward to the brief respite.

As I laid there, I began to practice some very slow deep breathing to recharge. I focused energy on the area of the tailbone. It was an enjoyable feeling as I laid there practicing the slow, deep, rhythmic breathing. Eventually fell into that twilight peacefulness between sleep and consciousness. However, I was suddenly awakened by an enormous electric shock as it coursed through my entire body.

In no more than a fraction of a second, without any conscious attempt to move, my body responded to the electrical-like force by flipping me over from face down to face up in that fraction of a second.

I was stunned by the sudden violence of the flip and for a while a laid there unmoving and staring at the ceiling. Whoa—what was that! Although I can't say whether the experience had anything to do with *kundalini* or other form of energy, nevertheless the experience was quite profound. To this day it serves as testimony to the presence of some kind of dormant power residing in the tailbone that has the power to awaken, surge, shock, and physically move the entire body in a surprising way.

JB

Dangers

The preceding paragraphs touch on some of the difficulties associated with *kundalini* awakening. In Krishna's experience, *kundalini* activation produced side effects ranging from the benign to the bizarre, including twelve years of extreme physical pain.

Researchers, as well as authentic teachers of the *kundalini* tradition, emphatically warn of the dangers of sudden, full awakening. They universally stress that the student must be properly prepared and guided for the experience. As Krishna puts it, if the person's "system wasn't ripe for the experience," he doubted that an unprepared individual could survive the ordeal. [86] This kind of extraordinary warning is well understood in India, where "kundalini clinics" operate to treat those afflicted with disorders related to full *kundalini* crisis. Fortunately, and contrary to advertised claims sometimes associated with the term *kundalini*, few Western teachers offer authentic "kundalini" meditation or yoga. This watered-down instruction has a positive side; it helps to prevent an excess of potentially potent and dangerous *kundalini* experiences.

Emotional disturbances associated with full *kundalini* activation can be either acute or chronic. During one period, Krishna described himself as being constantly disturbed, [87] and feeling as though he was "heading toward a lunatic asylum." These experiences persisted on and off for years. [88]

Other writers on the topic describe the psychological dangers of the more intense energetic-meditative states. Insight into the potential of highly concentrated internal energy on the nervous system is reflected in a story by Ram Dass, formerly Dr. Richard Alpert, and an associate professor of psychology at Harvard. In *Miracle of Love,* Dass describes his guru's warnings about intense energetic experiences during meditation states called *samadhi*. In one report, Dass tells how his guru, Neem Karoli Baba (Maharaji), would interrupt this meditation in order to preserve Ram Dass's psychological health.

> Maharaji's process of teaching concentration and meditation was unique. He'd somehow shake you out of it the moment you began to feel some pleasure. I once asked him why he'd stopped my Samadhi, and he answered that the mind has its limitations, that I was in a physical body, and that these things are achieved slowly, otherwise I'd become a lunatic. He understood the capacity of your body. [89]

Guru Baba Karoli "shook" Dass out of his deep trance because the teacher was aware of the potential dangers of some deep meditative states, even the pleasurable ones. His actions seem consistent with Gopi Krishna's descriptions of the dangers that one must be aware of while in these kinds of advanced states:

When aroused in a body not attuned to it, without the help of various disciplines, or not genetically mature for it, it can lead to awful mental states, to almost every form of mental disorder, from hardly noticeable aberrations to the most horrible forms of insanity, to neurotic and paranoid states, to megalomania, and by causing tormenting pressure on the reproductive organs, to an all-consuming sexual thirst that is never assuaged. [90]

The sentiment that premature *kundalini* awakening can be dangerous is also reflected in the advice offered by high lamas. For example, Rinpoche Chamgon Kenting Tai Situpa describes in an online interview how premature *kundalini* awakening can be especially dangerous:

Kundalini is a very serious business. This physical body with a spine, head and limbs, everything that a fully matured human body is supposed to have, Kundalini is its potential of experiencing the great non-dualistic joy, this ability. All have it, male and female. But Kundalini practice is reserved for a person who is totally dedicated for it. [91]

Situpa explains further that if an individual who is not ready for the experience, or is not living a spiritually-dedicated life, awakens *kundalini,* yet tries thereafter to lead a normal life, this poses difficulty for the individual because the experience:

...will not stop. and if you live an ordinary life it will drive you mad. It will cause you tremendous problems and it can practically make you mad. You won't be able to take it. Therefore, *Kundalini* practice is reserved for somebody who lives a yogic life and who is totally, totally dedicated for it. [92]

Because of the extreme effects on the nervous system, anyone considering working toward the goal of activating their *kundalini* should proceed with extreme caution and only under proper guidance. I advise students and clients never to attempt to "awaken *kundalini*" prematurely. *Kundalini* will awaken if and when it is supposed to, and according to its own timeline. The potential dangers associated with these kinds of intensive meditative practices are reflected in the experience of a well-known European writer:

I believe it started one day during meditation. I felt a tremendous release of energy around my sacrum, inside of my pelvis and hip joints, as if my bones and muscles felt like they had melted and changed into hot liquid. While in meditation, I perceived that my body had started to change its shape (into flowers animals etc.), and finally disappeared completely. I had experienced sensations like this before and I had always been very careful not to get attached to any kind of these so called "exalted states of mind." I don't meditate to get high, but this time it was different. It was very intense, very real. I was sure I had made some type of major breakthrough.

I woke up the next day with the same feeling I had after being beaten up by a gang of older teenagers when I was fourteen years old. My entire body was numb and swollen. Still, I didn't pay too much attention to it. I knew from previous experience that a release of energy is very often followed by temporary pain and even higher degree of stiffness, but it always disappears. And indeed, it did, at least for a while.

Shortly after this experience, I began to have a problem with my left leg. It was noticeably getting weaker. I also felt an occasional sharp pain in my left buttock. Again, I ignored it, there is always some kind of pain when you practice martial arts but when it became more serious I visited a chiropractor. I suspected I might have a trapped or pinched nerve, periformis syndrome, or sciatica. The chiropractor took an x-ray of my spine but didn't find anything abnormal. He performed some small adjustments to my back and afterwards I felt better. I thought that was it.

A few months later, the pain returned, becoming constant and unbearable. I went back to the chiropractor, but this time it didn't help. The pain became worse. After returning home my entire body went into a spasm (imagine the feeling of a Charlie horse that affected every muscle in your body). I couldn't move . . . I couldn't walk, I couldn't sit or lie down; all I could do was crawl on my knees and elbows.

That night I fell into kind of liquid hallucinatory dream state. In it, I was scanning my body from the inside, observing places of tension and sending mental instructions to muscles to release and relax. Suddenly, I noticed something arising from my perineum. The object looked like a compressed ball made of extremely fine golden wires or soft hair. When I focused my attention on the ball, I was shocked. It felt as if I had run into an incredibly strong force field. The small bundle of golden hair seemed to have the energy of a black hole.

Then the ball started to move. First traveling up and into to my coccyx, next through my sacrum and spine, exactly as it is described in old Indian literature on Kundalini. I remember saying to myself: Thank you very much, whoever you are. Excellent timing! That's exactly what I need right now. But it wasn't funny. My spine felt like a hose swollen under pressure or vibrating string ready to break. The ball behaved like liquid metal; it was changing shape going through, and the same time, outside of my spine. When it reached a thoracic area, I sensed that something was wrong, and instead of going up, was aiming for my heart. I got scared. And I mean scared. I was pretty much sure that my heart was going to explode. So, I decided to stop it, using all attention and breathing tricks I learned during my meditation training and I succeeded. The ball stopped just above a diaphragm, returned down to perineum and disappeared.

I felt completely burnt out, as if my nervous system was short-circuited. I crawled under a hot shower, gently moving my spine trying to release it from its twisting grip. Finally, I managed to stand up, for the first time in the twelve hours.

That night I lost twelve pounds, and all my strength, flexibility, speed, balance, everything. My spine was shot, my ribcage was shot, my abdomen muscles and diaphragm were partially paralyzed, there was no knee reflex and my shoulders were frozen; I couldn't lift my right arm above my head without screaming. I sought medical help, however no one really knew what had happened to me. An MRI scan revealed only a small disk herniation between S1 and L5 juncture, but the doctor told me that it was too small to cause such serious effects.

Although extremely painful, I tried to return to my usual exercise routine almost immediately. Despite the pain, I knew I had to do something. Otherwise, I was certain I would be crippled for the rest of my life. Strangely enough, my overall physical condition improved very fast, at least on a superficial level, but that was all. Everything else was getting worse. I felt that initial damage I suffered was spreading like a chain reaction through my nervous system on a very deep level. I thought that meditation would help, but that was out of the question. Whenever I tried to meditate I immediately felt energy rising again, twisting and crippling my body, sending shock waves of heat, cold and pain into every cell. I was not able to concentrate, write, work or sleep. I went through a period experiencing symptoms of various diseases such as arthritis, digestion problems and so on. During the same period, I also had episodes of terrible depression. I saw my life as a chain of mistakes, defeats, and blunders and I saw the entire Universe as a stupid nonsensical shit hole.

To make the story short, with all my experience in martial arts, yoga, energy work, meditation and so on, it took me almost five years, to get myself back into reasonably functional state. Nowadays, I rarely have any pain. I am flexible and almost as strong as I used to be. I can meditate again but I am very careful. Whenever I feel energy rising too strongly, I stand up and disperse it with gentle movements. In other words, I am still scared.

(Name withheld by request)

Kundalini **Syndrome**

Some researchers interested in psycho-physiological effects of *kundalini* are beginning to study the phenomenon in terms that they call "kundalini syndrome." In one study, Bruce Greyson, MD, looked at psycho-neurological changes associated with the phenomenon. Researchers found characteristics related to *kundalini* arousal to be associated with fantasy proneness, dissociation, absorption and a temporal-limbic brain (TLB) hyper-connection. [93] Since a relationship exists between TLB hyper-connection and previously neutral events eliciting strong emotions, Greyson's findings suggest that those prone toward *kundalini* experience possess stronger than normal connections between the limbic lobe, the "seat of emotions," and the cerebral cortex.

Itzhak Bentov also studied the psychoneurological effects of the *kundalini,* and in 1977, he described what he referred to as the "physio-kundalini syndrome." Bentov identified biological markers of aroused kundalini that include the brains of subjects possessing unique patterns of acoustical standing waves in the cerebral ventricles, which, Bentov explains, "depolarized the sensory and motor cortices of the brain." [94]

Other research supporting the notion of *kundalini* activation as both a physical and mental phenomenon was conducted by Greyson. He identified a series of markers suggestive of *kundalini* arousal, including the body assuming and holding strange positions for no apparent reason. Other markers include spontaneous body movement, spontaneous ecstatic tickle or orgasmic feeling, extreme sensations of heat or cold moving through the body for no apparent reason, and the reported sensations of internal lights or colors.

Conclusion to *Kundalini* Section

Of particular relevance to the present discussion are the possible relationships between *kundalini*, Taoist energetic meditation, and *tantric* sexual yoga. These relationships provide more insight into the meaning of "internal energy," and prominent among them is the belief that describes a potent psychobiological interaction between sexual energy, creativity, advanced spiritual awareness, enlightenment, and genius.

Of special interest to our inquiry is the role of the spinal column in each of the traditions just cited. All three posit that because of the connection between the brain and the sexual centers, the structure, or parallel energetic structure, of the spine helps initiate those attributes. *Kundalini* appears as an example of a potent force linking sexual energy to the most etheric aspects of human experience, which, as suggested by Gopi Krishna, "stands in urgent need of investigation." [95]

Chapter 32

Tibetan Tantric Sexual Practice

Section V introduced the Tibetan Buddhist yogic practice of *tummo,* or "inner heat," meditation. There, the doctrine of "transforming poison" was described as a *tantric* energetic-meditative practice, based on the notion that pleasure can be converted into transformative wisdom. The present section takes a closer look at this esoteric Tibetan *tantric* practice, as well as the relationship between pleasure and wisdom. In this regard, particular focus is placed on the Tibetan Buddhist *tantric* doctrine of *bliss,* how *bliss* converts into wisdom, and how these issues relate to sexual union. Note that Indian and Tibetan *tantra* are complex practices. The brief discussion presented here is not intended to be a comprehensive statement on these nuanced subjects; rather, the material that follows serves only as an introduction to how practitioners in these traditions view sexual-*tantric* practice.

Of particular interest is the claim that pleasure can be converted into spiritual advancement. Although *ecstasy* in sexual *tantra* is most often compared to the pleasurable sensations of orgasm, *tantric* practitioners emphasize that their experience of *ecstasy* is quite different. As reflected by sampling the instructions of the *tantric* masters cited below, and applied to dual practice, pleasure associated with ordinary orgasm is only a hint of the experience of *bliss* that can be attained through sexual *tantric* practice.

Part of the explanation for this is that instead of "sexual energy" being "lost" in ejaculation, through paired *tantra* sexual union it is redirected into the central channel — the previously described energy channel that runs along the spinal column — for the purposes of consciousness raising.

Transforming Desire

The core tenant of *tantric* sexual practice is the *transformation of desire.* Applied to partner practice, there are four levels. The first involves the initiate transforming desire when they gaze at a lover or someone to whom they are attracted. The second progresses through several levels of interacting with a partner, called "laughing with the lover." The third involves embrace, and the fourth and final stage is the channeling of sexual unity "into the path of spiritual evolution energies as intense as sexual union itself." [96] Lama Yeshe, who was cited earlier, discusses the four classes of *tantra:*

> Each of the four classes of *tantra* is meant for a particular type of practitioner. What differentiates one class of tantra from another is the intensity of the desire energy used in the path to enlightenment. In Action *Tantra*, great bliss is aroused by simply looking at all the beautiful deities; in Performance *Tantra*, smiling and laughing is used to energize bliss; in Yoga *Tantra*, blissful energy is generated from holding hands; and in Highest Yoga *Tantra*, the energy of the sexual embrace is used. .... The result of successful practice is the experience of clear-light during orgasm. [97]

Tantra developed as an organized movement in India, in the middle of the first millennium CE. Translated from the Sanskrit word for "woven," the terms *tantra* and *tantric* refer to several disciplines that include prayer, visualization, and physical yoga. Regardless of the specific practice, *tantra* is used as an empowering method directed toward the disciple's progressive realization of *mind* and the achievement of buddhahood, a state believed by practitioners to be of ultimate benefit to living beings. To emphasize an earlier point, *tantra* in the Buddhist tradition is considered a transformative path whereby human energies are focused on the achievement of advanced spiritual understanding, rather than being stifled, ignored, or used for selfish purposes.

Tantric practices, especially if undertaken prematurely or incorrectly, hold potential dangers. For these reasons, *tantric* practices are treated as secret.

Due to a combination of inherent dangers and secrecy, [98] reliable information on *tantric* sexual practice is limited and difficult to find. Furthermore, the reader is advised not to attempt any of the advanced methods of sexual yoga discussed below without proper preparation under the guidance of a qualified teacher. Sexual *tantric* yoga involves long and specialized training with a qualified guide.

There are many types of *tantric* practice, and the general overview of *tantric* sexual yoga introduced here covers only one of them. Other examples of *tantric* practice include the use of empowerment ceremonies, specially prepared amulets, and the placement of mandalas or *yantras* — individually prescribed wall hangings — believed to issue a vibrational energy that attracts blessings.

Through empowerment ceremonies, the novice obtains blessings and permission to arise meditatively as a deity, [99] with proponents believing that participation in an empowerment ceremony develops wisdom and compassion *through* visualization and ritual practice. By participating in the empowerment ceremony, the practitioner believes that they will one day achieve a state of consciousness identical to the enlightened being for whom the ritual was performed.

Tantric sexual practices are reserved exclusively for the most advanced adepts. For practitioners seeking to practice sexual yoga with a consort, the list of obstacles to overcome is lengthy, and includes the realization of "emptiness" [100] and the ability to transform desire, delusions, and selfish motivations. [101] It is useful to note that in the Tibetan *tantric* tradition, the practice of taking on a consort was emphasized by *tertons* (treasure revealers) as a process to unveil treasures *(terma)*. According to tradition, many had to take them, otherwise they would become sick and die.

According to Ian Baker, the Dalai Lama states that the inner teachings of Tibetan *tantra* have traditionally been kept secret because "to engage in them without proper guidance can lead to misunderstanding." [102] However, the Dalai Lama goes on to explain that "in the right context," *tantric* techniques are "held to lead speedily to the total liberation of the body, mind, and spirit." [103] As with the examples of intensive practice provided earlier, *tantric* sexual yoga is considered a two-edged sword that can either speed up the training of one's consciousness or, if the protocols and disciplines are not carefully followed, hasten one's demise.

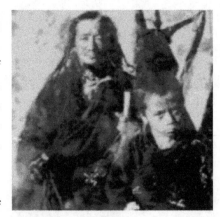

Photo 6-5

Like Father, Like Son

The young Buddhist tantric master and Acharya, * Dawa Chödak Rinpoche, with his father, Kathak Rigzin Dorje Rinpoche.

* An Acharya has completed formal advanced training in Tibetan Buddhism

Of particular focus for the *tantric* yogi is the conscious management of *thigle* "droplets" within the body's energy channels. It should be noted that *thigle* has other translations, but in the context applied to this chapter covering sexual *tantra*, it refers to subtle energy "droplets" contained within the body's energetic channels, which in Sanskrit are called *nadis*. * Section V cites the Tibetan lama Namkhai Norbu Rinpoche, who explained that *thigle* is not separate from *lung* "wind" energy that moves through the channels, but rather "one is the essence of the other." According to Norbu, "When the *prana [lung]* is brought into the central channel, its essential nature — *thigle* — is activated."

Through *tantric* practice, sexual essences are redirected through a subtle channel that runs parallel and in front of the spinal column. This is the central channel, which responds to the *thigle* directed there by leading one to a blissful state that subsequently reveals the "empty and luminous nature of reality." [104]

* Introduced in Section V, in Sanskrit, *nadi* (नाड़ी) translates as a tube or channel. The *nadi* are channels which transport the body's subtle energy. These are the subject of traditional Indian medicine and spiritual sciences.

Like most *tantric* teachers, Lama Yeshe emphasizes the importance of gaining control over the *thigle* in the body. Yeshe explains that the *thigle* activated through yogic practice must be controlled and directed into the body's central nervous and subtle energetic systems, otherwise it can be "dangerous and can produce illness if it becomes blocked in any one place." [105]

From an interview with Shenphen Dawa Rinpoche

"I had one especially qualified tutor named Lachung Apo who I studied with for a couple of years. He had studied in Mendro Ling monastery and almost became the abbot there, but instead he lost his vows. After that he went totally into secret tantric practices. He was a very realized teacher."

S: He lost his vows?

SDR: "Yes. It's a stage of development where he felt that he wanted to transcend the monastic path and become a yogi. Also, he lived with this lady who was a prostitute, who was in fact a dakini. She gave up her body and left one day, without leaving any trace behind. My tutor was involved with her."

Source: www.tersar.org/continuity.html

*Female angelic-like entity

Tantric sexual practices are restricted to advanced non-monastic yogis (Photo 6-5), who marry or take on consorts. *Ngakpas* are one type of yogi that train in the Tibetan *tantric* tradition to master the *tsa-lung* "channels and wind," and practices like these take many years to master, with the preparation alone requiring a long period of training. Moreover, a qualified lama will impart the teachings only to disciples possessing the requisite character, compassion, and capacities.

Master Padmasambhava brought *tantric* practice to Tibet in the eighth century. Known popularly as "Guru Rinpoche," Padmasambhava is regarded as a "second Buddha" among his disciples, and within *tantric* circles he is considered the quintessential *tantric* master. His teachings included the doctrine of "experiencing all appearances as innately pure," [106] and, as an example of his instruction, below are his words to the king of Tibet, Trisong Detsen:

> Your majesty... gain certainty in the fact that since the very beginning, your own mind is the awakened state of buddhahood. Gain certainty in the fact that all phenomena are, in essence, the magical display of the mind. Gain certainty in the fact that the final goal is already present within you and is not to be sought elsewhere ... unless you experience the innate nature of phenomena and mind as beyond thought and conception [you will suffer when] your kingdom and worldly power, which are as insubstantial as a rainbow, fade and vanish. [107]

The doctrine of *transforming desire* is central to *tantric* practice, and Baker describes this teaching as transforming "turbulent psychic forces into the energies of wisdom and compassion." [108] On this point, Baker quotes the Dalai Lama's description of the nature of *tantra:*

> In the early Buddhist traditions, desire was viewed as a poison to be avoided. The later Mahayana view was not to avoid the poison, but to antidote it with the appropriate remedy. In tantra, desire is seen as a potent energy to be used on the path to enlightenment; just as peacocks in the jungle thrive on poisonous plants and transform them symbolically into the radiant plumage of tail feathers.

> ...However, due to unconventional perspectives and because of the danger of subtle misinterpretation, the innermost teachings were traditionally presented only to those of refined sensibility, and only after many years of monastic study. [109]

Baker stresses that *tantra* is not the rejection of agitated mental states, but rather the transformation of them. He emphasizes the point with a citation from the *Hevajra* tantric text: "What for others is the source of bondage, in *tantra* is the cause of liberation." [110]

Yeshe explains that in *tantric* sexual practices, it is the seminal essence not released during intercourse, but instead redirected and then dispersed throughout the body, which leads "to [the ultimate] blissful state [that] reveals the [simultaneous] empty and luminous nature of reality." [111]

Dakini

Referring to an angelic, feminine being, the term *dakini* (in Tibetan, *khandro ma,* མཁའ་འགྲོ་མ) is found throughout *tantric* transformational literature. Sometimes she appears in the context of the conversion of consciousness practice expressed through sexual intercourse, [112] but *dakini* most often refers to an etheric female being, or fairy, which can also appear in human form. In either case, they are viewed as assistants that aid the individual toward enlightenment. The non-incarnate *dakinis* are said to reside in the etheric realm and appear as "protectors of the teachings," and in some cases, male adepts have been cited as invoking *dakini* feminine energy. Consider the use of the term *dakini* in light of the following report of Tibetan Buddhist practice:

> It's a whole training on its own. [It is included in] the monastic tradition as well as in the lay tradition. In that, we have two approaches, which are "penetrating through somebody else" and "penetrating through self." It may be in the other traditions, but I would think that most profoundly, this is a Nyingma [113] [secret] teaching. It deals with the dakini practice and the terms of dakini practice. It ... is the core of realization. [114]

Bliss, Orgasmic Experience, and *Tantra*

Tantric practice relies on the power of pleasure as a transformative agent. This is a special kind of transformation, involving the practitioner's control over sexual energy in the central channel, which leads "to a blissful state that reveals the empty and luminous nature of reality." [115]

The sense of pleasure described in both *tummo* inner heat meditation and *tantric* sexual yoga is sometimes compared to that of orgasm. However, it is important to distinguish between types of orgasm. As Lama Yeshe explains, ordinary sexual orgasm does not arise from the central channel, but from the *thigle* touching the outside of the central channel. [116] Yeshe elaborates on the relationship between bliss, orgasm and channel energy in the following way:

> In the logic of tantric yoga, if the *[thigle]* generates such bliss when it touches the outside of the central channel, there is no question that it will generate incredible bliss when it flows inside the central channel. Bringing all winds [subtle energies] into the central channel gives rise to an experience of incomparable super-bliss. [117]

Yeshe emphasizes the importance of not having sexual release during practice:

> Because [thigle] is the main resource that we use in inner fire meditation, it is important for both male and females not to lose their sexual energy. Naturally, as beginners, we find it difficult to control the energy when we experience it strongly; we have limited concentration we have not yet learned to bring the airs [lung/wind] into the central channel. [118]

Sexual Energy and Advanced Consciousness

When, and under what conditions, is it appropriate for an advanced yogi to take on a sexual consort for the purpose of *tantric* sexual practice? The question pertains not only to a yogi, but sometimes challenges the monk and his vow of celibacy. In this light, the general assumption is that a monk who participates in sexual acts would no longer be considered a monk. A story concerning celibacy and monastic vows tells of a *tantric* monk named Lama Tsongkhapa, the founder of the Gelug sect, who lived from 1357-1419 in the northeast Tibetan region of Amdo. Upon his death, he was perceived as having attained a high state of spiritual development called the "illusory body"(*gyu-lus*), and *tantric* practitioners believe that during his lifetime he had achieved a level of development so advanced, it would have been appropriate for him to engage in sexual yoga with a consort. However, he declined to take a consort, and his reasoning sheds light on our discussion.

According to tradition, Tsongkhapa was concerned about the volatile and potentially dangerous nature of consort practice, and the example he would be setting. He worried that future monks might abuse the practice by prematurely taking on consorts and engaging in union. Thus, he chose to set an example of pure monasticism, declining to take on a consort and keeping his celibate vows. Tibetan Buddhists believe that Tsongkhapa attained final buddhahood at the time of death. [119]

The Non-Celibate *Ngakpa* Tradition

In contrast to monastic celibacy, sexual *tantra* may be practiced by yogis of the non-celibate *Ngakpa* yoga tradition, where an advanced *Ngakpa* yogi can take a consort in order to achieve "buddhahood" more quickly. To reemphasize the main point, this form of paired practice is based on neither interest in procreation nor pleasure; it is practiced in order to attain the most sublime spiritual states. Since a yogi participating in this form of *tantric* practice must be free of selfish desire, few are qualified to undertake the practice.

Of the non-celibate yogis in the Tibetan Buddhist tradition, the Nyingma sect is known for many such adepts. Advanced *tantric* masters in the tradition include lamas such as Dudjom Rinpoche and Mindrolling Trichen Rinpoche, who, despite being married and raising families, were nevertheless renowned for their consummate spiritual power. Although we cannot say for certain, these are most probably two examples of lamas who chose to take consorts and practice sexual yoga in order to embody a practice that would benefit others. Within Tibetan Buddhist circles, it is believed that through *tantric* sexual yoga, they are able to direct their internal energy and "wind" to transform their physical being and experience of the world. [120]

Both men and women should learn to work with their desire and control their sexual energy, rather than losing it. This is not just a question of breaking samaya [the yogis pledge to keep their vows and commitments.] The point is that we lose the strength of our [thigle] and that is not good.

Lama Yeshe [121]

> **SIDEBAR/**
> Actually, real tantric liaisons are extremely rare.
>
> I once asked Khamtrul Rinpoche, "Seeing as sexual yoga is such a fast way to Enlightenment, how come you are all monks?"
> And he replied, "It's true it's a quick path but you have to be almost Buddha to practice it."
>
> To have a genuine tantric relationship first there must be no feeling of lust. Then there must be no emission of sexual fluids. Instead you must learn to send the fluids up through the central channel to the crown while doing very complicated visualization and breathing practices. All this requires tremendous control of body, speech, and mind. Even yogis who have practiced *tummo* [inner heat yoga] for many years say they'd need one or two lifetimes of practice to accomplish sexual yoga. So, these tantric weekends on offer in the West these days may give you a jolly good time, but little else!
>
> Vicki Mackenzie,
> *Cave in the Snow: On the life of Tenzin Palmo*
> Bloomsburg Publishing, London. 1998, p. 182

Conscious Control of Sexual Energy

A clue to the relationship between *tantric* yoga and the yogi's control over sexual energy is found in the poetry of the Sixth Dalai Lama (1683-1706). The former Buddhist monk gave up his vows and monk's robes, and as a young man chose frolicking with women and enjoyment of wine. However, his poems suggest that while he became dedicated to the pursuit of pleasure, he still practiced the discipline of non-ejaculation during intercourse:

> Never have I slept without a sweetheart
> Nor have I spent a single drop of sperm. [122]

The Sixth Dalai Lama left other clues to the nature of yogic sexual energy. Consider where, in the following poem, the image of the *vajra* refers to the "lightning bolt" implement used in *tantric* ritual:

> Visualize yourself as Heruka [123] with consort,
> Body clear yet empty,
> Energy channels ...vibrating within ...
> Place the tip of the *vajra* [lightning bolt] firmly in the lotus
> And in the mind, the letter *HUM* in the central channel;
> Drink, drink the essence of nectars
> Ecstatic with innate unmoving joy. [124]

Through this poem on the matter, the Sixth Dalai Lama emphasizes the importance of conservation of sexual energy, even while one engages in sexual intercourse.

Lay Practice of Sexual Yoga

The yogic arts of transforming sexual energy are not limited to the monk, and both non-celibate yogi and lay practitioners are encouraged to practice basic forms as well. Lama Yeshe offers the following advice:

> Lay people with a regular sex life should use the force of inner fire meditation to hold [thigle] in the secret chakra [base of the penis] for as long as possible during intercourse. Imagine that you experience simultaneously born great blissful wisdom before you release the energy.[125]

Yeshe explains that the ability to control sexual energy brings even greater bliss and satisfaction when matched with strong generation of internal energy due to "magnetic attraction" to the other person. Yeshe calls this approach the "secret path to liberation." [126]

> You cannot experience bliss if you cannot control thigle
> Lama Yeshe [127]

Energy Channels

Although the secrecy surrounding paired yogic tantric practice limits access to reliable information, a few clues are still available. Other pieces of the puzzle are found in the way that consort practice is said to activate specific energetic centers. For example, as explained by Lama Yeshe, while attention to the area of the lower abdomen is useful for tummo inner heat training, the crown chakra at the top of the head is important in consort practice. Yeshe emphasizes control over the flow of thigle subtle energy "droplets," and offers the following advice to lay practitioners: "The lower down the thigle flows, the more difficult it is to control… especially if it flows below the navel chakra." [128]

Chapter Conclusion

*A*lthough the present discussion introduced sexual yoga in the context of the Tibetan *tantric* tradition, it is important to keep in mind that there are a wide range of *tantric* practices besides the sexual. The purpose of *tantric* practice is to transform subtle energies.

In the *tantric* view, actions of body, speech, and mind produce subtle vibrations that, in turn, influence one's mental and physical states. Not only every action, but every thought creates an energetic ripple on the pond surface of one's experience. The ripples and waves represent *karmic* forces that make up the "water," or "conditions," of life. Through *tantric* practice, whether prayer, devotion, ritual physical yoga, or sexual yoga, the devotee's goal is to stir and manage subtle energies to transform their inner and outer worlds for the benefit of all living beings. The perceived link between *tantric* sexual practice and the awakening of advanced consciousness offers further insight into the meaning of subtle human bio-energy, beyond presently understood physiology.

Conclusion to Section VI

*T*he chapters in this section looked for clues that might reveal the meaning of internal energy in traditions that focus on the transmutation of sexual energy. It was also considered how, despite being often thought of as an Eastern tradition, the genesis of many of these ideas can be traced to the earliest periods of Western Civilization.

In both East and West, the transmutation of sexual energy was believed to be responsible for a number of powers. As with related topics considered in Section V, the ancient Greeks believed that seminal energy contributed to both one's lifespan and intelligence. As practiced in disparate traditions, ranging from the earliest organized Christian religions to ancient Tibet, India, and China, numerous practitioners have devoted tremendous amounts of resources to the study of how to capture and optimize the sexual energy related to two-person practice. Emperors kept concubines to use as medicine, Tibetan yogis studied the mind-altering states expressed through dual practice as a potentially dangerous shortcut on the road to enlightenment, and Taoist men and women engaged in a "battle of the sexes" to acquire the quintessence of human emotion and energy in order to attain immortality. These are but a few examples of how various traditions and cultures sought to master and willfully direct the volatile power of sexual energy.

The shared belief between those traditions cited is the recognition of the magnetic power of sexual energy. It is testimony to the power of this magnetic super-charged energy that, through the most intimate relationships, it can potentially be so strong that it can cure disease, prolong one's lifespan, and perhaps, if mastered, even assist one on the road to enlightenment.

Endnotes

1 Ni, Maoshing, *Yellow emperor's classic of medicine: A new translation of the neijing suwen with commentary,* Shambhala, Boston 1995, p.3.

2 Consistent with comments in the opening pages of the present work, for the most part, Chinese characters are transliterated using the *pinyin* system of transliteration. However, there are a few exceptions where Chinese is romanized in the Wade-Giles style. Examples of Wade-Giles transliteration in this section include Taoist, Taoism, *t'ai-chi,* and P'eng Tzu.

3 Hoare, Philip "Some very unreasonable erotic practices," A review of Schuchard, Marsha Keith, *Why Mrs. Blake cried: William Blake* and *the sexual basis of spiritual vision, The Telegraph,* April 30, 2006

4 Hoare

5 This point is disputed by scholar Brian Talbot in "Schuchard's Swedenborg," *The new philosophy* July -December 2007.

6 Ibid. p. 190.

7 Adams, Jad, "Blake's big toe," A review of *Why Mrs. Blake cried: William Blake* and *the sexual basis of spiritual vision,* The Guardian/Books Saturday 1 April 2006.

8 The Liver Meridian starts from the top of the great toe and crosses the top of the foot. After crossing the inner ankle on its upward journey, it continues upward along the inner side of the lower leg and the thigh, until it reaches the pubic region. It then circulates around the external genitalia and enters the lower abdomen. Afterward, it goes up the abdomen and reaches the lower chest to connect with the liver and gall bladder. From there, the meridian continues upwards along the throat and connects with the eyes. Finally, it emerges from the forehead to reach the vertex of the head. One of its internal branches originates internally from the eye and moves downwards to the cheek where it curves around the inner surface of the lips. Another branch starts from the liver and passes through the diaphragm to reach the lung, where it connects with the lung meridian and completes the cycle of the twelve meridians.

Based on the description by Angelo Chung, B Pharm, Integrated Chinese Medicine Holdings Ltd.

9 Swann, Ingo, *Psychic sexuality: The bio-psychic "anatomy" of sexual energies,* Panta Rei/Crossroads Press, 1998/2014 *Psychic sexuality,* Panta Rei, [Crossroads Press digital edition] Retrieved from Amazon.com Kindle Reader location 1058-1060.

10 Swann, Kindle location 1433.

11 Ibíd., Location 1156.

12 Ibíd., Location 1164.

13 Ibíd., Location 1433.

14 Wile, Douglas., *The art of the bedchamber: The Chinese sexual yoga*
classics including women's solo meditation texts, State University of New York (1992), p.59.

15 Wile, p. 60.

16 Adams Kristian, *et al.,* Neuroscience of sexual desire, http://neuro-sciencefundamentals.unsw.wikispaces.net

17 Raghavendra, BR et al, "Voluntary heart rate reduction following yoga using different strategies," *Int J Yoga.* 2013 Jan-Jun; 6(1): 26–30.

18 Wile, Douglas, *The art of the bedchamber: The Chinese sexual yoga classics including women's solo meditation texts,* State University of New York, 1992 p. 42.

19 Wile, p. 28.

20 http://newsroom.uvahealth.com/about/news-room/missing-link-found-between-brain-immune-system-with-profound-disease-implications

21 Internet Archive Book Images, via Wikimedia Commons.

22 Ware, James R. (translator), *Alchemy, Medicine, and Religion in the China of A.D. 320: the Nei P'ien of Ko Hung (Pao-p'u tzu),* Cambridge, MA and London, 1966, p. 122

23 Wile, Douglas, *The art of the bedchamber: The Chinese sexual yoga classics including women's solo meditation texts,* State University of New York (1992), p.11.

24 Wile. p. 60.

25 Ibid., p. 39.

26 Ibid., p. 56.

27 Ibid., p. 39.

28 Ibid., p. 16.

29 Miller, James, "Chinese sexual yoga and the way of immortality," adapted from the translation by Paul R. Goldin, 2006. "The Cultural and Religious Background of Sexual Vampirism in Ancient China." Theology

30 Wile, Douglas, *The art of the bedchamber: The Chinese sexual yoga classics including women's solo meditation texts,* State University of New York, p. 16.

31 Wile, p. 20

32 As translated by Douglas Wile, *Art of the bed chamber,* p. 9.

33 Wile, Douglas, *The art of the bedchamber: The Chinese sexual yoga classics including women's solo meditation texts,* State University of New York (1992 p. 46.

34 Wile., p. 13.

35 Ibid., *p.* 15.

36 Ibid. p. 13.

37 Ware (translator), Ko Hung, *The Pao Pu Tzu of Ko Hung*, p. 138.

38 Hsi Lai, *The sexual teachings of the white tigress*, Destiny Books, Vermont, p. 7.

39 Hsi Lai

40 Wile, Douglas, *The art of the bedchamber: The Chinese sexual yoga classics including women's solo meditation texts*, State University of New York, 1992, p. 20.

41 Wile, p. 48.

42 Ibid., p. 16

43 As translated by Douglas Wile, *The art of the bedchamber*, p. 20.

44 Wile, Douglas, *The art of the bedchamber: The Chinese sexual yoga classics including women's solo meditation texts*, State University of New York (1992) p. 16, p. 20.

45 The exception being where male adepts use techniques during sexual intercourse to "steal the woman's *qi*"

46 In the study, subjects' blood was analyzed for concentrations of adrenaline, noradrenaline, cortisol, prolactin, luteinizing hormone and testosterone concentrations. The study found that, "although plasma testosterone was unaltered by orgasm, higher testosterone concentrations were observed following the period of abstinence. These data demonstrate that acute abstinence does not change the neuroendocrine response to orgasm but does produce elevated levels of testosterone in males."

Exton, M.S., et al, "Endocrine response to masturbation-induced orgasm in healthy men following a 3-week sexual abstinence," *World journal of urology*, 2001 Nov;19(5) ,pp. 377-82.

47 Wile, p. 15.

48 Ibid., p. 7.

49 Ibid. p. 6.

50 Ibid. p. 56.

51 Ibid. p. 14.

52 Blofeld, John, *Taoism: The road to Immortality*, Shambhala, Boston, 1978, pp. 140-141.

53 Blofeld.

54 仙人 Literally, *xian ren*, or "immortal," see Section V

55 Blofeld, John, *Taoism: The road to Immortality*, Shambhala, Boston,

1978, pp. 140-141.

56 Ware (translator) Ko Hung, *The Pao Pu Tzu of Hung*, p. 140.

57 Lowenthal, Wolfe, *There are no secrets: Professor Cheng Man-ching*, North Atlantic Books, Berkeley, p. 104

58 Yang, Jwing-Ming, *Qigong: The secret of youth*, YMAA publications, Boston, MCA 2000 pp. 213, 243-245

59 Blofeld, John, *Taoism: The road to immortality*, Shambhala, Boston, 1978, p. 115.

60 Blofeld

61 Chang, Stephen T., *The complete system of self-healing*, Tao Publishing, Tao Longevity, LLC, Reno, NV, p. 26.

62 Wile, Douglas, *The art of the bedchamber: The Chinese sexual yoga classics including women's solo meditation texts*, State University of New York, p. 50.

63 Wile, p.55.

64 Ibid. p. 50.

65 Ibid. p. 55.

66 According to the report, the genesis of the incident was an unintended insult by the brother toward the fox spirit, who thereafter initiated a successful revenge plot that culminated in the brother's death. This was said to be attributed, at least in part, by the *hulijing* depleting the brother's life energy. The youth, captivated by the beauty of the fox spirit appearing as a rapturously beautiful woman, began a love affair that lasted several months. There were unsuccessful attempts at intervention. Alerted by the youth's change in appearance from one of vitality to that of pale lifelessness, the abbot of the monastery eventually learned of the affair and tried to intervene using a variety of methods that included locking the young hermit in his bedchamber. However, the measures could not prevail against the fiery passion that surged through the youth's body. In the end, all that was left of the Taoist recluse was a life-drained and a blood-soaked body. Blofeld, John, *The secret and sublime: Taoist mysteries and magic*, E.P. Dutton & Co., New York pp. 81-88.

67 Ibid.

68 Hsi Lai, *The sexual teachings of the white tigress: Secrets of female Taoist masters*, Destiny Books, Rochester, VT

69 Lai. pp.2-5.

70 Ibid. pp. 46-47.

71 Ibid. p. 94.

72 "Melancholy Man," The Moody Blues, lyrics by Michael Thomas Pinder.

73 https://en.wikipedia.org/wiki/Kundalini

74 Kieffer, Gene (Editor), Kundalini: *Empowering human evolution: Selected writings of Gopi Krishna*

75 Krishna, Gopi, *Kundalini: The evolutionary energy in man*, Shambala, 1997, p. 51.

76 Krishna, p. 56.

77 Ibid., p. 48

78 Ibid., 60

79 Krishna, Gopi, *The biological basis of religion and genius*, New York, Harper & Row, 1972

80 Krishna, Gopi, *Living with Kundalini*, Shambhala, Boston, 1993, as cited in *Kundalini: Empowering human evolution*, selected writings of Gopi Krishna 1996; edited by Gene Kieffer, p. 21

81 Krishna, Gopi, *Kundalini: The evolutionary energy in man*, Shambala Publications, 1970 p. 4

82 Krishna, p. 241

83 Ibid., p. 165

84 Hawkins, David, MD, *Power vs. force: The hidden determinants of human behavior*, Hay House, 1995 p. xvii.

85 Hawkins, p. 384.

86 *Krishna, Gopi, Kundalini: The evolutionary energy in man*, Shambala Publications, 1970 , p. 167

87 Krishna, p. 166.

88 Ibid., p. 159.

89 Ram Dass, et al., *Miracle of love: Stories about Neem Karoli Baba*, E. P. Dutton: New York. 1979. pp 243-244,

90 Dass, p. 161.

91 http://www.greatliberation.org/library/tai-situpa-library/Sadhana_Practices/Chenrezig%20Practice%20-%20December%202009.pdf

92 http://www.greatliberation.org/library/tai-situpa-library/Sadhana_Practices/Chenrezig%20Practice%20-%20December%202009.pdf

93 Greyson, Bruce, MD, "Some neuropsychological correlates of the physio-kundalini syndrome," *The journal of transpersonal psychology*, 2000, Vol. 32, No. 2.

94 As cited by Bruce Greyson in "Some neuropsychological correlates of the physio-kundalini syndrome" *The Journal of Transpersonal Psy-*

chology, 2000, Vol. 32, No. 2 Bentov, I., *Stalking the wild pendulum: On mechanics of consciousness* New York: Dutton, 1977.

95 Krishna, Gopi, *Kundalini: The evolutionary energy in man*, Shambala 1997 p. 55.

96 Ibid., p. 162.

97 Ibid.

98 Baker, Ian A., *The Dalai Lama's secret temple: Tantric wall paintings from Tibet*, Thomas & Hudson, NY, 2000, p. 9.

99 In the Tibetan Buddhist *tantric* tradition, this approach involves the use of the "fruit" as the path, where the practitioner visualizes him / herself as a deity, although he / she has not yet reached that state.

100 Yeshe, Lama, The *bliss of inner fire: Heart practice of the six yogas of Naropa*, Wisdom Publications, Sommerville, MA 1998, p. 166.

101 Baker, Ian A., *The Dalai Lama's secret temple: Tantric wall paintings from Tibet*, Thomas & Hudson, NY, 2000, p. 8.

102 Baker, p. 9.

103 Baker

104 Norbu, Chögyal Namkhai, *The crystal and the way of light: Sutra, tantra, and dzogchen*, Shambhala, Snow Lion Publications, 2000, p. 124

105 Yeshe, p. 150.

106 Baker, Ian A., *The Dalai Lama's secret temple: Tantric wall paintings from Tibet*, Thomas & Hudson, NY, 2000, p. 49.

107 Baker, p. 50.

108 Ibid.

109 Ibid. pp. 50-51.

110 Ibid. p. 51.

111 Yeshe, p. 33.

112 *Dakini* translates as "moving through space." It is the feminine principle associated with wisdom. This term has several levels of meaning. There are ordinary *dakinis* who are beings with a certain degree of spiritual power, and wisdom *dakinis*, who are fully realized. See Patrol Rinpoche, *Words of my perfect teacher*, Vistaar publications, New deli, India 2004, p. 409

113 The Nyingma is the oldest of the four schools of Tibetan Buddhism.

114 Norbu, Chögyal Namkhai, *The crystal and the way of light: Sutra, tantra, and dzogchen*, Shambhala, Snow Lion Publications, 2000, p. 124

115 Baker, Ian, *The Dalai Lama's secret temple: Tantric wall paintings*

The Search for Mind-Body Energy: Meditation, Medicine & Martial Arts *from Tibet,* Thames & Hudson, NY, 2000, p. 33.

116 Yeshe, Thubten, Lama, *The bliss of inner fire: The heart practice of the six yogas* of *Naropa,* Wisdom Publications, 1998, p. 49.

117 Yeshe, p. 148.

118 Ibid.

119 Tsenshap, Kirti, *Principles of buddhist tantra,* Wisdom Publications, Somerville, MA 2011, p. 204

120 As explained by Keith Dwoman, even when the "Fulfilment Phase" of *vajrayana* is practiced, the consort may be internalized. However, the maxim "No *mahamudra* without *karmamudra*" is taught in some lineages, particularly in the Kagyu school. See Glen Mullin "The Six Yogas of Naropa" or Keith Dowman, *Masters of Mahamudra* (SUNY).

121 Yeshe, Thubten, Lama, *The bliss of inner fire: The heart practice of the six yogas* of *Naropa,* Wisdom Publications, 1998, p. 101.

122 Baker, Ian *The Dalai Lama's secret temple: Tantric wall paintings from Tibet, Thames* & Hudson, NY, 2000 p. 33.

123 Wikipedia's entry on Heruka begins: **Heruka** (Sanskrit; Wylie: *khrag 'thung*), is the name of a category of wrathful deities, enlightened beings in Vajrayana Buddhism that adopt a fierce countenance to benefit sentient beings. In East Asia, these are called Wisdom Kings. https://en.wikipedia.org/wiki/Heruka

124 Baker, Ian *The Dalai Lama's secret temple: Tantric wall paintings from Tibet,* Thames & Hudson, NY, 2000 p. 34.

125 Yeshe, Thubten, Lama, *The bliss of inner fire: The heart practice of the six yogas* of *Naropa* p. 177

126 Yeshe

127 Ibid., p. 148.

128 Ibid., p. 149.

Section VII
The *Qi* in *T'ai-chi Ch'üan*

One day a monk arrived unannounced at Master Yang's doorstep in Peking. Powerfully built and over 6 feet tall, the monk saluted and expressed his great admiration. But during Yang's reply, the monk suddenly shot at him like a cannonball with clenched fists. Master Yang evaded with his chest and lightly patted the attacker's fist with his own soft palm, and as if struck by a bolt of lightning the monk flew back to land behind a wall-screen. Taking a long amount of time to get up, he said very solemnly: "I've been extremely rude, please forgive me!" Master Yang still invited the monk in for a chat.

— A story about Yang Lu-chan, Founder of the Yang Style [1]

VII

The *Qi* in *T'ai-chi Ch'üan*

Introduction to Section VII

Some of the proposals that follow will be controversial; they will challenge the conventional narrative that describes the origins of *t'ai-chi ch'üan*.[2] These alternative views will question not only the traditional story of the art's origins, but its traditional birthplace as well. The discussions that follow are based on the notion that the art which has come to be known as *t'ai-chi* might not have been passed down from a long line of wizened sages. Instead, the practice was more likely more recent, and the product of accidental discoveries leading to a more efficient way of engaging an opponent. Following this, the pioneers of the art systematized what they had discovered as a training method. The tradition that emerged was profound. It manifested as the practitioner's ability to merge technical skill with an altered, and super-efficient, mind-body state.

It will also be argued that the art could only have evolved in the context of specific social, psychological, and neurochemical influences. Thus, the pages that follow also describe how the new style could only have developed under conditions that fostered those innovations. To accomplish this, we suggest that the practitioners engaged in a type of martial play.

Many *t'ai-chi ch'üan* practitioners believe that the genesis of their art can be traced to a secret. Most often, that secret involves the sudden realization by a founding master of how to subdue an attacker while employing no more than the slightest touch. Thus, a martial discipline emerged based on the promise that an individual could attain a kind of superpower. Instead of relying on gross physical strength, the new art incorporated subtle, but no less powerful, forces of intention, and even more so, the enigmatic force known to the Chinese as *qi*.

The present section comprises two interwoven themes. The first considers the meaning of *qi* internal energy as perceived by the founding masters of the martial art of *t'ai-chi ch'üan*, hereafter most often abbreviated as *t'ai-chi*. The second is an alternative theory for how the martial art might have developed. This alternative origin theory may shed light on the meaning of "internal energy" in the martial arts. It may also shed light on the question of why out of hundreds, if not thousands, of Chinese martial art styles, *t'ai-chi* stands above most others, not only as a remarkable close combat art, but the gateway to the systematic teaching of "internal energy" principles in all forms of close combat.

Why is the subject of *t'ai-chi* central to a book on internal energy? The answer comes in four parts. The first has to do with the way sophisticated skill associated with the art is linked to the practitioner's mind-body state, while the second involves the practitioner's reliance on biofeedback sensations that allow the art to be effective as a close combat skill. Later, it will be explained how attention to these biofeedback sensations, rightly or wrongly identified as *qi* internal energy, were, and still are, used to activate superior athletic abilities.

The third part considers *t'ai-chi's* unique approach to resolving physical conflict. If indeed it can be utilized as an unusual way of engaging an adversary, it advances our discussion of "internal power," as it describes how brain-cognitive training develops alongside the practical / combat side of one's physical practice. This new model incorporates principles from neurophysiology that highlight the relationship between brain structures and how a person responds to stress.

Later, the co-influences of brain structures and the stress response will be considered in light of a particular training environment. Could it be that these are factors that also contributed to the development of *t'ai-chi?*

"Internal energy" may one day become scientifically measurable, or perhaps it will remain mysterious. In either case, one's ability to express the particular kind of athleticism associated with *t'ai-chi* will be shown to be inseparable from the synergism of experience, training environment, and the subsequent mental and emotional patterns that emerge from the training *milieu*.

The fourth and final part of the answer speaks to the *t'ai-chi* ideal of *minimal contact-minimal force*. *T'ai-chi* involves a particularly interesting way to engage an opponent. As *t'ai-chi* researcher and historian Douglas Wile suggests, this kind of engagement is sometimes referred to as the "softening of t'ai-chi." [3]

There are different ways to engage an adversary and resolve conflict, including physical combat, and contact with an adversary and "solutions" employed can be either "heavy" or "light." Where it might be possible for a person to utterly destroy an attacker, it is also often possible that a minimal, or in some cases even a non-aggressive, response can accomplish the same end. In this light, *t'ai-chi* provides a model to investigate the possibility of how a "light hand" is often superior to the use of a "heavy hand" in response to a physical challenge — and metaphorically, perhaps, to other forms of challenge.

Taken together, these four points seek to elucidate *t'ai-chi* as a close combat art. It is a practice that includes the induction of a specific mind-body state, biofeedback training, learning to access creative brain structures under stress, and the skill of "light touch," or "soft" problem solving. All of these contribute to the discussion of subtle energy and the possibility of something that might be called "internal energy in the martial arts."

The discussion that follows has implications for other styles of martial arts, as well as contact sports in general. The genesis of what we today know as *t'ai-chi* is based on the notion that a master practitioner can influence and defeat an opponent through the aforementioned minimal contact and physical effort. This goal, first systematized in the art of *t'ai-chi*, has broad implications for the way martial arts have been thought about and taught ever since.

Covered in this section:

- *T'ai-chi* as we know it: a nineteenth-century phenomenon
- The accidental discovery of exceptional efficiency in close combat
- The concept of using *qi* and mind to defeat an opponent
- A definable advanced mind-body state

Chapter 33

Harmony, Flow, and Power

*I*n the Introduction to Sections VI and VII, it was suggested that the secrets of *t'ai-chi* were probably <u>not</u> revealed by an alchemist monk living in the mountains of China hundreds of years ago. It is more likely that they are traceable to a more recent, accidental discovery of mind-body training principles in the late-nineteenth century.

However, although their discovery would forever change the way martial arts were thought of, the theme of the pages that follow is that *t'ai-chi* pioneers were not consciously aware of the significance of the art they were developing and systematizing. Their practice was group-oriented and social; they had no conscious awareness of the psychological, biofeedback, or neurophysiological mechanisms they had tapped. They could not explain why, when they entered a special, and now definable, mind-body state, they could so effortlessly defeat an adversary. In other times and places, proponents of the fighting arts might have attributed their newfound abilities to magic, but *t'ai-chi* pioneers believed the wellspring of their new skill was the powers of *mind* and *qi*.

> *Self-control is strength. Right thought is mastery. Calmness is power.*
> James Allen, *As a Man Thinketh*

Two key components form the center of this relatively recent form of close combat. These are the practitioner's ability to maintain a calm state under stress, and the ability to induce synchrony, or harmony, between the practitioner's biological rhythms. As with the principles of meditation described in Section V, these psycho-physiological states can be attained only when the practitioner is relaxed and has let go of all unnecessary tension in their body.

The pages that follow also provide insight into the larger discussion on the meaning of internal energy in other disciplines. For example, a trait shared between the energetic practice of Taoist yogis, * the energetic meditators, and *t'ai-chi* is that at the core of each tradition, practitioners are instructed to *pay attention to subtle cues within their bodies*. One's ability to attend to these cues is essential. The skill must be mastered to such an extent that the practitioner is able to perceive them, or their associated "background cues," even while under extreme stress.

* Discussed in Section V

In the Chinese traditions such as those just cited, whether correctly or incorrectly observed, practitioners learned to identify certain sensations within their bodies in the context of *nei qi,* or "internal energy." Thus, *t'ai-chi* pioneers, without knowing it, practiced a form of biofeedback training. For early practitioners of the art, this required a working theory to explain the discipline they engaged in, which in turn required a history. The best fit was one that drew from Taoist mysticism, and the result was a merger of Taoist philosophy, alchemy, and meditation principles with combat science. Subsequently, pioneers referred to their new art as "ultimate" boxing, or *t'ai-chi ch'üan.*

However, this alternative approach to martial arts did not emerge from a vacuum. Not only was a philosophical antecedent necessary, but the right training environment was also required. That special kind of training environment would be one that could foster an unusual — what some might consider an antithetical — approach to combat study. Such a martial art could only come to fruition under the perfect conditions, where the practitioner could embrace the right neuro-physical and psychological preparedness.

All societies have examples of remarkable talent expressed through individuals who achieve the highest level of performance. There is fighting, there are warrior disciplines, and then there are those rarer martial art disciplines where a spiritual practice merges with a fighting art. War dances have always been quasi-religious; the ancient Greek Olympics were religious festivals, and the warrior / athlete's training in the gymnasium was inseparable from philosophy. Other examples include Buddhism and Shaolin, and Shinto and *aikido,* as well as Zen and Japanese archery. They all cross the mind-body dichotomy. *T'ai-chi* is among those rarer fighting arts: part meditation, part Taoist inner alchemy, and partly a unique set of physical principles.

The Philosophical Antecedent

The notion of effortless skill has a long history in Chinese culture. For more than 2,000 years, Taoist philosophical principles describing the epitome of skill contributed to the development of Chinese arts and proto-sciences. The Taoist paragon is often described as a person who functions through a special mind-body harmony, with the prototype of such a master being the *Chuang Tzu's* story of cook Ting. As portrayed in the *Chuang Tzu,* the cook was so efficient that while butchering oxen, his blade touched neither bone nor sinew, and thus, never dulled. Through the story of cook Ting, Chuang Tzu presents a scheme of skill development that progresses from one's focus on cutting up the ox to achieving an effortless state, characterized by surrender and trust in the *Way.*

Cook Ting was cutting up an ox for Lord Wen-hui. As every touch of his hand, every heave of his shoulder, every move of his feet, every thrust of his knee — zip! zoop! He slithered the knife along with a zing, and all was in perfect rhythm, as though he were performing the dance of the Mulberry Grove or keeping time to the ching-shou music.

"Ah, this is marvelous!" said Lord Wen-hui. "Imagine skill reaching such heights!"

Cook Ting laid down his knife and replied, "What I care about is the Way, which goes beyond skill. When I first began cutting up oxen, all I could see was the ox itself. After three years I no longer saw the whole ox. And now — now I go at it by spirit and don't look with my eyes. Perception and understanding have come to a stop and spirit moves where it wants. I go along with the natural makeup, strike in the big hollows, guide the knife through the big openings, and follow things as they are. So I never touch the smallest ligament or tendon, much less a main joint.

"A good cook changes his knife once a year — because he cuts. A mediocre cook changes his knife once a month — because he hacks. I've had this knife of mine for nineteen years, and I've cut up thousands of oxen with it, and yet the blade is as good as though it had just come from the grindstone. There are spaces between the joints, and the blade of the knife has really no thickness. If you insert what has no thickness into such spaces, then there's plenty of room — more than enough for the blade to play about. That's why after nineteen years the blade of my knife is still as good as when it first came from the grindstone.

"However, whenever I come to a complicated place, I size up the difficulties, tell myself to watch out and be careful, keep my eyes on what I'm doing, work very slowly, and move the knife with the greatest subtlety, until — flop! The whole thing comes apart like a clod of earth crumbling to the ground. I stand there holding the knife and look all around me, completely satisfied and reluctant to move on, and then I wipe off the knife and put it away."

"Excellent!" said Lord Wen-hui. "I have heard the words of Cook Ting and learned how to care for life!" [4]

Did *t'ai-chi* emerge as an expression of cook Ting's effortless flow? Is it possible for a martial artist, under the stress of close combat, to express the effortless skill that Chuang Tzu describes? We suggest that not only is it possible, but that this epitome of adeptness can be achieved by all martial artists who learn to bring their biological rhythms into synchrony.

The cornerstone of this alternative view is that a person can function from a state of exceptional efficiency by learning to invoke, and pay attention to, specific feelings in the body. In turn, the ability to attend to these kinds of subtle cues can induce a <u>definable</u> mind-body state. When linked to physical training, it becomes a form of biofeedback that produces martial magic.

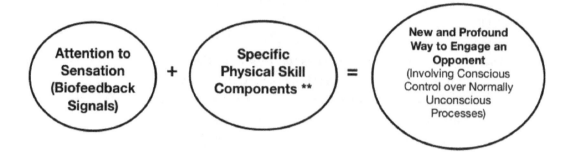

Diagram 7-1

Biofeedback training model applied to *T'ai-Chi*

Illustrated in the diagram, the training of athletic skill sets associated with *t'ai-chi* involves the pairing of skill, or skill sets, with biofeedback sensations. In turn, these become cues that can be relied on to trigger superior athletic skill. As an alternative way to appreciate *t'ai-chi*, biofeedback signal becomes so closely associated with skill that the practitioner's ability to pay attention to a particular "feeling" in the body can activate a superior and hyper-coordinated mind-body state.

**These are the biomechanical principles of the art, such as maintaining a natural vertical spine, not allowing the knees to go past the toes, Empty-Full weight distribution, etc.

Chapter 34

Biofeedback and the Development of Sophisticated Skill

Sensations identified as *Qi* are linked to Profound Abilities

*I*t is possible to place some aspects of normally unconscious physiology under conscious control. This chapter considers whether conscious control over some of those normally unconscious processes can trigger an altered, and more efficient, mind-body state. In this light, a more complete understanding of *t'ai-chi,* "internal energy," and the relationship between the two must include consideration of those consciously triggered, and exceptional, mind-body states.

As suggested by the scheme presented in Diagram 7-1, under some conditions, conscious control over normally unconscious processes can induce an especially coherent mind-body state. When engaged, this special mind-body state allows the practitioner to move more efficiently, and in an exceptionally coordinated way, against an opponent.

The easiest way to gain some degree of conscious control over one's physiology is through biofeedback training. Biofeedback involves the pairing of a cue (which acts as a signal) with a physiological effect (such as the lowering of blood pressure). Through biofeedback training, a cue can become so closely tied to a physiological phenomenon that the mere presentation of the cue can produce the targeted (trained) physiological effect. A common example of biofeedback training involves working with a machine-generated tone that is paired to, and becomes associated with, lowering blood pressure. Through clinical training, a patient might learn to trigger changes in their body when a tone is presented in order to keep blood pressure in the acceptable range. In this example, an association is made between the tone and control over blood pressure, which in turn leads to some conscious control over normally unconscious physiology.

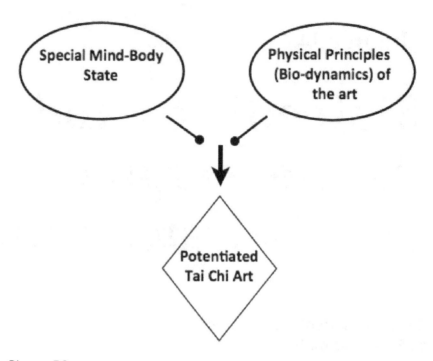

Diagram 7-2

The Merging of a Special Mind-Body State with Physical Principles Potentiates the Martial Art of *T'ai-Chi*

You can practice t'ai-chi ch'üan while you are walking, standing, sitting and laying. The method is to use your mind to circulate the "qi" and find the feeling.

Tung Ying Chieh
T'ai-chi ch'üan master

The linking of biofeedback with physical skill begins to explain some of the more remarkable abilities of accomplished *t'ai-chi* masters of the past, whose attention to biofeedback cues allowed them to focus on sensations. In this example, the cue was, rightly or wrongly, believed to be the coursing of *qi* energy through the body. For founding masters of the art, mental attention to these sensations acted as a biofeedback "tone" that initiated a psychophysiological state known as *entrainment,* which in turn allowed *t'ai-chi* pioneers access to that exceptionally efficient skill.

T'ai-chi is more than a series of choreographed postures and movements. It is a complete mind-body art brought to fruition not only through the application of correct bio-mechanics specific to the internal arts — for example, the knees not passing on a vertical line beyond the toes, the empty-full body weight principle, and so forth [5] — but also through the simultaneous *induction* of a specific mind-body state (Diagram 7-2).

Is it possible that this mind-body state of entrainment, when matched with correct physical principles, potentiates a highly efficient / minimal effort art like *t'ai-chi?* Accordingly, if one of these components is missing, movements become ineffectual, with minimal, if any, realistic self-defense application. In other words, without the practitioner being in a state of physiological harmony, the art becomes "empty." Furthermore, without attending to correct physical principles, such as "empty-full" weight distribution and avoidance of overextension in stances, the physical-mechanical power and technique of the art cannot be expressed. The correct mix of these two — the physical principles and the inner harmonious state — is necessary to initiate the most optimal way to engage an opponent.

To understand, and then recreate for oneself, the experience of effortless power, whether in close combat training or other physical discipline, it is useful to consider how the founding masters of *t'ai-chi* might have first discovered and systematized their observations.

Chapter 35

A Revolutionary Approach

"Use the mind and not force to defeat your opponent."

When my *t'ai-chi* ancestor Li Yi-yu (1832-1892) espoused what was to become the *t'ai-chi* ethos, it was revolutionary. Although Li was not the first to write about *qi* and mind in the martial arts, he left us the first detailed descriptions of an organized system where subtle power, *qi energy*, and *mind* were described as being able to overcome brute force. [6]

Over subsequent centuries, first in China, then Japan and Korea, and ultimately the rest of the world, the ethos of "using the mind and not force" pervaded martial arts culture, and, in modern times, television and motion pictures. Going beyond strictly physical skill, without the notion of a mysterious power directed by *mind* and *intention* that could be accessed in combat, it is unlikely that the idea of the *Force* –- the life energy an initiated warrior accesses, as imagined in George Lucas's *Star Wars* — would have come to fruition. Whether one believes in the power of human will to influence the physical world through "internal energy" or not, the ethos is so powerful and pervasive that even today, more than one hundred years after Li wrote those words, these principles continue to influence how the martial arts are perceived.

T'ai-Chi as a New Discovery

Expanding on some of the observations of martial arts scholars, and presented through layers of discussion, here we explain how *t'ai-chi*, and in particular the Yang style, can be understood as a series of evolutionary steps traceable to a group of individuals, their discoveries, and their subsequent application to a systematized way of study in the late-nineteenth century.

Figures 7-3

Comparison of the Chinese characters for T'ai-chi and *Qi* **/** *Ch'i* **Energy**

Left: Chinese Characters for "T'ai-Chi" or Grand Ultimate

Right: Chinese Characters for *ch'i* / *qi*, as in nei qi "internal energy"

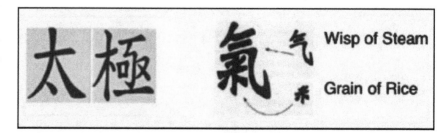

Wisp of Steam

Grain of Rice

First, clearing up a Basic Point

However, before presenting the alternative model that describes the remarkable development of *t'ai-chi* as a close combat art, it is important to clear up a basic point in regard to the use of the terms "chi" and "ch'i." The majority of the present work is concerned with discussion of what the Chinese refer to as *qi,* and also transliterated as *"ch'i."* However, as illustrated in Figure 7-3, it should be noted that the two Chinese characters for *ch'i / qi,* internal energy, and *chi* as in *t'ai-chi ch'üan* (also written *taijiquan*), appear near identical in Wade-Giles renderings.[7]

However, these two characters and their denotations are completely unrelated. Where *"qi,"* as used in *nei qi* (內氣) (Box 7-4), has to do with the internal energy of Chinese yoga, meditation, and medicine, the character for *chi* in the Wade-Giles transliteration of *t'ai-chi* refers to "the ultimate," a philosophical principle for which the art was named. These points on the distinction of Chinese characters for *ch'i /qi* noted, it is ironic that the present chapter has more to do with the notion of internal energy in *t'ai-chi ch'üan,* or, more accurately, what founding masters of the tradition *identified* as internal energy. More discussion on contrasts between the "ch'i/qi" terms appears in Endnote.[8]

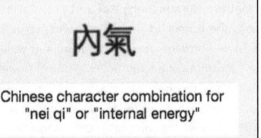

Chinese character combination for
"nei qi" or "internal energy"

Box 7-4

The Archetype of *Qi* in the Martial Arts

In Chinese culture, the notion that *qi* energy is essential to life and personal empowerment has a long history. As covered in Sections II and III, the belief in *qi* as a form of internal energy within the body can be dated to at least the dawn of the first millennium of the present era. Furthermore, both Confucians and Taoists referenced the more abstract notion of *qi* as a primordial, effervescent substance that could influence health as far back as the sixth century BCE. However, more relevant to the present discussion is how the notion of *qi* became germane to the practice of martial arts.

Although the oldest reference to the use of internal *qi* for martial purposes is suggested by Chuang Tzu's (Zhuangzi) fourth century BCE "Discourse on Swords," a more direct reference to how the merging of mind and *qi* allows a person to achieve superiority in combat is found in the literature of China's classical period. There, in *The Annals of the State of Wu and Yueh,* a dialog between the King of Yueh and a woman warrior named Yüeh Nü is striking in how it describes the merger between martial arts and internal energy. Yüeh Nü tells us her secret of superior combat:

> The art of swordsmanship is extremely subtle and elusive; its principles are most secret and profound. The *tao* has its gate and door, its *yin* and *yang*. Open the gate and close the door; yin declines, and yang rises. When practicing the art of hand-to-hand combat, concentrate your spirit internally and give the impression of relaxation externally. You should look like a modest woman and strike like a ferocious tiger. As you assume various postures, regulate your *qi*, moving always with the spirit. Your skill should be as obvious as the sun and as startling as a bolting hare. Your opponent endeavors to pursue your form and chase your shadow, yet your image hovers between existence and non-existence. The breath moves in and out and should never be held. Whether you close with the opponent vertically or horizontally, with or against the flow, never attack frontally. Mastery of this art allows one to match a hundred and a hundred to match a thousand. If your Highness would like to test it, I can demonstrate for your edification.[9]

Yüeh Nü's description of her combat art provides early and powerful evidence for the cultural archetype of *qi* as a martial art enhancement. Yüeh Nü discusses the connection to the nameless spiritual source of the *Tao,* secrets mustered through application of *yin* and *yang,* how concentration empowers *nei qi* internal energy, and the primal power harnessed through secret breathing techniques. This amazing collection of requirements formed the bulb of a flower, which waited for the right time and place to bloom and spring forth from the fertile ground of China's martial arts lineages.

Important contributions to *t'ai-chi* theory appear in the sixteenth and seventeenth centuries, in the martial arts literature by Huang Tsung-hsi and Chang Naizhou (more on those later). However, it was not until what was most probably an accidental discovery by a group of martial artists in the late-nineteeth century that the potential of "*qi*" as a force to be reckoned with would change the martial arts world.

Chapter 36

Mind-Body State and Physical Skill

*T*he premise of this chapter is that a special mind-body state called *entrainment* constitutes the cornerstone of the special abilities described by *t'ai-chi* pioneers. Entrainment is not synonymous with biofeedback, but biofeedback can induce entrainment.

Entrainment occurs when a person's biological oscillators — another term for "body rhythms" — become harmonious, or "in phase," as the term applies to a special kind of synchrony between one's natural bodily rhythms. There are a number of body rhythms, and some, such as breathing, are easily observed. Others, such as a measure of stress vs. non-stress management of the heart known as heart rate variability, or HRV, are extremely subtle, and thus require laboratory instruments to reliably measure. Another example of a physiological oscillator is the profusion of blood through arterial vessels, a measure referred to as *pulse transit time,* or PTT.

Upon attaining this special kind of harmony between biological rhythms, a martial arts practitioner (or other athlete) becomes more efficient. Later, it will be described how some of my martial arts students and I tested entrainment in mock combat. The results that we observed through our informal research suggest that this bio-rhythm harmonic state allows an individual with at least moderate skill to prevail against an opponent in an exceptionally efficient, often expert way, as if the former had studied a decade, or more, longer.

If this observation is supported by further research and experimentation, it is revolutionary for two reasons. First, because of the way that the mind-body state, when linked with physical skill, defines the abilities of the top athletes, and second, because it functions as the long sought-after secret of advanced performance, allowing medium and high-level athletes to quickly advance to world-class status in their respective endeavors. In short, it becomes a state of internal harmony that allows a person with only a modicum of skill to perform in a masterful way. A video demonstration of the principle, applied to mock combat practice, can be viewed from the link shown in Box 7-5.

For the practitioner or close combat fighter engaged in the state of entrainment, and, importantly, who is able to maintain the state when in contact with an opponent, the experience can be extraordinary. At times,

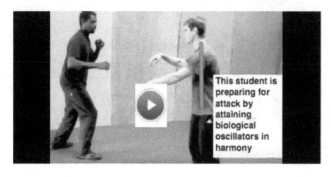

This student is preparing for attack by attaining biological oscillators in harmony

Box 7-5
Links to video of demonstrations of practitioners using *entrainment* in close combat practice

http://youtu.be/uVhkCtUav4g

or

https://chiarts.com/7-5

the practitioner will experience what might be described as moving in a time warp or other-dimensional state, and while engaging an opponent from this elevated position, sometimes they will experience the sense of being a move ahead. Other experiences related to this state are neutralizing, or countering, the opponent's move before he has initiated the attack, or performing a strike before the opponent can even think of blocking. These experiences are difficult to explain, but, at the same time, incredibly exhilarating.

It is our contention that these were the kinds of exceptional experiences that led late-nineteenth century *t'ai-chi* pioneers to describe their combat engagement as "effortless." Later, we will recount how their interaction with an opponent was so profound that new terms were needed to describe this remarkable way of engaging an adversary. Searching for expressions that might match their experience, they would apply phrases such as "use the mind and not force" and "four ounces of strength can defeat a thousand pounds." Here is how Li Yi-yu details the essence of *t'ai-chi* in the late 1800s:

> How wonderful is *t'ai-chi ch'üan*, whose movements follow nature!
> . . . the whole body is filled with one unbroken *ch'i [qi]*
> Above and below are without imbalance .... moving the *qi* feels like coiling silk
>
> .... Raise the back and relax the chest. When the *wei-lü* is naturally vertical, †
> the body feels relaxed and the *qi* lively
>
> Use the mind and not strength
> .... There is a slight feeling of swelling in the fingers,
> For wherever the *qi* goes there is a manifestation in the body
> All of this is a function of the mind,
> And has nothing to do with brute force.
>
> .... Movement arises from stillness, but even in movement there is stillness
> The spirit leads the *qi* in its movements.
>
> .... Speed or slowness follows the opponent's movements;
> .... Without losing contact or grappling, every posture must anticipate the opponent.
>
> After drawing the opponent in and neutralizing his energy,
> We issue power like a bubbling well.
> Let the strongest aggressor attack us,
> While four ounces deflects a thousand pounds.[10]

† The *wei-lü* (尾闾; *pinyin: weilü*) *translates* as the tailbone. "Naturally vertical" refers to maintaining the natural curve of the lumbar spine without "tucking the tailbone." (Also, see notes on the distinction of the *wei-lü* as a physical structure or energy center in Chapter 25)

The above sample from Li Yi-yu's *Song of the Essence of T'ai-Chi* describes a new order of systematized training. Although, as suggested in the Introduction to Sections VI and VII, foundational aspects of what would become known as *t'ai-chi* existed earlier,[11] according to Wile, Li's was the first detailed description of an internal martial art, emphasizing both the central role of mind and spirit and incorporated principles of *qi* energy and Taoist alchemy.

However, the most important of Li's instructions were the hints that he left regarding the key to unlocking *t'ai-chi's* remarkable abilities: **the practitioner must pay attention to sensations within the body.** Referring to those sensations as the "flow of *qi*," Li's instructions warrant a closer look:

.... the whole body is filled with one unbroken *ch'i [qi]*
Above and below are without imbalance .... moving the *qi* feels like coiling silk

For wherever the *qi* goes there is a manifestation in the body
All of this is a function of the mind,
And has nothing to do with brute force.

In today's language, Li was describing the merging of biofeedback with specific physical skill sets. Sense the feeling, move with it, and observe it throughout the body, but as you move, treat it as if you were "reeling silk," and don't lose touch with that feeling.

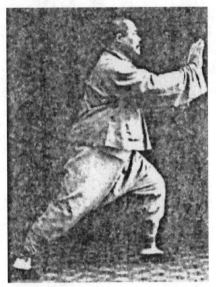

Photo 7-6

Yang Cheng-fu in a *T'ai-Chi* Posture

At this juncture, it is important to ask whether Li's description of a martial art that relied on only "four ounces of strength" to defeat an opponent was only metaphor? If it was indeed an accurate portrayal of the practitioner's engagement with an opponent, and if the minimal contact of four ounces could really defeat an adversary, this would go a long way toward explaining why *t'ai-chi* became so respected as a fighting art.

Furthermore, if Li's description of minimal effort control over an opponent were true, it would be evidence that a "soft power" art — described by seventeenth-century Huang Pai-chia and his father, Huang Tsung-hsi — that could counter the "hard Shaolin" had been realized. [12] The sudden appearance of a new kind of ability in close combat would also validate descriptions of the abilities attributed to the person who would become its primary advocate in the early 1900s, Yang Cheng-fu. (Photo 7-6).

<u>**Chapter 37**</u>

An Accidental Discovery

*T*he mind-body principles delineated by Li Yi-yu in the late-nineteenth century represented a radical approach, at least in a systematized way, of how to interact with an opponent. However, there is a serious issue that needs to be addressed. In many cases, knowledge of the realistic fighting applications of the art have not been fully transmitted to the present generation of *t'ai-chi* instructors. As noted in the Introduction to Sections VI and VII, in many cases today, even in China, knowledge of *t'ai-chi* as an effective self-defense art has, for the most part, been lost. ‡ This makes it especially urgent for the serious student of the art to investigate the possibility that those late-nineteenth and early-twentieth-century masters might have discovered something profound that led to the creation of the art we know as *t'ai-chi*. We need to know what they knew. The art needs to be rediscovered.

‡Also see Wang Xiangzhai's comments on this point, referenced in Section VIII

Roots: Counter to the School of Shaolin

As was mentioned earlier, the notions of an "internal martial art counter to the school of Shaolin" and "internal boxing" date from the writings of Huang Tsung-hsi (1610-1695) in the late-seventeenth century. However, as Wile points out, the combat disciplines Huang described bear little resemblance to the art we identify as *t'ai-chi* today. [13] This point demonstrates the difficulty encounterd when trying to establish a reliable history of the art. Wile discusses the problem of tracing *t'ai-chi's* roots for both theory and principle in the following way:

> Thus, tracing the history of *t'ai-chi ch'üan* at the level of theory and principles shows considerable intellectual continuity but no historical lineage to connect the literary dots. [14]

The lack of traceable lineage is a curious thing. The point supports the suggestion that *t'ai-chi* as we know it may actually be a relatively new, as opposed to an ancient, practice. The concept of "invented traditions" may go a long way to explaining why the nineteenth-century pioneers of this art might have attributed its origins to earlier sources. If indeed something radically "new" (especially in a martial context) emerged, to add credibility, its founding authority would not ascribe the brilliant new discovery to a group of gentlemen experimenting with new ideas and training together — essentially, a men's martial arts practice club. [15] Consider that, in the late-nineteenth century, a group of individuals might have been practicing together and, through experimentation, made some remarkable discoveries. To add authority to whatever amazing breakthrough they might have made, the origins of the new concept and training method would, as was the Chinese custom, be credited not to a contemporaneous, but to an ancient and mysterious source. [16]

Furthermore, such an origin story would increase in potency if the legendary person to whom the art was credited had removed himself from society. For those writing their art's myth of origin, the ideal progenitor would be a quasi-historical person who could be claimed as being the source of the ancient wisdom. The most suitable candidate would be one who, for example, lived high atop a sacred mountain, since according to Chinese cultural beliefs, only such an environment could provide the requisite conditions whereby one might tap into perennial wisdom. [17] Prof. Wile offers tacit support for such a thesis, and the appeal to Chang San-feng and Wang Tsung-yüeh may also be an attempt to give the art deeper roots and make it seem less like a contemporary creation. [18] On the assertion that the Ch'en family of Ch'en-chia-kou (Ch'en Village), Henan, is the place of origin, Wile notes, "the paucity of pre-twentieth century theoretical writings in Ch'en Village."

Other *t'ai-chi* origin stories are equally dubious. As was mentioned in the introduction to Sections VI and VII, these include Yang Chen-fu's grandfather, Lu-chan, spying on Ch'en village members in order to learn the secret of a complex training system surreptitiously, and the tale of the art's origins resulting from the discovery of an ancient manual found in the back of a salt shop. Both stories lack credibility, as an art like *t'ai-chi* is a highly refined skill derived from many years of intense, practical work, and *tactile*, dual-person training is essential to grasp its essentials. Consider the artful neutralizing of an opponent's force, which includes instruction in the subtle shifting of weight, matched with the slightest turning of the hand, to thwart the opponent's grasp with, of course, correct placement of mental focus. It takes years of training before skill like this can be transferred from master to disciple.

Significantly, sophisticated skill of this order requires *physical contact* and interaction with fellow martial arts "family" members. Since *t'ai-chi* is more than a series of movements, it is believed to be impossible to learn such a complex skill from either surreptitious observation or through the sudden discovery of a previously lost manual. Wile's comments are apropos, ".... the difficulty in dating and authenticating genealogies and form manuals there leaves the door open for questions of which Ch'en created the art or whether it was transmitted from the outside." [19]

Consider again the significance of directing one's attention inwardly while learning to attend to sensations within the body. In his manuscripts on t'ai-chi, Li was describing a close combat training system based on the practitioner's ability to become mentally aware of subtle internal signals. As described earlier, for the more experienced practitioner, these act as bio-feedback signals.

Other nineteenth-century exponents also described the importance of attending to sensations within the body. For example, Wu Cheng-ching, a Yang style pioneer, * also wrote about the importance of paying attention to one's "internal sensations," and not the external form. However, in keeping with traditional Chinese theory, t'ai-chi practitioners would describe their inner subjective experience of these sensations in terms of qi energy (See Box 7-7).

"Within the framework of Chinese thought, no notion may attain such a degree of abstraction from empirical data as to correspond perfectly to one of our modern universal concepts. Nevertheless, the term qi comes as close as possible to constituting a generic designation equivalent to our word "energy". When Chinese thinkers are unwilling or unable to fix the quality of an energetic phenomenon, the character qi (氣) inevitably flows from their brushes."

Manfred Porkert
The Theoretical Foundations of Chinese Medicine

Box 7-7
Note on the Chinese use of the term Qi

* Discussed in more detail later

Those skilled in the art, no doubt then, as now, experienced sensations that came along with slow, moving meditation-style training. Examples of those kinds of sensations might, at times, include the feeling of an electrical current moving through the body. This is a crucial point, which forms an interesting parallel with observations by current researchers that describe the power of human consciousness to influence the physical world — a point that will also be returned to later.

Li Yi-yu helps us to understand the late-nineteenth century t'ai-chi theory as a novel approach to training, describing a martial art that can access the secrets of yin and yang. Li's description foreshadows the secret of "softness" as a category of athletic and personal empowerment. The notion that it is possible to defeat an opponent by "using the mind, not force" represented a revolutionary paradigm shift.

Chapter 38

The Power of Intention and *Entrainment*

The Power of Intention

*F*or a moment, let us step away from our discussion of the history of *t'ai-chi* to look at the psycho-physiological foundations of the art. Over the last twenty-five years, a new category of mind-body research has emerged which demonstrates that when one's bio-rhythms attain a state of synchrony, one can non-physically influence an external physical target. This groundbreaking research suggests that human *intention* may soon be recognized as a *force of nature*, but then, why is this discussion relevant to the topic of *t'ai-chi*?

Here, we will describe how this special mind-body state, when matched with the power of intention, adds a kind of magic to athletic performance. In the examples that follow, that magic materializes as the ability to control an opponent with the most minimal touch.

> For me, the heart-pulse and entrainment technique has been life changing. I use it to deepen awareness of my energetic body, ground myself, and open channels of empathy and patience. It also helps me stay poised and clear headed in stressful situations and when I perform. It is really something.
>
> —David Walton, actor

Introduction to Entrainment

The practitioner's ability to entrain biological rhythms may be a new way to investigate the genesis of *t'ai-chi*. As introduced earlier, *entrainment* refers to the ability to synchronize one's biological rhythms. Applied as the key to unlocking *t'ai-chi's* highest secrets, entrainment involves the unconscious pairing of skill with a type of biofeedback training.

T'ai-chi pioneers would not have understood the psycho-physiology of biofeedback training. However, they would have noticed how the power of attention could merge with physical skill in a special way that produces a more advanced level of performance. In the current vernacular, this would be called being "in the zone."

Clues to this kind of superior performance are provided by scientific studies of the power of intention. To demonstrate that human potential could be awakened through the synchronization of one's biological rhythms, in one of his experiments, Stanford University *professor emeritus* William Tiller relied on a gas-discharge device to test whether a person could influence the apparatus through *intention* alone. Results showed that when a person attained the entrained mind-body harmonious state, and then **intended** to interact with the gas-discharge device, they could cause the device to generate an electrostatic discharge. This occurred when the individual was standing next to, but not making contact with, the device. [20] In other words, the experimental results suggest that *intention* acted as a physical force! Expanding on his intention experiments, Tiller conducted many other kinds of studies to test and verify that *intention* could act as a real force. [21] Some of these are described in Section X.

However, although studies describing the potential of entrainment are impressive, some evidence suggests that the physiological state may be even more powerful in settings that demand optimal human performance. The relationship between the harmony of mind-body states and the power of intention as a demonstrable force made me wonder if this insight into human potential could provide a new way of unlocking some of the secrets of the early *t'ai-chi* masters.

Diagram 7-8

When two pendulum clocks are mounted side by side on the same wall, they gradually come to swing in synchrony (becoming "in phase" or "in sync"). In this state, the two clocks generate the wave in the right-hand panel. This is a classic example of the phenomenon of *entrainment*, which occurs throughout nature (both in nonliving systems and in living organisms). In general, when systems entrain, they operate with increased efficiency. In the human body, the heart--as the body's most powerful rhythmic oscillator--is the central "pendulum" that sets the stage for entrainment of other physiological systems.

Source: HeartMath Foundation Illustration based on the one provided by the HeartMath Foundation

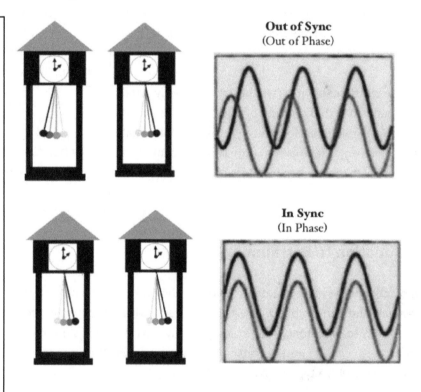

Out of Sync
(Out of Phase)

In Sync
(In Phase)

Advanced Mind-Body States in Contact Sports

With the participation of our organization's martial arts students, we began informal research to investigate how entrainment might be applied to mock, but aggressive, close combat. However, there was a hurdle that had to be overcome. Since the literature describing the induction of entrainment was based on a time-consuming relaxation process,[22] we needed a faster, near instantaneous, way to induce the entrained state in athletes while they were performing. We needed to develop a technique that could quickly induce synchrony between a practitioner's biological rhythms under the stressful conditions of aggressive mock combat.

Consider the illustration presented in Figure 7-8, which defines entrainment as the ability to bring various biological oscillators into "phase," or harmony. The figure shows a drawing based on one from the HeartMath Institute that illustrates how the pendulums of two grandfather clocks, set side-by-side, will synchronize with each other. Applied to human beings, entrainment describes how various biological rhythms also synchronize and, like the swinging pendulums of the grandfather clocks, can also entrain, or synchronize, with each other.

> **Box 7-9**
> **The Freeze Frame ® Technique**
>
> One technique used by the HeartMath Foundation is Freeze Frame ®. The technique teaches clients to mentally disengage the mind from attending to negative emotions and instead focus attention to the area of the heart. One reason this might work is since the mind, when engaged in negative emotions, tends to focus either in the past (regret, anger) or future (anxiety, fear), and by placing awareness on the heart, one puts oneself in a state of present tense. This is the goal and result of most meditation and stress reduction programs.

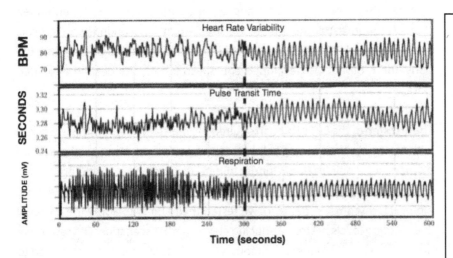

> Diagram 7-10
> **Three Biological Oscillators Becoming in Sync**
> The figure depicts three biological oscillators, HRV (Heart Rate Variability), pulse transit time ** and respiration becoming synchronized in one subject before and after use of an emotional self-management technique. Compare the left side of three graphs (before application of the emotional management technique) to the right (after application).
>
> From William Tiller, et al, "Cardiac coherence: A new, non-invasive measure of autonomic nervous system order," [24]
>
> ** Pulse Transit Time (PTT) is the time it takes the pulse pressure waveform to propagate through a length of the arterial tree.

Entrained Pulse Training (EPT)

Before we could find out if the ability to synchronize rhythms might influence the practitioner's effectiveness in mock combat, we had to develop a technique that would allow the individual to attain synchrony between biological rhythms *instantly,* and especially while under stress. In Tiller's study of individuals in the state of entrainment, investigators relied on a self-management technique known as "Freeze Frame" ® (Box 7-9) to entrain biological rhythms. However, as mentioned earlier, that technique requires the individual to maintain a calm and relaxed state and relies on them practicing a meditative-cognitive process that involves mental disengagement from negative emotions. At the same time, positive emotions are focused to the area of the heart.

For our purposes, it seemed significant that researchers observed how the ability to attend to one rhythm could bring the other rhythms into harmony. This inspired us to develop a new way to induce entrainment, based on attention being focused on a different rhythm: the pulse transit time (PPT).

The protocol we developed is called *entrained pulse training*, or EPT. As with the Freeze Frame technique, EPT also requires the practitioner to maintain a positive emotional state. † Drawing on the principle that attention to one oscillator could bring others into harmony, we relied on *pulse transit time*, or PTT (the middle-graphed oscillator in Diagram 7-10).

> † Significantly, as confirmed though research described in Section IX and our own experience working with athletes, a person who dwells on negative emotions, or is in a state of fear or anger, is unable to attain synchrony between biological rhythms.

As described in the heart-pulse protocol included in Section III, my students and I were very practiced in placing attention on the heartbeat and pulse at various locations throughout the body. Thus, it was natural for us to test whether attention to heartbeat and pulse could also induce the entrained state. Through experimentation, we found that by working with specific sequences involving attention directed to the feeling of the pulse within the body, the protocol we developed could also induce the desired entrained state.

The first step of the EPT protocol required the martial arts students we worked with to entrain their biological rhythms while relaxed. Next, they practiced harmonizing their rhythms under different conditions, including sitting, talking, and walking. Once they were confident in their ability to entrain their biological rhythms on demand, we tested their ability to apply the protocol in ascending levels of stress-inducing close-combat scenarios. The results we obtained exceeded our expectations; we found that an individual trained to observe and work with the biological oscillator associated with the transit of the pulse could dramatically improve their performance against an opponent.

Both at work, in an uncompromisingly stressful environment, and in my meditative prayer life, exercising, wherever practicable, entrainment and/or heart-mind path awareness, has been a great mental and spiritual instrument for re-centering my mind, positive intention, focus, and peace.

—Senior U.S. Political Official, Washington, D.C.

Significantly, we found that a practitioner trained in EPT could induce and maintain the requisite harmony of biological rhythms even while under stressful conditions of aggressive mock combat (some video demonstrations of our work with the EPT protocol can be viewed at the web address included in Box 7-5). When entrainment is induced and maintained during mock combat, an individual becomes more coordinated, is better able to quickly counter an opponent's attacks, and is more creative in their own attack. In most cases, a practitioner applying the technique while being challenged by an opponent could apply what could be called "effortless control" over the opponent, *as long as the entrained state was maintained.* [23]

While engaged in the entrained state, our students consistently exhibited superior abilities. Often, they seemed to be "a·move ahead" of their attackers, and their ability to control an opponent so effortlessly supports the notion that *t'ai-chi* pioneers might well have stumbled upon the same psycho-physiological principle. Later, we will consider how, using their own cultural terms, *t'ai-chi* ancestors applied this principle in a systematic way. To emphasize an earlier point, using the words and concepts they had available, they stressed the importance of becoming sensitive to the "flow of *qi*" within the body. But first, an introduction to EPT.

Chapter 39

Introduction to Entrained Pulse Training (EPT)

*B*efore returning to our discussion concerning the development of *t'ai-chi*, it is useful to introduce the basics of *entrainment*. This chapter includes a brief overview of the protocol I developed to teach a student or client to harmonize their biological rhythms, known as Entrained Pulse Training, or EPT.

Reverse Engineering: The EPT Protocol

Since many of our group's martial arts and *qigong* practitioners had previously spent a good amount of time learning to work with their heartbeat and pulse as biofeedback signals, ‡ it was an easy step for them to apply their practiced observation of the profusion of blood through arterial vessels as a measure of a biological rhythm.

‡ Described in Section III

For this purpose, we relied on the pulse transit time (the middle of the three oscillators graphically depicted in Diagram 7-10). We found that when the practitioner mentally attended to this rhythm, this would, in turn, bring other biological rhythms into synchrony, and thus allow the individual to achieve the entrained state. As an example of athletic performance illustrated in the video available at the web address included in Box 7-5, the EPT protocol improved student close combat performance to a such a remarkable degree that it has since become the cornerstone of our programs.

While the EPT protocol is useful as a way to instill a sense of peace and wellbeing, the technique also tends to induce remarkable efficiency of movement that can be applied in athletic performance. Currently, many of our students and clients, whether business professionals, pain patients, or professional fighters, include EPT as a regular part of their practice.

EPT Protocol Basics

As introduced above, the physiological measure students and clients learned to consciously observe in order to induce physiological harmony is pulse transit time (PTT). PTT refers to the time it takes blood to propagate through an arterial vessel from the heart to a specific point in the extremities, with the most common measuring location for laboratory purposes being the tip of a finger. In this way, the body rhythm of heartbeat-pulse transit time becomes useful as a measure of a biological oscillator. There are several steps involved in learning to apply the EPT protocol to close combat sports, athletics, and other situations. Although only briefly reviewed here, these are explained in more detail in Appendix B.

The goal of EPT training is for the individual to become confident enough in their awareness of the feeling of the pulse (or pulse related secondary signals) through the body that entrainment can be induced at will. The practitioner must be able to gain awareness of the subtle bodily cues and induce entrainment under any conditions. In the real world, this kind of mind-body synchronization presents as calm and coolness under pressure.

The four steps to the EPT protocol are:

1) Learning to mentally attend to signals associated with the profusion of blood through arterial vessels.

2) Learning to observe these same signals while sitting in a chair or on a meditation cushion.

3) Learning to observe these same signals, or associated signals, while standing or moving about, with or without being engaged in a conversation.

4) The ability to *entrain* biological oscillators at will, even when the practitioner is under extreme stress.

Note that during athletic competition, at levels three and four the individual learns to remain aware of the sensation as a sort of background feeling. [25]

The EPT Protocol

Note: Because the EPT protocol relies on the practitioner's ability to mentally attend to the heartbeat and profusion of blood through arterial vessels, it is recommended to <u>first</u> become proficient with the Heart-Pulse method described in Section III.

Before the EPT can be applied in mock or real combat, the awareness of pulse as a signal must be studied in a relaxed and meditative way. With practice, the ability to feel the pulse at specific locations throughout the body becomes a skill that can be transferred to other scenarios. Initially, the individual learns to become aware of, and then attend to, the heartbeat while relaxed. For new practitioners, this is often a challenging task, as sometimes even experienced meditators have difficulty with this first step. As with the heart-pulse method described in Section III, the goal is to become not only aware of the heartbeat at will, but also the pulse at various locations within the body, also at will. Thus, the opening stages of training often involve lying flat and face-up in a comfortable position. Begin by becoming as relaxed as possible, and, when ready, turn your attention inward to become aware of the heartbeat.

For beginners, it is helpful to place your relaxed hands on your chest as you search for the sensation of the heartbeat. For individuals who cannot easily feel their heartbeat in the thoracic cavity, the relaxed fingers and palms can act as a kind of sensor. If you have difficulty observing your heartbeat, refer back to the suggestions in the Heart-Pulse lesson provided in Section III.

After learning to observe the heartbeat at will, next practice paying attention to the pulse at distal locations throughout the body. This, too, may be challenging at first, but with time and practice you will be able to sense the pulse at will, wherever you focus attention within your body. As you learn to attend to your pulse, you will find your preferred pattern of working with your pulse sequences. Although this varies between individuals, a typical pattern involves being able to mentally attend to the heartbeat, and then observing the pulse in the abdomen or pelvic region, followed by a more distal pulse signal in the legs and / or feet. You will need at least two locations to entrain, e.g. the heartbeat and then the pelvic / abdominal area.

Once you can successfully observe the pulse at distal locations, next pay attention to the heartbeat / pulse locations as a sequence, e.g. heartbeat-pelvic or heartbeat-pelvic-feet. Just focus on the heartbeat, and then notice the pulse at the other location(s). As long as you maintain a positive attitude while gaining mental awareness of these sequences, attention focused in this way will begin to synchronize your bodily rhythms. Note, it can sometimes take several weeks, or longer, of regular practice before a new practitioner is able to track the heartbeat and profusion of blood through several pulse points. Initially, the technique requires commitment to the practice in order to "get it." With regular practice, the ability to entrain gets easier, and, ultimately, it can become virtually instantaneous. The benefits derived from the practice make it well worth the time and effort.

As mentioned earlier, entrainment is induced by paying attention to the interval between the heartbeat and pulse. When you are able to apprehend the sequences just described, you may notice that the breath will suddenly relax and deepen. This is a sign that your biological rhythms are becoming entrained **due of your attention** to the targeted rhythm. "If you do not breathe correctly, you do not move correctly." [26]

Also as mentioned earlier, not everyone feels the pulse throughout the body in the same way, and this is especially true for more experienced individuals practicing at more nuanced, and increasingly subtle, levels. Although the heartbeat is most often felt as a distinct signal, instead of a pulse at a distal location, those with more experience may also discover the sensation of a *swish*. This level of sensitivity indicates that the practitioner is actually sensing the flow of blood through the arterial vessels. The experience is enjoyable and is an especially good sign of progress.

Although briefly mentioned above, it is worth noting that there is a mental-emotional component to this training that cannot be neglected. It is essential that positive attitudes and emotions are maintained during the EPT practice, even if one is under stress or is facing a dangerous opponent. This point is covered in more detail in Section IX, but as a general guideline, emotions and attitude influence the sympathetic vs. parasympathetic (stressful vs. non-stressful) regulation of the heart (and subsequently the entire nervous system) through a measure of heart health known as HRV. Earlier, it was described how HRV is an important body rhythm that contributes to entrainment. Since the mind-body response to emotions is reflected in a person's HRV profile, as suggested by the HeartMath Foundation research, individuals in states of fear, anger, or any other negative emotion cannot entrain.

EPT stages two and three involve learning to first attend to heartbeat and pulse signals while sitting, and later while moving and walking about. Through experience and practice, the practitioner learns to pay attention to signal while engaged in more intense activities, such as participating in an athletic competition. However, in this case, the heartbeat-pulse signals will no longer be present in the foreground, but instead observed as a background impression that the practitioner increasingly learns to become aware of and trust.

Chapter 40

More Efficient Mind-Body States:

Play and the Development of "Soft" Martial Arts

This chapter returns to speculation on the genesis of *t'ai-chi* and several key points of that theory are explored in greater detail. One of these topics has to do with how brain physiology may have contributed to the development of *t'ai-chi* as a martial art. Social interaction and the training environment, which contribute to mental states and habits, are also considered.

Three questions are at the forefront of this part of the discussion. The first has to do with what it is about *t'ai-chi*, and by extension, other Chinese "internal" martial arts, that makes it distinct from other forms of close combat training? The second asks, which aspects of that uniqueness might provide more insight into our questions concerning the meaning of *internal energy*? The third line of inquiry considers how a notion called the *softening of t'ai-chi* might contribute to the first two questions.

The answer to the first question relates to the art's particular way of engaging an adversary. If it is possible for a person to defeat another using no more than what Li describes as "four ounces of strength," it would be remarkable. If this is more than simply a metaphor, it means that conventionally understood athletic power and body mechanics can be replaced with *something else* — but what exactly is that *something else*?

However first, another element needs to be factored into the equation. Although the prospect that a highly-trained practitioner can defeat an opponent while applying only the most minimal contact is worthy of a closer look, *t'ai-chi* involves an even more radical idea; one which distinguishes the art as a unique way of blending combat skill with meditation. For that reason, we must also consider what evidence there may be to support the development of a new tradition, based on a martial art incorporating meditation, and meditation inhabiting a martial art.

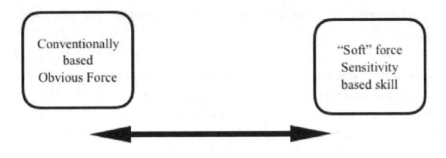

Diagram 7-11

Conventional vs. "Soft" Force Sensitivity Skill

As Li Yi-yu was writing down the principles that were to form the essence of the new approach to martial arts, he carefully included the single most important clue that might lead one to master mind-body harmony: pay attention to internal cues. He didn't use those exact words; he used the theoretical constructs that were available in the Chinese language to best describe his experience. He believed that the sensations he and fellow practitioners experienced during practice were the coursing of *qi* energy through their bodies. They had discovered that paying attention to those sensations could unlock remarkable power and ability.

Li left other clues about how to attend to those sensations during practice. He tells us that, when rich and full, the sensation that emerged was *one* of *unbroken qi.* He also informs us how he and his fellow pioneers of the art learned to work with those sensations. They discovered that the subtle and elusive bodily sensations they identified as the flow of *qi* through the body could be disturbed by choppy movements. In Li's words, the correct way to work with those subtle bodily sensations was to be very "smooth," as if *reeling silk.*

The Softening of *T'ai-Chi*

At first blush, the idea that one could be soft and relaxed amidst the stress of close contact combat is a radical idea. On its surface, a relaxed attitude seems incompatible with the instinctive response to the pressure of being under attack. The following paragraphs look for clues to that puzzle. A key component of that puzzle: did the art we today refer to as *t'ai-chi* undergo a "softening" process.

However, first, it should be noted that support for many of the assertions made in the next few paragraphs having to do with "the softening of *t'ai-chi*" is weak at best. It is problematic that there is little scholarly evidence to support the notion of how and when *t'ai-chi* and the internal martial arts went through a "softening" process. As was discussed earlier, there was the theoretical foundation put forward by Huang Tsung-chi in the seventeenth century, which suggested that softness and stillness could overcome hardness and movement, but no historical line whereby such principles could be demonstrated and reported continued into the nineteenth century.

On a related note, there is the old axiom in Chinese culture that refers to the merging of hardness and softness, known as *gangrou xiangji* (刚柔相济), or "hard and soft in combination." Again, though, there is little tangible support for the notion of "softness" as a category of close combat effectiveness.

There are, however, clues that hint toward a kind of softness, and one in particular which alludes to *play* becoming an aspect of *t'ai-chi*. This came in the appearance of a two-man practice of a style that is considered a sister art to *t'ai-chi, xingyiquan (*形意拳, also written *hsing-i ch'üan)*. The two-person form is named *an shen pao* (安身炮), or "peaceful body cannon," and its first confirmed appearance in print was in Ling Shanqing's 1929 *Xingyi Wuxing Quan Tuishou*. It may be more than just a coincidence that Ling's book was published during the same period that the so-called "classic" internal martial arts were undergoing what might well be described as a "softening" process.

As with the principles of *t'ai-chi's* two-person forms, first recorded by Wu Cheng-ching in the late-nineteenth century, another "internal martial art," *baguazhang,* was also developing its dual-person practices. *Rou shou* (柔手), or "soft hands," being one example. Further evidence is found in the two-person practice known as *tiao da* (tentatively believed to be represented by the Chinese characters 調打, and meaning "blending and striking" or "adjusting and striking"),[27] as well as an unnamed practice thought to be part of the curriculum of the Central Martial Arts Academy in Nanjing during the late 1920s and 30s. [28] Representing a merger of *t'ai-chi ch'üan* with *pa-kua chang (baguazhang)* training methods, it might have developed as a collaboration between Sun Lu-tang and Yang Cheng-fu, * who were renowned instructors at the academy.

Box 7-12
A video demonstration of
Eight Diagram Palm's "Soft Hands" can be viewed at

https://www.youtube.com/watch?v=RRYS0fWDEIU
or
https://chiarts.com/7-12

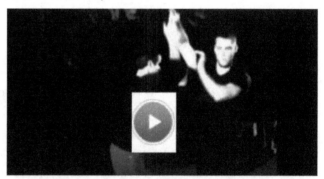

Box 7-13
A brief clip of Baguazhang tiao da practice in Beijing can be viewed at

https://youtu.be/1qpl1a4l8jA

https://chiarts.com/7-13

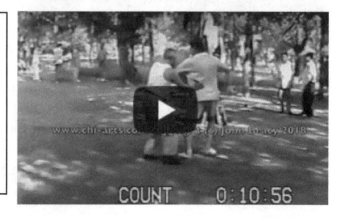

* Yang Cheng-fu was introduced earlier. Sun Lu-tang, his writings and contribution to the internal martial arts are discussed below.

An example of *bagua's* "soft hands" video can be viewed via the link in Box 7-12, a brief example of *tiao da* practice in Beijing can be viewed via the link in Box 7-13, and the partner training routine of the Central Martial Arts Academy can be viewed via the link provided in Box 7-14.

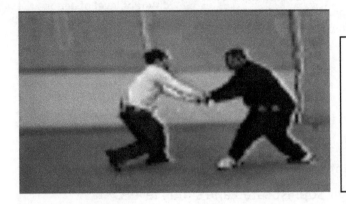

Box 7-14

The Two-Person routines Nanjing Central Martial Arts Academy, circa 1930

https://youtu.be/A1qrgVQXu_0

https://chiarts.com/7-14

Another clue suggesting that a new genre of internal martial artists was developing a distinct set of body mechanics is found in a training concept known as *wai san he* (外三合), or "three outer relationships." As discussed in Sections II and III, the term refers to a holistic set of body relationships that can be applied for therapeutic and yogic purposes. However, the term also refers to a particular set of coordinated body mechanics relating to the timing of a hand strike, for example, that is deployed in perfect coordination with the practitioner's footwork. [29] [30]

Wai san he as a set of body mechanics contributes to the argument that the internal martial arts may have been undergoing a "softening" process (Diagram 7-11) since the technique allows torque and normally accessed shoulder-based fulcrum power to be replaced by whole-body coordination and precise timing of a movement. In this way, the technique illustrates how sophisticated coordination of movement can trump gross physical power.

Another thread of evidence in support of the "softening" thesis appears during the same period. Although lacking scholarly confirmation, this clue is found in training guidelines attributed to the noted *xingyiquan* master Guo Yunshen. Citing Guo's protocol presented in Box 7-15, Robert Smith describes the progression of soft power from "obvious" to "peaceful" to "mysterious."

Guo Yunshen's
Three Levels of Power

MingJin	$\rightarrow$	AnJin	$\rightarrow$	HuaJin
"Obvious Force"		"Peaceful Force"		"Mysterious Force"

Based on specific sets of physical principles	Bio-mechanics merging with biofeedback signals the practitioner identifies as the presence, or use of *qi* internal energy	Presentation of an entirely different level of action that is difficult to explain or understand

Adapted from Robert Smith's scheme of internal power development in the martial arts attributed to the famous *xingyiquan* (hsing-I chüan) master Guo Yunshen (Kuo Yuen-shen). This scheme of development describes "soft" skill on a continuum that ranges from "internal martial art bio-mechanics" to increasingly sophisticated and subtle levels. *

Box 7-15

* Scheme of Power Development in the Internal Martial Arts Attributed to Guo Yunshen (1829 – 1898), in the context of Taoist inner alchemy, the scheme describes the development of internal power through three stages: overt, covert and mysterious. At the overt level, *jing* converts into *qi*. At the covert level *qi* converts into *shen,* and at the final stage of "mysterious energy," *shen* converts into *emptiness.*

Appearing to reference Guo, Smith explains, "...the way to mysterious (*hua*) energy is through the obvious and concealed energies. To get obvious energy you must be centered and balanced." Citing the Taoist alchemical model, Guo states that through this energy, sperm [*jing*] converts into the *qi,* which then infuses and changes the bones. (Some additional points by Guo is included in Endnote [31])

How significant are those threads of evidence suggesting that the internal martial arts were undergoing a "softening" process during the late-nineteenth and early-twentieth centuries? As mentioned earlier, to "soften" means giving up one's reliance on crude physical effort. However, to be effective in combat, the normal rules of force and typically understood body mechanics must be replaced with something else. This is a key point; this "something else" must be a new element. Is it possible that it is the majestic, but nearly lost, secret of *t'ai-chi?*

We do know a few things about that nearly lost "something else." We know that the lost element has something to do with what pioneers referred to as *mind,* but then what does *mind* truly mean? One definition most probably refers to an increased reliance on the use of sensitivity, which then merges with physical skill. It reminds me of a training point Ho Shen-ting taught me about striking with a relaxed hand. At first, the instruction seemed counterintuitive, but over the years, the point increasingly made sense. Any body part that is used in a tense way is little more than a cudgel, whereas a relaxed state — in this example, a relaxed fist — under stress brings with it the possibility of ever-increasing bio-mechanical ranges of motion. Even more significantly, a relaxed hand contacting the adversary offers the potential, through sensitivity, to instantly adapt and vary the strike against a human target.

In the example of the closed-but-relaxed fist, a relaxed punch can instantly adapt at the point of contact in ways that are minute, but also hugely effective. On one level, it converts the striking instrument from a cudgel to a sap or blackjack (a leather pouch, filled with marbles or lead, which police officers used to carry in the old days to "softly" break bones), while at the same time, a soft hand is better equipped to transfer what has been previously described as "information." **

> ** *Information* as an explanation for "internal energy" in the context of healing was introduced in Section IV, *information* as a model of "internal energy in the martial arts" will be introduced in the next section.

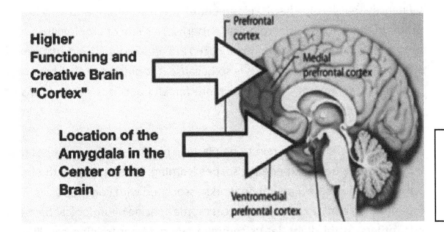

Diagram 7-16
Brain Structures and their Reaction to Stress
Source: Wikipedia Commons

The Role of Play and the Softening of *T'ai-Chi*

The relationship between brain structures and the learning process is not completely understood. [32] However, enough is known to contribute to our understanding of the development of a martial art such as *t'ai-chi*. For example, it is understood that learning a physical skill involves recruitment and functional integration of different brain regions. [33] It is also known that a person's mood affects learning, and this is especially true in the acquisition of complex skills. [34] [35] [36] This background information supports the argument that *t'ai-chi* might have developed in the context of an enjoyable learning experience, with participants engaging in a kind of "game."

Consider the idea that a person who is fully immersed in an entertaining game enters an altered state. Under these conditions, the prefrontal cortex (indicated by the top arrow in Diagram 7-16) becomes more active. By contrast, when performing an activity while in a fearful or stressed state, the amygdala (indicated by the lower arrow in the diagram) not only becomes more active, but also tends to become dominant. Furthermore, recent brain research shows that the prefrontal cortex responds in different ways to stress, and that emotion acts as a rudder in guided learning: [37] [38]

> When events are positive, the left prefrontal cortex shows more activity, with higher-frequency brain waves. By contrast, when events are negative, activation in the prefrontal cortex occurs dominantly in the right. [39]

When the amygdala becomes more dominant, a "fight or flight" nervous system response is triggered that affects the entire body. When this happens, there is less access to refined muscle control, and one's ability to access creative solutions is lessened.

> *Flow doesn't come to those who try to do things well... it comes to those who try to do things freely.*
> — Barry Michaels

The question of whether or not neuro-physiology might have contributed to the development of *t'ai-chi* provides an interesting way to think about influences that led to the development of the martial art, and which also promote these specific neurological patterns. This line of inquiry also helps us to understand how something practiced in a relaxed way (e.g. "soft") could still be effective in combat. This is so because it is presumed that creativity and subtle techniques can replace more forceful and less subtle forms of attack in close combat.

New research shows the brain to be plastic. This observation suggests that a person's emotional experience shapes learning. When positive, the brain tends to lay down new neural networks associated with complex skills. This requires the ability to selectively access some specific neurological patterns over others. In this light, let us compare two different training conditions, and then consider how each triggers a distinct neurophysiological response.

First, imagine a teenage basketball player performing in front of his overbearing and judgmental father. In this scenario, the father yells at his son whenever he misses a shot, and in response, the boy's feeling of stress is reflected through a specific "fight or flight" profile. In this example, the amygdala tends to become dominant, while the "flow" and creative centers of the brain are less available.

Contrast the above scenario with one where the boy plays basketball with a sense of freedom and joy. In this setting, the teen's father is encouraging, but not overly demanding. Here, because of his total commitment to the practice and love of the sport, the boy unconsciously engages the prefrontal and creative centers of his brain. When this happens, the "flow potential" is enabled as a result of the merger of the nervous system with brain creativity centers, which then translates into greater proficiency.

Although the sport is the same, the different ways of engagement demonstrate how the brain responds differently to various kinds of training environments. Emotions experienced during practice influence skill development because of the way the brain responds to different emotions during the learning process.

This way of looking at the merging of creative brain centers with physical performance gives rise to that interesting question of the influence of the training environment, and prompts us to consider how the training environment experienced by *t'ai-chi's* ancestors might have contributed to the development of their art. The experience of many decades of teaching close combat has taught me that training in the context of play is the most effective way for an athlete to awaken their potential. When things are fun, a person's higher potential is more likely to emerge. Thus, more fun means more mastery.

For these reasons, play — in the sense of total immersion in a joyful activity — would have been essential to both the development of *t'ai-chi* and the subsequent formation of a new approach to relaxed "soft-style" practice. The antithesis of a soft approach is military-style training, where fear and stress are the norm, and the trainee can easily become fearful of the teacher or of getting injured. Under these conditions, the individual tends to be tense, and subsequently performs in more cautious and less creative ways. In other words, the brain is not free to explore alternative possibilities. In this scenario, the amygdala, near the brain center, takes over the nervous system and limits response options. By contrast, when training is conducted under conditions emphasizing a sense of lightness and playfulness, the practitioner is more likely to access skill sets associated with the brain's creative centers.

However, some challenges to the **play thesis** need to be addressed. For example, the martial arts literature does not include descriptions of "play" as a contributing factor in the development of *t'ai-chi*. Thus, it is likely that if the play thesis is true, then practitioners did not think of, nor describe, their own practice in such terms. The absence of the discussion of play makes one wonder if *t'ai-chi* pioneers, even if they did engage in a kind of playfulness, might not have thought about their practice as an enjoyable game. Nevertheless, because of the effects of play on neurophysiology, along with other environmental factors, it is worth considering its role — i.e., participation in a pleasurable and safe activity — as a contributing factor in the development of what we today know as *t'ai-chi*.

In this light, *t'ai-chi's* partnering practice of "push hands" performs a central role. It is the perfect example of how non-aggressive cooperative play between two practitioners might have contributed to the development of the art. Among other factors, the non-violent, and often non-aggressive, practice of push hands allowed *t'ai-chi* to develop as a sublime mind-body discipline akin to dance, with participants engaging in martial arts **without the fear of injury.** More on push hands later.

However, when considering the role of play in the development of *t'ai-chi*, three major challenges to such a proposal must first be addressed. The first has to do with the question of whether or not there was the possibility of close combat play and playfulness during the trying times of late-nineteenth century China. The second looks at whether the play theory might be the product of *presentism* and *culture-bound syndrome*, which means falsely attributing present day experiences based on one's own culture to a past way of life. The last of the three challenges is the lack of scholarly support for the notion that *t'ai-chi* could be linked to play.

You go for it. All the stops are out. Caution is to the wind and you're
battling with everything you have. That's the real fun of the game.
—Dan Dierdorf

1. The Role of Play and *Playfulness*

T'ai-chi and "push hands" may be *fun* for us now, but was it fun for early pioneers of the art? The nineteenth century gave rise to some of the most painful and trying times in Chinese history, such that, generally speaking, no one was having fun. The many challenges to the Chinese of the period included the Opium Wars, the Sino-Japanese War, the Boxer Rebellion, warlords, crop failures, and natural disasters. Thus, it is important to consider whether or not play as we know it could have even been possible during such a painfully difficult period. Having said that, many sociologists believe that not only is play possible during times of social stress, but that it is necessary as a means of coping.

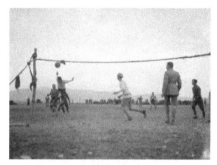

Photo 7-17
Christmas Football (Soccer) Match
Between Opposing Forces in WWI
Photo: Football in WWI [44]

Two of my teachers, Ho Shen-ting and Chang Shr-jung, were Chinese air force officers during the period when Japan's military was threatening to take over their entire country. Despite this external threat, they both managed to practice the complex forms of their internal martial arts daily, not because they expected to ever use the complicated twists and turns of the practice against an invading foe, but for exercise and as a way of maintaining their sanity. Similarly, my father served on patrol torpedo boats early in the WWII Guadalcanal campaign, at a time when things were looking precarious and uncertain for the U.S., yet he still had time to play cards and master sleight-of-hand magic tricks. Likewise, in England, children played together during the Blitz; the BBC's WWII archives even include photos of children playing games while wearing gas masks! Games are created and played during the most extreme times of national crisis. Baseball was invented just before the American Civil War but was popularized in the prisoner of war camps on both sides. To maintain morale, general officers encouraged the troops in the camps to play the game. [40]

However, the most dramatic example of play in the midst of conflict came during the Christmas truce of 1914, when opposing German and British troops ceased hostilities and engaged in a football (soccer) match (Photo 7-17). [41]

2. Presentism?

It is sometimes a mistake to assume that our own experiences, and the way we view the world of today, are comparable to those of past cultures. Consider, for example, the role of the two-person *t'ai-chi* exercise of "push hands." For many who engage in the practice now, push hands is considered fun. However, is it presentism to think that early *t'ai-chi* pioneers would have experienced push hands as an enjoyable game, in the same way that practitioners do today?

3. Scholarly Support for the Play Thesis?

If it is true that play contributed to the development of *t'ai-chi,* then it seems logical that there would be references in support of such a theory in the academic martial arts literature. There doesn't appear to be any such reference, but there remains two possible explanations for how *t'ai*-chi might have developed from two-person play without ever being described in those terms.

It is conceivable that martial arts historians searching for the origins of *t'ai-chi* might not have considered whether or not brain neurophysiology contributed to the development of the art, as their research often focuses on lineage. In most cases, they look for the secret form or transmission from some mythical creator who developed the art, and, relying on this criteria, their research focuses myopically on the search for founders who might have created a new approach or method that evolved into modern *t'ai-chi.*

This category of investigation emphasizes the search for long-lost manuals, stone etchings, and local gazetteers of bygone eras for clues that might reveal the true founder of a tradition. Their engagement in this line of investigation sometimes yields new documents and conflicting theories regarding the genesis of an art, but, as evidenced by more recent finds, there remains no consensus among scholars as to how *t'ai-chi* actually developed. [42] Thus, it is time to consider the possibility that *t'ai-chi* as we know it did not evolve as an art with a traceable lineage. Instead, we suggest that the art emerged serendipitously, perhaps a century or two ago, from the shared training of a group that practiced in an unusual way, which just so happened to link the practitioner's creative neurophysiology to a physical discipline.

If this is true, then the search for t'ai-chi's roots must be studied using a different set of research tools and criteria. One of these new methods would involve considering the types of practices and influences that contributed toward creating a unique training environment, which subsequently led to the development of t'ai-chi as an enjoyable activity. Another potential consideration is that although pioneers of the art might have begun to enjoy their participation in a martial game, it might not have occurred to them to write about their practice in this way. Is it possible that they might have participated in a game without knowing or writing about it in this way? A rose by another name?

Brain Structures and an Evolved Martial Art

(Removal from the battlefield and associated psycho-physiological changes)

On the importance of play, Professor Ruth C. Engs writes:

> Play is not just a pastime activity; it has the potential to serve as an important tool in numerous aspects of daily life for adolescents, adults, and cognitively advanced non-human species (such as primates).

Dr. Engs goes on to cite Johan Huizinga's classic on play, *Homo Ludens*:

> Summing up the formal characteristic of play, we might call it a free activity standing quite consciously outside 'ordinary' life as being 'not serious' but at the same time absorbing the player intensely and utterly....

In a related point that applies to the development of the art, Engs, again citing Huizinga, seems to support the proposal that t'ai-chi as play developed as a secretive subculture:

> ... [play] promotes the formation of social groupings that tend to surround themselves with secrecy and to stress the difference from the common world by disguise or other means.

American education philosopher John Dewey writes: "Play is a source of freedom when it is enriched by authority of outcome or purpose." He follows with: "It is possible to be playful and serious at the same time, and it is the ideal mental condition." [43] Certainly, early t'ai-chi pioneers would have appreciated the sense of joy and momentary escapism while participating in t'ai-chi, as a kind of inoculation against the tremendous stressors afflicting late-nineteenth century China.

An Evolved Martial Art?

An evolved martial form, if it exists, would be one that incorporates the full range of human potential. Whether one day shown to be the product of "internal energy" or something else altogether, an evolved practice would be one that activates both the participant's entire nervous system and the brain's full potential.

All training is not the same, and different training environments affect the brain differently. How the brain learns also affects how the brain responds.

When training is undertaken in ways that promote access to the brain's creative centers, the interaction between practitioner and opponent looks different to that seen in typically understood fighting situations; there is less struggle and more flow. Often, for a practitioner operating in such a state, everything seems to come together perfectly. At times, the practitioner's skill against an adversary may even appear magical. Examples of this kind of elevated performance are represented in Michael Jordan's most memorable basketball shots and Muhammad Ali's effortless dance-like flow while facing the world's most dangerous boxers. Neither of these exceptional individuals could have honed their remarkable skills without total joyful and playful emersion in their respective disciplines during their formative years.

Still, the question remains, can skill of this kind be utilized in a *real* close combat situation against a dangerous opponent? One incident in particular serves as testimony that it can and does happen, when I myself was the target of a surprise attack by a highly trained martial artist.

Years later, when looking back on that unfortunate encounter, I remember clearly my body's response to the attack. It was as though my brain said, "Oh, we are playing the grab to the throat game. I know that game, and this is how we play." Of course, these situations happen so fast that you can't think about it at the time, but to this day, that dangerous interaction, and my mind-body answer to it, serves as evidence that the mind-body can process and respond in the "real world" based on training that took place under the conditions of play. In such scenarios, the mind-body simply performs as taught. Your job is to stand back, trust, and watch the events transpire as if an objective observer. Truly a taste of the miraculous.

When applied to actual close combat, brain training that merges activity with the creative centers of the prefrontal cortex allows the practitioner to stay detached while functioning at a higher level. Under these conditions, a light touch placed at exactly the right spot at a precise moment can influence an aggressive and angry opponent intending to harm you. To cite another true example, there may be the full power charge of an angry person coming at you out of nowhere. In this situation, maintaining a playful style of engagement enables you to set your conscious thought processes aside and, as in the first scenario, also allows your brain's creative centers to take over. For the practitioner, the experience is that of being "out of body." From such a vantage point, one is able to sit back and watch the application of the well-honed defensive tactics apply on their own. These outcomes are reminiscent of Chuang's Tzu's description of Cook Ting's effortless skill.

As described above, the brain's architecture allows it to respond to stress in different ways (consider again the brain structures illustrated in Diagram 7-16). When a person operates under fear, anger, or just plain raw aggression, the amygdala near the center takes over much of the decision-making. In no more than a fraction of a second, the amygdala can trigger a range of survival and "fight or flight" responses in the body. T'ai-chi, and for that matter any physical discipline that is "evolved" — as defined here, involving creativity, subtlety, and access to normally unconscious bio-mechanics — could develop only under conditions where the fight or flight instinct was **not dominant.** At this juncture, it is useful to consider how the art might have developed in the context of play and cooperative learning.

If such a brain neurochemistry/ architecture profile was linked to the development of a physical discipline like t'ai-chi, these relationships could answer some of the questions about how such a unique art might have developed. This hypothesis suggests that skills were honed alongside brain chemistry not dominated by stress-related cortisol and amygdala control. Instead, participants would have engaged in brain learning patterns characterized by joy, triggering distinct neuro-chemical constituents, especially monoamine neurotransmitters like serotonin, which is a neurotransmitter associated with arousal, positive emotions, and skill-specific memory.

If true, it would mean that the fighting art was developed in concert with the presence of pleasure-related brain chemicals and higher brain prefrontal lobe functions associated with creativity. † Like the fight play between two wolf pups, who learn to kill prey through joyful play, similar responses would have been trained through "combat play" in "push hands" practice, where amygdala fear-based activity is replaced by higher brain processes associated with the neocortex.

> † On a related note, because of the way creative skill-solutions depend on access to particular parts of the brain, and especially the prefrontal cortex, the fighting posture of the "internal martial arts" tend to be more upright compared to their "external" counterparts. It is probable that the vertical orientation of the base of the brain in relationship to the upper part of the spine co-developed with that art, which in turn also promotes quicker reactions and more creative brain function. These observations are expanded upon in Sections VIII and XI.

Chapter 41

An Alternative Theory of *T'ai-Chi*

*T*he origin of *t'ai-chi* is controversial, and there are several ways to date its beginnings. [45] However, first one must consider an important question which will set the stage for this inquiry: is *t'ai-chi* principally a set of principles derived from psycho-biological insights, or a systematized series of movements passed down generations ago from an unknown source? What follows favors the former hypothesis.

For the purposes of this chapter, two qualifiers characterize the origin of the art. The first of these involves insights derived from training that availed the practitioner of new vistas of emotional and psychological experience. Linked to our earlier discussion of *entrainment,* here a definition of *t'ai-chi* is suggested that merges psycho-physiological influences with bio-mechanical principles.

The core of those derivatives involves learning (because of the way the brain's prefrontal cortex is accessed / jointly trained along with physical principles) to problem solve. "Problem solving" applies to both daily life challenges and one's response to an attack. In this scenario, the potential of the "soft" *t'ai-chi* art emerges when crude force is replaced by subtlety. This sets the stage for a "light touch" that can neutralize a threat. However, in this model, the practitioner must engage specific brain-neurophysiological components before they are able to express refined physical skill.

The second qualifier is related to the first, but is more pragmatic. It refers to a style of practice that fulfills the stated goal of Li Yi-yu, where only four ounces of strength are necessary to defeat an opponent. In other words, if a **realistic** self-defense application of the art cannot be completed with very little effort, it does not meet this definition of *t'ai-chi*. Physically, this is an easy test to try out. Either a practitioner can neutralize and counter a forceful attack using minimal effort, or they cannot. Together, these two distinct, but related, qualifiers define the psychological prerequisites that reveal the "secret of four ounces" to form a new mind-body art.

Linking inner experience to physical skill, pioneers observed that when they paid attention to subtle "internal" cues, focused attention could influence technique. When one pays attention to the "internal," over time, the body relaxes. Unnecessary tension disappears, and the problem-solving creative

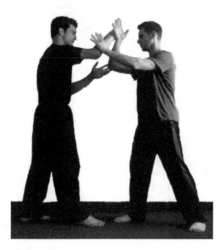

Figure 7-18

Two-Person "Push Hands" Practice

centers of the brain are more engaged. In partner training, when highly practiced, relaxed movement produces the simultaneous sensation of a current, or tingling, throughout the body; sensations that *t'ai-chi* pioneers identified as *qi*. Our thesis, then, is that this non-violent, dual-person practice was critical to the development of a new style that allowed the brain to function in more coherent ways.

Distance from the opponent

Another factor contributing to the development of the art was the distance between training opponents (Photo 7-18). With just the right amount of space between partners, skill developed in the context of separation that was neither too close nor too far away. Being just far enough away minimized reliance on hand and foot striking, while at the same time, not being too close discouraged use of grappling, such as Chinese forerunners of judo-like techniques and Greco-Roman wrestling; skill sets favoring youthful attributes of physical strength, quickness, and agility.

We are concerned with internal skill and not the external form.
—Wu Cheng-ching

Internal Martial Arts Understood in Terms of *Inner Focus*

Wu Cheng-ching was the first to define what I call internal principles in partner practice. Described by Wile as "an active participant in the formulation of theory," [46] Wu's training manual, *Treatise on Boxing*, emphasized the importance of developing "inner skill" *(nei kung / neigong)* in order to interpret force *(tung chin / dong jin)* [47] and thus defeat an opponent. Significantly, Wu describes an approach to martial arts training "concerned with 'internal skill' and not with the 'external form,'" and includes what Wile calls the "earliest description of push hands practice." Wu left other clues to the thinking of the nineteenth-century *t'ai-chi* masters about their art. In describing his theory of *tung chin,* or "interpreting force," ‡ and the development of *nei kung / neigong* "inner skill," Wu explains, "if you are unable to develop inner skill, how can you interpret the opponent's incoming force?"

‡ Where Dr. Wile translates *tung chin* as "interpreting energy," due to reasons which will shortly be made clear, and so as not to confuse the word *chin/jin* (force) with *ch'i /qi* (energy), I translate *tung chin* as "interpreting force."

Both Wu Cheng-ching's pragmatic approach, and his description of "inner skill" in the context of "interpreting force," are intriguing. Without adding mystical meanings, and strictly on the basis of a literal understanding of his words, the statement "if you are unable to develop inner skill, how can you interpret the opponent's incoming force" simply means, that if you are unable to "tune in" and develop sensitivity, you will not be able to counter the opponent's attack. For the moment, let us analyze Wu's primary instruction: direct your attention inward, not outward.

Three Conditions

For practical purposes, the internal martial arts, as known today, begin with the merging of three conditions: _proximity_ to the opponent, _enjoyment_ of safe combat training, and an _inward shift_ in mental orientation by participants. Is it possible, then, that these three conditions merged in just the right way to create a new approach to practicing close combat in a rich and fulfilling way?

The convergence of these three conditions allowed practitioners to merge physical skill with the earlier described more creative mind-body state. Their new art looked and felt effortless. As it _softened,_ it awakened new power and hitherto unknown abilities that gave rise to an entirely new approach to combat training. _The secret: pay attention to subtle biofeedback signals; use the qi and mind, not force, to defeat your opponent._

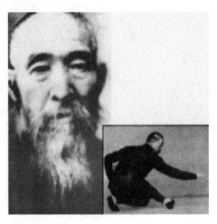

Figure 7-19
Authored books on _nei jia quan / nei-chia ch'üan_ (内家拳) internal martial arts In the 1920s.

Insert at right: Younger Sun in _xingyiquan's (hsing-i ch'üan's)_ "Dragon Style" posture

New Terms and Concepts

Changes in martial arts terms and language in the late-nineteenth and early-twentieth centuries suggest that participants believed they had discovered something new and profound. Some of the best examples of these are found in the books of Sun Lu-tang (Figure 7-19). For example, although the term "internal martial art" had been used in a non-specific way much earlier, it was in his books published during the 1920s that Sun popularized _nei jia quan / nei-chia ch'üan_ (内家拳) as a distinct class of training.

Sun strove to explain how these martial practices were more than simply self-defense techniques; he promoted the idea that they could simultaneously initiate Taoist spiritual wisdom. To this end, he believed that these arts functioned as forms of yogic-alchemy, describing how they operated as relaxed and "soft" technologies. He also described how they represented a distinctive class of training, where mind and _qi_ were at the center of practice.

At times, Sun was remarkably candid about his personal experiences with what he perceived as the movement of internal energy within his body:

> Tao embodies the universe and is the foundation of the _yin_ and the _yang_. In boxing, Tao symbolizes the [internal martial arts]. The forms of these three are different, but the principle is the same: everything begins and ends in emptiness. The _Yuan-ch'i_ [original energy] must

be maintained. This force that keeps the sky blue and the earth calm also makes for achievement in man .... I had always heard that boxing is Tao, but I could not really understand it until I learned secret energy. In our training we combined hard and soft tactics and became light, dexterous, and natural. But when we learned mysterious energy we did not tell each other the sensations we felt. But I want to write of it now. After practicing one form or style, I would stand upright and calm, collecting my *ch'i [qi]* and intent. Then I would feel something in my genitals. I felt it every day. From action came inaction. When I stopped practice, I felt everything outside and within me was empty. At this time the real *yang* felt as if it wanted to discharge. If you moved, the true *yang* would discharge [spontaneous seminal release]. I used the boxing way to curb this: I sank the insubstantial spirit to my navel and at the same time moved the *yang* upward from my genitals to the navel. My genitals thus shrank, the sperm moved to my *tan tien* [lower abdominal energy center / *dan tian*], and I could feel continuous circulation throughout my body. After four or five hours of being in a near coma I would become normal again. Boxing is difficult at first; later it becomes easy. When you sink the *ch'i*, it will cure everything. Therefore, boxing and Tao are the same. [48]

Sun's account describes how the practice stimulated sexual centers, and how the overpowering experience sometimes left him in a dissociative state. His description of the experience included his report of how the practice was sometimes so intense that it affected his nervous system in remarkable ways. As Sun explains, the sensations could be so overpowering that he felt they might trigger spontaneous seminal emission.

Although an attempt to describe an art that incorporated Taoist alchemy, traditional medicine, and the use of *qi* energy was provided by Chang Naizhou (苌乃周) a century earlier, Chang described such knowledge only for the purpose of enhancing fighting ability and to injure an opponent. * In contrast to Chang's exclusive focus on fighting, later nineteenth century *nei jia* "internal family" arts promoted the use of specific skill sets, such as minimal touch control over an opponent coupled with *changes within the practitioner*. [49] Thus, for the advanced practitioner, demonstrations of skill became paired with a particular kind of inner experience.

* More on Chang in Section VIII

Two-Person Exercise

It seems more than just a coincidence that terms referring to "soft" and "peaceful" power were becoming popularized at the same time that the internal martial arts in the late-nineteenth century were being codified. Significantly, at the same time, systematized, two-person martial *push hands* training "games" were being developed.

The systematized teaching of push hands was a crucial contributor to the development of *t'ai-chi, a martial art based on the imitation of nature.* Just as in nature, where a cat or wolf doesn't learn to conquer the prey through anger or fear, but through play fighting, this same principle applies to the development of *t'ai-chi* as a game. Like young wolves engaged in the joy of combat games, in the new practice of push hands "combat games," aggression and fear are minimized. These emotions are replaced by the prioritization of inner stillness, *"listening" and staying relaxed.*

Significantly, in the emerging discipline, the role of spiritual experience was not neglected. No doubt some believed then, as now, that their new art had become a form of mystical practice. These observations leave one to consider what masters like Guo *Yunshen* meant by their use of terms such as "mysterious force" (Box 7-15).

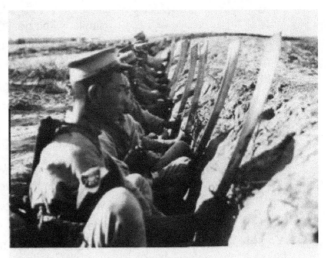

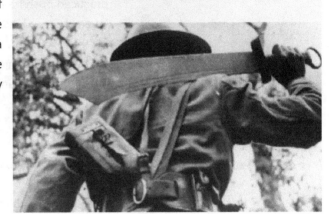

Photos 7-20

Chinese Military use of Curved Swords in the Modern Period

1930s photos credited to the Republic of China Ministry of Defense

An Intellectual's Game?

When some members of China's upper-class elite became interested in *t'ai-chi* in the late-nineteenth century, their participation also contributed to the development of the art; most important among these being the evolution of the goal of practice. It changed from a discipline meant to destroy the opponent to participation in a martial arts game, with an emphasis on non-violence toward their fellow practitioners. Their adoption of the straight saber as the iconic *t'ai-chi* weapon came at a time when practical military swords featured curved blades, and Western firearms were prevailing on the battlefield (see Photos 7-20). For close troop combat, the straight sword, like the Western foil, had no place and was a gentleman's adornment; one that demanded more sophisticated knowledge in its application. [50]

Furthermore, in a martial "game," the risk of potentially harmful techniques is minimized in favor of skills such as pushing and controlling. This method of practice would further eliminate the practitioner's experience of fear during training, while at the same time promoting creative brain responses associated with play. The enjoyable participation in a martial arts game, as opposed to the desire to physically harm or kill, allowed brain changes to be engaged as an aspect of training.

The result of training in this way is observed in *t'ai-chi's* "push hands," and in sister styles such as *baguazhang's rou shou* "soft hands" (Box 7-12), where similarly, the goal of training is not to injure, but to neutralize the opponent through subtlety in a *game* of inner stillness and minimal effort. In both examples (push hands and soft hands), new terms based on *sensitivity*, like *ting chin* "listening," and *lien*, "connecting," [51] identified the skills necessary to defeat an opponent.

The development of *t'ai-chi* is intimately tied to the practice of "push hands." In the twilight years of the nineteenth century, Wu Cheng-ching was the first to describe the two-person exercise. The practice was a kind of chess game, where participants learned to sense, neutralize, and counter each other's movements. The goal: conquer your opponent with subtlety, not with force; destabilize the opponent while keeping your center. In traditionally practiced push hands, soft control that manipulates the opponent is a win, whereas a hard, aggressive push is considered a losing move. [52] When the ideal is exhibited, crude force is avoided, replaced by light, non-forceful contact applied through flowing, relaxed movements. Again, this is a kind of interaction that cannot be realized if fear and tension are present.

Other Contributing Factors

Appeal to an Educated Class

The following tangential point supports the thesis that *t'ai-chi* underwent a "softening" process. Although there is an older body of Chinese martial arts literature that suggests it was possible to defeat an opponent with a *soft* method, for practical purposes, the internal martial arts phenomenon was largely unknown before the late-nineteenth century. This leads one to consider what other factors, beyond those already discussed, could have contributed to the development of a "soft" style internal martial art. One contributing factor might have been the sudden participation of intellectuals in the practice, a question that led Wile to ask why:

> ....certain members of the intellectual and political elite so bent on dis-
> covering, mastering, and elaborating the ultimate martial art at a time
> when gunboats, cannons, and rifles were determining the fate of the
> nation? [53]

Wile proposes a number of reasons to explain why intellectuals might have suddenly become interested in the martial arts. These included escapism, practical need for militia training, a psychological defense against Western imperialism, and a subtle spiritual practice based on returning to natural principles. [54] While each of these no doubt contributed to the appeal that led intellectuals to become involved in martial arts, the final point may offer the best clue to explain why a more educated class would be attracted to a new "soft" martial art. More appealing to an intellectual class would be an approach not based on magical powers derived from an external source, such as the Buddha or a god, but a practice based on self-empowerment and natural principles. Those participants would not frame their experiences in terms of positive bio-chemical changes, but they would have been aware of the feelings triggered by such an empowering mind-body state; one based on an internal *locus of control*.

Keep in mind that, for the practitioner, this kind of practice produces an array of sensations that are useful as biofeedback *signals*. Sometimes, these come in the form of electric-like tingling throughout the body. At other times, they are experienced as the spreading of warmth throughout the body.

Regardless of which particular *signal* an experienced practitioner of moving meditation learns to "get in touch" with, these are almost always accompanied by a deep sense of peace and relaxation. This is the most probable reason why late-nineteenth century *t'ai-chi* practitioners believed that they were experiencing the flow of *qi* throughout their bodies. No doubt, through their practice, some believed it brought them into mystical union with the *Tao*. A new kind of student was ready for a new kind of practice

Together, *signal* and the experience of the flow of "internal energy" had the potential of inducing what we would today call the "psycho-physiological benefits" of practice. In general, intellectuals then, as now, are less inclined toward a practice that occasionally involved blows to the face. To them, a moving meditation practice / martial art experienced through playfulness, whether consciously understood this way or not, would be infinitely more appealing.

Here, a further point relating to the involvement of intellectuals in the development of *t'ai-chi* is also worth noting. Based on my experience teaching a variety of Chinese martial arts over many decades, medical doctors, college professors, engineers, and similarly well-educated students are less inclined to participate in a rough and tumble martial study that occasionally includes the breaking of bones and rearrangement of facial characteristics. However, if *t'ai-chi* did develop as an enjoyable, safe, and interactive game, this kind of training would have appealed more to that class of student. This is one of the key reasons why a softer and gentler combat art would have been more inviting to an intellectual class.

Inner Alchemy, Calmness, and the Taoist

Li Yi-yu and Wu Cheng-ching, along with other members of their clan, would have noticed that access to the new skills they practiced depended on the practitioner working on their inner self. As discussed earlier, skill sets like these are linked to management of the nervous system, which is trained through emotional centeredness and equanimity. No doubt experiences like these contributed to the notion that the study of the art could function as a self-cultivation practice. Like Sun, other intellectuals would have begun to think of the practice as a form of inner alchemy, capable of initiating changes within the individual.

When actualized, "inner alchemy" allowed the practitioner to engage an opponent from a more evolved state of mind. Internal work like this brings about the strange sensation of forgetting the opponent. This is more than avoidance of self-consciousness; it entails a complete lack of self-awareness. *T'ai-chi* became a special medium whereby one could simultaneously work on oneself while learning to perceive and join with the flow of the *Tao*, and occasionally even experience the transcendent state of *wu xin,* or "no mind."

Conclusion to Section VII

*T*he chapters in this section have traced how *t'ai-chi*'s use of "mind and not force" developed in response to a number of specific influences. This included *enjoyment of safe practice, an inward shift in orientation*, and *physical proximity to the opponent.* It was suggested that these influences combined in just the right way to permit the practitioner to focus not on the "external," but on one's inner experience. The experience was heightened through sensations elicited by the unique characteristics of moving meditation. When paying attention to these sensations, identified by the Chinese as *qi*, founding masters developed a physical form intimately connected to the power of harmony between biological rhythms.

Without conscious awareness, they engaged in what we would today call biofeedback training. When skill became closely linked to the ability to reproduce *signals* — warmth, tingling, pressure, and electric-like sensations — a new way of mastering martial arts was born. Based on the principle of what practitioners referred to as using "mind and intention" to defeat an opponent, this experience gave birth to the *t'ai-chi* formula, "use no more than four ounces to defeat an opponent."

Contributing to the development of the new *t'ai-chi* model, proximity to the opponent, an integral part of push hands, played a part in the maturation of the art. Push hands provided the perfect distance between opponents, neither too close nor too far away, and this set the rules for engagement. The distance was one that was close enough to decrease reliance on launching long-distance strikes, while at the same time just far enough to discourage games of grappling that favor youth, agility, and muscular strength. Conditions were created that allowed the process to slow down; as practitioners relaxed, a new kind of learning took place in the midst of enjoyable conflict training. As the creative centers of the brain became unfettered, practitioners were free to explore new vistas in problem solving. They could start to make their own magic.

> *Flow can only be achieved when we are*
> *willing to let go of the outcome and just play.*
> Sandra Taylor Hedges

The art of *t'ai-chi* as we know it could not have evolved without the ability of practitioners to relax during their practice, as it was relaxation that awoke their latent power of higher brain function. Pioneering masters discovered that in place of normally expected fight or flight responses, they learned to focus within, "listen," and release what we today refer to as mental and physical tension. Suddenly, a martial arts practice became a psychological and physical tool for self-healing.

This model of *t'ai-chi's* genesis suggests that the participant's mind and body were invited to cooperate in a new venture, changing their physical state in order to change their mental state, and then discovering that the principle worked both ways: through mental attention, one could awaken the latent power of the body.

T'ai-chi's ancestors left clues to the potential of special mind-body states as means of responding to challenge. Their message was about problem solving, not with a forceful approach, but with a sense of subtlety and lightness. This evolved as an expression of calmness in motion, permitting martial arts to merge with the deeply personal work of moving meditation. The founding masters also left us an example of how to access higher brain potential under stress and *choose* the way we respond to external stressors, based on creativity instead of knee-jerk reaction.

Endnotes

1 From the website, http://www.tai-chi.co.za/taichi/stories.htm

2 Consistent with comments in the opening pages of the present work, for the most part, Chinese characters are transliterated using the *pinyin* system of transliteration. However, there are a few exceptions where Chinese is romanized in the Wade-Giles style. Examples of Wade-Giles transliteration in this chapter include *t'ai-chi ch'üan*, Chuang Tzu, cook Ting, Li Yi-yu, Ch'en Village and Huang Tsung-hsi.

3 Wile, Douglas. 2016. "Fighting words: Four new document finds re-ignite old debates in taijiquan historiography", *Martial arts studies* 4, pp. 17-35.

4 Burton Watson translation, *Chuang Tzu: The basic writings*, Columbia University Press, 1965.

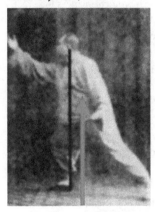

5 This point refers to definitions by some schools, particularly Yang, which describe unique bio-mechanics of *t'ai-chi* and the internal martial arts. This way of applying force and effective technique is not over reliant on large muscle groups, for example, the use of fulcrum/shoulder-based power of the trapezius muscles. This otherwise (for most individuals), habitual pattern of movement is replaced with integrated athletic connection expressed through a movable center vertical line called "empty-full". The included photo of Yang Cheng-fu captures this principle in the "diagonal flying" posture. The photo indicates the forward of center "full" front leg weighting. The arrow in the middle of the photo indicates Yang's center of mass. Related to the empty-full principle, "Base of the skull and the neck: The suboccipital triangle" and "The "Open" and "Vertical" in Contact Sports" are discussed in Section XI.

A YouTube video presentation of Empty-Full in close combat can be viewed at https://www.youtube.com/watch?v=B-DvtxpAHYw

6 There is, however, some mention of "internal" martial art and sparse literature describing the notion that *qi* internal energy could optimize the warrior's potential in combat. These references date back to at least the mid 1600s. Of particular note is Huang Tsung-hsi's philosophical discussion regarding cultivation of *qi* energy (*Tai Chi Ancestors*, p.41), the notion of coordinating the entire body (*Ancestors*, p. 43), and description of an "internal art" being counter to the brute force of Shaolin (*Ancestors*, p. 47). Huang writes: "Now there is another school that is called 'internal' which overcomes movement with stillness. Thus we distinguish Shaolin as 'external.' " As translated and quoted by Wile in *Tai Chi Ancestors*, p. 51. More on Huang in Endnote 12.

Contributing to our discussion of disciplines purported to merge "internal energy" or "*qi* cultivation" with ancient Chinese yoga and martial arts is the mid-eighteenth-century writings of Chang Nai-chou, who created a style that intertwined martial art with meditation, and which Professor Wile describes as "all but extinct." (*Ancestors*, p. 71). Chang's art placed priority on *qi* development, (*Ancestors*, p. 76), qi circulation (*Ancestors*, p. 77) — instructing that stagnation can be removed by movement (*Ancestors*, p. 77) — and emphasized the importance of focusing the body's qi to a single point. (*Ancestors*, p. 78). (More on Chang later and in Section VIII).The internal martial art development described in this section is suggested as an "evolutionary advancement" since the "new" way of *t'ai-chi* practice in the late nineteenth century emphasized "use of the mind" and "minimal strength" to defeat the opponent in a *systematized way* that remains the goal of practitioners to the present.

7 To avoid confusion for uninitiated readers, the present work most often refers to *pinyin* "qi," however, at times, especially when citing the works of other writers, the Wade-Giles transliteration *ch'i* is used. In either case, the Chinese word is pronounced "chee." Note, in the Wade-Giles system, when *chi* is used without an apostrophe, it would be pronounced "ghee"

8 The below is adapted from John Voigt's definitions. **Qigong** meaning "Energy Work" theoretically may include Chinese traditional medicine, martial arts, visual arts and certain Asian spiritual practices. However, as commonly used *qigong (ch'i kung)* is a set of breath, body positions and movements used to cultivate and balance life energy, especially for health. Its practice grows richer when mental focused intention leads and guides the *qi*, even more so when visualizations are added.

"T'ai-Chi" is a common expression in the Western world, which refers to **"Taijiquan."** However, most Americans improperly call **qigong** "t'ai-chi." These malapropisms may lead to misunderstandings; e.g., the "chi" in "tai-chi" does not mean "energy" or "life energy."

Taijiquan / T'ai-chi ch'üan [太极拳 - tài jí quán] literally means "Supreme Ultimate Fist" or "Grand Boxing." Originally it was (and still is) a martial art developed for self-defense—although now it is more often practiced as a kind of moving meditation.

Source: Qi: Journal of Traditional Eastern Health & Fitness

9 *Annals of the State of Wu*, as cited by Douglas Wile in T'ai Chi's *Ancestors: The Making of an Internal Art*, Sweet Chi Press, 1999, p. 3.

10 Selected portion of Li Yi-Yu's, *Song of the Essence of T'ai-chi Chüan*, Translated by Douglas Wile, Ibid., pp. 50-51

11 According to Douglas Wile, *t'ai chi's* postures and framework can be traced to General Ch'i Chi-kuang, its philosophy and ideology to Wang Chen-nan, and theory to Chang Naizhou (苌乃周). See Wile, Douglas, *T'ai Chi's Ancestors: The making of an Internal Martial Art*. Sweet Ch'i Press, Brooklyn, New York, 1999.

12 The term "internal boxing" (*nei-chia ch'üan fa*) was used to describe the art of Huang Pai-chia and his father, Huang Tsung-chi in the seventeenth century. Douglas Wile references Huang Tsung-chi as the

founder of, if not physical form and movement, "a theoretical line of internal martial arts" with a distinct theory of "softness overcoming hardness," "stillness overcoming movement" and "reversing the principles of Shaolin" On this "style," Wile writes, "The internal form, as described by Pai-chia, bears little resemblance to t'ai-chi forms, and it is not until a century later that we have a similar statement of soft-style principles." Note, that Pai-chia stated the line as abandoned and not further transmitted.

Wile, Douglas, *Lost T'ai Chi Classics from the Late Ch'ing Dynasty*, State University of New York, 1996 p. xvi.

13 Wile

14 Wile further describes the problem of the paucity of *t'ai-chi* documentation, stating: "When specifically t'ai-chi texts do appear, it is with Wu Yu-hsiang in the nineteenth century, and his editor and mouthpiece Li Yi-yu, who attributes them not to Ch'en Village, but to an accidental manuscript find in Wu-yang County, Henan, and to a mysterious master, Wang Tsung-yueh." Wile, *Lost tai-chi classics*, p. xvi.

15 Principal members of the club would have been Wu Yu-hsiang, his son, Wu Cheng-ching, Wu's nephews, Li Yi-yu and Li Chi-hsuan and associates from the Yang family.

16 Here is a personal story that illustrates this point. When I lived in Taiwan, I once heard about a martial art school that was represented as having original secrets and lineage passed down from an ancient source. One day, my teacher and friend, Yi Tien-wen and I decided to visit the local branch of this mysterious school. The martial art practice we observed while visiting didn't seem particularly impressive, but the ritual and uniforms certainly were. According to the style's origin story, the martial art was created by the legendary Yellow Emperor himself! Consistent with their "tradition," the students paraded around the studio in a kind of formal ceremony, wearing gowns and ancient official head-ware of the ancient ruler. The students wore a characteristic Yellow Emperor headpiece, the top of which was a platform that extended forward and back in the fashion of paintings of the legendary emperor. Attached to the platform were little strings of beads like those you might sometimes find on the shades of antique lamps.

17 For example, in "The origin & evolution of taijiquan", Michael De-Marco writes on the practice of ascribing the origin of *t'ai-chi* to an ancient authority:

The technique of attributing the origin of Taijiquan *[t'ai-chi ch'üan]* to Chang San-feng is just one illustration of the Chinese use of antedating. In so doing, Taijiquan is given the respect of antiquity and the sacredness of a para-normal manifestation. Chang represents an ideal boxing master with super-normal abilities.

DeMarco, Michael A., "The origin & evolution of taijiquan, " *Journal of Asian martial arts*, 1992, p. 9

18 Wile, Douglas, *Lost T'ai Chi Classics from the Late Ch'ing Dynasty*, State University of New York, 1996, p. 16.

19 Wile

20 In his research Tiller investigated the power of intention to influence the external world via a gas-discharge device experiment. The gas-discharge device was designed to investigate intention as a real world force of nature (as opposed to theoretical or conceptual). Tiller and fellow investigators found that when a practitioner was next to the device while and in a state of biological harmony and then *intended* to interact with the device that the device registered the intention. Tiller et al conducted numerous tests with multiple individuals between 1977 and 1979.

Tiller, William, *Science and human transformation*, pp. 5-7.

21 Tiller, pp. 222-224.

22 The induction technique used in Dr. Tiller's studies of entrainment could not be applied to our mock combat studies because first the method requires more time for the individual to attain the entrainment mode. Second, Dr. Tiller's research protocol involves the practitioner working through a calm, meditative state, obviously unattainable in the circumstance of stressful mock combat.

23 We found that the use of entrainment in mock combat could be "broken" when a practitioner experienced fear or self-doubt while employing the skill.

24 *Tiller, William, et al,* "Cardiac coherence: A new, non-invasive measure of autonomic nervous system order," *Alternative Therapies*, Vol. 2:1 1996.

25 Under extremely stressful conditions of close contact with an opponent it might be difficult to attend to some specific criteria such as the heartbeat or feeling or feelings associated with the propagation of blood through arterial vessels. Subsequently, those trained in the EPT protocol learn to identify other sensations, such as a heavier feeling in their legs and rely on that as a biofeedback signal. My personal and most favored technique is to mentally attend to the sense of warmth-tingling-relaxation feeling in the back of my neck. As will be shared later, this technique has been successfully employed in some real close-combat situations.

26 Instruction from Chiun, master of *Sinanju*, to his disciple-assassin trainee in the *Remo Williams* 1985 action-adventure film.

27 The practice was taught to the author years ago in Beijing, but the characters for the name of the practice were lost. Thus, the characters for *"tiao da"* and their suggested meanings are a best guess.

28 The curriculum of the Nanjing Central Martial Arts Academy appears to have included the merger of *t'ai-chi ch'üan* and *pa-kua chang (baguazhang)*. The two-person forms of the academy suggest this, and that the internal martial arts were undergoing a "softening" during the 1930s. Some of the dual-person training routines can be viewed from the link in Box 7-14.

The material was taught to the author and his students in the early 1980s by Ho Shen-ting, who was trained in the martial arts by Cheng Huai-hsien (Zheng Huaixian), student / disciple of Sun Lu-tang). Some of Master Ho's background relates to the discussion. Ho was a retired general of the Chinese (Nationalist) Air Force. By training, Ho was an aircraft maintenance officer. He had an engineer's mind for detail and memorization, and he graduated at the top of his officer academy class (and, because of this, was presented a gold watch by Chiang Kai-shek during the graduation ceremonies).

This is an important point since it illustrates Ho's attention to detail. For these reasons, the routines are believed to accurately represent the instruction of Cheng HS and the curriculum of the "internal" methods that academy members referred to as the Wu-tang (Wudang) arts.

SEE ALSO, https://www.quora.com/What-style-of-Chinese-martial-arts-was-demonstrated-in-the-1936-Berlin-Summer-Olympics-closing-ceremony

29 For example, if the practitioner's foot is weighted even a fraction of a second before the upper body punch, push, or other move is expressed, this is not a *wai san he* application. It took the author a year's worth of training in Taiwan to master this, and years more to fully appreciate the principle.

30 According to martial arts historian Douglas Wile, Li, Yang, Ch'en, and Sun publications yield few clues to the earliest references to the *wai san he* term applied to physical training.

31 Guo explains the use of *xingyiquan*'s power through three stages: overt, covert and mysterious:

"How is *xingyi* used in the three stages? In the first stage it is like a steel chisel, which goes out strongly but falls like a light piece of bamboo. In the second, it starts like an arrow, and falls weightless like the wind. In the highest stage, it follows the wind and chases the moon. An outsider never sees it hit; if he does, it does not belong to this stage."

Smith, Robert, *Hsing-I: Chinese mind-body boxing*, North Atlantic Books, 1974, p. 92-94

32 Cohen, Dayan E, "Neuroplasticity subserving motor skill learning." Neuron. 2011 Nov 3; 72(3):443-54. As cited by Danielle S. Basset, et al, in "A Network Neuroscience of Human Learning: Potential To Inform Quantitative Theories of Brain and Behavior," Trends Cogn Sci. 2017 April; 21(4): 250–264.

33 Learning involves integration of motor cortex, visual cortex, basal ganglia, precuneus, dorsolateral prefrontal cortex, and cerebellum all show changes in their activity levels during motor skill learning. Telesford, Qawi K, et al, Neuroimage. 2016 Nov 15; 142: 198–210.

34 Richard F. Betzel, *et al*, "A positive mood, a flexible brain" arXiv:1601.07881 01/2016

35 In Betzel's study of global (brain) flexibility, results implied that positive emotional states correspond to a more flexible brain.

36 It is also germane to note that self-affirmation tasks have been shown to parametrically alter brain activity to a degree that predicts individual differences in future behavior. Falk, E.B., *et al, Proceedings of the National Academy of Sciences* 112, 1977 (2015).

37 Frijda, N.H. *The Laws of Emotions*. New York, NY: Erlbaum. Fuster,

J.M. (2008). *The Prefrontal Cortex*. London, UK: Academic Press, 2006

38 The brain uses emotion to tag experiences as either positive and worth approaching, or as aversive and worth avoiding. www.howyouthlearn.org

39 Hinton, C. & Fischer, K.W. "Learning from a Developmental and Biological Perspective." In H. Dumont, D. Istance, & Benavides, F. eds. *The Nature of Learning: Using Research to Inspire Practice*. Paris, France: OECD, 2011

40 On the history of baseball, Terry Bluett writes that during the Civil War, New Yorkers started teaching baseball to comrades from other states. They loved it and played as often as they could. Commanding officers sent reports encouraging the playing of baseball in the P.O.W. camps since it promoted "good health and keeps the mind off of the war." For a baseball they employed a walnut wrapped with yarn and covered the ball with tightly fitting horsehide, while carved oak limbs were employed as bats. Bluett, Terry, http://www.pacivilwartrails.com/stories/tales/baseball-and-the-civil-war

41 http://www.cnn.com/2014/12/23/sport/football/christmas-truce-football-match/index.html

42 Of recent document finds in China, one describes the founding of the art as derived from the teachings of Li Chunmao (1568-1666), who is said to have studied with a Taoist priest, Bogong Wudao. The newfound documents are believed by some to support the notion that t'ai-chi principles were written down by Li in a manual called *Wuji yangshenggong shisanshi quan (Infinity health cultivation thirteen postures boxing)*. However, some scholars challenge the authenticity of the supporting documents. Other examples of recent document finds pertaining to the contested origin of *t'ai-chi* state that the roots of the art can be traced to the Wang Family of Wangbao Village. Critics challenge these claims as unconvincing. Other theories attest to a manual purported to be a deathbed transmission of a training manual which states that Ch'en Wangting brought the Thirteen Postures to Ch'en Village. This thesis also has its detractors. Detailed discussion of these new finds and origination theories is provided by Douglas Wile in "Fighting Words" and is highly recommended for anyone interested in the historicity of *t'ai-chi ch'üan*. See Wile, Douglas, "Fighting words: Four new document finds reignite old debates in taijiquan historiography," *Martial Arts Studies* 4, 2016, pp. 17-35.

43 As cited by Rajagopalan, Krishnaswamy, *A Brief history of physical education in India* (New Edition), Authorhouse, UK, Ltd, Bloomington, IN. p. 202.

44 http://www.openuniversity.edu/news/news/football-in-world-war-1-photo-gallery

45 According to Professor Wile, although the origins of *t'ai-chi* as a martial art are controversial, he suggests four ways that one can determine the origin of the art: 1) Through analysis of postures and forms, (2) training techniques, (3) internal "soft" style combat strategies, and (4) links to Taoist philosophy and legend (see Wile, *Lost T'ai-Chi Classics*, p. xv). Disregarding the legendary and fanciful, if evaluated from the standpoint of postures, the art can be traced to General Chi Chi-kuang's sixteenth century boxing classics and postures, which were adopted by Ch'en Village boxers in the seventeenth or later centuries. However, if viewed in terms of "internal training

and soft strategy," which includes principles of stillness overcoming movement and reversing the principles of Shaolin, although superficially mentioned earlier, these were first described in detail by Huang Tsung-chi, who lived until nearly the end of the seventeenth century. (Noteworthy despite Huang's son, who received the transmission of the art from his father, stating that he abandoned the practice and the transmission was terminated.) (Wile, *Lost T'ai-Chi Classics* p. xvi). The first detailed description of an art linked to Taoist alchemy and traditional medicine is provided by Chang Naizhou (Chang Nai-chou) in the late-eighteenth century. Although not similar in appearance to known *t'ai-chi* forms, Chang describes an internal art that emphasizes "slow movements during training, sticking to the opponent, concentrating, and circulating the qi." However, Chang's art was not passed on. For the purpose of the present chapter, which is concerned with psychological and neurophysiological changes within the practitioner that led to the development of the art, an additional way to date *t'ai-chi* is forwarded. The suggested way of looking at the development of the art defines it as a "soft art" practice that induces specific mind-body state which, when sufficiently mastered, promotes a kind of super-efficiency. Thus, it requires "only four ounces" of strength to control an opponent. Such an approach is that believed to have partly resulted from two-person practice developed in the late-nineteenth century that can traced to the writings of Wu Cheng-ching (discussed later) and other Yang School authors.

46 Wile, p. 41.

47 Wile, pp. 41-42.

48 As translated and quoted by Robert Smith in *Hsing-I: Mind-Body Boxing*, Smith, Robert w., *Hsing-i: Mind-body boxing*, Kodansha International, New York, 1974, p. 103.

49 In order to "feel the flow of *qi*," the practitioner is required to relax any excess physical tension. In modern parlance, there is a well-established link between physical tension and bio-chemistry. The practice of relaxation produces marked changes in the blood chemistry profile of the individual, which includes decrease in cortisol stress hormone in blood serum.

50 This introduces a tangential, but no less interesting, question about the late (at least through the early 1940s) use of bladed weapons by a formal army. This, especially for China, seems counterintuitive. Not only had China invented gunpowder, but by the 1800s, the Chinese had experienced a long history with muzzle-loading firearms.

Until the Nationalist Revolution of the early-twentieth century, China was an empire under a Manchu emperor and not a "modern" nation-state. In addition to the central government, there were bandits, rebels, and paramilitaries, all armed with an eclectic assortment of traditional and modern weapons. After the founding of the Republic of China in 1911, a Communist insurgency arose, capable of challenging the central government and ultimately defeating and replacing it. This peasant army was equipped with even less "standard issue" weapons, including pitchforks and hoes.

51 Referring to the term, *zhan lian gen sui* (粘连跟随), some Chinese commentators interpret it as four distinct concepts, and some as two compounds. If you take it as four, it is usually translated as, "adhere, connect, stick, and follow," otherwise, the compound school just interprets it as "stick and follow."

52 However, the principle of subtle technique during contest is currently in rapid decline. Many push hands competitions today allow aggressive judo-like contact and forceful pushing.

53 Wile, Douglas, *Lost T'ai Chi Classics from the Late Ch'ing Dynasty*, State University of New York, 1996, p. 23.

54 Wile pp. 23-26.

Section VIII
Internal Energy in the Martial Arts

A practitioner in Beijing could not press anything with his hands. When he was shopping for a baby carriage, he was surprised that the baby carriage would collapse with a crash when he checked its sturdiness with his hands. When he went home and sat in a chair, he could not press it with his hands. If he did, the chair would break. He asked me what was going on. I did not tell him because I did not want him to develop an attachment. I just said that it was all natural, let it be, and ignore it since it was all good.

— Master Li Hongzhi, speaking on his advice to a student

VIII

Internal Energy in the Martial Arts

Introduction to Section VIII

*T*he previous section considered the genesis and fulfillment of the ancient Chinese archetype of *qi* in the martial arts. There, it was discussed how the art we know today as *t'ai-chi*[1] might have emerged from an accidental discovery. That discovery: how to subdue of a means of subduing an opponent using superior efficiency. Influences contributing to the discovery included training environment, social interactions, and brain physiology. The section described how the art's unique strategy of "minimal contact" with an opponent was facilitated by the practitioner's ability to attain synchrony of their biological rhythms.

However, these factors contribute little to our understanding of how "internal energy" can be used for self-defense purposes. The present section takes a closer look at that controversial question, asking if something that can be called "internal energy in the martial arts" may objectively exist. Later, a new theory will be advanced to explain at least some examples of "internal power" in martial arts and contact sports.

Can Internal Energy be Used for Self-Defense?

Is it possible to rely on "internal energy" in close combat and contact sports? If so, this would mean that a yet-to-be-identified force could be deployed against an opponent in ways that are as yet unknown to orthodox science. It would also mean that a category of "energy," "force," or "influence" exists that may be demonstrated to exceed, or contribute to, the level of skill presently understood within the context of accepted bio-mechanical forces. If proven to be true, this hypothesis would challenge the known boundaries of human potential.

Since the question of whether "internal energy" can be used for martial arts or self-defense purposes is disputed, it is necessary to consider carefully how, and under what conditions, the use of "internal energy in the martial arts" *might* be possible. Understanding how this phenomenon could manifest in hand-to-hand combat would contribute toward our knowledge of human potential in the narrow application of fighting arts and beyond.

Chapter 42

Three Categories of Internal Power in the Martial Arts

Introduction to the Three Categories

There are three types of claims regarding internal energy in the martial arts. The first has to do with secret knowledge and magical abilities, the second focuses on training that allows the practitioner to attack an opponent with a concentrated reserve of focused energy. The third category is new to the literature, and is based on the notion of "energy as *information*."

Category 1: Special Powers: Magic and Feats of Strength

Asian culture has long had a fascination with magical powers and abilities. Legends of individuals purported to possess supernatural powers are found throughout lore dating back to ancient times, and in Chinese culture, many of the stories that describe an individual endowed with extraordinary abilities credit this advancement to the awakening of an inner power. In many of these fables, the individual's exceptional abilities are said to have been initiated through secret yoga and /or magical practices.

Examples of the special powers described in such stories include accounts of individuals who could jump onto roof tops or fly, while in other tales, the initiate gains the ability to resist tremendous force without harm. In Chinese culture, the acceptance of many of these capacities was supported by the tradition of itinerant martial art troupes, who went from town to town demonstrating amazing feats that seemingly defied ordinary human limits.

At least until the founding of the Republic of China in the early-twentieth century, martial arts troupes presented their performances in open public spaces. Often, the centerpiece of their demonstrations included exhibitions of "inner strength," intended to represent the martial artist's mastery of *qi*. These might have included anything from a performer being unaffected by a car or truck that ran over his body as he lay on the ground, to sword

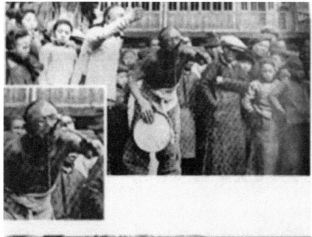

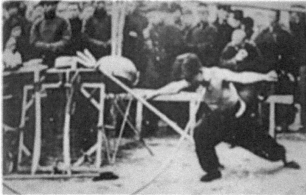

Figure 8-1

Beijing 1900: Exhibition of Special Powers and Abilities

Members of a traveling martial art troupe demonstrate
their skills, represented as "mastery of internal power."
Upper photo: Sword swallowing. Lower photo: A master
demonstrates resisting the force of a spear placed against his
throat. (Note the reaction of the young man in the top photo,
center-right.)

Source: Wikipedia Commons

swallowing or resisting the pressure of a spear-point placed against the neck. Photos 8-1 depict two of these demonstrations, captured from photographs taken in Beijing *circa* 1900. It is interesting that these same exhibitions of "internal power" can still be witnessed in martial arts demonstrations to this day.

Sometimes, the performer's superior physique was credited with allowing them to perform special feats. In many of these examples, the ability was attributed to the performer's ingestion of a special elixir; this being a secret formula that had been handed down within the tradition. Often, and to the spectators' great fortune, such magical potions would conveniently be offered for purchase after the show, so that members of the audience, too, might enjoy the benefits of a super-human body. The tradition of a secret elixir formula passed down from master to disciple over many generations still exists. This is a fascinating subculture in East Asia, often associated with drinking vile-tasting substances, sometimes prepared with compounds from snake gallbladders and other exotic sources. I myself imbibed a few of these in hidden corners of dark and dank East Asian alleyways back in the 1980s.

The tradition of special powers and abilities, then as now, distinguishes one master and school from another. During the Boxer period of the late-nineteenth and early-twentieth centuries, feats of "skill and strength" (the meaning of the term, *kung fu)* served as popular street entertainment in Chinese towns and villages, and while some of the more spectacular demonstrations were doubtless the work of charlatans, other demonstrations were, and still are, extremely impressive. The latter includes acts such as breaking stacks of tiles with one's palm or fist, or having them held over the top of one's head while an assistant smashes them with a sledgehammer. However, demonstrations of these kinds of remarkable skills, stunning though they may be, do not necessarily prove mastery of *qi* energy; at least not as defined as a human-directed subtle bio-energetic force.

Since the time of Bodhidharma, supposed founder of the Shaolin monastery in the fifth century, and the individual traditionally credited with introducing Indian martial arts to China, an association has existed between martial arts and the ability to perform supernatural feats. However, mastery over internal energy, at least in terms of a bio-energetic force, should not be confused with the ability to perform amazing physical feats. Skills such breaking bricks or pounding nails into boards with one's bare hands are no doubt examples of exceptional physical training, but they do not necessarily meet the definition of "internal energy in the martial arts."

Category 2: Attacking with Directed Internal Force

Proponents of the second category believe that skilled initiates, possessing special knowledge of the body, are able to direct concentrated energy against their opponent. Explanations offered as to how this might occur vary in sophistication, ranging from superstitious to scientific. The former, as in the first category, most often involve secret initiation.

More sophisticated explanations can be traced to the writings of eighteenth-century Chang Naizhou (苌乃周). Chang's mid 1700s training manual is a blend of traditional Taoist meditation, alchemy, and martial arts, which Professor Douglas Wile describes as a "fully mature synthesis of martial arts with military strategy, medicine and meditation." [2]

The Chang manuscript details how to train one's internal energy for martial arts purposes. It includes what Wile calls a heterodox description of the way *qi* responds to body movement (i.e., moving forward when the body arches backward, and reserved when moving forward [3]), along with a description of how to "issue *qi*;" a three-step process of concentrating, withdrawing, and then releasing *qi*, training the *qi* by combining softness with hardness, and the importance of focusing the body's energy to a single point.[4]

Two points regarding Chang's manuscript are relevant to our discussion of *qi* in the context of martial arts. The first concerns Chang's concept of using *qi* energy to attack an opponent. If it is true that an invisible force can be consciously directed against an opponent, it would mean that this example of "internal energy" is activated through destructive intent. This runs counter to the notion, to be discussed in this section, that in order to gain access to the human potential involving the individual's conscious "extension of influence," a practitioner must cultivate a mental state characterized by inner calm and benevolent intent.

Second, in contrast to some twentieth-century masters such as Wang Xiangzhai [5] and Morihei Ueshiba, whose exploits are discussed later, there is no evidence that Chang himself actually possessed special abilities that might be characterized as "mastery of internal energy in combat." [6] Thus, it is not clear whether Chang was only theorizing, or if he was describing martial skills that he actually used in combat. This makes it impossible to say whether the Chang manuscripts are merely speculative, or if he is writing from personal experience. Finally, except for its value as an historical document, Chang's writings tell us little about *qi* internal energy and body mechanics. There are no extant forms of the style he created, or any practical ways of evaluating his ability to apply internal energy to martial arts. With that in mind, although Chang's manual remains invaluable from a historical perspective, the material makes a limited contribution to the discussion of internal energy in the martial arts.

Our working assumption is that if something that can be classified as *"qi* energy" exists and can be deliberately deployed against an attacker, then there will be shared attributes between internal martial artists and other practitioners of internal energy, such as meditators and healers. The most important of these shared characteristics is the practitioner's ability to attain a synchronized and internally harmonious state.

Is it possible that authentic "energetic practitioners" share mental–emotional-neurological characteristics associated with *coherence* and internal order? [7] As previously introduced in Section VII, and covered in more detail in Section IX, coherence refers to the practitioner's ability to attain synchrony between various biological oscillators, or bodily rhythms. A surprising source contributes to this discussion, from the literature on Taoist sexual practices. As described by Wile, the instruction includes "the ability to simultaneously relax and mobilize *qi*," which "sets the stage for inspiration, while technique channels the energy and ensures it is not dissipated." [8] This rule can also be applied to the models of internal energy in the martial arts: relax, mobilize *qi*, and then consciously direct its power.

This is a good juncture at which to introduce the relationship between the ability to express internal energy and a phenomenon known as "noise level." [9] In this context, "noise level" refers to relative harmony, or disharmony, between one's biological rhythms. More harmony equates with less noise; when noise levels reduce, things become clearer. When sufficiently reduced, it is possible for a person to extend will and influence, and thus affect the physical world in measurable ways.

It has been proposed that decreased "noise level" functions as an essential precondition for expressing non-physical influence. The concept of decreased noise level provides another lens through which to examine the meaning of "internal energy" in martial arts, healing, and other applications. However, before introducing Category 3, and an alternative definition of internal energy in the martial arts, let us first consider the meaning of the "reduction of noise" in another way.

What it is Not

High in the mountains of Wu Tai Shan, a crisp autumn breeze blows past a rock cave as a monk sits in deep meditation inside. The most probable goal of the monk's practice is to attain profound peace and understand the nature of mind. Examples of practices like this, which trace their origins back more than two millennia, are still found throughout the East. However, the image depicted in comic books and movies stands in sharp contrast to the model just presented. In real life, we do not find a monk who spends years in meditation as a means of transforming himself into the ultimate fighting machine, capable of dispatching an opponent with a single touch.

Category 3: Transmitting Disruptive *Information*

Many martial arts apply size, speed, and aggression to injure or subdue an opponent. However, these attributes would rarely be described as skills that merge physical technique with internal energy. At this juncture, it is useful to consider another theory that might explain how an advanced practitioner, while employing only the most minimal of physical contact, can weaken and control an opponent. This model of "internal energy" suggests that a person's ability to extend non-physical influence, combined with physical skill and a deep understanding of body mechanics, is the most likely explanation for at least some examples of the use of "internal energy" in the martial arts.

Brief Introduction to *Information Theory*

This category of internal energy extrapolates from Kenneth Hintz's *information theory*. It is based on the notion that *information,* or more specifically, *disruptive information,* such as Master Bao's ability to annihilate bacteria in a Petri dish, * when applied against an opponent, can disrupt their structural and psychological integrity.

> * *Information theory,* as well as Bao's ability, was described in Section IV

In this application, "internal energy" does not refer to a super charged bio-electrical force. Further, it does not describe a person's access to an energy reserve that lies dormant within the confines of the human body, waiting to be unleashed. Instead, information, as it pertains to "internal energy," is a more subtle and *interactive* force. It is best thought of in terms of *influence.*

Just as with research which suggests that some *qigong* masters are able to weaken bacteria in a Petri dish,[10] is it possible that some exceptional martial arts masters are likewise able to project a weakening, or disruptive, influence against their opponent? If so, this would add credence to the idea that a minimum, or "soft," contact martial art could still be effective under the extreme stress of close combat. The center of the model is the notion that this kind of influence can have a disruptive effect on the opponent's balance, while simultaneously producing a weakening influence on their ability to resist a strike or pressure point attack.

The information model suggests that the opponent becomes vulnerable in response to the disruptive information, and that subsequently he is less able to resist a relatively gentle but well-placed physical technique. The new model suggests that technical skill, executed by a person knowledgeable regarding exactly where and when to place the precise pressure, merges with the extension of disruptive energy. The result is an effect against the opponent that cannot be explained by technique alone.

In this information model for internal martial arts, three preconditions are believed to be necessary in order to produce this effect. First, the practitioner must be sufficiently trained in skills such as balance and leverage in close combat, so that they will intuitively know exactly where and when to place the right pressure against an opponent. ** Second, the practitioner must attain, and maintain, a reduced "noise level;" this refers to the harmonic state associated with an *entrained* electrophysiological condition. Third, the expert practitioner must *intend* to extend the "energy / *information*" against an opponent. [11]

* The meaning of *entrainment* was introduced in Section VII. The state is characterized by the practitioner's ability to attain a specific electrophysiological profile. This principle is covered in more detail in Section IX.

** Sufficient skill level provides confidence and a platform wherefrom the practitioner is able to "let go," "get out of the way," and trust in the use of subtle influence.

To restate, when applying these principles against an opponent, a master-practitioner, operating against an opponent while in a harmonious entrained mind-body state, need only apply intention, along with a slight touch to just the right joint or pressure point, in order to send the adversary flying. More details on this process will be forthcoming, but first, consider the roles of emotional state and attitude, and how these relate to the ability to use internal energy against an opponent.

Diagram 8-2
Model for Internal Energy
in the Martial Arts

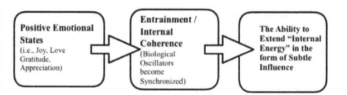

Illustrated in Diagram 8-2, the information theory explanation for internal energy in the martial arts is closely tied to the practitioner's ability to maintain a positive psychological state. This prerequisite allows an individual to manage their electrophysiology and thereby entrain biological oscillators. Entrainment, and the resulting coherence, allow the practitioner to project disruptive information against an opponent. [12]

However, the ability to preserve a calm inner state while under attack presents a challenge for martial artists. The model suggests that optimal ability, augmented by something called "internal energy," can be accessed only when one is calm, non-reactive, and emotionally detached from what would otherwise be a threatening situation. This may seem counterintuitive, since it means that one must be able to access calmness and inner harmony, again characterized by synchronized biological rhythms, even while performing under stressful conditions.

For most of us, the ability to maintain a peaceful state under stressful conditions, like those just described, is difficult. Feeling calm is not the normal "state" when a person suddenly must defend themselves against a surprise attack. Nonetheless, calmness in the midst of violent conflict is exactly the inner state demanded of the new information model of internal energy in the martial arts. Thus, before we describe information theory in the martial arts in greater detail, first consider two examples of martial arts masters who are believed to have met the demanding challenge of a peaceful demeanor in the midst of conflict.

No matter how many times I tried to get the better of him, the results were always the same. Each time I was thrown, he tapped me lightly on my chest just over my heart. When he did this, I experienced a strange and frightening pain that was like a heart tremor.

— Kenichi Sawai describing his interaction with Wang Xiangzhai

Chapter 43

A Tale of Two Masters

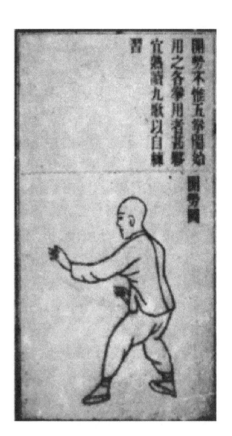

Figure 8-3
"San Ti Shi" Posture
From an Old *Xingyiquan* Manuscript

A Search for the Masters

At this juncture, examples are needed of individuals who possessed the ability to control their opponents with minimal contact. These examples may serve as evidence that something beyond obvious force and skillful technique exists, as they are expected to yield more clues to the meaning of "internal energy in the martial arts." The "light touch"/minimal contact part of the formula is essential to this discussion, as it assumes that something extraordinary is occurring beyond the range of normal body mechanics and technique.

Another point to be considered is that due to the need to validate reports of claimed "internal energy" skill, it is necessary to avail ourselves of reliable evidence attesting to such a master's ability from multiple sources. Furthermore, it is also necessary for the candidate to be either currently alive or to have lived in recent times, since legends of a master from a hundred years ago or longer are too difficult to examine with any degree of reliability. With this in mind, there are two famous masters who meet our criteria.

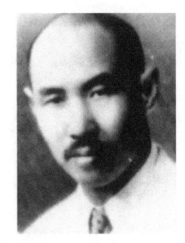

Wang Xiangzhai (王芗斋, 1885-1963) founded the art of *Yiquan* (also written, *I Ch'üan*), or "Mind Boxing," while Morihei Ueshiba (植芝 盛平, 1883-1969) founded the art of *Aikido*. In each example, reliable reports suggest that these exceptional practitioners were able to control an opponent while using no more than a slight touch. For reasons that will shortly be made clear, it is believed that a centerpiece of their martial practice was their ability to cultivate the previously described reduced "noise level."

Reports provided by their opponents suggest that both Wang and Ueshiba were known not only for their consummate skills, but also for their compassion, playfulness, and the gracious way they treated their defeated challengers: an essential element. For these reasons, and because of reliable third-party reports (and in the case of Ueshiba, film records), masters Ueshiba and Wang are two of the best examples of individuals who were able to influence an opponent in an unknown way beyond physical technique.

Photo 8-4
Wang Xiangzhai
1885-1963
Founder of *Yiquan*, "Mind-Boxing"

Wang Xiangzhai

Kenichi Sawai's description of his encounter with Wang Xiangzhai (Photo 8-4), which introduces this chapter, is one of many credible reports documenting Wang's ability to control an adversary while expending only minimal effort. Among other testimonies are those of opponents who met with Wang in response to his offer to "exchange opinions," which was published in a 1940 Beijing newspaper:

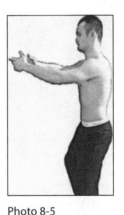

Photo 8-5
"Open Embrace" Posture
Posture Holding and "Standing Practice" was Central to Wang Xiangzhai's Training

> The founding master of *"Da Cheng Quan,"* † Wang Xiang-Zai, [Wang Xiangzhai] who is famous in the north and south and praised by the martial arts circle of the whole county, has recently moved to Beijing. For the exchange of knowledge and opinions among the practitioners of different martial arts, he has arranged for people to meet every Sunday afternoon from 1:00 pm to 6:00 pm, at Dayangyibin Alley No. 1, where he acts as the host, and exchanges opinions with other famous experts of boxing, carrying forward and promoting the martial spirit of our nation as his sincere wish.[13]

> † "Great Achievement Boxing," an earlier, alternative name for Wang's art of Yiquan, or "Mind / Intention Boxing."

Note: The historical account of Wang's early martial arts training is disputed. What follows is one version.

Although Wang had been involved in some aspect of martial arts for most of his life, it was his uncle, Guo Yunshen, a highly regarded *xingyiquan* teacher, who would have the most profound influence over his development. In the late 1800s, Guo [14] took nephew Wang under his wing, with *stillness training* being the focus of his practice. Illustrated in Photo 8-5, *stillness,* or "standing" practice, involves holding specific postures for long periods of time (usually 20-45 minutes per session) while remaining as motionless as possible. Consideration of Guo's training routine yields important clues to how Wang might have developed his exceptional ability to effortlessly control attackers.

Lineages representing Wang's teaching, with emphasis on stillness practice, are still found today, not only in China and Japan, but throughout the world. A curious question concerns *why* Guo might have emphasized this training method, and it is noteworthy that their training took place when Guo was semi-handicapped and relied on a cane to walk; after all, you don't have to chase your student around the room if he is standing still. Regardless, the practice of stillness training was a significant part of Wang's martial arts development.

For a martial artist like Wang, already possessing a background in the martial arts, standing practice — what his Japanese disciple Sawai would later call *Standing Zen* — allowed him to go deep into his physical and psychological interior to perfect his skill.

"Standing Practice"

Correctly performed, standing practice places the burden of carrying the body's weight onto the body's soft tissue support structures. Instead of relying on poor posture habits to do the job, the muscles, ligaments, tendons, and fascia support systems are engaged, and as the body "drops" into the practice, excess tension releases. The practitioner will notice that relaxation begins to merge with strength in a new way; these conditions are ripe for the expression of total-body connected power.

After a few minutes of posture holding, the discipline begins to work its magic. Since the body, mind, and emotions are all intimately linked, not only physical tension, but emotional and mental tension releases as well. With tension release comes an increase in tactile strength and sensitivity, and this increase in tactile sensitivity is one reason why stillness training translates so well into the ability to control an opponent. Thus, when physical contact is made, the practice develops the ability to know instantly where the adversary is storing his tension and "blocks." This is important information that can be turned against the adversary.

In application, when an experienced practitioner initiates the lightest physical contact with an opponent, the adversary's body structure is instantly "read." For example, when only slightly touching an opponent's arm, an experienced practitioner is able to sense tension in the adversary's shoulder, hip, or knee. In another example, the skilled practitioner, when applying the slightest hand contact to the opponent's wrist or forearm, instantly senses the opponent's weight distribution. These factors contribute to the practitioner's ability to control an opponent using minimal contact.

With stillness practice forming the core of his training, Wang Xiangzhai's martial arts assignments were far from ordinary. Instead of conventional combat training, which might include jump kicking, heavy bag punching, weight training, or learning to subdue an opponent with an arm twist, Wang rose early in the morning to begin his daily "standing practice." Upon rising a bit later than his nephew, Guo would go to the place where Wang was engaged in his standing; then, touching the ground under where he was standing, Guo checked to see whether it was dry or wet with sweat. If dry, Wang was instructed to continue the holding posture practice a bit longer.

For those unfamiliar with this practice, at first glance, "posture holding" may seem unimpressive. However, those familiar with this style of training understand the challenge of holding correct postures for a prolonged period. Correctly performed, posture-stillness training releases reliance on large muscle group / fulcrum-based movements * and integrates the fascia, or connective tissue, "soft tissue" support of the body. The result is a full-body sense of "springiness," a principle referred to as *peng*.** A comedic representation of this training method is portrayed in the movie *The Peaceful Warrior*, where the character Dan is instructed by his teacher "Socrates" to hold a specific posture for a few minutes on a table top, as a challenge to Dan's smug view of his superior athletic condition, and one which he fails after only a few minutes.

* Covered in more detail in Section XI

**Also covered in Section XI

Upon completing his training with Guo, Wang traveled across China to challenge other teachers. In 1928, he issued the following public statement:

> I have traveled across the country in research, engaging over a thousand people in martial combat, there have been only a few people I could not defeat. [15]

A decade later, Wang arrived in Beijing. However, upon observing the teachers there, he became disillusioned by the poor quality of instruction offered in the capital. It was then that he issued the challenge to martial artists to meet him at his residence, "to discuss" the martial arts.

In Beijing, Wang received numerous challenges, and, according to reports,

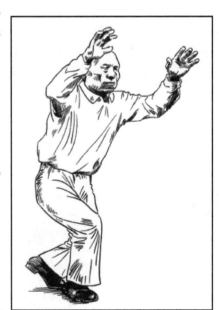

Photo 8-6
Kenichi Sawai (1903–1988)
Illustration by Sergio Verdeza

was defeated only once. Supporting the contention that one's attitudes and emotions play a role in the ability to control an opponent with minimal contact, Wang often dispalyed playfulness. An example is illustrated in the way he tossed his opponents across the room, onto a specific place on his couch.

It is often challenging to determine the veracity of reports of a past master's martial arts skills, including those proclaiming Wang Xiangzhai's prowess in particularly glowing terms. For this reason, one report is particularly noteworthy. It is the description of a match between Wang and a challenger, written by the challenger-turned-disciple, Kenichi Sawai.

Sawai met Wang when he was serving as a Japanese military officer in China during the war. He was an accomplished martial arts master of both *kendo* (wooden sword art) and *judo.* Thus, Sewali's description of the match provides a powerful testimony:

> At that time, I was a fifth dan in judo, and I had a degree of confidence in my abilities in combat techniques. When I had my first opportunity to try myself in a match with Wang Xiang-Zai, [Wang Xiangzhai], I gripped his right hand and tried to use a technique, but I at once found myself being hurled through the air.

> I saw the uselessness of surprise and sudden attacks with this man. Next, I tried grappling. I gripped his left hand and his right lapel and tried the techniques I knew, thinking that, if the first attack failed, I would be able to move into a grappling technique when we fell. But the moment we came together, Wang instantaneously gained complete control of my hand and thrust it out away from himself.

> No matter how many times I tried to get the better of him, the results were always the same. Each time I was thrown, he tapped me lightly on my chest just over my heart. When he did this, I experienced a strange and frightening pain that was like a heart tremor.

> Still I did not give up. I requested that he pit himself against me in fencing. We used sticks instead of swords; and, even though the stick he used was short, he successfully parried all of my attacks and prevented my making a single point. At the end of the match, he said quietly, "the sword—or the staff—both extensions of the hand."

> This experience robbed me of all confidence in my own abilities. My outlook, I thought, would be very dark indeed, unless I managed to obtain instruction from Wang. I did succeed in studying with him; and, acting on his advice, I instituted a daily course in standing Zen [standing practice].

> Gradually I began to feel as if I had gained a little bit of the expansive Chinese martial spirit. [16]

It is unclear how long Sawai studied with Wang, but we do know that upon returning to his home country, he founded a new style based on what he'd learned in Beijing. In Japan, Sawai's variation of Wang's protocols was presented as *tai ki ken,* and as with the original system, his own instruction was also based on the practice of standing and stillness.

In the early-twentieth century, Wang Xiangzhai had established himself as one of China's leading martial artists, and his new style of *Yiquan (I Ch'üan)* was gaining popularity. However, Wang continued to become increasingly vocal in his criticism of the popular "form training" (as oppose to "principles training") that was being increasingly emphasized in the first decades of the new century. His criticism of this "forms" approach to *t'ai-chi ch'üan* training appeared in a 1940 newspaper article:

> As for its method of training, a punch with a fist here, a slap with the palm there, a kick to the left and another one to the right, this is pitiful and laughable. As for dealing with an enemy in a fight, against a mastery-hand [expert], please do not even consider it. If the adversary is not stiff and sluggish, even the famous masters of this boxing have no chance to apply their skills. These abuses are so big that *taiqiquan [t'ai-chi ch'üan]* might soon become just a mere form comparable to a chess manual. For the last twenty years, most people who have studied this boxing have not been able to differentiate right and wrong, even if someone has been able to differentiate these, he has not been capable of putting it into practice. [17]

Subsequently, Wang recommended that teachers of the art correct the deficiencies that were "ruining" the discipline:

> So ruined is this boxing that it has become useless. This is really deplorable. I wish that the powerful members of this school would promptly and strictly clean it up and attempt to develop it in the future. When the day of success comes, they will be held as the bosom friends of all boxing fans. [18]

Wang was dedicated to the rehabilitation of the Chinese martial arts.

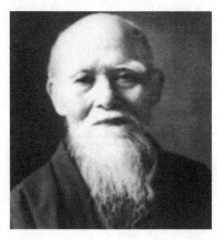

Photo 8-7
Morihei Ueshiba
1883-1969
Founder of Aikido
Source: Wikipedia Commons, Photo by Aikishihan

Morihei Ueshiba

Morihei Ueshiba shared a few things in common with Wang Xiangzhai's disciple, Kenichi Sawai. Both were martial arts experts before WWII, both were Japanese military officers, and both were influenced by Chinese martial arts during their military service in China.

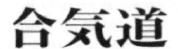

Figure 8-8
Characters for Aikido

After witnessing Japan's defeat and the devastating effects of the atomic bomb on his homeland, Ueshiba renounced violence, and his subsequent dedication to peace led to his greatest contribution to the martial arts: *aikido*.

Literally, the "art of harmonizing," or "merging" with internal energy, *aikido* is based on nonviolence. The essence of the art is not to resist, but to instead control an attacker by blending with their oncoming force. Ueshiba's skill was extraordinary, and his expertise at effortlessly controlling one or more simultaneous attackers became legendary. John Stevens describes Ueshiba's abilities:

> [He] manifested powers that can only be described as miraculous. He could throw ten attackers at once, pin huge sumo wrestlers with a single finger, even dodge bullets when challenged by a military firing squad. (Many of these amazing feats were recorded on film). [19] [20]

A Smiling Old Man

Jay Gluck's 1963 *Zen Combat* includes one of the earliest accounts of Ueshiba's exceptional abilities to be published in the West. Based on interviews and film recordings, Gluck detailed the master's nonviolent martial art and documented some of his more remarkable demonstrations. Two included the participation of five U.S. military policemen (MPs), who agreed to attack Ueshiba. In the first demonstration, the MPs were instructed to grab the old man in any way they could, but despite trying with all their might, they failed to get any effective grab or control over him.

The next demonstration was to become Ueshiba's trademark. First, he allowed several of the larger and younger Americans to grab him in any way they wished, and, holding tightly, the MPs prepared themselves with strong, solid stances. However, their combined strength and youth were ineffective, and with a flick of Ueshiba's arms, the attackers were sent flying. Neither Gluck nor the airborne MPs could explain how it was possible for a seemingly frail old man to dispatch his opponents so easily, and this was just one of many examples of Ueshiba exhibiting abilities beyond what could be explained in terms of size and strength. His remarkably light touch, which so easily control his opponents, makes him a prime example of the manifestation of "internal energy" in the martial arts.

Gluck, for his part, could not comprehend the source of Ueshiba's uncanny abilities. Searching for clues that might reveal the master's ultimate secret, he employed the best motion camera technology available at the time. Gluck filmed these demonstrations using hi-speed 64 fps film, only for his attempt to decode Ueshiba's hidden skill to fail to reveal anything more than:

> A smiling old man moving unconcernedly amidst intense, charging GIs, seemingly unaware that they existed—indication that Ueshiba was, in effect, moving in a different time continuum. [21]

Is Gluck's description of Ueshiba's ability to move "in a different time continuum" another clue to how some might be able to use internal power in combat? Ueshiba left other hints as to the source of power, such as his description of the relationship between martial arts prowess, use of *ki* internal energy, and emotional self-management:

> There are two types of *ki* [internal energy]: Ordinary *ki* and true *ki*. Ordinary *ki* is coarse and heavy: true *ki* is light and versatile. In order to perform well, you have to liberate yourself from ordinary *ki* and permeate your organs with true *ki*. Strength resides where one's *ki* is concentrated and stable; confusion and maliciousness arise when ki stagnates. [22]

Here, Ueshiba is telling us that the key to his remarkable ability is emotional self-management.

Chapter 44

Information Theory

*I*nformation Theory in the Martial Arts represents a new way of thinking about how human-directed, non-physical *influence* can be used against an adversary. This alternative model is not based on the notion of a mysterious, super-human force. Accordingly, that super-human force is replaced by *influence,* which refers to the expert practitioner's ability to extend, or transmit, *information;* more specifically, *disruptive information.* The model describes how information may be able to influence the opponent's nervous system in subtle ways, making them unstable and less equipped to resist a physical technique.

"These aren't the droids you are looking for." [23]

When joined with a technique, such as a strike, joint lock, or takedown against an opponent, disruptive information adds a bit of extra "juice." The working model is that disruptive information degrades an attacker's *coherence,* and that as a result, they are less able to move or resist effectively. A comparison with the application can be made using the fanciful "Jedi mind trick," which, as described in George Lucas's *Star Wars,* is an essential part of the Jedi's power. [24]

Information Theory in the Martial Arts suggests that disruptive information extends through electromagnetic (EM) and electromagnetic-like [25] fields, in concert with physical contact and techniques. Before examining this concept in greater detail, let me share some personal anecdotes that prompted me to consider the possibility of *information* in the context of martial arts.

During a class in the late-1970s, a group of students sat in a semi-circle, cross-legged at the side of the training area. I had been telling stories about some famous masters who could throw an opponent with no more than a touch, and, attempting to convey what such a demonstration might look like, I asked for a volunteer. An athletic college student promptly bounced to his feet and took a strong stance. Truth be told, I wasn't expecting anything special as I tried to imitate how the exhibition of such skill might appear. With the volunteer in his solid stance in front of me, I made a relaxed motion with my hand that lightly brushed against his upper body.

What happened next was shocking, not least to me. Just as my hand made the most minimal contact, the individual was shot violently backward. Our jaws froze in open amazement, as it appeared as though an invisible cannonball had hit the student and knocked him back several feet. This was a lot of fun, and we immediately wanted to repeat it! However, after that first invisible *qi* cannonball, subsequent attempts failed to reproduce the magical opponent toss and I was unable to effect anything more than a conventional push. Rule one: the magic is elusive.

The experience of being able to produce such a strange effect left an indelible impression on me in terms of what may be possible. Rule two: if you can do something once, eventually you will be able to do it again.

This was my introduction to the puzzle of *effortlessness,* which is summed up by a riddle: *Whenever one tries to manifest an advanced order of power, it is impossible to do so.* Like the proverbial advice of a "Twelve Step" program, the only way to access this skill is to surrender completely to the process. This principle is also expressed in the *Tao Te Ching:*

The Highest Power does not strive to be powerful, therefore attains true power.
Lower power is forever trying to be powerful, therefore never attains true power.
The Highest power is attained through non-action. [26]

If I grasp, I lose; to manifest power, don't try; to gain, let go. Like the experience of invisible energy hitting the opponent, the expression of this category of power in internal martial arts appears quite different from normal physical force.

When a practitioner first projects this category of influence against an opponent, it's often hard to understand the results, as the experience may or may not make sense. It doesn't seem possible that little more than a light touch could throw an attacker, or that a mere poke could drop someone to the ground. Years later, it is still hard to explain.

Teaching a student to apply the principle is even more challenging, and although the teacher may try very hard, it is often difficult to teach someone to apply *information* against an opponent:

"Just do the technique without trying to put any effort into it."

This always seems counterintuitive.

Or:

"Maintain your proper orientation and let go."

This one makes a lot of sense to the teacher, but the words are often lost on the student.

Or, even better:

"Just laugh when you are doing 'it,' and one day it will happen."

Accordingly, the theory holds that as long as you pay attention to certain feelings in your body and have faith, something magical will eventually take over and the effortless technique will appear.

In this model, the "transmission of disruptive information" merges with physical skill. However, to manifest a technique where minimal contact can influence an attacker significantly, a combination of factors must be precisely timed. It may be significant that the application of this kind of skill is accompanied by a vague emotional component; especially in the early stages of the practice, performing a "transfer of information" technique can be emotionally unsettling. The experience evokes feelings that cannot easily be put into words.

My working hypothesis to explain this experience, seemingly beyond the temporal dimensions is that each day offers unlimited opportunities to transcend the mundane realm, though we might not be consciously aware of it. The musician, dancer, athlete, or artist trains to regularly access this state of exceptional body-mind, whole-field integration, but even the accountant may find themselves totally absorbed in their numbers and ecstatic when the balance sheet shows a profit! Indeed, the mysticism of the ordinary was precisely Chuang Tzu's point in the parable of Cook Ting, the chef who wields his kitchen knife with the same grace and effectiveness as the expert martial artist wields his sword.

Do phenomena such as these offer a glimpse into the mystical state that forms the kernel of all religious experience? Part of the explanation for these feelings of absorption and awe lies in surrender, "going with the flow," or finding "the path of least resistance." Moreover, consummate skill in any art leads to a sense of freedom, playfulness, and joy. For the martial artist, this kind of spontaneous improvisation may be expressed in the following formula: skill + surrender + jo y= effortless neutralization and powerful projection.

Information Theory: An Alternative Explanation

I first began to rely on *information theory* as an explanation for internal energy in martial arts in the early 1990s. Through a private client who worked as a neurosurgeon, I was introduced to a former researcher of human bio-energy and a doctor of traditional Chinese medicine, and during our subsequent conversations I became acquainted with the theory of internal energy. To honor their request for confidentiality, I will refer to them as Dr. Smith (researcher / health practitioner) and Dr. Jones (client / neurosurgeon).

Hintz's *information theory* was presented in Section IV as an alternative explanation for energetic healing. The theory holds that non-contact healers are able to assist patients through the transmission of anti-entropic *information*. Accordingly, anti-entropic *information* is encoded and then transferred from healer to patient via the most minute, but measurable, bio-electrical fields. These are exchanged, or merged, between the two participants in the transaction.

In response to the anti-entropic *information*, the receiver-patient's mind-body nervous system reacts to the *information* and generates a healing response. In practitioner-patient terms, "transfer of *information*" does not involve the transmission of a healing force per se, but rather coded "instructions," which are interpreted by the patient's nervous system. Significantly, according to Omura's description of *"energy"* as "+ / positive" and "- / negative," *information* appears to be *selectable* from two types. If, as suggested by Omura and other researchers, positive or negative *qi* is *selectable*, it makes sense that while one type of energy / *information* can promote healing due to its anti-entropic properties, then the other type, which can annihilate bacteria in a Petri dish, might also be "selectable."

When utilizing such methods against an opponent in a contact sport, *disruptive information* is applied; in this case, the *information* produces a weakening or disordering influence on the target. Like the emitted "energy" described in the Seto studies, † the application of *disruptive information* also involves the practitioner's emission of a very minute bio-electric (and / or bio-electrical-like ‡) field. According to the model, the EM field is the medium that allows the encoded *information* to transfer to the opponent. As mentioned earlier, in most cases, the receiver responds to the *disruptive information* by becoming just a bit weaker and less stable, and is therefore more easily controlled. When this happens, the opponent is less able to resist a throw, push, or joint lock.

† Discussed in Section IV

‡ The suggestion that "internal energy" might be explained as the merger of electromagnetic and electromagnetic-like fields was introduced in Section II, and is expanded in Section XII. A video demonstrating this interaction against an opponent is also included in Section XII.

I first learned about the *information* model through my contact with Drs. Smith and Jones. After completing his doctorate from the Massachusetts Institute of Technology in a field involving human bio-energy, Smith subsequently accepted a position at Stanford University. There, he participated in classified government-sponsored research with a group of scientists who investigated various phenomena, such as human potential, remote viewing, extra sensory ability, and human-directed subtle bio-energy. However, Smith's fate was not to remain in bio-energetic research; that prospect was unexpectedly altered one morning when, upon arriving at work, he discovered that the Stanford research program had been terminated, and that the doors to the "paranormal" labs were padlocked. Nevertheless, his interest in human bio-energetics continued as he shifted his focus to the study of traditional Chinese medicine. His new course of study led to him becoming a licensed TCM practitioner, and it was a few years later that we met and discussed the emerging field of medical intuition, as well as the relevance of *information theory* in the martial arts. Together, these might be thought of as a continuum through which to explore the meaning of "subtle energy."

My initial meeting with Smith began with us talking about how internal energy might be applied in the context of martial arts, traditional medicine, and energetic healing. Eventually, he brought up the TCM diagnostic procedure known as "pulse reading," which involves diagnosis based on "reading" the body's internal organ system through six pulse *signals*, with three located on each wrist. [27] Inquiring about my skill with the technique, he asked, "How is your pulse diagnosis?" I responded by admitting that since I didn't practice it very much, my skill wasn't especially good.

"Well then, how do you diagnose?" Smith asked. "I just sort of look at the patient and see what's wrong," I replied. On the spot, he stood up and challenged me to diagnose him. As he faced me, my first impression was that he had something wrong with his spleen, and at the conclusion of my diagnosing him, he confirmed that he did in fact have some "spleen issues," a condition described in TCM terms as "a chronic spleen deficiency."

Smith remained standing on the opposite side of the room as we continued. I provided a list of his present and past health issues, which included an old knee injury, shoulder pain, and a "tightness" on one side of his lower back, immediately adjacent to the lowest lumbar vertebrae. When I had finished, Smith told me that I was correct about everything except the last issue, referring to the tightness in his lower back. However, I was certain that I had sensed a knot or "imbalance" at the indicated spot, so I asked him to remain standing where he was, and then requested that neurosurgeon Jones cross the room with me.

Standing behind Jones, and making no contact with Smith, I guided the surgeon's hand to two different spots on Smith's lower back. First, to the normal-healthy side for comparison, and then to where I had perceived the "knot." Through palpation — using pressure from the hand to sense physical change to the target area of Smith's back — Jones compared muscular tension between the two sides of the spine. Although Smith was unaware of tension at the indicated point, Jones confirmed that there was indeed significant physical tension at that location on the lower back.

The ability to read an "energetic imbalance" like this is not difficult. Most individuals with an open mind can learn the basics of "seeing" an energy imbalance fairly easily. I regularly teach classes in how to do this, and over the years I have taught hundreds of people of varying ages and from all walks of life, from young to old, from high school kids to scientists, to "read energy" in the same way. The tool is sometimes useful for helping pain patients and training athletes. [28]

Returning to *information theory* as an explanation for "internal energy" in the martial arts, our next interaction is more to the point. Before my meeting with the two doctors, I believed that "internal energy," when applied to both the martial and healing arts, must involve the practitioner's ability to generate a surge of bio-electrical energy. My thinking was that the ability must be akin to the way an electric eel can store and then release a bio-electric charge. That belief was about to change.

Toward the end of our meeting, I was asked to demonstrate something "energetic" in a martial way. We went outside to find one of Smith's assistants handy, and the young man kindly volunteered his mid-torso as the target for my demonstration. My challenge was to demonstrate something that might provide evidence of internal energy in the martial arts — in other words, a martial art application involving some unknown factor beyond bio-mechanics — and, of course, to do it without injuring the volunteer. I prepared to demonstrate a light "internal strike," since, in theory, this is a type of minimal contact skill application which generates effects that cannot be explained by the normal rules of size, force, and speed. The demonstration would have to be done just right: effective enough to illustrate something different, and presumably "energetic," yet at the same time gentle enough so as not to injure the volunteer.

It was a bit on the cold side, and the volunteer was wearing a medium-weight parka jacket. The "tap" I executed was delivered from about two inches away from his body; he was asked to breath out as I delivered the blow without tension, torque, or weight transfer. In other words, it looked like a light touch with a closed fist. We got the results we had hoped for, as although uninjured, the volunteer was knocked backwards a foot or so. To us, his body's reaction to the "tap" seemed beyond what the light punch should have been able to produce. Sometimes, this type of demonstration leaves a special type of trace evidence. In this case we were lucky, and it did.

At the point on the volunteer's body where contact was made, discernable through his parka, a spot of concentrated heat radiated from his body. Sometimes, as in this demonstration, other evidence also remains, and radiating warmth could also be detected from the volunteer's back, exactly opposite from where the strike was delivered on the front side of his body. We stepped behind him and asked him to lift up his jacket and shirt, so that we could see the source of the heat, and at the point where the warmth radiated, there was indeed a reddish welt. Something had not only caused heat to emit from the target on the front side of his body, but apparently all the way through his body to a spot on the exact opposite side as well, even leaving a mark. To us, this was evidence that "energy," or another unknown agent, was involved.

As mentioned earlier, I previously believed that the effects of such a demonstration must somehow be related to the person's ability to muster and project a burst of bio-electrical energy. However, Smith disagreed with this idea and suggested another explanation. He stated that if someone was able to generate and release that degree of electrical energy, the demonstrator's "head would explode." As an alternative theory, he suggested that the volunteer's bodily response to the strike could be accounted for by *information*. Smith believed that the sudden appearance of the radiating points of heat on the volunteer's body had nothing to do with the force of the strike itself, and instead proposed that both the emitted heat and the markings were the result of the assistant's reaction to *disruptive information.*

The suggestion that minute, *information*-containing bio-electrical discharge might be transferred between practitioner and opponent can be compared to the workings of a telephone. In telephony, the actual voice of the person at the other end doesn't transfer through the phone line; it is a *representation* interpreted by the phone receiver that translates the *information* — in this case, also involving a minute degree of electrical energy. Applied to a martial arts demonstration like the one just described, the bio-mechanical force associated with a punch, push, or joint lock becomes less relevant to the ultimate effect. More important is the ability to convey *information.*

Calmness in the Midst of Movement is the Secret to all Power

As suggested by the stories of Wang and Ueshiba, before a person can encode and transmit information to an opponent, the practitioner must function through a state of equanimity. The attainment of such a state, with its characteristically calm mind-body attributes, represents the practitioner's experience of increased coherence and "decreased noise." The ability to combine information with skill explains many examples of what are referred to as "internal energy in the martial arts."

Calm under Stress

One's ability to maintain calmness while under attack is the cornerstone of the model of *information* as "internal energy," but what then is the evidence for the possibility of calmness and inner peace, or even joy, in the midst of combat? Author John Blofeld offers evidence of such a possibility. Among the acquaintances he made while traveling through the mountains of pre-communist China was a group of warrior-monks, and an observation that he made during his time with those recluses illuminates our discussion.

While visiting a Taoist hermitage, Blofeld witnessed a ferocious swordfight between four monks. The event left him disturbed, and, at the same time, puzzled. Writing that the battle possessed "the aspect of a frenzied ritual in which the contestants were determined to die beneath one another's swords." [29] The ferocity of the encounter left him gasping for breath:

> By the time it ended, I was sweating with anxiety and could scarcely believe my eyes when the four recluses walked towards the Abbot smiling and unscathed. [30]

While discussing the savage confrontation with Blofeld, the leader of the monastery, the abbot, described the attributes that influenced the swordfighters' abilities:

The principle of void-ness and passivity must be carried over into all affairs. As Lao Tzu says:

> He who excels in combat is one who does not let himself be roused. That the warriors of old flocked to our peaceful hermitages to foster their martial skills is no paradox; they came to learn how to apply the secret of emptiness, how to ensure that the enemy's sword, though aimed at flesh, encounters void, and how to destroy the foe by striking with dispassion. Hatred arouses wrath; wrath breeds excitement; excitement leads to carelessness which, to a warrior, brings death. A master swordsman can slay ten enemies besetting him simultaneously, by virtue of such dispassion that he is able to judge to perfection how to dodge their thrusts. A swordsman or an archer's aim is surest when his mind, concentrated on the work in hand, is indifferent to failure or success. Stillness in the heart of movement is the secret of all power. [emphasis added] [31]

The abbot stressed that the adepts' high-level performance was linked to their ability to attain a specific mind-body state. Thus, detachment was the most important attribute. As the monk explained, skill of that level could only be fostered through dispassion; while the warrior-monks had sword battled, their thoughts and emotions were equanimous. [32]

The sword practice of the young warrior-monks can be compared to the combat-play of young predatory animals; the highest proficiency in close combat and the subduing of prey is best learned through play. The principle is reminiscent of Wu Cheng-ching's instruction not to not pay attention to the "external form," but instead focus on one's *internal mind-body state*. * The master warrior is one who is not roused by external events.

*Included in Section VII

Chapter 45

Power vs. Force

*A*n additional lens through which the meaning of "internal energy in the martial arts" can be evaluated is through a continuum called power vs. force. As illustrated in Diagram 8-9, this continuum was delineated by psychiatrist David Hawkins, MD. Based on Hawkins's research, he developed a hierarchy designed to study all forms of human interaction, from athletics to personal relationships, to business. According to the model, *every aspect* of a person's rational and emotional life falls somewhere on the scale of either *power* or *force*.

Diagram 8-9 **Power vs. Force Continuum**

Power ⟵⟶ **Force**

More Subtlety, "lightness," and positive emotions

Raw Force and aggression. Neutral or negative emotions

As shown in the scale depicted in Table 8-10, the hierarchy is based on calibrations derived from muscle testing. The system was designed by Hawkins as a means of investigating mental-emotional states and their attributes, with the result being a "calibration" that he believes applies to specific aspects of human behavior. For example, reason and acceptance fall on the power side of the continuum, whereas anger and fear come under *force* side of the hierarchy.

If Hawkins's *power vs. force* continuum is useful as a measuring stick to determine the mental-emotional level that one is functioning at, then it is reasonable to explore whether the calibrations might apply to questions having to do with "internal energy in the martial arts." Applied in this way, the scale might be used to consider whether a technique is more or less efficient; in other words, either relying more on *power* or more on *force*. In this context, efficiency, characterized by *flow* and minimal effort, can be thought of as representing skill that falls on the power side of the equation.

The Hawkins Scale

Level	Calibration	Emotion	
Enlightenment	700-1000	Ineffable	
Peace	600	Illumination	
Joy	540	Transfiguration	
Love	500	Reverence	
Reason	400	Understanding	
Acceptance	350	Forgiveness	
Willingness	310	Optimism	
Neutrality	250	Trust	
Courage	200	Affirmation	**Power**
Pride	175	Scorn	**Force**
Anger	150	Hate	
Desire	125	Craving	
Fear	100	Anxiety	
Grief	75	Regret	
Apathy	50	Despair	
Guilt	30	Blame	
Shame	20	Humiliation	

Table 8- 10

Seventeen Strata of the Power vs. Force Continuum

Delineated in levels from a low of 20 to a high of 1000, the table shows Hawkins's 17 levels with corresponding emotions.

Applying the Hawkins hierarchy proved helpful to me in my own study. In my experience, attention to the strata helps to decrease reliance on "forceful" movements, such as torque-based techniques, in exchange for increasing degrees of subtlety, such as taking down an opponent with well-placed finger pressure. The hierarchy also provides another means of investigating the notion that *information* might merge with, or replace, physical skill. In this sense, the model can also be applied to the exploits of masters such as Wang Xiangzhai and Morihei Ueshiba, who were presumed to have engaged their opponents in terms of the power – and, perhaps, *informational* — side of the hierarchy.

The Hawkins scale also serves as a lens through which to evaluate the different styles of fighters in various combat sports, such as boxing. For example, when applying the scale to the skill level of some famous boxers, it suggests that Muhammed Ali often exhibited skill that could be characterized as belonging to the *power* side of the *power vs. force* continuum. However, in boxing, like other contact sports, Ali's style of fighting is not the norm. Ali was not known for raw aggression, but rather, a level of subtlety and finesse that was often accompanied by a sense of lightness and play. Thus, if we were to contrast Ali's style with the aggressive, raw power of some other well-known boxers, we can compare different types of fighters in terms of the *power vs. force* scale. With this in mind, some of Ali's most famous "light touch" knockouts might be best understood as his ability to convey *disruptive information* from the power side of the scale.

The same cannot be said for more aggressive boxers, however. In those cases, the view through the lens of the *power vs. force* hierarchy suggests that many successful boxing styles fall on the *force* side of the continuum. Note, this observation does not imply that the *power vs. force* model could serve as a predictor of which athlete will emerge as the victor in a contest. Its value is simply as a tool for looking at different fighters and their varying ways of engaging an opponent.

Conclusion to Section VIII

*I*f proven correct, the *information* model is testament to the human potential, through intention, to influence an opponent. If one day validated by modern science, internal power in the martial arts will no longer be thought of as a martial artist's ability to project an invisible energy beam against an opponent. Instead, it will be understood as another example of the power of human intention to interact with the world in subtle ways.

In terms of the ability to disrupt an opponent's defensive systems ("Aye captain, the shields are down"), *information theory* posits a new way of looking at the meaning of "internal energy" in the context of contact sports. Citing the rare and exceptional skills of more recent martial art masters, such as Morihei Ueshiba and Wang Xiangzhai, is it possible that at least some of their exploits could be explained in terms of their ability to access and optimize *disruptive information*?

The information theory described here has implications beyond the martial arts. Our premise is that if something which can be called "internal energy" in the martial art exists, then it is believed to be related to energetic healing, energetic meditation, and other modalities. In this light, it is hoped that what follows will demonstrate how it might be possible for a person to achieve greater human potential through learning to achieve and practice more "harmonious" mind-body states.

In sharing my first experience of what I call "internal energy in the martial arts," I described how my assistant was thrown in response to a minimal contact technique. However, subsequent attempts failed to reproduce the desired effect, as I had not yet learned about the mind-body state that Chinese philosophers call *wu-wei*, or "non-action." This state represents more than just a *state of mind*: it is a *state of being*. Perhaps, the ultimate goal of a master-in-training is to learn to embody that principle of non-action. When achieved, it is one wherein a practitioner becomes so detached that they are barely aware of their own actions. Thus, the art of non-action is really the art of forgetting the self, letting go, and allowing one's *qi energy* to flow effortlessly.

The late Alan Watts (1915-1973), philosopher and writer on Eastern philosophy and religion, described the merging of *wu wei* ("non-action") and the flow of *qi* as a type of intelligence. To Watts, it represented a particular type of intelligence that translated into efficiency of movement. His description of non-action provides an appropriate conclusion to this section:

> *Wu-wei* [non-action] is thus the life-style of one who follows the *Tao* and must be understood primarily as a form of intelligence — that is, knowing the principles, structures, and trends of human and natural affairs so well that one uses the least amount of energy in dealing with them. But

this intelligence, as we have seen, is not simply intellectual; it is also the "unconscious" intelligence of the whole organism and, in particular, the innate wisdom of the nervous system. *Wu-wei* is the combination of this wisdom with taking the line of least resistance in all one's actions....This may be illustrated with the Aikido exercise of the unbendable arm. The right arm is extended to the front, and the opponent is invited to bend it. If the arm is held rigidly, a strong opponent will certainly bend it. If, on the other hand, it is held out easily, with the eyes fixed on a distant point, and with the feeling that it is a rubber hose through which water is flowing towards that point, it will be extremely difficult to bend. Without straining, one simply assumes that the arm will stay straight, come what may, because of the flow of *qi*.[33]

Afterword to Section VIII

On Kong Jin, "Empty-Force"

*K*ong jin (空勁), translated as "empty-force," is viewed by some as a martial practice that allows a trained practitioner to throw or subdue an opponent without making any physical contact whatsoever. This practice is the martial arts cousin to *wai qi* (外氣) non-contact healing in traditional Chinese medicine. As with non-contact healing, proponents likewise believe that an attacker can be influenced, without physical contact, through a master's projection of an invisible force, like *qi* or *ki*. Originally, I had wanted to avoid discussing *kong jin* in the context of martial arts in the present work, but I continue to be approached with questions about the nature of "empty-force." So, it is with some hesitation that I am compelled to share my thoughts on the practice.

Earlier, I described three categories of internal energy in the martial arts. *Kong jin* "empty-force" falls into Category II, which is "secret knowledge" passed from master to disciple. In *Ba Gua: Hidden Knowledge in the Taoist Internal Martial Art,* I describe my interaction with the late master Shr Ming, who, at the time, was regarded as one of the leading exponents of *kong jin* in Beijing.

In the late 1980s, a few years before Shr and his students were featured on Bill Moyer's PBS show *The Mystery of Chi*, one of my contacts at Beijing University introduced me to Master Shr. In a park on the north side of the city, I enjoyed watching demonstrations with Shr and his students, which were very similar to those featured in the Bill Moyer program. One of these can be viewed here: https://www.youtube.com/watch?v=HOpXpQGoub0 .

However, one of the more fantastic of Master Shr's demonstrations was not included as part of the Moyer program; one which involved subduing and throwing one of his students through the medium of a leaf. In response to light contact made by the leaf held by the master, the "opponent" lapsed into a violent electrocution-like spasm that rendered him unable to effect an attack against the master.

I am occasionally asked if *kong jin* "empty-force" demonstrations like the one just described are "real," but the answer depends on what "real" means. In my experience with Shr, it was curious that while he performed numerous *kong jin* demonstrations on his students, he refused to demonstrate anything on me. Master Shr's explanation was that before he would demonstrate on me,

399

I would be required to become his disciple and apprentice for three years. Only then would I be permitted to experience his "empty-force" skill.

I am convinced that a yet-to-be-named "energy" can be emitted and willfully directed. However, I believe it is rare, if it ever happens at all, that a **non-contact technique** can influence an opponent who has not been properly conditioned by the master or fellow students. At the same time, it is possible that the conditioning can be performed unconsciously, and that even the most sincere students and masters can fall under the spell of their desire to believe in the power of the unseen force.

My first personal experience with *kong jin* practice was in the 1980s. Dan Miller, the editor / publisher of the now defunct *Pa Kua Chang Journal*, shared some *kong jin* training techniques he had picked up with us during a visit to our school. The first stage of training involved one student acting as a receiver and another as the sender of invisible energy. The instructions were for the recipient to close their eyes and learn to feel the *influence*, or non-contact *pressure*, exerted by the empty-force practitioner. Through this process, an open-minded receiver learns to be moved by the empty force. This is a fun exercise, and there is a tactile sense that comes with the practice.

The enjoyable practice allowed us to learn to move with the feeling of the non-contact force. Years later, another *kong jin* practitioner shared a variation, which included feeling the top of a doorway as you pass through blind-folded or sensing one's proximity to a wall. These are amusing exercises that are valuable in terms of sensitivity training, and I invite the reader to try them out with a friend or training partner. In my experience, most people can fairly quickly learn to throw each other around a bit by directing and becoming sensitive to this invisible "energy."

However, there is a dark side. Some online video demonstrations provide an example of a master who has come to believe so strongly in his invisible power of non-contact energy that he challenges a trained fighter who is not his student. I've never seen an example like this come to a good end.

So, is "empty-force" real? Yes, in a way, but will it work as a non-contact defense against an uncooperative (non-conditioned) attacker? Probably not.

My personal belief is that Shr would not demonstrate on me because, without the requisite years of experience studying with him and participating with his group, I had not been properly conditioned; I was not brainwashed to respond to his "empty-force" power. In any martial arts practice, there is a tendency for students to wish to please their teacher. Unless carefully monitored and corrected, it is easy for unconscious conditioning to take place, involving students learning to respond in the expected manner. In systems that emphasize sensitivity and response to the invisible *kong jin* force, a "good student" will learn to respond to the subtle force and / or psychological cues that are presented by the teacher.

It is instructive to observe how the concept is applied, to at least some degree, in the Russian martial art of *Systema*. A good example of responding to the teacher can be viewed in this video clip: * When watching, pay particular attention to the opening non-contact "punch," where the person being demonstrated on begins to fall away from the attack before the punch is thrown by *Systema* expert, Mikhail Reebok.

*https://www.youtube.com/watch?v=i3wVSys7cwo [34]

Training to be a student of *kong jin* requires reciprocal practice with a senior student or master, in order for the student in training to adopt the expected feeling and response. A good example of the back-and-forth sensitivity and response to *kong jin* practice can be viewed here: https://www.youtube.com/watch?v=n5qSwPlyX5U

As described earlier, subtle *information* can be useful in an adjunctive way when making physical contact with the opponent. However, without the opponent having the requisite conditioning, it is unlikely that a non-contact force can be used effectively against a real attacker.

Kong jin training is usually harmless, and, by learning to respond to subtle cues, the practice may enhance the student's ability to sense and work with very subtle physical forces. However, there have been a few instances of individuals who presented themselves as transmission holders of a secret lineage of invisible non-contact power. When a student is asked to spend many thousands of dollars to be initiated into a cult of a secret internal power, this is fraudulent, and perhaps even psychologically dangerous to the practitioner.

Endnotes

1 Consistent with comments in the opening pages of the present work, although for the most part Chinese characters are transliterated using the *pinyin* system, there are a few exceptions where Chinese is Romanized in the Wade-Giles style. Examples of Wade-Giles transliteration in this chapter are *t'ai-chi*, and *Tao Te Ching*.

2 Wile, Douglas, *Tai-chi ancestors: The making of an internal martial art*, Sweet Ch'i Press, New City, NY 1999 p. 196.

3 Wile, p. 78.

4 Ibid., p. 79.

5 For the most part, this transliteration of romanized script for Master Wang's given name is used in the present work since most sources rely on this version. The exception is when other sources are cited.

6 There are, however, fanciful stories describing Chang's super human abilities which lack credulity. Those reports include a description of his steps which shattered stones (Wile, Ancestors, p. 72), smashing two-foot stone steps, and walking on water (Wile, p. 73).

7 Note, this bias does not necessarily apply to "energetic technologies" that interact with the unconscious internal energy processes of the body, which for example are addressed through acupuncture or massage.

8 Wile, Douglas, *Art of the bedchamber: The Chinese sexual yoga classics including women's solo meditation texts*, State University of New York, 1992, p. 72.

9 An interview by Dr. Tiller, where he discusses reduction of the practitioner's "noise level" and its relationship to "internal energy," can be viewed at: https://www.youtube.com/watch?v=fO4vcxD2_Wg&feature=youtu.be

10 In studies conducted by researcher Feng and colleagues, a *qi* master named Bao, emitted *qi* for one minute toward a test tube held in her palm, and between 44%-89.8% of *E. coli* and 66.7%-98% of *Shigella* were dead after being subjected to a *qi* emission with "termination" intention.

Xin Yan, et al. 1999 Mat Res Innovat (1999) 2:349-359.

11 "Intention" can be extended on a subconscious level.

12 As with Tiller's gas-discharge experiment described in Section VII, which documents the ability of non-physical influence, the extension of *disruptive information* is presumed to occur when the same two conditions are met. First, the individual must attain the state of *entrainment* (or the related state of *internal coherence**), then there must be the intention to influence. More discussion on this topic is included in Section X.

13 "Wang Xiang–Zai discusses the essence of combat science," *Shibao* Newspaper, Beijing, 1940, translated by Timo Heikkila and Li Jiong.

14 Citations attributed to Guo regarding levels of internal energy development were included in Section VII.

15 "Wang Xiang–Zai discusses the essence of combat science," *Shibao* Newspaper, Beijing, 1940, translated by Timo Heikkila and Li Jiong.

16 Sawai, Kenichi, *Taiki-ken: The essence of kung fu*, Japan publications, 1976, p. 10.

17 "Wang Xiang–Zai discusses the essence of combat science," *Shibao* Newspaper, Beijing, 1940, translated by Timo Heikkila and Li Jiong, p. 7.

18 Wang, p. 7.

19 John Stevens, *The philosophy of Aikido*, Kodansha America, New York, 2001 p. 24.

20 Some of these films are available on YouTube, and can be found by searching Morihei Ueshiba.

21 Gluck, Jay, *Zen combat*, Ballentine Books, 1962 (1976 edition), pp. 177-188.

22 Stevens, John, *The philosophy of aikido*, Kodansha America, New York, 2001, p. 35.

23 *Star Wars: Episode IV - A New Hope* (1977).

24 The on-line Star Wars fan site, Wookieepedia, describes the Jedi mind trick in the following way:

"The Force can have a strong influence on the weak-minded." - Obi-Wan Kenobi to Luke Skywalker. A mind trick was an ability of the Force that allowed the practitioner to influence the thoughts of the affected, to the user's advantage.

Mind trick | Wookieepedia | FANDOM powered by Wikia
starwars.wikia.com/wiki/Mind_trick

25 The new model of a yet-to-be-measured electromagnetic-like field as explanation for "internal energy" is provided in Section XII.

26 *Tao Te Ching*, Chapter 38.

27 As introduced in Section II, there are six organ pulses, three on each wrist, which in the traditional model is said to reveal the conditions of the patient's *qi* energy of the visceral organs. Note that one tier of diagnosis in traditional Chinese medicine is the evaluation of psychological "excesses," which relate to imbalance in specific visceral organs and are reflected through the pulses. An example is "spleen deficiency," which, according to the traditional model, is related to excess "dwelling." In this example, the emotion of excess dwelling is said to harm the spleen and is reflected through specific pulse representations.

28 The ability of an intervention specialist to "see" energy imbalances is the basis of an emerging field called "medical intuition." The principles are outlined in Carolyn Myss's *Anatomy of the Spirit: The Seven*

Stages of Power and Healing, wherein Myss describes her role as a medical intuitive in the following way: "Since that autumn day in 1983, I have worked wholeheartedly as a medical intuitive. This means that I use my intuitive ability to help people understand the emotional, psychological, and spiritual energy that lies at the root of their illness, disease, or life crisis. I can sense the type of illness that has developed, often before the individual is even aware of having an illness at all. The people I work with usually are aware, however, that their lives are not in balance and that something is wrong."

Myss, Carolyn, *Anatomy of the spirit: The seven stages of power and healing*, Three Rivers Press, 1997, p. 5.

29 Blofeld, John, *The secret and sublime: Taoist mysteries and magic*, E.P. Dutton, 1973 p. 122.

30 Blofeld, pp. 122-123.

31 Ibid., p. 125.

32 The *New Oxford American Dictionary* defines equanimity as "Mental calmness, composure, and evenness of temper, especially in a difficult situation."

33 Adapted from Alan Watts, "Chapter 4: Wu Wei," *Tao: The watercourse way*, pp.76, 77.

34 I have never studied with, nor worked under, a Systema master, and I do not mean to imply that "empty-force" is the total explanation for this interesting martial art. I am only referring to the unconscious suggestion aspect, which seems to have been, to some degree, involved in the demonstrations I have witnessed.

Section IX
Three Rules of the Heart

Calmness in the heart of movement is the secret to all power [1]

IX

Three Rules of the Heart

Introduction to Section IX

*T*he present section focuses on two opposing mind-body orientations viewed from three perspectives: *open-closed, love-hate,* and *growth-defensive.* Whether in the context of body orientation and the thymus gland in the center of the chest — the body's major immune system regulator — or heart electrophysiology, each perspective offers its own way of interacting with, and triggering responses in, the body's nervous system. Each has its own way of responding to, and managing, stress, and each contributes to our understanding of internal energy.

Common to each perspective are the *instructions* that they present to the immune system. Within each perspective, one orientation promotes healing, access to love, and personal power. However, in each case, the opposing orientation, if habitually dominant in one's life, can inhibit full health and energetic potential. In some ways, the two opposing orientations can be said to represent the "light" and "dark" sides of our nature, a principle explained through the Cherokee story of an old man teaching his grandson about life:

> "A fight is constantly going on inside of us," the grandfather told the boy.

> "It is a terrible fight between two wolves. One represents anger, envy, sorrow, greed, arrogance, self-pity, guilt, resentment, inferiority, lies, false pride, the need to feel superior, and ego."

> The old man continued, "The other represents joy, peace, love, hope, serenity, humility, kindness, benevolence, empathy, generosity, truth, compassion, and faith."

> The grandson thought about it for a minute and then asked his grandfather,

> "But, Grandfather, which wolf will win?"

> The old Cherokee simply replied, "The one you feed the most." [2]

Mindset and the Body's Response to Stress

In the fourth century BCE, the Taoist philosopher Chuang Tzu[3] observed that a person's mental-emotional state could influence the body's response to stress. Noting the power of our mental orientation in responding to physical challenge, Chuang reflected that, while a sober person falling from a carriage is often seriously injured, a drunk man experiencing the same calamity is rarely hurt. This led the philosopher to ponder that if such an "elevated" mind-body relationship could be effected through over-imbibing, how much greater could the result be for someone consumed by the *Tao*?

Since Chuang's time, philosophers and scientists have sought to understand the optimal ways to deal with life's challenges. One way of examining this question is in terms of open vs. closed posture "configurations."

Chapter 46

"Open" vs. "Closed"

*P*osture is usually characterized as a physical attribute. However, one's posture can also be mental or emotional. Shared in common between each of these orientations, whether physical, mental, or emotional, is how one's bearing influences the immune system and a person's ability to project power and influence.

Diagram 9-1

The Interrelationship Between Posture, Immune System, and "Subtle Energy Influence"

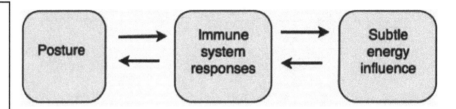

One illustration of the power of posture is observed in the expression of *openness*. Here, openness can refer to a physical orientation, but it can also describe a person's attitude. As an example of the power of openness, *both* the physical and emotional "posture" of openness can influence the immune system, while at the same time boosting one's personal store of "life energy."

As described in the chapters that follow, some postures promote growth, strength, and openness to love, while others signal protective responses. In the latter case, the mind-body system is so interconnected that a mental or emotional protective response can instantaneously trigger a protective physical orientation, such as a startle response. Due to the intimate and highly responsive nature of the nervous system wiring, when a person is presented with a real or imagined threat, a physical protective response is instantly matched with a protective "fight or flight" response. Physiologically, this response is generated by the amygdala, near the brain center, and reflected through the entire nervous system. However, a response like this becomes problematic when these patterns develop into habits.

Closed vs. Open

Providing more clarity on the meaning of "open" vs. "closed," biologist Bruce Lipton's observations of endothelial cell behavior is especially enlightening:

> When I was cloning human endothelial cells, they retreated from
> toxins that I introduced into the culture dish, just as humans retreat

from mountain lions and muggers in dark alleys. They also gravitated to nutrients, just as humans gravitate to breakfast, lunch, dinner and love. These opposing movements define the two basic cellular responses to environmental stimuli. Gravitating to a life-sustaining signal, such as nutrients, characterizes a growth response; moving away from threatening signals, such as toxins, characterizes a protective response … It turns out that mechanisms that support growth and protection cannot both operate optimally at the same time. In other words, cells cannot simultaneously move forward and backward. The human blood cells I studied at Stanford exhibited one microscopic anatomy for providing nutrition and a completely different microscopic anatomy for providing a protection response. What they couldn't do was exhibit both configurations at the same time. [4]

The intersection of human behavior and a person's physical and emotional "configurations" can be compared with Lipton's observation of endothelial cell behavior, with an example of this being the varying pugilistic styles of different combat athletes. Just as with the cell behavior observed by Lipton, it may be that a deep evolutionary link also exists between a fighter's posture and the mind-body system. Accordingly, a more "open" orientation will tend to produce specific mind-body and nervous system responses, while a "closed" orientation will tend to produce quite different responses.

It is speculated that, along with one's posture and orientation, a cascade of nervous, emotional, immune, and homeostatic responses occur that are associated with a person's posture. In other words, an upright body with open arms will trigger certain kinds of nervous system responses, while a chin-down, crouched posture, typical of a boxer, will initiate a significantly different set of mind-body and nervous system responses. As with cell morphology, a person may also adopt physical orientations that influence their physiology. These "configurations" demonstrate a person's dominant orientations, or "configurations," that respond to openness or closedness.

An individual who tends to "configure" more toward openness and growth is more likely to receive sustaining growth influences from the neurology and electrophysiology of the heart, such as openness to love and nurturance. Extrapolating from Lipton's observation of cell behavior to the larger human form, the growth potential of humans who maintain primarily defensive postures is likewise limited. Lipton's observations of endothelial cell behavior can be instructive in our discussion of the meaning of "internal energy" in the following relationships:

Openness = Growth

Defensiveness = Retraction

Openness = Energy flowing outward

Defensiveness = Energetically constricted inward

These aspects of openness vs. closedness provide another way of viewing the human energy-endocrine-immune system that, like endothelial cell "configurations," might also represent different kinds of human "configurations."

Lipton's description of cellular behavior in bipolar terms of either open-growth or closed-protective shares a remarkable resemblance to human motivation forces, described as the bi-polar / bi-direction possibilities of the forces of *love* or *fear* discussed in Neale Donald Walsch's *Conversations with God:*

> Every action taken by a human being is based in love or fear, not simply those dealing with relationships. Decisions affecting business, industry, politics, religion, the education of your young, the social agenda of your nations, the economic goals of your society, choices involving war, peace, attack, defense, aggression, submission; determinations to covet or give away, to save or to share, to unite or to divide—every single free choice you ever undertake arises out of one of the only two possible thoughts there are: a thought of love or a thought of fear.
>
> Fear is the energy which contracts, closes down, draws in, runs, hides, hoards, harms. Love is the energy which expands, opens up, sends out, stays, reveals, shares, heals.
>
> Fear wraps our bodies in clothing; love allows us to stand naked. Fear clings to and clutches all that we have; love gives all that we have away. Fear holds close; love holds dear. Fear grasps, love lets go. Fear rankles, love soothes, fear attacks, love amends.
>
> Every human thought, work, or deed is based in one emotion or the other. You have no choice about this, because there is nothing else from which to choose. But you have free choice about which of these to select. [5]

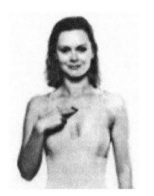

FIGURE 9-2

Location of Thymus Gland

Located behind the sternum and in front of the heart, John Diamond describes the thymus as "the gland most responsive to stress."

From Dr. John Diamond's *Life Energy*.

Posture, Life Energy, and the Thymus

In some ways comparable to Lipton's observation of endothelial cell behavior, John Diamond, MD, also describes the influences of posture on a person's "life energy." In this context, he focuses on the way open vs. closed posture and attitude affects the thymus gland in the center of the chest.

Illustrated in Figure 9-2, the thymus is the gland most responsive to *stress*. The meaning of stress, as currently used, derives from research conducted by late endocrinologist Hans Selye, [6] whose seminal work in the 1930s came at a time when there was little understanding of the impact of *stress* on physical health. Subsequent research has demonstrated that the human body responds to real or perceived *stressors* by the swelling of the adrenal glands and shrinking of the thymus; this is important since the thymus is the source of the body's immune fighting "T-Cells," hence the name for this component of the human immune system.

Although the thymus is often described as atrophying and shrinking in adulthood, recent research has shown that the immune response of the thymus continues into adulthood. [7] However, its function in the realm of mind-body energy may be more profound, as according to Diamond, the role of the thymus is actually much broader, especially as an aspect of what he calls "life energy."

The notion that the thymus continues to play a role much later into life than previously suspected is supported by research demonstrating that it can be reinvigorated in order to restore immune function in older adults. [8] It is also worth noting that the thymus is of special concern in alternative health practices, an example of this being the practice of "thymus thumping," which proponents claim promotes immune system enhancement. [9] Diamond, who incorporates management of "life energy" in his work with patients, sees the thymus as the "master controller" of both the body's life energy and the acupuncture meridian system. [10]

Diamond believes that the thymus is critical to the body's ability to balance the flow of life energy, explaining that it "monitors and regulates energy flow throughout the body's energy system, initiating instantaneous corrections to overcome imbalances as they occur so as to achieve a rebalancing and harmony of life energy." [11]

Reminiscent of Lipton's description of microscopic cellular anatomy and configuration, other comparisons can be made between a person's posture, the thymus, emotions, and the immune system. Diamond introduces us to these relationships:

> As the thymus emotions are predominantly love and hate, it is not surprising that the supreme gesture of love, the open-armed embrace of a mother toward her child [Left image of Photos 9-3] is a thymus-strengthening gesture. I call it the thymus gesture. Whenever this heart-opening gesture is adopted and held for a brief period of time, it will be found that the energy imbalances throughout the body will be corrected and the thymus will test strong and active. . . Conversely, if we close in our arms to ourselves and refuse to put ourselves out we would be "turning away without love." This negative gesture diminishes our life energy. [12]

Echoing the Greek philosopher Empedocles, Diamond defines these bipolar orientations in terms of *love* and *hate:*

> While there are many emotions, there are essentially only two primary ones. These are love and hate in their various and deepest manifestations. [13]

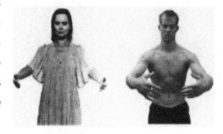

Photos 9-3
The Influence of Posture on the Thymus and "Life Energy"
These images compare John Diamond's "High Thymus" "Mother's Gesture" with a common qigong "Open Embrace" posture. According to Diamond, the "high thymus" gesture shown on the left strengthens the body's immune system and balances the body's *life force* energies. Illustrated by the right photo, *qigong* and *t'ai-chi* practitioners often use variations of the posture shown as a standing meditation, or as a *t'ai-chi* preparatory exercise. (Note: since preparing this section of the present work, the standard "open embrace" posture shown on the right has been modified in our organization's classes to reach more outward and, thus, be more "open.")

Left image from John Diamond, MD's Life Energy

415

Diamond continues:

> Beneath the more superficial emotions such as joy and happiness there
> will be love, and beneath sadness and unhappiness there will be a latent
> deep fear or hate. [14]

Comparing Lipton's observations with insights provided by Diamond suggests new clues to the meaning of "internal energy." Where Lipton describes cell behavior in terms of a bifurcated choice between open or closed, growth-oriented or defensive "posturing," Diamond describes "openness" and "closedness" as defining attributes of a person's *life energy*. Describing the influence of these on mental health, Diamond sees them in terms of the life enhancing energy he calls "love," and the force that drains a person's energy system he calls "hate." [15]

Love, Hate, and Mental Illness

Diamond developed his understanding of the influence of attitude and emotions on physical and mental health through his experience with patients. As his writing explains, the most profound impact a patient could have on their own psychological and physical health was the choices they made in terms of love and hate. He found this to be so true that he was able to predict which patients would return to health and which would fail to recover based on the decisions they made in terms of love and hate. His observations included the effect these emotions had on the thymus gland.

According to Diamond, the strength or weakness of the thymus gland determined why some individuals could successfully fight and recover from diseases such as cancer, while others were unable to do the same because of their dominant attitude and emotions, which negatively affected their thymus. One sad, but poignant, example illustrates the point:

> A young male patient who had been "given" a diagnosis of cancer came
> to me for help. In the course of the interview, I asked him, "Do you hate
> anyone?" He said, "I loathe and detest my mother." When I test-touched
> his thymus, it was weak. I said, "As long as you hate your mother, this
> hatred will so diminish your thymus activity, your life energy, that you
> will never get completely well. The patient's response: "I would sooner
> die than give up hating my mother." [16]

Other researchers support Diamond's views on the effect of negative emotions on health. An example is found in Andrew Newberg, MD's *How God Changes your Brain,* which describes how anger and chronic negativity is cognitively, emotionally, and spiritually destructive. [17] Many spiritual healers share similar beliefs, especially in regard to the thymus. For example, psychic and energy healer Barbara Brennan describes the role of the thymus as "a place holding 'sacred lodging… very specific to our life task.'" [18] Diamond explains the relationship between ill-health and negative emotions:

> The underlying specific emotional state in most if not all such cases of psychiatric illness is that of anger—chronic, ongoing, festering anger. This anger is often conscious, but also frequently unconscious—that is, not known to the patient. I say unconscious because he is so unable to deal with it that he represses it, pushes it down, out of his mind. [19]

Other health practitioners describe the destructive effect of negative emotions on the body in similar ways. The noted chiropractor Dr. Thurman Fleet taught his patients that negative emotions affected their digestion. Fleet explains: "Our mind plays an important role in the source of constipation. Destructive emotions such as worry, hatred, fear directly interfere with digestive organ's normal functions, thus paving the way for an unwholesome internal condition." [20]

As Diamond sees it, a person with lowered thymus strength has less access to available power, whereas a strong thymus response promotes recovery from illness. A weak thymus leads to illness and is the "precipitating factor causing the initial energy imbalance." [21] Referring once again to the relationship between stress and the thymus, Diamond explains that stress *always* results in the reduction of *life energy*, and that this can be evaluated based on the status of the thymus, [22] which forms the core of a mind-body-energy principle he calls "psychobiological harmony;" the place where "all parts of mind, body and spirit join together for the good of the whole." [23]

Psychobiological Harmony

By drawing parallels between the Greek philosopher of medicine Hippocrates's *Vis Medicatrix Naturae,* the Indian concept of *prana,* and the Chinese concept of *qi,* and then integrating these with Western concepts of spirit, Diamond explains that only *life energy* can evoke "true healing" — the healing that occurs from within. "True healing" has to do with the **flow of energy** and an **"energetic balance,"** where "all parts of our psychological functioning are coordinated, whole within themselves and where the energy flow through our bodies is balanced, coordinated … [and in a] state of perfect health, happiness, and love." [24]

"Psychobiological harmony [25] *is* the state where one's "ch'i [qi] flows, brain hemispheres are balanced and where all parts are joined together for the good of the whole." [26] *Psychobiological harmony* manifests as a vibrant life energy flow and is expressed by the overall strength of the body. This model suggests that balanced flow is power, and balanced power is flow.

Poison to the Energetic Field

While energetic balance determines overall health, according to Diamond's model, some mental-emotional influences produce an especially weakening effect; the most harmful of these being envy. Speaking here of narcissistic envy, Diamond explains it as the underlying negative emotion in _almost every psychiatric and many physical disorders._ [27] As Diamond explains, envy is an underlying, often unconscious, destructive force, citing experiences with his patients to illustrate the link between envy and mental illness.

Diamond was intrigued to learn that many of his patients _envied_ his sanity, and wished that he _would not be mentally well_. Their attitudes represent the destructive nature of narcissistic envy, which is the wish to destroy, sometimes confused with jealousy, which is the will to possess. [28] As Diamond explains, his patients manifested poisonous envy not because they were hopeful of becoming well themselves, but because they wanted the doctor, who had been devoting much of his life to their care, to share their misfortune:

> They did not wish that they were sane but wished me to be crazy, recognizing of course that if I were crazy as well, I could do nothing to help them. This is the basic expression of envy. Rather than wishing to be sane, as they presumed I was, and rather than wishing that my sanity could help them regain theirs, they became envious of my sanity and wished to destroy it. It was more important to them for me to be insane than for them to be sane. [29]

The underlying drive of the envious person is: "If I can't have it, no one will," a thinking pattern which develops into a deep-seated psychological obsession. Representing "not a wish to possess, but a wish to destroy," vandalism is an example of envy. [30] Another example illustrating the way envy impedes psychiatric healing was presented when Diamond assumed duties for another psychiatrist who had suffered a mental breakdown. Diamond was puzzled by the reactions of most of his new patients, who were not sympathetic to their former doctor's condition, but who, in many cases, were elated. Some even laughed out loud when they learned of their former caretaker's situation. Diamond reports that he was distressed:

> By [the] lack of compassion toward the doctor who had done a great deal for them over the years, who had worked with them and cared for them and worried over them. Most of them openly expressed delight. Many of them smiled, and some even broke into laughter. It was then that I started to see why at least some of these patients were still in the hospital even after many years. They had, in a sense, resisted every effort on the part of the doctor to help them. They preferred the doctor be a "nut case" like them than to allow him to heal them. Their envy had destroyed them. [31]

Another Kind of Block

Not only the words you use, but your innermost thoughts, affect your ability to embody power, health, love, and support on multiple levels, both seen and unseen. Whether expressed through the spoken word or silence, *dialog* represents an individual's psychological-energetic "set point." This principle speaks to a tangential, but no less important, point about the body's unconscious and limiting visceral response, which is produced when a person makes negative statements about others.

In the case of an athlete or a martial artist, whether spoken or unspoken, *dialog* habits influence athletic skills and success. The principle is particularly applicable to any activity where a high level of mind-body integration is required; the greater the degree to which mind, intention, and subtlety are required in a particular discipline, the more the principle applies.

In American football, the principle applies more to a quarterback than a lineman, where total functioning-coherence and 360-degree awareness in the heat of competition is imperative. However, the rule is even more applicable for those studying subtle physical and energetic skills like *qigong* and the internal martial arts, such as *t'ai-chi* and *aikido*. This is because the spoken and unspoken dialog interacts with that person's energy-consciousness field. In turn, that inner dialog is reflected in the degree of sophisticated skill they can apply under stress.

As discussed in Section VII, judgment and negative statements produce a disordering influence on the individual's coherence and the synchrony of biological rhythms known as *entrainment*. Negative emotions like these also produce a disruptive effect on heart electrophysiology, important because, as will be discussed later, optimal heart electrophysiology is a critical element in a person's ability to realize full power and potential.

Whether directed toward oneself or others, a person's inner dialog, when obsessively negative, produces a disorganizing and thus limiting influence. In these cases, poisonous negative attitudes and emotions, like the envy described by Diamond, act as a "governor," [32] limiting the person's ability to achieve more advanced levels of mastery.

Applied to the study of energetic martial arts, when a teacher or fellow student belittles another practitioner, their words create an invisible ceiling limiting the speaker's access to greater skill, and this applies especially to the specific skill being mocked or belittled. When we dialog in this way, an energetic-emotional block forms within the psyche-energy structure of the person demeaning that individual. *Aikido* master Morihei Ueshiba seemed to share this belief:

> As soon as you concern yourself with the 'good' and 'bad' of your fellows,
> you create an opening in your heart for maliciousness to enter. Testing,
> competing with, and criticizing others weakens and defeats you. [33]

Chapter 47

Thymus Energy Exercises

Photo Series 9-4

Thymus Strengthening Exercise

Feeling or imagining that one senses an "energy ball" in front of the center chest/thymus location will increase the sensation of "energy," both outside the body and in the area of the thymus. Notice the changes in hand position and shape in this photo series. After developing the feeling of electrical-like buzzing feeling in front of the thymus, aim the hands inward to the center of the chest to stimulate electrical-like sensations in the middle of the chest.

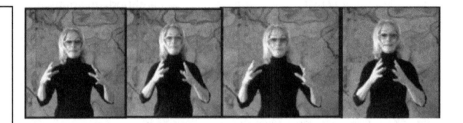

*B*oth mental attitude and physical practices, such as *qigong* and yoga, can strengthen the thymus. Just as chronic stress weakens the thymus and its immune system function, the practice of its antithesis, relaxation, is the most obvious way to promote thymus health. However, learning to maintain a calm state is often easier said than done. Because of the thymus's response to mental and emotional stress, it means that positive thoughts also have an influence on thymus function; thus, striving to maintain an overall positive disposition is a profound health practice. A related practice, that of changing negative into positive thoughts through such methods as the Freeze Frame® technique, * can also help reduce stress. There are also several *qigong* and yoga exercises that, when directed to the area of the thymus, can also strengthen the gland.

*Covered in Section VII, Box 7-9

This chapter describes three thymus-strengthening exercises:

1) A basic thymus-energetic *qigong* practice.

2) A more advanced Interactive-Detector exercise series.

3) Heart-Thymus Myofascial Band *Qigong.*

A Basic Thymus-Energetic *Qigong*

In Chinese *qigong* and *hatha* yoga, as well as various other practices, there is a class of energy work that is specifically directed to the thymus. The method involves focus of one's attention on the anatomical location of the gland. For example, the technique shown in Photo Series 9-4 is a thymus-strengthening practice, which also serves as an excellent way to begin any *qigong* or meditation routine.

When practiced with a calm mind and positive intention, the sensations associated with the technique balance the *"qi"* energy of the left and right sides of the body. This strengthens the thymus, and, with a little practice, creates the experience that practitioners identify as the sense of balanced *qi / prana* circulating through the entire body. The practitioner shown in the photo series is working with the feeling of "energy" in the empty space between her palms, and this *qigong* exercise can be performed while sitting, standing, or while lying down, face up.

Begin the exercise by holding your hands at the center of the chest, four to six inches in front of the thymus, as illustrated in Photo 9-2. Hold your open palms and facing each other in a stretched but relaxed position and, while making small adjustments to the shape of your hand, follow the guidelines described in Section III for working with *signal*.

As with other *qigong* exercises, with regular practice, most individuals develop a sensation between the open palms that is not dissimilar to the feeling one experiences while holding the positive sides of two magnets near to each another. When searching for these kinds of magnetic-repulse-interactive sensations, hold the intention that your hands are "communicating" with each other. With experience, this creates a palpable energetic cross-communication between opposing sides of the body. In practice, imagine that your right hand is "listening" for feedback from the left, and then simultaneously do the same with the left. Be especially attentive to changing "energetic" sensations you note while making very slight movements and hand shape changes.

With continued practice, most will notice how just the right amount of tension, or stretch of a finger on one hand, can stimulate a pressure or electromagnetic (EM) change on the other hand. Pay attention to these subtle changes in sensations between your palms, and when you feel the sense of magnetic energetic-pull and push interactions between your open palms, form the intention to build upon and increase these sensations. With practice, most individuals will be able to experience these sensations, which will feel like pressure, tingling, or warmth in the "empty space" between the two hands, especially when attention is focused on the space between the palms.

The Next Level: Three Interactive-Detectors

A variation of the thymus-*qigong* practice just described involves three "interactive-detectors." These are ways of exploring the magnetic-like sensations in the space between the open palms. They are:

- Signal

- Breath

- Fascia / muscle stretch

These three interactive-detectors represent distinct pathways to detecting and enhancing one's awareness of *signal*. When used together, these different approaches synergistically form a more powerful experience of "energy" practice.

Breath

The second interactive-detector involves awareness of *breath* as it interacts with the feeling of *signal* between your open palms. For best results, add breath as an interactive-detector only after you have confidence in being able to detect and engage with *signal*. (If you are having trouble working with *signal*, first develop confidence by revisiting the "working with *signal*" portions of Section III.)

Add breath as an interactive-detector first by maintaining the sensation of *signal* between the palms of your hands, as shown in Photo Series 9-4. Then, while focusing on the sensations you feel between your open palms, begin deep, rhythmic breathing. Pay close attention to any changes in the sensations between your open palms; they are clues that will help you gain greater success with the exercise. As you slowly and rhythmically breathe in and out, continue to pay attention to changes in the empty space between your palms. Mentally encourage your breath (through your body's reaction to the breathing technique) to interact with that "empty space," and look for changes that might appear in the form of a feeling of the open space between your palms becoming denser, or an increase in EM activity between the palms.

Progress with breath as an interactive-detector begins when you notice that the *signal* changes between your palms coincide with your inward and outward breath. This is an important step that shows you have linked intention and *signal* with breath, and you will know that you're really "getting it" when you experience the sensation of your breathing no longer seeming to originate only from the normal movement of air moving through your nose and mouth, but also from the space between your open palms. When you feel an especially dense feeling in the space between your palms that feels like an "energy ball," it is an especially good sign that the practice is going well.

Note that the length of time it takes to master both this and the subsequent interactive-detector varies between individuals. Where someone with considerable meditation and / or *qigong* experience might immediately sense one particular field (e.g., breath or *signal*), for a newer practitioner, the process could take weeks or even months. Either way, the skill of mastering any interactive-detector is increased through regular practice and patience.

Fascia / Muscle Changes

The third interactive-detector involves mastering small stretchy movements of muscle and fascia in the palms of your hands, with the goal being to observe and engage with the same kind of sensations that you did with breath. In this aspect of the exercise, the interactive-detector is the interaction between muscle / fascia changes in the fingers and palms, and the corresponding "energy ball" sensations between the open palms.

Begin this aspect of the exercise by making slight, stretchy changes to the shape of your hand and fingers as you attend to the sensations between your palms. Examples of these kinds of small changes in hand shape, along with the experience of changes in the space between the open palms, are illustrated in Photo Series 9-4. These subtle hand shape changes are not performed passively, as though one were merely opening and closing the hand. Instead, the exercise is practiced slowly, and executed with purposeful and gradual *differential* stretching which stimulates the deep muscles and myofascial bands of the hands. When performed correctly, these movements actuate slight changes in the shape of the hand, as well as changes in the perception of the "energy fields." Be patient, as in many cases, this level can take weeks, months, or sometimes even years to master.

In working with this interactive-detector, the goal is similar to the merging of the breath with *signal* into a single unit in the space between the palms. Here, the method focuses on the same space, but now with the addition of a third interactive-detector: muscle and fascia movement.

In this part of the exercise, continue to notice the merging between the previous interactive-detectors with small changes in your hand shape, as you activate tensional stretching in the palms. Maintain awareness of both *signal* and breath in the space between your palms, and then add the slow stretching hand movements to the exercise. As before, the goal here is to develop the feeling that small stretching movements in the palms are producing an enhanced feeling of interaction with the empty space between your hands.

Once you are able to feel the interaction with the "energy ball" between your hands, which coincides with the stretchy feeling of your hands, practice simultaneously feeling or merging all three interactive-detectors until they ultimately merge into a single unit. Work toward feeling the reaction simultaneously with fascial-muscle stretch, breath, and *signal,* combining all three and allowing them to grow, merge, expand and shrink together. When successful, the experience should be that of a pulsating ball of energy that changes in shape and intensity. By being sensitive to direction from these feelings, and allowing your body to respond to them, they can initiate a stretching and healing yogic movement throughout the entire body.

Each individual's experience of this kind of yoga / *qigong* will vary. However, they will all involve attending to the confluence of these sensations, initiated through very slight stretches between the open palms. With practice, the slight feeling of fascial stretch within the hands should extend into the forearms, the upper arms, and then finally to the center of the chest.

After you successfully merge the three interactive-detectors, continue with the practice by experimenting with the feeling of slight changes in your breath and muscle / fascia, remembering that you should never practice in a forceful way. Ultimately, when you open the palm, you will feel flushing through the entire hand and beyond. While playing with this sensation, simultaneously incorporate more slight movements through the palms, anticipating the experience of an unusually deep pulling feeling in your palms, as compared to the regular feeling of your hand opening and stretching. One client reported that he was more successful with the exercise if he imagined he was easing *qi* deep into the bones of his hand.

With continued practice, train to notice the feeling that every opening of the hand, flex of the fingers, or smallest change in hand position triggers the awareness of "energetic" sensation in other areas of the body. This integration is an essential component of *qigong* and the internal martial arts, and the ability to integrate this "total system connection" is considered one of the markers on the path to mastery.

When these sensations are especially strong, it means that you have integrated the three elements of *signal, breath,* and *fascia* between the palms. At this point, continue to build the sense of energy in front of the chest by turning the palms inward while mentally directing the "energy" to the thymus at the center of the chest. Many practitioners notice that this generates not only the feeling of warmth in the area, but that it also produces a deep sense of peace.

Heart-Thymus Myofascial Band *Qigong*

The correlation between myofascial structures and the energetic meridians of TCM was described in Section III. This new exercise is based on that convergence, with particular focus on the "heart meridian." As illustrated in Figure 9-5, one of those stretchy myofascial physical structures runs from the fingers and palms to the area in the center of the chest. The following exercise is designed to address that myofascial band along with the meridian associated with the heart channel and myofascial network, which Thomas Myers refers to as the "superficial front arm line" (SFAL). [34]

As suggested by the diagram, the exercise is based on gentle stress being applied to the myofascial line that runs between the myofascial structures in the palm and the center of the chest. Directed tension along this connective tissue meridian / myofascial band provides an additional approach to providing healthful stimulation to the thymus. The exercise is based on the principle that movements in some parts of the body — in this case, the palms and fingers — can be stimulated to direct beneficial stress through the entire channel, and ultimately, to the target organ.

The following exercise also introduces what is sometimes regarded as a secret martial art training technique; one that is also useful as a *qigong* routine for thymus strengthening. The martial arts application of the exercise increases power and effectiveness in styles such as *t'ai-chi* and *baguazhang*, providing more clues to the meaning of "soft power" in the martial arts.

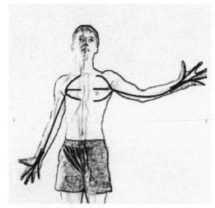

Figure 9-5
Myofascial Bands of the "Heart Meridian," Thymus, and Fascia
Illustration inspired from Peter Dorsher MD's image in "Myofascial Meridians as Anatomical Evidence of Acupuncture Channels." [35] (Repeated from an image presented in Section II for the convenience of the reader.)

This exercise involves incorporating deeper than normal stretching, and other movements of the hand and arm that are reflected through tensional changes in the center of the chest. Because of its total system integration, it addresses the bad habit many of us have of moving the arm in a segmented way that is not optimally moved in relation to the body's core.

Begin the new exercise by lifting your hand away from your body as shown in Figure 9-5. As you arrive at this position, work to develop the feeling of stretching deep into the palm while opening and closing the hand. Now experiment with subtle changes to your opening / closing hand, and then, making a slight bend at the elbow, find a place where you feel the stretch extend into your upper chest. That is the myofascial stimulation that will be your focus. When practicing, the goal is to move the hands and arms so as to induce that feeling in *every* movement, no matter how slight, creating a responsive slight stretch at the center of the chest. When performed correctly, which takes some practice, the slightest stretch of the small finger, or the stretching of the metacarpal tendons in the hand, should simultaneously be reflected in a tugging feeling in the upper-center part of the chest.

After establishing this tensional relationship, try to establish the same interaction in other areas of the body. When you can successfully feel these tensional relationships at will, try applying the principle to movement practices such as *t'ai-chi* or *baguazhang*. After you become familiar with the feeling of activating the fascial band from the palms to the chest, try applying the exercise to daily activities, from lifting a cup of tea to picking up something from the table. This will serve as your own secret body integration practice.

Applied to the internal martial arts, the small movements initiated in the palms, and expressed through the myofascial lines to the muscles at the center of the chest, adds more "energy" and power to techniques. This is through the use of refined physical movements that incorporate the entire fascia band from the palms to the chest.

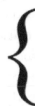

Heart electrophysiology

(Stress vs. Non-stressful regulation of the heart)

One of many natural rhythms or "oscillators"

Other oscillators include breathing, propagation of blood through arterial vessels, etc.

Chapter 48

Heart Electrophysiology and Conscious Influence

*T*his chapter describes how heart electrophysiology contributes to the discussion of internal power. It addresses the body's single most important rhythm, which is the regulation of the organ. It will look at the heart as a natural oscillator, the rhythm of which is determined by the interaction between two antagonistic aspects of the autonomic nervous system (ANS). This chapter will also consider how the roles of heart electrophysiology and rhythm increase our understanding of one's ability to direct conscious influence, which is an important aspect of "internal energy."

The heart's rhythm can be observed through a phenomenon known as heart rate variability (HRV). [36] This is the rhythm that is governed by the two competing aspects of the ANS, and the stress vs. non-stress management of the heart's pulse regulation. The two primary reasons that HRV is covered here are:

HRV as a way of observing heart regulation is, arguably, the single most important oscillator, or rhythm, studied by scientists to investigate human potential. Measured in terms of stress vs. non-stress regulation of the heart, this particular rhythm can be consciously directed to help one gain more control over otherwise unconscious factors. This control can, in turn, improve sleep, digestion, openness to love, and attributes associated with mastery of one's internal energy. [37]

HRV can be measured and compared with other natural body rhythms to determine whether or not a person has attained *entrainment,* or synchrony, between rhythms; the present work includes numerous citations referring to special abilities that emerge when an individual is able to synchronize their rhythms. A person's ability to attain synchrony, characterized by frequency "locking" when various biological oscillators become "in phase," is the single most important attribute that might explain the ability to mentally project subtle influence to another person or object, which is one expression of "internal energy." This suggests that HRV is extremely relevant to our exploration of consciously directed "influence."

Since HRV discriminates between stress vs. non-stress regulation of the heart, it also serves as a useful lens for looking at the influence of attitude and emotions on heart health. By extension, these same influences may also apply to one's overall energy field. The scheme of relationships between attitude / emotions, heart health, and a person's overall energy field can be illustrated in the following way:

Diagram 9-6

Attitude and Heart Health

Contribute to a Person's Overall

"Energy Field"

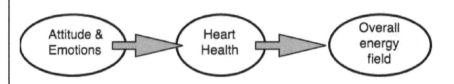

One day, the ability to consciously influence the external environment may or may not be understood as the effect of an as-yet-unidentified subtle energy. Regardless, **consciously-directed influence** will be shown to be related to the attainment of harmony between various biological oscillators, and in particular, the specific oscillation, or rhythm, relating to stress vs. non-stress governance of the heart. I had mixed feelings on whether or not to include this chapter in the present work, as the material addressing aspects of heart physiology could be challenging to those unfamiliar with the technical language of neurology. That challenge increases exponentially when the discussion includes analysis of data in the form of x-y graphs.

When presented with these kinds of discussions, it is difficult for many of us to avoid having our eyes glaze over in response to statistical formulas, plots, and graphs. That said, the material is included here because of how important the heart — in particular, its electrophysiology — is to the discussion of "internal energy," personal empowerment, and general health. Moreover, it is important to the present discussion because mastery of HRV as a biological rhythm is directly related to our ability to exert a measurable influence on an external target, and hence provides meaning to the whole subject of "internal energy."

If this section is too challenging, pass over it for now, and then return when it beckons to you. For many, it is sufficient for the time being to know that attitude and emotions influence the heart's energy field, and that positive thoughts and emotions are an important aspect of a person's journey to mastery.

Two Competing Aspects of the Nervous System

Two competing forces govern the electrical regulation of the heart. These involve the two branches of the ANS: the sympathetic and parasympathetic systems. Those competing branches advance our understanding of consciously-directed "internal energy" because one of them can, within a fraction of a second, take control over the entire nervous system. When this happens without us having made any conscious choice, that aspect of the nervous system can excite the fear and terror pathways of the brain's architecture. In response, the ANS suspends life-sustaining functions, such as healing, digestion, and libido. At the same time, the system dumps tremendous amounts of adrenaline and stress-related hormones such as cortisol into our bloodstream.

Significantly, when the sympathetic, or "fight or flight," aspect of the ANS is dominant, the individual has less access to creative problem-solving. Thus, by comparison, this may go a long way to illuminating those enigmatic qualities associated with "high functioning" and "internal energy."

These two competing branches of the nervous system are independent but interrelated. The balance between the two heart-regulation systems has a lot to do with how a person manages stress, the degree to which one is more protective or open to love, and even the kinds of hormones that are secreted into the bloodstream. However, most importantly, the relative balance of these two competing systems determines the level of stress and the degree to which the person is at peace with themselves and others.

Conscious Control Over the Normally Unconscious and "Habits"

Unconscious practices turn into unconscious habits. However, some conscious practices can also influence the development of unconscious nervous system habits. This principle applies to many areas, but here we will address habits related to the stress vs. non-stress regulation of the heart. For some, their heart-mind-emotion health habits may express themselves as the tendency to make fear-based choices ("It's dangerous to go outside!" or "I must constantly be on the alert for people trying to steal from me," etc.). By contrast, those with less stress-dominant nervous system habits, when faced with a serious challenge, have confidence that they will be able to arrive at the right solution at the right time. This is an attitude that has profound implications for how one "trains" their nervous system. However, to train the nervous system in such a way, especially under pressure, requires attention to one's emotions and attitudes.

Although possessing the same brain and nervous system architecture, the two examples of nervous system responses drawn from two different individuals illustrate how each develops unique nervous system response pattern "set points." They represent different ways a given individual's nervous system learns to respond to both real and perceived threats. While the first case illustrates a dominant sympathetic nervous system stress response, the second illustrates a more active parasympathetic profile, which allows for the creative engagement of neocortex regions of the brain.

A poignant example of the ability to maintain calmness under extreme stress came to my attention during my final assignment in the U.S. Marine Corps. One of my duties each morning was to prepare the overnight messages for the group's commanding officer, which involved prioritizing the messages based on urgency vs. routine. Because we were part of an air wing, a lot of the message traffic had to do with aircraft issues, and one day, a sad but remarkable message came through. It contained details of a fighter pilot and his attempts to save himself and his aircraft as the engine malfunctioned, sending the plane spiraling toward the ocean.

The first part of the message included the pilot's attempts to restart his plane's engine, and then, as it approached contact with the water, the priority shifted to his effort to eject. After the ejection system failed, his transmissions recorded his attempts to activate various other emergency protocols, which the pilot continued with until the moment the plane plunged into the sea.

What struck me most — and this was also the impression of the senior officers that later read and commented on the message — was how the fighter pilot remained extremely calm throughout the entire, ultimately futile, process. It was a remarkable example of calmness under stress. No doubt, that calmness under stress was due to his well-practiced training, but it was also testimony to the way he trained his brain to respond under extreme conditions.

The mind-body habits that a person forms will guide them through life's challenges. They will determine which part of the brain and nervous system tends to become dominant in response to a potentially stressful event.

In Section VII, HRV was described as one of the body's natural rhythms. There, techniques were discussed that could help one attain harmony (frequency locking) between biological rhythms that characterize the state of *entrainment*. As was discussed there, harmony between various body rhythms is a pretty important thing, and one's ability to attain that kind of biological rhythm synchrony can be empowering on several levels. For example, some scientists have documented how *entrainment* — that psycho-physiological harmony of various biological rhythms — when linked to intention, allows a person, without physical contact, to influence the external environment in measurable ways.

Some examples of non-physical abilities, such as Tiller's gas-discharge experiment, were described in earlier chapters. Other examples included research documenting the ability to influence the growth rate of plants, or "condition" a room, along with other non-physical contact abilities. ‡ Furthermore, as was suggested in Section VII, it is believed that the ability to entrain biological rhythms could also explain high-level athletic ability, superior coordination, and control over an opponent in contact sports. These are only a few examples of why the balance between dueling sympathetic-parasympathetic (stress vs. non-stress) regulation of the heart is so important to the development of at least some conscious control over the nervous system.

‡ The last two examples are included in Section X

To emphasize an earlier point, many individuals, including some medical doctors, [38] energetic healers, and shamans currently believe that consciously-directed non-physical influence can affect the physical world in measurable ways. However, at this point, the accepted scientific paradigm holds that this kind of interaction is impossible. Still, for those outlying researchers who are documenting non-contact influence, there is a consensus that there are two requirements for manifesting this ability.

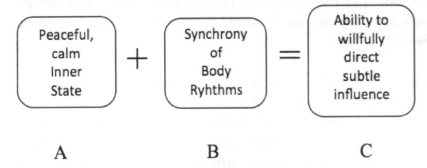

Diagram 9-7

A Peaceful and Calm Inner State, Plus Synchrony of Body Rhythms, Leads to the Ability to Direct Subtle Influence

A   B   C

Illustrated by Boxes A and B in Diagram 9-7, A represents a person who, after having attained a positive emotional-psychological inner state, is then able to B, attain harmony over one's biological rhythms. Note that in the proposed model describing influence, it can be extended only **after** the person has attained the state associated with feelings of inner peace. In other words, the state of calm, characterized by the sense of inner peace, allows for the possibility of B, the ordering of various biological oscillators (rhythms), which after becoming in-phase (harmonic) allows for the individual to exert C, a measurable influence on the external world.

Referring primarily to the stress vs. non-stress regulation of the heart, the two competing aspects of the ANS that control the electrophysiology of the heart are measured by electrocardiograph equipment. An important measure of relative stress vs. non-stress regulation of the heart is HRV, which, for clinicians and researchers, acts as a useful tool for predicting a number of health consequences.

Electrophysiological balance is described in terms of sympathetic (stress) vs. parasympathetic (non-stress) regulation of the heart. [39] Parasympathetic aspects of the ANS are primarily governed by the vagus nerve (Diagram 9-8), which governs control over relaxation and healing, and primarily functions to slow the heart rate. [40]

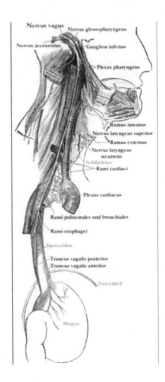

Diagram 9-8

The Vagus Nerve

Source: Wikipedia Commons

By contrast, although it is always active to some degree in maintaining homeostasis — the body's natural tendency toward balance — one of the primary functions of the sympathetic nervous system is to activate the body's "fight or flight" response. This reaction accompanies fear, anxiety, or stress, and is characterized by an extreme hormonal output of the adrenal glands following activation by the amygdala, near the center of the brain. Keep in mind that this is an **emergency state,** triggered by the perception of real or imagined danger.

As an emergency response to a real or perceived threat, the fight or flight response tends to become dominant. This is an important part of our physiology, which is invaluable in situations such as when walking around the corner and suddenly coming face-to-face with a grizzly bear. However, most of us rarely encounter grizzly bears on a daily basis. At the same time, many of us, way too much of the time, signal our body to release these same kinds of emergency stress-survival signals in response to an **imagined** danger. To reemphasize a point made earlier, this system is incapable of determining if those darn flying monkeys are real or not — in either case, it acts as though they are.

When the "fight or flight" survival response becomes habitual, the stress-survival aspects of the ANS achieves dominance too much of the time. Keep in mind that the "fight or flight" state elicits powerful adrenaline and cortisol stress releases, and that because of this adrenaline and other stress-related hormones, as well as the sudden experience of a flood of dopamine in the blood stream, some individuals learn to prefer the feeling of the "rush," and may habitually try to recreate the stressful *signals* / situations that produce that exciting feeling. As a result, a chronic state of stress exhausts the body's adrenaline system, which can be compared to running an engine at full throttle for long periods. Neither engines nor human nervous-immune-endocrine systems are meant to handle this kind of prolonged "emergency," so, unless actually faced by a grizzly bear, or comparable life-threatening challenges, it is helpful to offset these emergency responses with parasympathetic nervous system influences that promote sleep, digestion, healing, love, and, as discussed here, masterful control over one's internal energy.

Although the meaning of internal energy is not yet clearly defined, it is believed that the attributes associated with masterful control over enigmatic force are at least partly determined by the individual's ability to access creative centers of the brain while under stress. If true, it would mean that although adrenaline produces a gross kind of power, a person in a chronic state of anger, anxiety, fear, or any other negative emotion is denied, or has limited access to, superior mind-body abilities that are associated with inner harmony and creative problem-solving. Keep in mind that it is impossible for a person to entrain / harmonize biological oscillators while that individual is in an angry, agitated, or fearful state.

The Effects of Attitude and Emotions on the Heart

Since HRV can discriminate between stress vs. non-stress regulation of the heart, it is useful to examine how attitude and emotion can affect its electrophysiology. For example, HRV can be used to observe the effects of anger and other negative emotions on heart health. Consider the four statistically treated HRV profiles in Diagram 9-9.

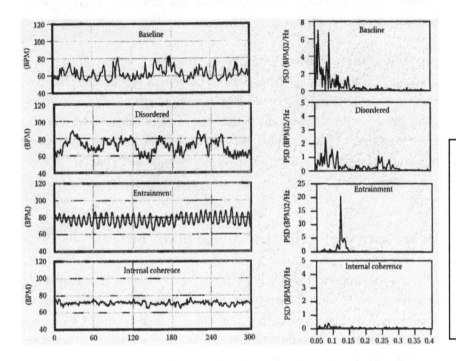

Diagrams 9-9
Four Heart Rate Variability (HRV) Graphs Derived from the Statistical Treatment "Power Spectral Density" (PSD)
From William Tiller, et al., "Cardiac Coherence: A New, Noninvasive measure of Autonomic Nervous System Order."

The four HRV profiles illustrated in Diagram 9-9 are from a study where researchers relied on electrocardiogram readings to evaluate the sympathovagal ** regulation of the heart. The plots that comprise the diagram illustrate the statistical treatment of four HRV profiles, including *normal*, *disturbed* (anger), *entrainment*, and an electrophysiology state that was new to the literature at the time, referred to as *internal coherence*. †

> ** Vagus nerve related stress vs. non-stress regulation of the heart

> † *Internal coherence* is described in Section X.

The graphs shown in Diagram 9-9 represent a mathematical conversion of HRV into a statistical treatment known as power spectral density (PSD). A graphical depiction of the way raw data is derived from sympathetic and parasympathetic regulation of the heart, [41] and an example of how raw ECG data is converted into PSD, is shown in the Endnote. Relying on PSD, Tiller identified three distinct modes: *normal*, *entrainment*, and a new mind-body mode which he labeled *internal coherence*. [42] Diagram 9-9 illustrates the HRV plots of these three distinct modes. (Note that the diagram includes an additional HRV "Disturbed" graph, where the experimental subject was asked to evoke the emotion of anger).

The Negative Impact of Anger and Agitation on Heart Electrophysiology

Consider the "Disordered" HRV plot illustrated in the second box of Diagrams 9-9, which visually demonstrates how persistent negative emotions such as anger affect heart health. The graph shows an HRV profile characterized by an increase in sympathetic (stress-based) influence over the heart, while at the same time indicating decreasing parasympathetic (non-stressed healing and restful) activity. [43] [44] [45]

Supporting the relationship between disturbed HRV profiles and psychological illness, research has shown that this HRV profile, when habitual, can predict psychologically-based illnesses, such as major depression and panic disorders. In other words, in the case of an individual who tends to present an erratic HRV, not only does such a profile indicate excessive stress regulation of the heart, it also suggests psychological disturbance. [46] [47] [48]

Heart Rate Variability (HRV) and Emotion

Tiller studied the effect of emotions on heart health, [49] and in that study, researchers relied on HRV status as one of three objective measures of entrainment that are associated with the synchronization of biological oscillators (rhythms). The study considered the effect of positive emotions on the electrophysiology of the *entrainment* mode, and subsequently the stress vs. non-stress regulation of the heart. As previously described in Section VII, to study these effects, experimental subjects were required to achieve states associated with calm and inner peace.

By way of review, researchers relied on the Freeze Frame ® emotional self-management technique. As discussed earlier, Freeze Frame was developed by the HeartMath Institute to teach clients how to disengage mentally from negative emotions by focusing on the feeling of positive emotions directed to the area of the heart (See Section VII, Box 7-7). The graphical depiction of the HRV profile associated with *entrainment* — a state characterized by frequency locking (harmony) between the HRV waveform and other biological oscillators — is illustrated in the third box of Diagrams 9-9.

Noting how emotional self-management and positive thinking leads to *entrainment*, Tiller states, "In general, we have found that sincerely experienced positive emotional states, such as appreciation, care, and love lead to the entrainment mode." [50] This is an important point that will be returned to later.

Tiller's definition of the phenomenon clarifies how *entrainment* can be understood when HRV attains frequency locking with other biological oscillators:

At the electrophysiology level, the experimental data shows that there is an abrupt shift… [in an individual's] fairly erratic HRV-plot with time to an almost pure sine-wave type of HRV-plot with time, indicating a special type of entrainment of heart and brain. If one is simultaneously measuring body respiration and pulse transit time for blood flow from the heart to the fingertips, one also notices that these rhythms also entrain to the new HRV rhythm; that is, the electrophysiological state of the body is becoming coherent. [51]

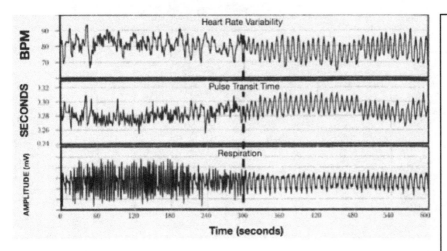

Tiller's description of how paying attention to one biological rhythm tends to bring other rhythms into harmony confirms my experience teaching *entrainment* to athletes. As described earlier, while attending to another biological oscillator (in that case, pulse transit), the practitioner could induce the same kind of synchrony between biological rhythms that Tiller's subjects relied on using the Freeze Frame technique.

While studying the relationship between mental-emotional states and the effect they have on heart health, Tiller was particularly interested in the therapeutic benefits of positive emotion. He points out that although the detrimental effects of negative emotional states on cardiovascular function have been known for some time, benefits associated with positive emotional states have not been well studied. Looking at the link between mind-body state, emotions, and heart health, researchers were able to demonstrate that while emotions such as anger negatively impact the heart health, certain positive emotions, for example how, like love and appreciation, protect the organ.

Diagram 9-10

Synchronization of Three Biological Oscillators (in Phase) First introduced in Section VII, and repeated here for the convenience of the reader, the diagrams show three biological oscillators: Heart Rate Variability (HRV), pulse transit time, and respiration becoming synchronized. The graphs illustrate the attainment of synchrony between three biological oscillators when a study participant practiced an emotional self-management technique. Compare the left side of three graphs (before application of the emotional management technique) to the right (after application). From William A. Tiller, "Cardiac Coherence: A new, Noninvasive Measure of Autonomic Nervous System Order."

Positive Emotions in a Heart Emergency

Observing the effect of attitudes and emotions on heart health, Tiller also observed that learning to change negative emotions into positive ones provided a protective advantage to the heart. Upon examining how the electrophysiology of the heart responds to emotional states, Tiller found that the use of positive thoughts and attitudes not only provided a protective influence, but also suggested that techniques designed to alter an individual's attitude and emotions could be useful as first aid in a heart-related emergency. These thoughts are reflected in Tiller's belief that intervention like Freeze Frame could be "beneficial in the treatment of hypertension and reduce the likelihood of sudden death in patients with congestive heart failure and coronary artery disease." [52]

Chapter 49

Three Rules of the Heart and Magnetic Power

*L*ike the old Cherokee man teaching his grandson about the competing wolves in our hearts, each of us has a dark and a light side. It is empowering to often remember and reflect upon those competing traits, because they remind us that choices are constantly available to us. We make choices throughout the day, every day, sometimes in conscious ways, but often through small, barely conscious acts.

Calmness in the heart of movement is the secret to all power. [53]

This quote, adapted from the words of the Taoist abbot to John Blofeld (cited in Section VIII), was offered as an explanation of how two warrior-monks could have escaped unscathed from the violent sword contest that Blofeld had witnessed. The match between the two swordsmen had been so ferocious that it left Blofeld "sweating with anxiety," as he expected the contestants to be torn apart as a result of their mutual combat. Not only does the instruction hold one of the most important secrets for practitioners of the fighting arts, but it is equally instructive beyond the study of close combat.

The aphorism represents the optimal way to handle any difficult situation. It expresses a masterful ideal to aspire to: the ability to maintain the state of equanimity when under stress. It allows us to more easily access creativity and to problem-solve, and it is the key to attaining the state of flow. However, in order to reach this level, the individual must remain emotionally detached and clear-minded. It is a lofty goal that few of us can naturally attain, although most of us can learn, to some degree at least, to attain this state through practice. Then, it will be available in an emergency. It is a habit that develops like a muscle. The more we practice the skill, the more natural it becomes.

Habits that help develop the art of calmness in the "heart of movement" require the training of one's nervous system to respond to small challenges in a calm way. Such a habit is developed slowly and gradually, until eventually one is able to actuate the mind-body magnetic field.

The Mind-Body Magnetic Field

Although a clear definition of internal energy is not yet available, one day, part of its definition will be shown to be related to the body's electromagnetic fields. Our ability to work with these fields has been a consistent theme throughout the present work; the power of one's magnetic field is reflected in Valentine Greatlakes's healing art of "magnetic stroking," introduced in Chapter One. It was the underlying principle of life energy that fascinated the nineteenth-century magnetists, and it remains the focus of the esoteric yogas of the Tibetan lamas and *neidan* Taoist alchemists / meditators. The common link between these disparate traditions is the participant's ability to observe and work with sensations within the body that feel, and often act, like strong magnetic energy.

At times, when we become aligned with the magnetic energy centers, healing can be administered via a simple touch. Likewise, its healthful benefits are employed by the master acupuncturist when a powerful effect is obtained by a single perfectly placed needle. Whether or not we are able to manifest this degree of magnetic alignment depends on the kind of habits we cultivate.

Like Blofeld's warrior monks, the potential of that sense of EM fields within the body is expressed by the person who is not swept up by the internal winds of emotion, but instead participates with the surrounding forces as though they are the calm and centered eye of a hurricane. At this juncture, it is useful to consider how the *three rules of the heart* and the principle of *calmness in the heart of movement* help provide a definition of internal energy and magnetic power.

A Magnetic Charge

A number of factors contribute to a person's ability to access the power of their body's magnetic fields. As will be discussed in Section XI, there are physical influences, such as posture, that contribute to the magnetic field. However, thoughts and intentions also produce subtle magnetic charges that affect one's overall magnetic field.

Earlier, I mentioned that I had the opportunity to assist Dr. Huy Hoang at the Natural Health Medical Center in Los Angeles. Although I had studied the power of intention through classes and seminars long before the "New Age" term had been coined, it was the briefest of interactions with Dr. Hoang that one day nudged me toward paying closer attention to the way one's thoughts produced an electromagnetic charge and response in the mind-body field.

That day, as I walked by the doctor's office while his door was open, I saw that he was sitting behind his desk eating lunch. I asked if I could step in and was invited to have a seat. I noticed that he had a little bit of the sniffles, and I said something like, "I'm sorry you're a little sick." Much later, I realize the power in his response: "I don't put any attention on it."

Over the years, his answer has stayed with me, serving as a constant reminder of how he refused to place a mental-emotional charge on his "being a little sick" because, integrated into the mind-body electromagnetic / neurological responses of the mind-body, less "charge" to the negative idea of being sick facilitates a faster positive ability to heal. It is a simple, but nevertheless important, lesson that is expressed in Matthew from the New Testament:

> For where your treasure is, there your heart will be also. [54]

In this context, I interpret the meaning to be: pay attention to every thought. Every little thought, attitude, opinion, and inner dialog produces a bit of electromagnetic charge. *Where you put your "charges" determines how your energy field develops.*

The beauty of this principle is that once you realize that your degree of personal power is reflected through "charges" and where you place them, just as with the choice of which wolf to feed in the old Cherokee's story, you become careful about where you place those little electromagnetic charges. How you think becomes important; how you judge or think about others becomes important; how you deal with pain, frustration, or being "under the weather" becomes important. Being aware of this rule allows you to more consciously choose where to put those "charges," and provides the ingredients for a powerful mental and physical medicine.

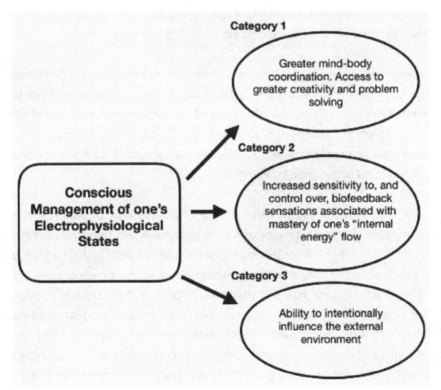

Diagram 9-11

The Conscious Management of One's Electrophysiological States

This section covered mind-body-nervous system habits, each of which, in their own way, concerns the conscious management of one's electrophysiological state. The management of that state can be viewed through three expressions, illustrated by the arrangement shown in Diagram 9-11. The three categories each represent a particular way of managing and consciously applying one's mind and body energy.

Category 1 includes aspects of the brain and nervous system that develop from habits related to the brain's creative centers; the skills represented by this category are not based on forcefulness. In athletics, it is epitomized by the skilled athlete's ability to implement the perfect skill at just the right moment. However, this category also represents problem-solving skills associated with the brain's prefrontal cortex. In contact sports, this category is expressed through "light touch" skill, and creativity when one is under the pressure of contest. It is a bit of the magic dust that creates legends.

Category 2 concerns the personal empowerment that emerges from the practice of regularly paying attention to one's biofeedback *signals*. Whether conscious or unconscious, or through the practice of meditation, *qigong*, or yoga, adeptness in this category expresses itself as the ability to synchronize one's biological rhythms. A common theme presented throughout the present work is that a special kind of power is awakened when a person pays attention to internal *signals*. This category is concerned with results, and since results are what matter, at this juncture, it is irrelevant whether the sensitivity in question is only attunement to one's inner rhythms or the flow of *qi*, or *prana*, through the body. However, what is of utmost importance is that the practitioner learns to pay attention to and then merge subtle *biofeedback sensations* with their "energetic" practices. In the practice of energetic meditation, for example, awareness of subtle sensations in the body becomes a valuable training aid.

However, if the energetic practice is in the context of a moving discipline, the most beneficial results are available when the practitioner attends to subtle biofeedback *signals* in the midst of moving practice, such as *t'ai-chi* or *aikido*, **while in motion.** In that case, it is the organizing effects derived from working with the mind-body system in a feedback-based practice that allows access to the greatest expression.

Category 3 has to do with that controversial question of whether it is possible for a human to produce a measurable effect upon an external target through non-physical means. Examples cited earlier include a *qigong* master's ability to influence the growth rate of bacteria in a Petri dish, the ability of an energetic healer or shaman to impact a patient's health through non-physical treatment, and the possibility that a group of meditators might be able to affect the growth rate of plants. Personally, I believe these are possible, and that, in some cases, credible evidence exists that suggests this is so. Whether the underlying cause of these kinds of demonstrations might one day be established as "internal energy," or some other form of yet-to-be-determined human influence, remains to be seen. That said, regardless of the explanation that will one day be forthcoming, what is clear is that the ability to demonstrate these kinds of remarkable feats will, in the future, be understood in terms of the individual's ability to harmonize their inner electrophysiological state. Whether actuated through ritual, prayer, *qigong*, or meditation, extended human abilities will be shown to be closely tied to the attainment of inner coherence and order.

An evolved level of mind-body mastery can come to fruition only when this advanced state of harmony can be summoned at will, having been forged into habit. This realization leads us to consider the words of Yoda:

> *Yes, a Jedi's strength flows from the Force. But beware of the dark side. Anger, fear, aggression; the dark side of the Force are they. Easily they flow, quick to join you in a fight. If once you start down the dark path, forever will it dominate your destiny, consume you it will, as it did Obi-Wan's apprentice.* [55]

Conclusion to Section IX

*T*his section considered two opposing mind-body orientations. Viewed through three perspectives: *open-closed, love-hate,* and *growth-defense.* The chapters in this section looked at the meaning of those orientations under different influences, such as the role of the thymus, posture, and heart electrophysiology.

The way we think affects our access to healing, power, and openness to love; a truth that is common to each of these orientations. Mental habits are not neutral; every one of them triggers electrophysiological and immune system responses that can be either positive and health promoting, or negative and restrictive. They also contribute to one's relative coherence or lack of internal harmony. As such, when "internal energy" is finally understood, it will no doubt be shown to be inseparable from one's spoken and internal dialog.

In many examples, true mastery of the more subtle arts, including examples from calligraphy and the internal martial arts, depends on the degree of communication the individual experiences between their heart and brain.

> Lately, I hear more and more people across different disciplines and walks of life talking about the heart. People seem to be waking up to the wisdom of letting their hearts guide them, finding it leads them to more joy and fulfillment. This is news that does my heart good.
>
> Deborah Rozman [56]

In an online article, Deborah Rozman describes how, in her former work as a psychologist, she would often ask her clients to dialog back and forth between their heart and their mind. Through this process, two different sets of ideas emerged. According to Rozman, "The heart spoke from genuine feeling and authenticity, in the present," while the mind "spoke from opinions, fears, shoulds and shouldn'ts." [57]

Through the back and forth process she used in her practice, her clients would eventually reach an epiphany, often, as Rozman explains, realizing that "their heart's voice was their true self, a voice that offered both more intuition and common-sense intelligence."

For Rozman, this wasn't surprising, since the heart has a brain of its own. She explains:

> Yes, the human heart, in addition to its other functions, actually possesses a heart brain composed of about 40,000 neurons that can sense, feel, learn and remember. The heart brain sends messages to the head

brain about how the body feels and more. When I first heard about this scientific research, it intuitively made sense. I had felt for a long time that the heart has its own mysterious way of knowing.

Rozman's therapeutic approach is based on research conducted by the HeartMath Institute. The institute, along with other researchers (some cited earlier in this section), has investigated how the heart contains a network of several types of neurons, neurotransmitters, proteins, and support cells, like those found in the brain proper. [58] Thus, for many applications, the answer to the question of full access to one's potential anti-aging factors and general success is found by attaining increased synchrony between the heart and the brain.

In summary, the three perspectives covered in this section — *open-closed, love-hate,* and *growth- defense* — can all be characterized in terms of a healthful and empowered relationship between the heart and the brain. In each of these examples, it comes down to choosing which wolf to feed.

Endnotes

1 Adapted from a quotation found in John Blofeld's, *The secret and sublime: Taoist mysteries and magic*, E.P. Dutton, 1973 p. 125.

2 Adapted from the Cherokee story, http://www.firstpeople.us/FP-Html-Legends/TwoWolves-Cherokee.html

3 Consistent with comments in the opening pages of the present work, although for the most part, Chinese characters are transliterated using the *pinyin* system of transliteration, there are a few exceptions where Chinese is Romanized in the Wade-Giles style. Examples of Wade-Giles transliteration in this section are Chuang Tzu and *Tao*.

4 Lipton, Bruce, *The biology of belief: Unleashing the power of consciousness, matter, & miracles*, Hay House, 2016, p. 146. See also, Lipton, B.H., K.G. Bench, et al [1991] "microvessel endothelial cell transdifferentiation phenotypic characterization." Differentiation 46:117-133.

5 Walsch, Neale Donald, *Conversations with God*, Penguin Putman, Inc., New York, NY pp. 18-19.

6 I was fortunate to have been able to attend a presentation by Hans Selye in 1979, a few years before he passed. Still, all these years later, I sometimes reflect on the things he shared with us at that time. Rest in Peace, Dr. Selye.

7 Although the thymus gland is understood as shrinking (involution) in adulthood, tissue function in the area of the gland continue to promote immune system-related functions, even through old age. See Mackall CL, Punt JA, Morgan P, Farr AG, Gress RE. "Thymic function in young / old chimeras: Substantial thymic T cell regenerative capacity despite irreversible age-associated thymic involution." Eur J Immunol. 1998; 28:1886–1893.

8 http://dev.biologists.org/content/141/8/1627.full

9 http://www.20somethingallergies.com/boost-immune-system-thump-thymus/

10 Diamond, John, MD, Life energy: *Using the meridians to unlock the power of your emotions*, Athena Books, Paragon House, NY, 1990, p. 20.

11 Diamond, p. 15.

12 Ibid., p. 16.

13 Ibid., p. 25.

14 Ibid., p. 26.

15 Ibid., p. iii, vii, xv.

16 Ibid., p. 26.

17 Newberg, Andrew MD, *How God changes your brain: Breakthrough findings from a leading neuroscientist.* Ballantine Books, NY 2010, p. 201.

18 Stein, Diane, *Essential psychic healing: A complete guide to healing yourself, healing others, and healing the earth.* Google e Book p. 48.

19 Diamond, John, MD, *Life Energy: Using the meridians to unlock the power of your emotions*, 1990, Athena Books, Paragon House, NY, p. 10.

20 Fleet, Thurman, DC, *Rays of the dawn: Natural laws of the body, mind, and soul,* Concept therapy Institute, San Antonio, TX 2000 p. 29.

21 Diamond, John, MD, Life Energy: *Using the meridians to unlock the power of your emotions*, 1990 Athena Books, Paragon House, NY, p. 10.

22 Diamond, p. 8.

23 Ibid., p. 10.

24 Ibid., p. 4.

25 Ibid., p. xiv.

26 Diamond describes *"qi* flow" to be indicative of balanced brain hemispheres. See Diamond, p. 93; see also Diamond, p. xiv.

27 Ibid., p. 42.

28 Ibid., p. 44.

29 Ibid., p. 43.

30 Ibid., p. 44.

31 Ibid., pp. 46-47.

32 In this usage, adopting the term for a mechanical device that limits speed by restricting the flow of gasoline to an engine.

33 Stevens, John *The philosophy of aikido*, Kodansha America, New York, 2001, p. 24.

34 Dorsher

35 Dorsher, Peter, "Myofascial meridians as anatomical evidence of acupuncture channels," *Medical Acupuncture*, Vol. 21, No. 2, 2009, p. 4

36 Detected as a measure of heart health called heart rate variability, or HRV, this is derived from analysis of beat-to-beat regulation of the heart, and can discriminate between sympathetic (stressful) vs. parasympathetic (non-stressful) regulation of the heart.

37 Heart Rate Variability (HRV) is viewed as a valuable resource for researchers, since it stands alone as a multi-faceted barometer of health and a predictor of mortality. Measured in terms of beat-to-beat variation (in R-R intervals), heart rate is regulated by sympathetic (stress-based) and parasympathetic (non-stress-based) input to the sinoatrial node of the heart. R to R variability refers to peak points of an electrocardiogram reading of heartbeat recorded by electrocardiogram. HRV is able to discriminate stress vs. non-stress regulation of the heart.

HRV is not determined by increase or decrease of heart rhythm, but by a statistically generated plot of sympathetic vs. parasympathetic regulation of the heart. One value of HRV is its usefulness as a reliable predictor of cardiovascular disease and likelihood of a second heart attack. In another application, it enables the clinician to predict the development of diabetic neuropathy sooner than with other available methods. (Comi G Sora, MGN, Cianchi, A, "Spectral analysis of short term heart rate variability in diabetic patients, J AUTON NERV SYSTEM 1990, 30:S45-S-50). Lowered HRV is also associated with aging, lowered autonomically mediated hormonal response, and increased incidence of sudden death. (Singer Dh, Martin, et al., "Lower heart rate variability and sudden cardiac death." J Eletrocardial. 1998). In other studies, reduced HRV predicted increased risk for all-cause mortality and in post-heart attack patients, studies have shown reduced HRV can predict risk for subsequent mortality. (From Circulation 1994-Tsuji 878-83).

38 Citations of medical doctors supporting this notion are included in Section X.

39 Purves, Augustrine and Fitzpatrick, in Neuroscience. 2nd edition, introduces the regulation of cardiovascular function in the following way:

"The cardiovascular system is subject to precise reflex regulation so that an appropriate supply of oxygenated blood can be reliably provided to different body tissues under a wide range of circumstances. The sensory monitoring for this critical homeostatic process entails primarily mechanical (barosensory) information about pressure in the arterial system and, secondarily, chemical (chemosensory) information about the level of oxygen and carbon dioxide in the blood. The parasympathetic [non-stressful] and sympathetic [stressful] activity relevant to cardiovascular control is determined by the information supplied by these sensors."

From Purves D, Augustine GJ, Fitzpatrick D, et al., editors., *Neuroscience*. 2nd edition, Sunderland, 2000. By agreement between the publisher and copyright holders, the more complete introduction to autonomic regulation of the cardiovascular function can be read at http://www.ncbi.nlm.nih.gov/books/NBK11075/

40 Also see, https://www.thecut.com/2019/05/i-now-suspect-the-vagus-nerve-is-the-key-to-well-being.html

41

A. Power in the low-frequency (LF) region indicates mostly sympathetic activity, with some hormonal influence on HRV; in the mid-range frequency (MF) region, power can be influenced by either sympathetic or parasympathetic activity, but is predominantly parasympathetic, whereas in the high-frequency (HF) region it is only a result of parasympathetic influence on HRV. The MF region, around the 0.10 region, is often referred to as the baroreceptor band because it reflects the blood pressure control feedback signals sent to the brain. B shows a typical power spectrum of the HRV waveform. Σ, sum of inputs; SN, sinus node.

Borrowed from Diagram 1, Tiller, et al., "Cardiac coherence: A new, non-invasive measure of autonomic nervous system order," *Alternative Therapies*, 1996.

42 Researchers used computers to evaluate stress vs. non-stress regulation of the heart, then data was collected and converted into PSD to create the HRV graphical representation of heart health.

43 Lindquist, A, et al., "Heart rate variability, cardiac mechanics, and subjectively evaluated stress during simulator flight." *Aviation and Space Environmental Medicine*, 1983; 54:685-690.

44 Kamada T., et al., "Power spectral analysis of heart rate variability in type As and type Bs in mental workload." *Journal of psychosomatic medicine*, 1992;54:462-470.

45 Kollai, M, "Cardiac vagal tone in generalized anxiety disorder," *British journal of psychiatry*, 1992;161:831-835.

46 Yeragani, VK, et al., "Decreased HRV in panic disorder patients: a study of power-spectral analysis of heart rate." *Psychiatric Research* 1993; 46:89-103 (As cited by Tiller in A., et al., "Cardiac Coherence: A new, noninvasive measure of autonomic nervous system order," Alternative Therapies, 1996, Vol. 2, No. 1 pp. 52-65).

47 Yeragani, VK, et al., "Heart rate variability in patients with major depression." *Psychiatric research* 1991; 37:35-46 (As cited by Tiller in A., et al., "Cardiac coherence: A new, noninvasive measure of autonomic nervous system order," *Alternative therapies*, 1996, Vol. 2, No. 1 pp. 52-65).

48 Thayer, JF, et al., "Autonomic characteristics of generalized anxiety disorder and worry," *Journal of sociology and biological psychology*. 1995; 37:1-11 (As cited by Tiller in A., et al., "Cardiac Coherence: A new, noninvasive measure of autonomic nervous system order, *Alternative therapies*, 1996, Vol. 2, No. 1 pp. 52-65).

49 Tiller, William A., et al., "Cardiac coherence: A new, noninvasive measure of autonomic nervous system order, *Alternative therapies*, 1996, Vol. 2, No. 1 pp. 52-65.

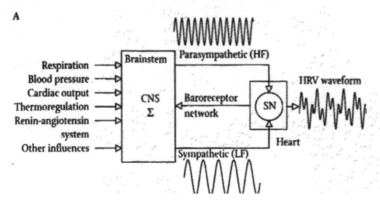

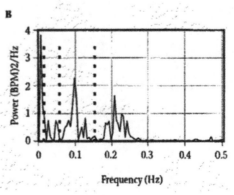

50 Tiller

51 Tiller, William, PhD, et al., *Some science adventures with real magic,* Pavior Publishing, Walnut Creek, CA 2005, p. 10.

52 Tiller, William A., et al., "Cardiac coherence: A new, noninvasive measure of autonomic nervous system order," *Alternative therapies,* 1996, Vol. 2, No. 1 pp. 52-65.

53 Adapted from a quote in John Blofled's, *The secret and sublime: Taoist mysteries and magic,* E.P. Dutton, 1973 p. 125.

54 Matthew 6:19-24.

55 http://thinkexist.com/quotation/yes-a_jedi-s_strength_flows_from_the_force-but/264916.html.

56 https://www.huffpost.com/entry/heart-wisdom_n_2615857

57 https://www.huffpost.com/entry/heart-wisdom_n_2615857

58 https://www.heartmath.org/research/science-of-the-heart

Section X
The Power of Intention

Where the mind goes, the qi follows; where the qi goes, the body follows.

— *The Guanyinzi* [1]

X

The Power of Intention

Introduction to Section X

*T*he Guanyinzi is among the oldest and most esoteric of Taoist alchemy texts. As suggested by the author, or authors, of the classic that introduces this section, they believed that *qi* is far more than just a bodily substance. For them, it was a force that responded to one's will and intention. This section looks at those interactions in the hope of finding more clues that could lead to a meaningful definition of "internal energy."

六內外合

Six Inner and Outer Relationships

Liu Nei Wai He

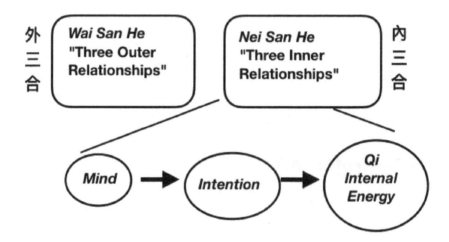

Diagram 10-1

The Six Inner and Outer Relationships

The three "inner relationships" are "mind," which leads

"intent," which in turn leads "qi" internal energy.

Chapter 50

Intention in the Traditional Chinese Model

*I*n traditional Chinese medical textbooks, *will* and *intention* are described as guiding one's internal energy, [2] [3] while references to the relationship between intention, "mind," and internal energy can be found in both ancient and modern sources (the principle is expressed through the *nei san he* (内三合), or "three inner relationships," formula shown on the right side of Diagram 10-1). These, together with the *wai san he* (外三合), or "three outer relationships," comprise the Taoist energy-alchemical formula, *liu nei wai he* (六内外合), or "six inner and outer relationships." [4]

The three outer relationships describe the diagonal holographic connections between various aspects of the body; for example, the right elbow holographically relates to the left knee, and the left wrist to the right ankle, etc. * In contrast, the "three inner relationships," shown on the right of the diagram, illustrate the relationship between mind, intention, and internal energy. That aspect of the formula describes how *mind* activates the source of *qi energy*, which then "leads" awakened *qi* energy through the power of *intention*.

    * These were described in Section III

Intention

When a more precise definition of "internal energy" becomes available, it will no doubt encompass the role of intention. However, the meaning of intention itself is so closely linked to internal energy in the context of subtle human-directed influence that the two become indistinguishable.

<u>Chapter 51</u>

Scientific Investigation of *Intention* in the West

*I*n the 1960s, Dr. Bernard Grad conducted the earliest modern scientific study of intention. His investigations focused on whether or not subtle, human-directed, "mental energy" could be used to influence plant growth. Relying on objective measures, such as increases in chlorophyll production, Grad documented how human intention could indeed influence plant growth. The first study considered whether "energetically charged" water could affect plant growth, assessing results in terms of chlorophyll content and other factors. Ultimately, Grad found that plants receiving the "treated" water flourished in comparison to other plants.

The "treated water" in Grad's experiments was stored in a container, and then handled by individuals who were instructed to send positive intention into it. Since the growth of these plants could not be explained as having occurred by any other influence, Grad concluded that the increase in plant growth had resulted from the power of positive intention produced by those handling the water.

With the treated water appearing to be the crucial variable, Grad's next study tested his hypothesis in a new way. Since the previous study had suggested that water in a closed container could promote vitality, he then wanted to find out if it could likewise be "negatively affected" by certain individuals.

In the subsequent study, rather than using "intention healers," Grad asked psychiatric patients to hold bottles of water, the contents of which were later fed to the plants in the experiment. With one puzzling exception, results showed that plants given water handled by mentally ill patients produced no, or marginal, improvement in growth rate, and in some cases declined. However, there was one notable exception, as one plant in the second study not only flourished, but accelerated in both seed germination and growth.

Looking deeper into the case of the outlier plant, Grad found that the psychiatric patient who had been assigned its water had learned the details of the experiment beforehand and had thus been inspired to handle the bottle in an untypical manner. The female patient cradled the bottle in her arms, as if it were an infant, and imagined sending "loving energy" into the water. Grad concluded that the improved plant growth was due to the patient's intention to "send love" into the water. [5]

Defining Intent

Intent is both powerful and important. Earlier chapters addressed the role of intention as it relates to a practitioner's ability to consciously direct an energetic force, and it has also been discussed how some energetic healers have the ability, based on their intent, to extend either healthful or negative energy. One definition of intent for research purposes is offered by Marilyn Schlitz, Ph.D., who defines intention as a "mental state directed toward achieving a goal." Schlitz further distinguished between intention and desire, defining intention as being based on "a certain amount of reasoning." [6]

Two Areas of Intention Research

1. Human-Directed Consciousness and Influence Over Electrostatic Inertial Forces

Support for the proposition that intention can function as a human-directed natural force has been the focus of classified U.S. Government research. According to one former researcher, investigators have been able to demonstrate that intention can be used for military and intelligence purposes. However, for obvious reasons, details are difficult to obtain. Nevertheless, in a July 2005 radio interview with retired U.S. Army Major Ed Dames, conducted by Art Bell, it was disclosed that an "operator's" focused intention may be able to affect electronics at a distance.

According to Dames, a researcher, author, and instructor in *remote viewing*, U.S. military intelligence experiments into the power of intention have successfully "affected" targeted electronics at a distance of hundreds, or even thousands, of miles away. The proposed theory for explaining this kind of interference is based on the notion that focused intention can influence the magnetic field of a "target." Describing the research that he conducted on behalf of various U.S. government agencies, Dames reports that those trained in the technique were able to weaken the electromagnetic field of targeted electronics. He also discloses that the magnetic fields of some electronic devices, such as pacemakers or clocks, are especially sensitive to this kind of influence, and explained that in these cases, the operator's interference "acts at the atomic level by influencing electrostatic inertial forces." [7]

It has been known for some time that certain individuals possess an especially uncanny, and unconscious, ability to influence electromagnetic instruments.

A notable example is the Nobel Prize winner in physics, Wolfgang Pauli (1900- 1958), who was known to project such a strong interfering influence on electronics by his mere presence that he had to stay at least 200-feet away from his laboratory, or else the electronic equipment would malfunction; hence the term, "the Pauli effect." [8] [9]

2. *Psychoenergetics*

"Psychoenergetics" is a new field of study, pioneered by Stanford University *professor emeritus* William Tiller. ** The term describes the study of intention, and in particular how it can be demonstrated to influence the physical world in measurable ways.

However, the claim that human, non-physical, influence can measurably impact the physical world has not yet been accepted by mainstream science, meaning that those involved in this area of research must continually navigate various hurdles. This is a result of the current accepted scientific paradigm stating that it is impossible for a person, through emotion, intent, or other non-physical means, to influence a well-designed experiment. Thus, any data from experiments that demonstrate the potency of intent, even in the most rigorous laboratory settings, are often ignored or dismissed out of hand by rigidly orthodox researchers.

> ** Aspects of Tiller's work on psychoenergetics and the power of intention were introduced earlier. For example, Section VII included a description of *psychoenergetics* research, which documented how an individual, who after having attained the requisite state of inner mind-body harmony (*entrainment* or *internal coherence*), could intend to interact with, and thereby initiate, an electrostatic response in a gas-discharge device. [10]

Conditioning Space

An intriguing area of study that investigates the ability of human-directed non-physical influence to interact with the physical environment involves "conditioning space" experiments. Tiller pioneered a number of studies in this area that demonstrated how a group of experienced meditators could alter the pH of water in a room, through a process he called *conditioning*. In their initial investigation and follow-up studies at external locations, Tiller and his collaborators documented how trained meditators, such as healers, engaged in deep, heart-felt prayer or meditation could alter or "condition" a room in measurable ways.

For investigative purposes, one criterion used to test whether the meditator's intention could influence a room's environment was the measurable change of the pH of water kept in the room. In the first instance, meditators were able to alter the levels to a 1-1.5 pH shift, and follow-up studies showed that this kind of remarkable influence by meditators could be replicated in experiments conducted in numerous other locations by other investigators. [11]

Commenting on Tiller's observation that a group of meditators could "condition space" in this way, author Lynne McTaggart, writing in *The Intention Experiment,* explains how meditators could create a 3-5 degree F oscillation in water or air temperatures, which persisted in the conditioned rooms for periods up to six months. [12] [13]

Another observation made by researchers in the experiment is worth noting. Scientists recorded that the degree of water oscillation that produced the 1-1.5 pH shift was dependent on whether or not the water was exposed to the magnetic North or South Poles. In the case of South Pole orientation, the pH went soaring upward (more base), whereas exposure to the magnetic North Pole caused the pH to decrease (becoming more acidic) and rhythmic changes in the pH to dwindle away (a pH of 7 is neutral). [14] Taggart records Tiller's reaction to the finding that meditators could induce these kinds of pH changes:

> Tiller felt as though he had somehow entered into a twilight zone of higher energy and that he was witness to a system with an extraordinary ability to self-organize. Indeed, the oscillations he had measured had all the hallmarks of a Bose-Einstein condensate — a higher state of coherence. Up until then, scientists had created a Bose-Einstein condensate only in highly controlled environments and at temperatures approaching absolute zero. But he had managed to create the same effects at room temperature and from a thought process captured in a rudimentary piece of equipment. [15]

Results of other psychoenergetic studies support the theory that intention can act as a *natural force.* One involved a trained meditator's ability to cause a strand of DNA suspended in an aqueous solution to move in a spiraling way. In that study, researchers found that "moderate to long-time practitioners of the [meditation / *entrainment* [16]] technique could *intend* to interact with an aqueous solution of DNA in a vessel several feet away from the body and cause the DNA to unwind or to wind more tightly by choice." In another study of intention, researchers demonstrated that focused intention could increase fruit fly larvae growth rate. [17] At this juncture, it is useful to note how results like these challenge the (current) conventional scientific model.

Physical Matter and Consciousness

The current orthodox scientific paradigm states that any carefully controlled experiment should be free from human "interference" produced by mind, intention, or emotion. Furthermore, the paradigm states that if any results are derived from subtle human mental-emotional interactions, they are considered irrelevant and dismissed as "artifacts," i.e. technical flaws that produce misleading or confusing data.

However, human interference can be subtle and pervasive, and accounting for this influence in scientific investigations is challenging. Consider the phenomenon called *expectancy*, which works on the principle that researchers tend to find whatever results they are seeking; the oft-cited example of this kind of unintended human interaction being the early discussions of the nature of light. There, it was problematic that whenever a researcher looked for evidence of light being a particle, data emerged in support of that hypothesis. Likewise, when a researcher looked for evidence of light as a wave, data emerged in support of that view, too. In other words, researchers tended to find evidence to support whatever their hypothesis happened to be.

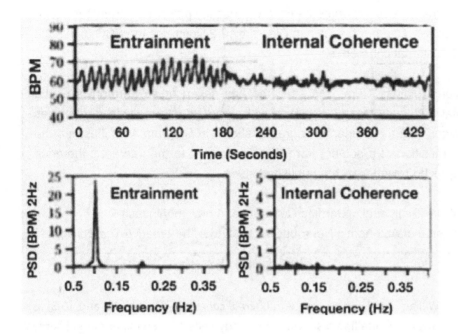

Diagram 10-2

Graphical Representation of One Subject's Transition from Entrainment to *Internal Coherence*

Internal coherence mode is identified by intentionally produced, very low-amplitude waves across the entire HRV [heart rate variability] spectrum compared with the baseline. The graph shows the ECG amplitude spectrum for internal coherence. (Note, supporting information on how this graph was produced is provided in the Endnote. [18])

Originally presented in Section VII, this graph is presented again for the convenience of the reader.

William Tiller, et al., "Cardiac Coherence: A new, noninvasive measure of autonomic nervous system order," *Alternative Therapies*

Chapter 52

Zen Mind?

*T*his chapter describes a special mind-body "flow" state that allows an individual to access the power of intention more effectively. The state is called *internal coherence*, and it is related to *entrainment*. By way of a brief review, *entrainment* was previously defined as the ability to bring one's biological rhythms into synchrony.

Internal Coherence

The Internal coherence mode is identified by an intentionally produced, very low-amplitude signal across the entire heart rate variability power spectrum compared with the baseline. The graph shown in Diagram 10-2 illustrates the ECG amplitude spectrum for internal coherence.

As Dr. Tiller explains: "Here, one sees the first seven or so harmonics of the fundamental frequency clearly displayed with very few intermediate frequencies having a significant amplitude." The graphs shown in Diagram 10-2 illustrate the conscious transition of a subject from the entrainment to the internal coherence mode. Graphs borrowed from the published study.

William Tiller, et al., "Cardiac Coherence: A new, noninvasive
Measure of Autonomic Nervous System Order," *Alternative Therapies*

Box 10-3

William Tiller coined the term *internal coherence* (Boxes 10-2 and 10-3) as a means of labelling a special mind-body state that an experimental subject could consciously shift into while in the *entrained* state. Represented in terms of the measure of heart health known as heart rate variability (HRV), Diagram 10-2 illustrates one subject's shift from the *entrainment* to the *internal coherence* mode. Characterized by a state of equanimity, an individual in the *internal coherence* mode exhibits a distinct heart electrophysiology profile.

While one is in the *internal coherence* mode, sympathetic and parasympathetic (stress and non-stress) outflow from the brain to the heart is reduced to such a degree that the oscillations in the HRV waveform become nearly zero. Electro-physiologically, the *internal coherence* state is characterized by an HRV profile within the frequency domain (amplitude) spectra of 10-second epochs of the electrocardiograph (ECG). The *internal coherence* state appears to be a special mode, exhibiting an HRV profile with a very low-amplitude signal across the entire HRV power spectrum compared with the baseline. *Internal coherence* provides electrophysiological evidence for what might be referred to as *Zen mind*. Tiller describes *internal coherence* as the state where:

> One's internal mental and emotional dialog is largely reduced, and one becomes aware of an inner electrical equilibrium ... In this state, the sympathetic and parasympathetic outflow from the brain to the heart is reduced to such a degree that the oscillations in the HRV waveform become nearly zero. [19]

When a person is engaged in the *internal coherence* mode, the heart's electromagnetic activity achieves a more stable pattern associated with increased parasympathetic (non-stress and mind-body healing) activity, and a host of health and rebuilding activities take place. These include an increase in DHEA and health-promoting hormones. Simultaneously, there is a decrease in stress-related factors in blood serum.

It is important to distinguish between clinical vs. research applications of HRV profiles. In this light, there are two different, and unrelated, types of "small" to "near zero" profiles. As described here, *internal coherence* refers to an experimental subject's ability to produce a very low amplitude *signal* across the entire HRV power spectrum compared with the baseline. In this application, the procedure refers to the low-frequency profile being exhibited by a trained, healthy individual who *consciously* shifts into the special mind-body mode. Significantly, a shift like this is associated with the subject's ability to induce the experiential state that Tiller calls *amplified peace*. However, it is important to note that such a state is distinct from the pathological patient's similar HRV profile. Discussion on this distinction is provided in the Endnote. [20]

For practitioners of mind-body disciplines, *internal coherence* is of particular interest because, while in this mode, an individual is able to achieve a special experiential state referred to as *amplified peace*. This experiential state is characterized by a reduction in "internal dialog" and a profound sense of peace. Could this be the same state described by long-time practitioners of meditation and contemplative prayer? Here is Tiller's definition of *amplified peace*:

> Amplified peace distinguishes an inner state in which a deeper than normal state of inner peace and centeredness is felt. In this state, one also has a sense of standing on the threshold of a new dimension of awareness, with a sense of inner electrical equilibrium and awareness that one has accessed a new domain of intuition. As with any experiential state, words do not adequately describe it. Also, one enters this state for relatively short periods. However, with practice of staying focused on the heart, time in this state can be increased. It may be similar to moments at the beach or in the forest when one feels an especially deep contact with nature or with oneself that is beyond one's normal experience. In such moments, one may find answers to life's deeper issues or problems. [21]

The potentially life-enhancing nature of *amplified peace* raises several questions, with first among these being whether this kind of physiologically triggered experiential state, might explain the timeless wisdom of the sages. Secondly, is it possible that a person who experiences such a state touches the hem of the atemporal and aspatial — the reported mystic's experiences beyond time and space?

Due to the potential of this state to provide insight and affect the practitioner in profound ways, one must wonder if it was this kind of experience that has impelled the most contemplative of our fellows, since the dawn of time, to leave society. Could the desire to dwell in this blissful state be the motivation to seek out the stillness and quiet of remote places like mountains or deserts? The third question has to do with whether internal coherence might be the source of the deep inner peace exhibited by holy persons.

The answers to these questions may help us understand the age-old quest of the saintly recluse, not only to commune with nature, God or the Tao, but perhaps also to experience the pleasurable state associated with optimized electrophysiology.

It is also useful to consider the meaning of the individual's sense experience while in a state of *internal coherence*, characterized by "an inner electrical equilibrium." Perhaps, as suggested in Section VII, early *t'ai-chi* practitioners might have linked their experience of sensations (feelings they identified in terms of the flow of *qi* through their bodies) with the ability to manifest more proficient skills. In this light, it is plausible that such sensations, similar to those reported by subjects in Tiller's study of an "an inner electrical equilibrium," could be of the same class described by pioneers of *t'ai-chi* and other forms of moving meditation? Although *t'ai-chi* pioneers did not have access to modern bio-physiological language, it is nevertheless possible that they experienced the same class of sensations. In fact, it is quite likely that late-nineteenth century Chinese martial artists would have identified their experience of "an inner electrical equilibrium" as the internal flow of their *qi*.

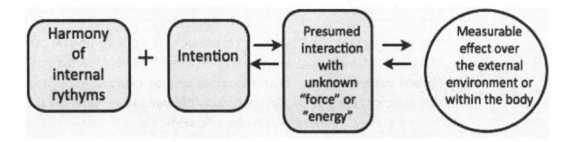

Diagram 10-4

Chapter 53

Is it *Energy* or *Intention?*

*T*his chapter considers distinctions and interactions between *energy* and *intention*. As an introduction to this discussion, it is useful to highlight two points that have been emphasized throughout the present work. First, a succinct definition of internal energy has so far not been forthcoming. Second, conclusive evidence that such a force exists as part of presently described physical reality is not yet available. However, some scientists have obtained strong evidence that the power of directed intention can indeed influence a physical target. At this point, it is useful to make a few more comparisons between intention and the notion of an invisible, human-directed force in the form of *qi, ki, prana,* or internal energy by any other name.

When the meaning of subtle, human-directed influence becomes clearer, another part of its definition will include reference to **use**. Consider how a battery has no purpose until connected to a light bulb. It has (unrealized) potential energy, yet this carries little meaning outside of the work that it can (potentially) perform. In other words, until it is brought into productive purpose, it is as if it doesn't exist. Likewise, whether in the context of *qi, prana,* internal energy, or intention, these terms have no meaning outside of the context of *use.* In all these examples, the phenomenon requires a human being to "get in touch with it" in order for it to enter the realm of "reality."

Some research examining the power of *intention* as a force of nature has already been discussed, including Grad's study of how directed intention could influence plant growth. Other studies describe how a practitioner, relying on intention, could direct a DNA strand suspended in an aqueous solution to spiral either clockwise or counterclockwise depending on the practitioner's intent.

Results like these suggest that intention research should be included as part of subtle or internal energy investigations. In terms of human-directed, non-physical influence, the two phenomena may be indistinguishable. Diagram 10-4 illustrates the sequence of consciously-directed human intention and "internal energy," with emphasis on the following areas:

1. Based on experiments described earlier, [22] in order to apply *intention* so as to influence the external environment, an individual must first harmonize their biological rhythms. The ability to attain synchrony between biological rhythms can be either conscious or unconscious. Methods employed to bring rhythms consciously into harmony include emotional self-management techniques like Freeze Frame ® and Entrained Pulse Training. †

Examples of unconscious entrainment include the contemplative practices of experienced meditators, such as Buddhist monks, who, as a result of their habit of non-judgment, inner peace, and stillness, naturally entrain their biological rhythms. However, whether purposeful or unconscious, the individual would be characterized as having attained a high degree of a practiced inner peaceful state associated with psycho-physiological rhythmic harmony. The harmony between biological oscillators is the necessary platform from which human intention can be extended to a target in the physical environment.

2. The second requirement is that the practitioner **intends** to influence the target. For example, as demonstrated in the intentional triggering of an electrostatic charge in a gas-discharge without physical contact, Tiller demonstrates that **both** synchrony of biological rhythms and the intention to interact with the device were necessary to influence the external target. [23]

The third box of Diagram 10-4 represents the point where an explanation for what is taking place in terms of *energy* becomes ambiguous. This represents the point where the practitioner feels certain conditions in their body, and, depending on specific cultural traditions, learns to identify these subjective feelings in terms of "conscious control over the movement of subtle energy within, or external" to the body. The equivalent sensations occur in Tiller's psychoenergetics (intention) experiments, where scientists noted that while in *entrained* or *internally coherent* modes, experimental subjects report similar sensations of "inner electrical equilibrium." [24] Unfortunately, it has not yet been established that there is, in fact, such a thing as "conscious control over internal energy," and wishing will not make it so. To restate, although there are reports of feelings associated with control over "energy," the meaning of these perceived sensations has not yet been determined.

† both techniques were described in Section VII.

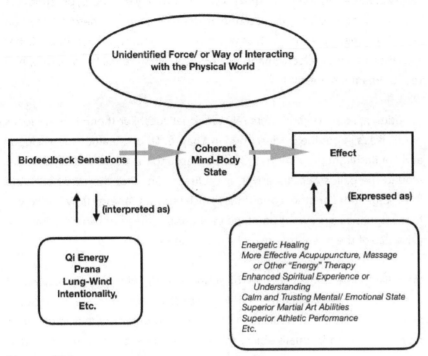

Diagram 10-5
Interpretation of Biofeedback Sensations and Effect

Chapter 54

Interactions with an Unidentified Force

*A*s suggested in Diagram 10-5, it is possible that the energetic "flow" reported by the *qi* master, yogi, and meditator may not actually be a measurable flow of energy within the body in terms of our common physical dimension, [25] but is instead sensory stimulation and feedback occurring in response to the practitioner's particular way of interacting with invisible / immeasurable elements. For the yogi, *qigong* master, or Tibetan lama, the interaction with this kind of feedback system may indeed feel like a "flow of energy." However, the meaning assigned to sensations such as the feelings of magnetic-like forces, pressure, and heat variations within the body are subjective, and vary depending on the practitioner's cultural beliefs. Those beliefs influence the practitioner to explain the sensations they feel in terms of *qi, ki, lung, mana* or connection with a sacred source.

No doubt the *qigong* master, the Tibetan lama, and the Taoist meditator truly experience sensations they identify as internal energy, and like the scientists Reichenbach and van Helmont, they, too, are convinced of the reality of these sensations as a *force of nature.* In many traditions, practitioners learn to identify what they describe as the flow of *qi* or "energy" based on sensations that they feel, such as warmth moving through their body. Other sensations may be electromagnetic, or electromagnetic-like, pressure, and real, or imagined, heat.

In addition, some practitioners rely on visual cues. For them, like the focus of Crookes's experiments described in Chapter One, the amorphous clouds and / or flashlight projections that appear around the body, and in particular around the palms and fingertips, are telltale signs that they are observing flow, stagnation, or other conditions associated with "energy flow." However, to reemphasize a previous point, perceptions like these still do not prove the existence of the phenomenon of internal energy.

Most likely, the perceived flow of subtle energy within the body, willful direction of non-contact healing to another, or even the ability of some martial arts masters to weaken an opponent through *disruptive information* represents the individual's ability to deploy a subtle dimensional force that is beyond our present comprehension. This may well be the grand mystery appreciated by the early Taoists, who expressed the elusive nature of the puzzle in the *Tao Te Ching:*

> The Tao that can be weighed and categorized is not the true Tao
> Whatever name you may give it, it is not its true name.

However, bodily sensations are one thing, and the ability to equate one's personal experience of sensation to what is, at least at the present time, an enigmatic and yet-to-be-documented force is quite another. Until we know more about the meaning of these sensations, it is good practice to be cautious of identifying them as *qi, ki,* or *prana.* These kinds of experiences may represent aspects of the life force, but then again, they may not. My preference is to minimize labeling that could limit future understanding and, perhaps, even greater experience. The quotation from the Taoist classic might be the closest description possible of a subtle, life-spiritual force that surrounds us, which can be breathed and swam in, but is never seen or grasped.

Conclusion to Section X

It is also ... consciousness-raising and a hope-raising ... for humanity in that it shows people how to use their own intentionality to bring about inner self-management at emotional and mental levels so that beneficial electrophysiological, hormonal, energy and structural changes develop in their own bodies. Such changes quite naturally lead to a significant growth in the individual's consciousness and have significant implications for human health and societal functioning.

—Ernest P. Pecci, MD [26]

There are strong experimental observations that support the notion that human will can interact intentionally with physical matter. In the above quote from the introduction to Tiller's work, Science and Human Transformation: Subtle Energies, Intentionality, and Consciousness, Ernest P. Pecci, MD describes the bio-physical and electrophysiological implications linked to the practice of intentionality.

<u>Afterword to Section X</u>

Infrastructure Changes Related to the Practice of Mind-Body Arts

*I*s it possible that one's intention can interact with the body in yet-to-be-understood ways? If so, what are the mechanisms that might promote this kind of function? Moreover, how does the nature of this interaction contribute to our discussion of "internal energy?"

The present section considered the meaning of intention through various perspectives, inculding the contexts of the traditional Chinese medical model, modern research, and the *"Zen mind"* state. However, what has not yet been addressed is whether focused intention, when matched with certain physical practices, might alter the practitioner's mind-body experience. This Afterword considers the possibility that intention could infuse the material constituents of the body to such a degree, that the physical body becomes altered. Based on this premise (of intention merging with, and altering, physical structure), the merging of intention with one's physical practice might aid in the ability to "get in touch" with, or master, the expression of *qi, ki,* or *prana*.

Although the cliché of "body-mind unity" is often repeated, there are few examples that suggest a mechanism by which to explain how these physical and amorphous entities interact. An alternative view of acupuncture meridians offers some insight.

The Commingling of Intention and the Meridians

Tiller suspected that acupuncture points and meridians may function as an embedded antenna array. Section XI will consider the physical structure of the meridians and how, due to their piezoelectric characteristics, they could be arranged in order to promote bio-electrical coherence. Section XII includes speculation on the nature of the myofascial meridians and their cross-dimensional interactions. However, at this juncture, it is useful to note another possible relationship between intention and the meridians.

It may be significant that when certain practices are done slowly, and with highly-focused concentration, the meridians, due to their piezoelectric characteristics, could interact with one's consciousness and intention in a special way. This may represent the merging between what could be thought of as an interstitial space between consciousness and the physical realm. Such a merging is presumed to take place in an

Is it possible that the practice of movement arts, for example *hatha* yoga, performed in "slow-motion" and involving the direction of focused concentration, coupled with the alteration of gentle stretching and applied tension along elements of the meridian system, allows intention to infuse with physical practice? If so, these modalities represent the fusion of intention with the meridians, which speaks to the possibility of the mind-body being defined by a third construct that is not quite physical nor mental / emotional.

Subsequently, if the meridians are responsive to focused intention, two things occur. Through the action of the meridians, not only is the power of one's intention enhanced, but the action would theoretically interact with an individual's psychoenergetic structures in a special way.

Psycho-energetic Structures?

Earlier sections described subtle body energy structures, such as the *chakras* and the *dan tian*. In keeping with the topic of the present section, it is useful to consider how focused intention might also influence those structures. For the moment, let us consider structures, such as the *chakras* and the *dan tian*, as places where the mind-body stores a kind of *template*.

Inspiration for this speculative model is derived from William Tiller's description of the way consciousness influences "structural changes." Tiller introduces us to the notion through his concept of "spirit interfacing with the physical:"

> It has often been said human evolution is characterized by and limited by the penetration of spirit into dense physical matter so that the more spirit there is present in the dense body of an entity, the higher is its consciousness. [27]

Psycho-structural Development

Tiller describes a relationship between what he calls "transformational changes" and a person's "dense and subtle matter of their body." In relation to this theory, it is useful to consider whether the advancement of an individual's subtle structures might be brought about through *intentionality*. In this light, the result would be development based one's actions, thoughts, and attitudes. Subsequently, this intentionality produces a more "refined structure" in which changes are induced. In turn, the refined structure allows a "greater inflow of spirit." [28]

An interesting thought exercise is to adapt Tiller's model of "consciousness (or 'spirit') influencing dense matter" to the theory that psychophysiological structures, acting as templates, exist and can be engaged intentionally.

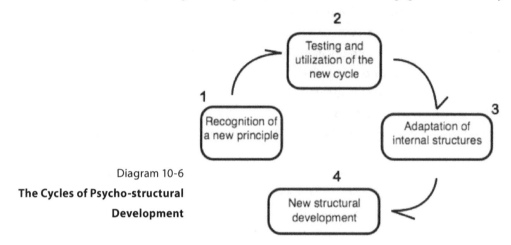

Diagram 10-6

The Cycles of Psycho-structural Development

Illustrated in Diagram 10-6, the model seeks to explain the influence of *intentionality* upon psycho-energetic structures through four steps:

1. Recognition of a new principle.

2. Testing and utilization of the new "cycle."

3. Adaptation of internal structures via the repeated utilization of the principle, which actualizes potential.

4. New structural development allowing a new level of function, which in turn leads to the recognition of another new principle, and so on.

Just as the model describes how intention might merge with meridians, in a similar fashion, intention might also influence those templates, offering justification for why practices such as *t'ai-chi* are often thought of as forms of "moving meditation." Regarded in this way, the effects derive not so much from the slow-motion execution, but as a result of the influence of the practice on one's psyche. Thus, when regularly practiced and matched with intention, they potentially exert a profound influence on the individual. Theoretically, that effect is due to the merging of intention practice with gentle and sustained myofascial tension. This is the action which acts upon, and builds, those psychophysiological infrastructures.

How, then, does this kind of practice influence changes in one's psycho-emotional, or "subtle energy," structures? Tiller suggests:

> The [human being] applies that in-dwelling consciousness, through its focused intentionality, in the various acts of its daily life.

Tiller goes on to explain:

> By the [person's] actions, thoughts and attitudes, transformational changes eventually occur in the dense and subtle matter of the body which can produce a refined structure allowing a greater inflow of spirit (or produce a degraded structure which does the opposite).

Templates

Psycho-physical-subtle energy structures involve the storing of "templates." If the mind and body are inseparable, then a mechanism is necessary to store and exchange information between the two entities. For this connection to take place, the medium of a psychoenergetic structure is required that is capable of sharing data with both aspects of the individual.

This view may provide more insight into the meaning of subtle energy structures, such as *chakras* and *dan tian*, and how they interact with mind-body subtle energy fields. Accordingly, this suggests that the body reflects the mind, and the mind reflects the body through templates inscribed in those centers.

Functionally, the templates represent a person's evolution and the ways that one sees, responds to, and interacts with the world. In psychology, this modeling of human experience, called *schema,* is a construct used to explain personal developmental and emotional progress.

Endnotes

1 From the *Guanyinzi* passage, 心之所之则气从之气之所之则形应之

2 Ishida Hidemi, "Body and mind: The Chinese perspective," Livia Kohn (Editor) *Taoist meditation and longevity techniques. Center for Chinese Studies*, University of Michigan, 1989, p. 55.

3 Essentially, the same formulation that describes the relationship between intention and *qi* appears elsewhere in the classics, such as, 意到氣到 (Where intention goes, the *qi* will follow), 氣到勁到 (Where the *qi* goes, strength goes), and 意領氣氣催形 (Where intention leads the *qi*, the body follows). Note, there is some lack of consistency in the use of the terms, "intention," 意, mind 心, and spirit 神. Also note that the polysemic nature of intention 意, which in different compounds and contexts would be translated as "meaning," "idea," "thought," and "intention."

4 The *liu nei wai he* (六內外合) formula first appears in print in 1927. Readers of Chinese can view a discussion comparing the "outer" with the "inner" relationships on the web page https://wenku.baidu.com/view/17e4a3ca31126edb6e1a10e1.html

5 As cited by Gerber, Richard, MD, in *A practical guide to vibrational medicine. Quill*, An Imprint of Harper Collins Publications, 2001, pp. 296-298.

6 Schlitz, M. PhD. "Distant healing intention: Definitions and evolving guidelines for laboratory studies." *Alternative Therapies in Health and Medicine.* May/June 2003. Vol. 9. No. 3., p. A31

7 Art Bell Radio interview of Edward Dames, Retired Major, U.S. Army, Coast to Coast AM radio show, July 19, 2005.

8 Swann, Ingo, *Psychic Sexuality: The bio-psychic "anatomy" of sexual energies*, Panta Rei/Crossroads Press, 1998/2014 Kindle Cloud Reader, Location 1211.

9 From Wikipedia: "The Pauli effect was named after Pauli's bizarre ability to break experimental equipment simply by being in the vicinity of the devices. Pauli was aware of his reputation and was delighted whenever the Pauli effect manifested. These strange occurrences were in line with his investigations into the legitimacy of parapsychology, particularly his collaboration with C. G. Jung on the concept of synchronicity." https://en.wikipedia.org/wiki/Wolfgang_Pauli

10 The earlier described "gas-discharge experiment" documented how a person physically separated from the device could "intend" to interact with, and cause, the instrument to register an electrostatic charge when a person, in a state of entrainment **intended** to interact with the device. See Tiller, William, *Some science adventures with real magic*, Pavior, Walnut Creek, CA pp. 11-12

11 Tiller, William, *Some science adventures with real magic*, Pavior, 2005, p. 28

12 McTaggart, *The intention experiment: Using your thoughts to change your life and the world*, Free Press: Simon and Shuster, NY, pp. 117-119.

13 Also see Tiller, William, *Conscious acts of creation: The emergence of a new physics*, Pavior 2001, 175, 180- 216.

14 McTaggart, *The intention experiment: Using your thoughts to change your life and the world*, Free Press: Simon and Shuster, NY pp. 117-119.

15 McTaggart, p. 121.

16 Entrainment is described in Sections VII and IX.

17 Since there is significant data available studying the rate of fruit fly larvae growth, it is an easily accessible and reliable factor to observe the effects of an experimental variables and compare results to a baseline.

18 From the published study. William Tiller, et al., "Cardiac coherence: A new, noninvasive measure of autonomic nervous system order," *Alternative therapies*, Vol. 2:1 1996.

19 Tiller

20 Tiller's comments from the cardiac coherence study are germane:

"In untrained individuals small to near-zero HRV, as just described, is an indicator of a potentially pathological condition or aging because it connotes loss of flexibility of the heart to change in rate or decreased flow of information in the autonomic nervous system. However, in trained subjects, it is an indication of exceptional self-management because their HRV is normally large and the shift into the internal coherence mode is a result of their entering the amplified peace state. This state is different from a pathological condition underlying lowered HRV (in such cases the HRV is always low). The connection between emotional state and HRV could account for the occasional observation of lower HRV in otherwise healthy individuals. This observation has detracted from the clinical utility of HRV analysis for unequivocally predicting disease."

21 From 'Glossary of New Terms," Tiller, et al., "Cardiac Coherence: A new, noninvasive measure of autonomic nervous system order," *Alternative Therapies*, 1996.

22 For example, Tiller's gas discharge device experiments.

23 As described in Section VII.

24 Tiller, William, et al, "Cardiac coherence: A new, non-invasive measure of autonomic nervous system order," *Alternative Therapies*, Vol. 2:1 1996.

25 Speculation on another dimensional model to account for "internal energy" is included in Section XII.

26 Ernest P. Pecci, from the introduction to *Tiller, William, Science and human transformation: Subtle energies, intentionality, and consciousness*, p. x, Pavior Books, 1997.

27 Tiller, William, *Science and human transformation: subtle energies, intentionality and consciousness*, Pavior 1997, pp. 145-146.

28 Tiller

Section XI
Energy and Form

Energy follows Form

XI

Energy and Form

Introduction to Section XI

Energy and Form

*T*his section addresses the intersection of "internal energy" and bio-mechanics, and some of the ideas that will be presented are unquestionably controversial. For example, it will be discussed how a fighter's ability to utilize "internal power" is not necessarily just a result of something that might be referred to as "energy," but is simultaneously related to the use of efficient bio-mechanics. Other aspects of our conversation on the relationship between "energy" and "form" will focus on how a person's morphology (body shape) influences access to power, conscious control over normally unconscious muscle groups, and an important principle of body suspension and support known as *tensegrity*.

When a person is said to have "strong energy" or an "energetic personality," these characterizations could be referring to several different things. For example, it may be that the individual is perceived as charismatic, or socially engaging and positive. However, a person who projects a powerful sense of presence might also be characterized as having strong energy due to their posture, or the way that they move with effortless grace.

This section considers how posture and bio-mechanics contribute to the meaning of "internal energy." Thus, in many of the cases that follow, it is difficult to distinguish what might be referred to as "energy" from efficient bio-mechanics. Consider, for example, the practice of holding one's head upright in correct "suspended" posture. * This posture habit is known to promote clear thinking, improved confidence, and an increased sense of well-being. Should such a practice be considered a postural influence, a bio-physical training method, a *qigong* exercise, or a combination of all three?

*Covered in Chapter 55

Another example of the relationship between posture and "energy" is found in John Diamond's description of how the way one holds their chest influences the thymus and thymus function, which in turn contributes to the balance and flow of *life energy*. **

There are more than a few examples like the one just mentioned, where the influences of posture and other bio-mechanical processes become indistinguishable from *qigong*, meditation, and yoga "energy" practices. Here, we take a closer look at those grey lines between internal power, life energy practices, and bio-mechanics, giving consideration to the adage found in internal energy literature that "energy follows form." This maxim is expressed through the masterful display of *t'ai-chi,* yoga, meditation, and numerous other disciplines, and the proceeding pages will examine the relationships between these practices and one's "internal energy," which can be expressed by the following two-way diagram:

** John Diamond's description of the relationship between posture, the holding of the chest in relation to the thymus, and "internal energy" was covered in Section IX.

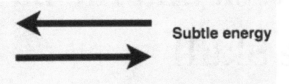

Diagram 11-1
The Relationship between "Form" and "Energy"

At this juncture, it is necessary to again consider the principal theme presented throughout the present work. Previous chapters have included suggestions that a definition for the term "internal energy" will one day be established, but, at present, a succinct definition is not available. While some suggested definitions describe the phenomenon to be electromagnetic, or a merger between various yet-to-be-defined electromagnetic-like interactions, other theories suggest that examples of "internal energy phenomenon" might be understood more accurately in terms of an individual's ability to attain a kind of body-mind super efficiency or synchrony.

Other proposed definitions include a model of "internal energy" for both healing and martial arts, which might be explained in terms of an exchange of *information* between the practitioner and another person. However, when a reliable definition is forthcoming, the attributes associated with an individual's "internal energy" will no doubt be understood in relation to the principle that:

"energy follows form"

It is easy to appreciate how good posture habits might lead an individual to be described as exuding strong and balanced "internal energy" and charisma. Based on my experience studying and teaching mind-body arts, and many years of working with athletes, pain patients, and my own continuing practice of self-healing following a debilitating back injury, I've learned an important lesson. It has to do with how attention to the mutual relationship between energy and form helps some individuals to succeed, others to recover from chronic pain, and, in the case of athletes, to realize their full potential.

Chapter 55

Energy Follows Form:
The Neck and the Base of the Skull

*T*his chapter considers the relationship between energy and form in the context of the soft tissue support at the juncture between the base of the skull and the top of the neck.

The discussion has been designed to address three key talking points:

1) An overview of new research which suggests that correct posture applied to this area may improve concentration and focus.

2) How one's attention to this area enhances athletic ability and improves reaction time.

3) A *qigong* / posture practice that detoxifies the upper lymphatic system.

The Structures and their Support

Figures 11-2
The Suboccipital Triangle
Indicated by the darkened areas on the skeleton drawing, these three pairs of small muscles manage the relationship between the cranial base and top of the cervical spine.
Image: *Wikipedia Commons*

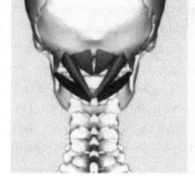
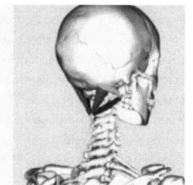

The Suboccipital Triangle

Correct support of the base of the skull above the neck increases mental and physical energy. This effect is due to the tensional soft tissue support provided by a unique set of structures at the base of the skull, known as the suboccipital triangle.

Shown in the illustrations provided in Figures 11-2, the three sets of small muscles that form the suboccipital triangle do more than just support the weight of the head; their shock-absorbing function also protects the area of the spine from stress or injury. The six muscles are also responsible for minute movements of the head over the top two of the neck's seven vertebrae, and the proper maintenance of this muscle group enhances one's athletic ability, meditation, "energy training," and mental focus in general.

It is important to understand that extreme movements of the head can temporarily compress or lengthen the sensitive structures that pass through this junction. Those areas include vascular, neural, and lymphatic elements that pass between the base of the skull and the neck. It is also worth noting that because of the twelve pairs of cranial nerves that travel through the area, improper posture can stress this very important passageway by reducing the available space for the spinal nerves and other conduits to pass through.

It is well understood that straining the suboccipital muscles with poor posture can result in headaches, [1] and that chronically poor posture can compress a nerve at the cranial base. However, if one maintains the correct degree of suspension-tension in the area, this aids in attaining full brain-spine physiological potential. Further contributing to the maximizing of one's potential is the ebb and flow of cerebral spinal fluid through the portals. Thus, as with the relationship between posture and energetic meditation that was described in Section V, the optimal rhythm of the cerebral-spinal fluid on its journey from the ventricles of the brain to the sacrum is also thought to be related to the "natural" athlete's unconscious access to superior performance.

Reaction Time and Athletic Performance

Diagram 11-3 depicts the posture of a mixed martial arts (MMA) fighter in the early days of our working together. His training goal was to incorporate internal martial arts principles that could add to his skill in fighting contests, and his head-forward posture was the first issue we addressed. Based on my coaching experience, his "head falling forward to the point of least effort" habit had prevented him from attaining his highest level of athletic performance. Becoming aware of, and then maintaining, the correct "naturally suspended" orientation at this location improves both one's ability to concentrate and reaction time. With a little practice, one can learn to observe this postural habit in oneself and others. ‡

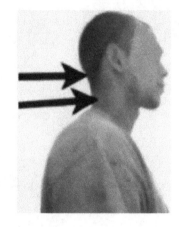

Diagram 11-3
Postural Support of the Base of the Skull above the Neck
Due to the unconscious tendency to succumb to the influence of a denatured † lifestyle, unless otherwise corrected for, the fascial-tensional support system of the head tends to collapse forward to the point of least effort. Arrows in the diagram indicate extreme lines from poor habitual posture that impede optimal nerve and blood supply between the brain and the top of the cervical spine.
† Referring to the pernicious influence of the "flat and level" - See Chapter 60

‡ To evaluate one's own posture, it is important to either have a photo taken from the side, at shoulder height, or to arrange a set of mirrors so that one can look forward yet see their posture from the side. Turning the head sideways to look in the mirror is not useful, since the muscles will alter head-over-shoulder relationships when twisting.

Photos 11-4
Three Presentations of the Head Support above the Neck
Left: A student's initial default posture. Middle: Working on it. Right: The student's default posture goal

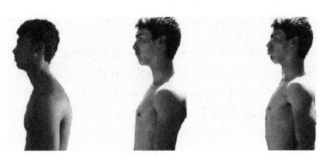

Photos 11-4 includes three images of a student early in his training. The left shows his "default" orientation at the start, the middle was the student's new "working" default posture a few weeks later, and the right represents the ideal orientation that he is striving to develop as his default. It is also useful to note that proper vs. less-than-ideal posture presents a strong, often unconscious, judgment-reaction by others.

After taking the photos, I sent a note to the student and asked him to imagine that he was an employer looking to hire a new employee; he was also to pretend that the three photos were of three different people. I instructed him to imagine that he didn't know the candidates in the photographs, and to choose which one would he thought might be more intelligent. Finally, still viewing himself from the perspective of an employer, he was asked to choose which individual he would be more likely to hire. The author now invites the reader to ponder the same set of questions in relation to Photos 11-4.

Especially prevalent in young people today, largely because of habits acquired from chronic smart phone use, the poor posture shown in Diagram 11-3 and the left of Photos 11-4 is, regrettably, becoming the norm. Unless corrected, an extreme forward collapse angle of the neck impacts optimal reaction time and performance in other areas. The inclined posture habits shown in those two examples is also found in many aspiring MMA competitors, who, without their conscious awareness of why, are unable to gain the success they seek. It is one of the hidden reasons why so many young athletes fail to achieve their potential, an idea that is supported by the comments of one exceptional athlete I worked with:

I have been training at Olympic / professional levels in sports for several years, and I have always been concerned with using every trick to improve my reaction time. It seemed like when participating in ball sports such as basketball or tennis, my mind would see the ball and would know where to go, but sometimes my body would take (what felt like) another half a second to react. I always attributed my slow reaction to a lack of training but seemed never able to improve. After the first week of posture-neck position training with Master Bracy, my athletic performance improved greatly. For some reason, by only changing the way I held my neck, I noticed a big change in that there was almost no mental effort to move to the ball. It also seemed like my body began to react without my mind even thinking about it. My physical response and reaction improved and became consistent. Those simple exercises increased my performance in several sports.

— Christian

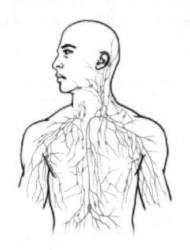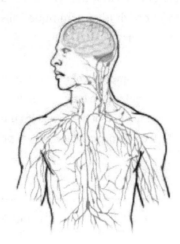

Diagrams 11-5

New Discovery: The brain connects and is integrated with the lymphatic system in a broader way than previously understood

Left: Architecture of the brain-lymphatic system as previously understood.

Right: Newly discovered relationship between the brain and lymphatic system. Previously, the two systems were viewed as separate entities. Image borrowed from University of Virginia Patient Services,

Newsroom June 1, 2015. [4]

Support for the notion that correct posture might promote brain detoxification and rejuvenation comes via a recent discovery, which demonstrated a new understanding of the brain's relationship to the lymphatic system. Researchers believe that the finding will have important implications for long-term brain health, describing it as a "game changer."

Consider the drawings of the upper torsos shown in Diagrams 11-5. Published in the journal *Nature*, they describe a new-found relationship between the brain and the body's major disease fighting network: the lymphatic system. According to the study, the discovery "opens new areas of research and transforms existing ones." Researchers characterized the discovery as filling a "major gap in understanding of the human body." [2]

The study details the discovery of functional lymphatic vessels that line the dural sinuses, thus enhancing our understanding of how the brain flushes toxins from the system, which authors of the study characterized as having "substantial implications for major neurological diseases." The research findings center on the way endothelial cells, carrying both fluid and immune factors, circulate through the deep cervical lymph nodes. As the researchers explain, this is an entirely new understanding that "may call for a reassessment of basic assumptions in neuro-immunology;" one which applies to the "study and treatment of neurological diseases ranging from autism to Alzheimer's disease to multiple sclerosis."

The article describes how scientists, while searching for T-Cell gateways into and out of the meninges, * discovered functional lymphatic vessels lining the dural sinuses that transported endothelial cells, which were demonstrated to carry both fluid and immune cells between the cerebral fluid and the lining of the brain. [3]

* Comprised of dura mater, arachnoid mater and pia mater, the meninges contain the brain and spinal cord. The previous understanding of the function of the meninges is that its purpose, along with the transport of cerebrospinal fluid, was to protect the central nervous system.

The lymphatic system, a system of lymph fluid and lymph nodes, is vital for:

- **Elimination of toxins**. The lymphatic system can be aptly described as the garbage disposal of the body, and is responsible for filtering and eliminating toxins.

- **The immune system.** The lymph nodes house a high concentration of white blood cells that increase when the body is fighting off illness or infection.

- **Weight loss and weight management**. Toxicity is a huge part of the weight loss puzzle. If you don't support your lymph system, you will have even more trouble losing weight and gaining muscle tone.

Source: Lauren Geertsen NTP [**]

Box 11-6

** Newsroom[5]

One Point Brain Clarity *Qigong*

The One Point Focus Qigong is based on traction and soft tissue support of the neck. It is an easy exercise that demonstrates the benefits of proper head-neck posture, and it is also useful as a brain detoxification technique. Illustrated by the skeletal drawing shown in Figure 11-7, the practice involves holding the head level and **completely still,** while focusing on a point in the distance for several minutes at a time. The exercise reliably improves focus, while simultaneously releasing tension in the shoulders, neck and other areas.

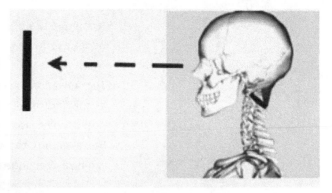

Figure 11-7

Base of the Skull and Spine Support *Qigong*

Begin the exercise by focusing on a single point in the distance. Although the initial practice time can be shorter, the goal is to be able to hold the head still with the eyes focused on a single point for ten minutes, or longer. While performing the technique, it is important to remain as still as possible. Allow your eyes to relax and the vision to "soften," as you direct your attention to the target.

Initially the exercise may be practiced while sitting, but with practice it can be performed while standing or "holding postures" (Section VIII). If possible, the focal point should be a natural object, like a flower or leaf; if focusing on a wall, imagine looking through it, into the distance that you imagine exists beyond. As you practice the exercise over the next few days or weeks, gradually increase the time spent in the posture, until eventually you can remain still and not move the eyes for ten minutes, and then a little longer again. Ten to twelve minutes are the magic numbers, where practitioners start to notice changes in their upper body, such as the shoulders relaxing, sinuses draining and the dissipation of neck tension.

After several minutes engaging the technique, practitioners will often report the feeling of tugging, or traction, in the muscles around the area of the neck and / or upper shoulders. As you continue the exercise, try not to allow even the slightest movement of your eyes off the target; this is important, as even the slightest eye movement will normally be matched with slight changes to those muscles of the suboccipital triangle.

As one approaches the ten-minute mark, other sensations will be noticed. First comes the release of shoulder tension, followed by an easing of tension throughout the upper body. Most practitioners are pleasantly surprised at the degree of tension release gained from such a simple exercise, and, taken together, these sensations suggest that the traction effects from the exercise are initiating the lymph detoxing process of the dural membranes.

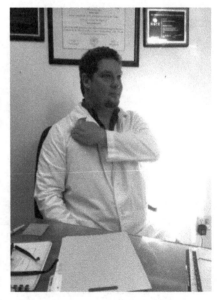

Photo 11-8

Dr. Michael Zalben Demonstrates the Point to Press that Helps the Body with Lymph Detoxification

An additional benefit of the exercise is that it promotes clear thinking. Michael Zalben, DC, who tried it out for himself, believes it is possible to increase the exercise's detoxing benefit by adding a hand pressure lymph-detoxing technique. Zalben suggests that pushing under the right clavicle (collar bone), as shown in Photo 11-8, will further promote brain detoxification.

The sensation of sinus draining while practicing the exercise is a good sign, as this indicates that the technique is working the way it's supposed to. Additionally, practitioners of the technique often report mood improvement. However, due to the habit of looking down at a computer or cell phone, it can be a challenge to maintain ideal neck and posture position at all times.

Try employing the exercise as a brain refresher while taking a break from reading or looking down at a computer for several minutes, and take it is an example of how a head-suspension posture exercise can function as a meditation or *qigong* practice.

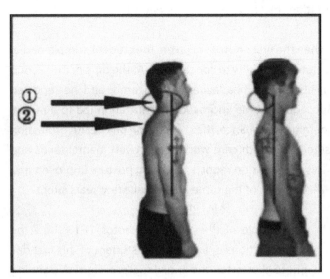

Diagrams 11-9
Neck and Body Alignment
These photos are taken of the same individual, one year apart (the right photo has been reversed for comparison).

In the left photo, arrow (1) shows too-forward neck position, where the muscles of the neck do not properly support the head. Arrow (2) indicates stress and habitual tension to the shoulders resulting from the poor posture habit. Compare with the more natural and free position of the spine and neck in the right and later photo.

Chapter 56

Optimal Balance = Optimal Performance

*A*nother aspect of the body's "default" habits concerns one's center of gravity, and the way in which the upper body is balanced in relation to the lower body. This a "cousin principle" to the structural support of the head and neck addressed in the previous chapter.

Consider the structural balance of the individual shown in Diagrams 11-9; the photos are of the same person and were taken around one year apart. The left image illustrates the individual's default orientation at the beginning of his training; the right image shows how his centerline changed, and his default posture improved over the period. In preparation for both photos, the individual was asked to stand naturally and not try to make any correction to his posture. Revealed by the vertical lines superimposed over the images, note how the person's centerline improved over the year.

Observing the change in the body's center, or plumb line, notice the line in the photo drawn from the bottom of the ear and vertically through the body; the position of the spine represented in the second photo illustrates the reduction in stress achieved by improvement in the posture. Moreover, the change in posture also triggered improved athletic ability.

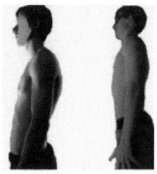

Photos 11-10

Standing: Before and After
Posture Correction

Posture changes on a student's first class

Similar reports are found in every case I have encountered where the practitioner has changed their default plumb line orientation. This observation suggests that reaction time and athleticism are more closely related to one's default spine-orientation than is generally understood.

On a related note, when the first photo was taken, the student complained of constant headaches and an inability to concentrate. At the time of the second photo a year later, his chronic headaches disappeared, and he reported improved focus. Subsequently, his improved concentration led to a radical upswing in his academic performance, the completion of a health profession degree, and licensure as a health care worker. Improved mental focus and concentration like this are common reports following posture improvement. (Note: Diagram 11-24, below, is of the same individual a few years later.)

Providing an additional example of the principle, Photos 11-10 show the before and after posture corrections of a martial art student on his first day of training. The left photo illustrates the individual's preferred standing postures before correction, and the right illustrates his initial correction. At the time the photos were taken, the individual performed poorly in high school and had a lazy left eye. Soon after engaging posture training as a regular practice, his focus and concentration increased, and the lazy eye stabilized to such a degree that he no longer required eyeglasses.

Three Contributing Principles

Since posture and performance are so interconnected, it is useful to consider what evidence might exist that supports the notion of this relationship. This part of the chapter presents both evidence for, and some speculation about, the relationship between posture and athletic performance.

1. Proper Posture and Internal Medicine

In the journals of modern medicine, the body's suspension-posture system as it pertains to health — and, by extension, to our discussion of human bio-energetics — was first described by Joel E. Goldthwait, MD, who developed his own system of healing based on attention to a patient's vertical relationship with gravity.

Goldthwait, a Harvard physician, observed that the way many of his patients held and moved their bodies was the root cause of some of the diseases they suffered. The inspiration for Goldthwaite's theory on the relationship between health and posture evolved from observations he made during surgery. In a paper published in 1934, Goldthwait shared these observations, stating that patients who habitually held their heads in a "bent" way had "stretching" and "kinking" of the cerebral arteries and veins. Similarly, Goldthwait observed that patients with cardiac problems had habitually poor chest posture. [6]

Among his observations, Goldthwait noted that the inordinate amount of stress to many of his patient's abdominal nerves and blood vessels was also due to their poor posture. Goldthwait discovered that both lack of proper balance in motion, and bodily misalignment related to poor posture, generally contributed to disease. Goldthwait subsequently developed a therapeutic approach based on his observations, which he used to demonstrate that many clinical conditions could be corrected without the need for drugs or surgery. [7] He presented his theory on health and posture in a 1911 article:

> The way we hold and move our bodies in our daily activities is more important than most people realize. It is desirable that we are able to stand erect and to have the parts of the body balanced so that easy and graceful movements occur. These ideas about how we stand and move are important for full health and economic efficiency of the body. The most economical way to use the body is with proper poise. This allows more energy to be available for whatever task is required. Any time structure departs from the balanced state, energy is wasted, and efficiency reduced. An imbalance can cause one part of the body to be strained more than another, but no one part can be strained without affecting the whole body. [8]

2. Posture and Brain Function

Other studies have confirmed the interactions between "energy," health, and posture in similar ways. In one such investigation, New Zealand researchers found evidence that good posture promoted healthful oxygen flow to the brain. The study not only showed that individuals who slump forward in their chair reduce the body's flow of blood and oxygen to the brain, but also that when the poor posture becomes habitual, it affects the person's psychological health and mental outlook in a negative way

In another study that compared psychological attributes of straight-sitters to those who slumped over, researchers found that subjects who maintained a straight posture while sitting showed greater self-esteem, improved mood, and lower levels of fear related to public speaking. [9] How, though, does this apply to our discussion of internal energy? Increased self-esteem and confidence are considered signs of high energy, and, in the same vein, investigators in New England hypothesized that increased oxygen to the brain, a byproduct of correct posture, is probably related to improvement in the self-esteem of test subjects.

Hoping to uncover the pernicious consequences of a slumped posture, the same study found that poor posture contributed toward a negative influence on a person's psychology, with subjects showing improvement in confidence and attitude after correction. In the next part of the study, those students with improved posture were compared to participants who did not change their "lazy" habits, and had instead maintained their slumped position, and it was found that the latter group fared much worse on scales of confidence and mood.

3. Posture and Adaptation to Stress

Another way to consider the meanings of "high" and "low" energies is expressed in the way posture can affect how a person responds to stress. In this context, "high energy" refers to the individual who is able to manage stress more effectively, while "low energy" describes a person with less adaptive responses to stress.

Researcher Elizabeth Broadbent explains that "Sitting upright allows the nervous system to respond to stressors" more optimally. Since terms like "strong" or "high energy" are also associated with positive emotions, it is interesting that in the same study examining the relationship between posture and "energy," linguistic analysis showed that individuals who maintained a slumped posture used more words associated with negative emotions compared to their upright-sitting counterparts. [10]

Chapter 57

Shape (Morphology), Nervous System Responses, and Contact Sports

*T*his chapter extrapolates from cell behavior research and applies other observations to human athletic performance. It includes speculation about an alternative way of thinking about the meaning of "internal energy in the martial arts." These extrapolations are based on research studies, anecdotal evidence, and my own experience as a trainer of athletes across several decades. The principles derive from attempts to explain how a person's "shape," or body orientation, might influence not only nervous system responses, but other responses as they apply to athletic performance. † These concepts are especially applicable to athletes who engage in contact sports.

> † Stress-sympathetic vs. non-stress and healing parasympathetic
> nervous system responses are also discussed in Sections VIII and IX

Inspiration for the suggestions that follow are based on observations of cell behavior by Stanford University professor Bruce Lipton, which were presented in Section IX. Lipton's observations of endothelial cell shapes, or morphologies, led him to describe cell orientations as either "growth" or "protective." Particularly relevant to the present discussion is Lipton's observation of cell characteristics after they assume a protective posture.

When an endothelial cell assumes a "protective orientation," important changes take place not only in its morphology (shape), but also internally. It is possible that these changes may also apply to large and complex organisms, such as humans. If so, those changes provide yet another clue to the meaning of "internal energy." When a cell is in a "closed" and protective mode, it is unable to access life-sustaining functions, such as growth and absorption of nutrients. In contrast, when the organism assumes an "open" orientation, the cells become responsive to the presence of nutrients.

Even more telling is Lipton's observation that a cell's morphology determines if it is in defensive or open mode. Significantly, and depending on the shape, a cell could engage in <u>only</u> one of these behaviors at a time; that is to say,<u> it could not do both simultaneously.</u>

Lipton's observations suggest that an organism's ability to present a physical shape, or "microscopic anatomy," co-evolved with microbiological and electrochemical presentations associated with either an "open" or "closed" orientation to the external environment. It may be enlightening to consider if these observations of the effects / responses to morphology might be applied to human behavior, as well as the kind of postural orientations athletes and martial artists adopt when in close contact with their opponents.

Co-evolution: Body Orientation and Nervous System Responses

Other observations support the notion that body orientation may have co-evolved with emotional experience and nervous system stress. Support for such speculation includes the role of instinctive protective reflexes; for example, the brain stem's reflexive function that causes one to suddenly pull the arms near and in front of the chest when surprised or frightened. By contrast, the co-relationship between some postures signal (to the person's nervous system) openness, safety and the availability of nurturance. An example of the latter is seen in the "mother's embrace" posture, and its subsequent influence on the immune system that was covered in Section IX (Photos 9-3). That example, provided by John Diamond, MD, describes how life energy is closely linked to certain postures and gestures –- particularly the open chest / thymus posture — and how these contribute to both a stronger immune system and an overall increase in body strength.

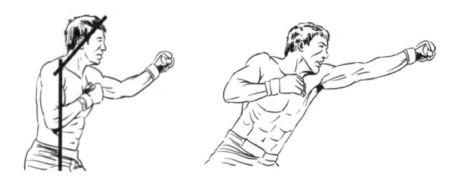

Diagrams 11-11
Disturbed (Non-vertical) Centerline
This drawing of an MMA fighter shows an interrupted (non-vertical) centerline.
Characterized by the forward hunching neck, the power of the punch is fulcrum-based. The right drawing is of the same fighter throwing a punch.
Illustrations by Sergio Verdeza

The "Open" and "Vertical" in Contact Sports

Now we will take a closer look at distinctions between two basic body orientations in contact sports and martial arts that, broadly distinguished, can be classified as horizontal and vertical. As discussed here, the illustration of the fighter shown in Diagrams 11-11 represents a horizontal orientation. It depicts how the fighter's upper body acts like a fulcrum (Diagram 11-12), with the large muscles of the upper body moving more independently from the lower body. In this example, the fulcrum and "horizontal" separation of the body is used to perform a leveraged strike. This is the most common martial arts and fighter orientation.

Diagram 11-12

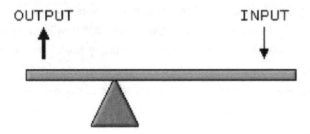

A Fulcrum

(Source: *Wikipedia Commons*)

In contrast to a fighter who relies on a horizontal orientation, illustrations of Aikido founder Morihei Ueshiba and *t'ai-chi* master Cheng Man-ching, shown in Diagrams 11-13, are examples of a fighting style in which one engages an opponent using a vertical orientation. In these examples, because of its "open" posture, the more vertical orientation offers another way to think about the meaning of "internal energy in the martial arts."

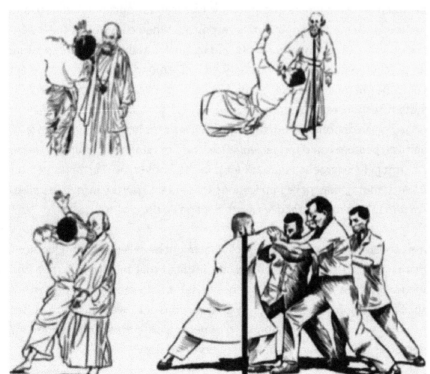

Figures 11-13
Vertical Fighting Orientations
First three images: Aikido founder
Morihei Ueshiba. Bottom right image:
t'ai chi master Cheng Man-ching.
Superimposed lines illustrate "vertical"
posture orientations. [12]

Reflecting once again on Lipton's description of cell behavior as either closed-protective or open, it is interesting to consider whether these definitions, when applied to an athlete's physical orientation, might contribute to not only a definition of a particular kind of athleticism, but also to the meaning of "internal energy in the martial arts."

To compare fighting styles, in general, a martial artist or contact sports participant who orients themselves with a typically jaw-forward and hands-forward guarding stance, as illustrated by the image shown in Diagram 11-11, can be said to fall into the category of a horizontal, or "closed / protective" posture. In contrast to this more common orientation, which is adopted by most fighters, the illustrations of Morihei Ueshiba and Cheng Man-ching (Figures 11-13) depict vertical and more "open" orientations.

It is easy to understand why the "crouched forward" orientations favored by most fighters is much more common. Sport fighting is stressful, and the fighter, along with their trainers, would naturally prefer the combatant to assume a protective posture while engaging an opponent. To be open and exhibit a vertical posture while under the stress of close combat represents a significant change from what might normally be regarded as a kind of default fighting orientation.

Compared to the closed, chin tucked and head forward protective stance of most fighters, the vertical orientation is rare in combat arts. However, as suggested by the illustrations in Figures 11-13, this mode of close quarter engagement is emblematic of the fighting styles of masters Cheng and Ueshiba, shown in the Figures 11-13, and it is also often the preferred orientation of styles such as *t'ai-chi*, *baguazhang* (八卦掌), and *aikido*.

For these reasons, it is useful to consider whether a link might exist between an individual's morphology (vertical vs. horizontal styles) and nervous system / hormonal / brain responses. When considering the "open" endothelial cell configuration observed by Lipton, and the effects of posture on psychobiological harmony described by Diamond, it seems an argument could be made that a link exists between physical orientation, nervous system responses and an individual's access to a more effective way of engaging an opponent. With this in mind, it is possible that a more open (e.g., vertical) posture could trigger, enhance, and / or reinforce a neuro-chemical / hormonal / energetic feedback loop in the body-mind. Furthermore, this understanding may have implications for contact sports, since it describes what may be a more effective way to engage an opponent.

It is conceivable that the founders of what might be called the more "vertical" martial arts, such as *t'ai-chi* and *aikido*, intuited that this type of open and vertical posture triggers not only specific sets of bio-mechanical power, but specific hormonal and nervous system responses as well. Taken together, could these, the combination of bio-mechanical power and hormonal / nervous system responses, be the secrets of mastery?

Another aspect of the vertical vs. horizontal orientation question has to do with the ability to relax when one is engaged with an opponent. Physiologically speaking, the ability to relax while under stress requires that the individual, consciously or unconsciously, activates just a bit more parasympathetic nervous system response. It seems likely, then, that this sympathetic-parasympathetic balance is an important part of the definition of "internal power" in the context of contact sports, since one's physical orientation can influence the sympathetic vs. parasympathetic balance.

There are a few examples of combatants who can maintain a more open and vertical posture under the extremely stressful conditions of close fighting. One example of this rarer type of fighter is MMA champion, Anderson Silva. Depicted in Diagrams 11-14, Silva had a very successful prize fighting career, holding, as of 2017, "the longest title defense streak in Ultimate Fighting Championship (UFC) history, which ended in 2013 with 16 consecutive wins and 10 title defenses." [11]

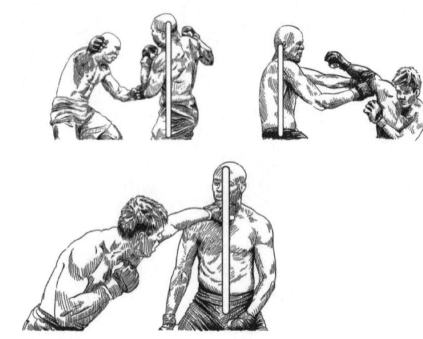

Diagrams 11-14

Illustrations Made of MMA champion Anderson Silva in a Contest
Note the vertical center line imposed over the image. To what extent did his vertical posture lead to his effortless control over an opponent?
Illustrations by Sergio Verdeza based on actual images from some of Anderson Silva's professional fights

As illustrated by the vertical lines superimposed over the three sketches modeled from video frame stills taken during actual matches, Silva's vertical and "open" fighting orientation is immediately evident. It is useful to consider to what extent Silva's postural orientation might have contributed to his unique style of "mastery" in the ring.

Bio-mechanical Advantages Associated with a More *Vertical* and *Open* Posture

Although posture, or physical orientation, alone can never predict who will win a match, it is possible to compare physiological differences between athletes based on the differences between an open (vertical) and closed (horizontal) stance. Adding to our discussion of "internal energy," we might consider how these differences inform our view of subtle or internal energy in athletic training. In the following chapters, three bio-mechanical processes: diaphragmatic breathing, "conscious control over normally unconscious muscles," and "attributes related to the vertical posture" are discussed in relation to efficient athletic training. We will investigate ways in which these factors could contribute to a definition of what is sometimes referred to as a "strong" or "high level" of internal energy.

Chapter 58

The Open Posture and Diaphragmatic Breathing

Good Mood, High Energy, or Serotonin?

It is instructive to compare benefits from diaphragmatic breathing (Box 11-15) to qualities associated with "strong internal energy." From lowered blood pressure to a "good mood," the effects of diaphragmatic breathing are often credited to the release of serotonin. [13]

Benefits of Diaphragmatic Breathing

- Helps lower blood pressure, and therefore the risk of heart disease.

- Helps lower blood sugar, and therefore the risk of diabetes.

- Releases serotonin, which not only makes you feel good, but can reduce cravings for processed carbohydrates and other junk food.

- Eliminates free radicals from the body, improving cellular function and lifespan.

- Increases the secretion of growth hormone and slows the aging process.

- Improves mental focus and clarity by increasing blood flow to the prefrontal cortex of your brain.

- Improves sleep quality.

- Facilitates weight loss by balancing stress hormones with anabolic hormones.

Source: Geoff Neuport, "The Most Important Exercise Missing from Your Workout," *Men's Health* October 29, 2014

Box 11-15

Comparisons between deep and "shallow" breathing are ancient. The Taoist philosopher Chuang Tzu informs us that while the common man breathes from his throat, an accomplished person, or "true man," ‡ always "breathes from his heels." [14] The fourth-century CE philosopher Ko Hung describes the relationship between breath and internal power as follows:

> Man exists in the mist of breath, and breath is within man himself. From heaven and earth on to all creation there is nothing that does not require breath to stay alive. The man who knows how to circulate his breath maintains his own person and banishes evils that would attack him.
>
> Among the people of Wu Yueh there is current a method for casting spells that is very effective; it consists merely of rendering breath more abundant. He who employs it can go even where there is plague and sleep with the sick without becoming infected … This is an example of the effectiveness of breath against natural disasters. [15]

‡ zhen ren, 真人

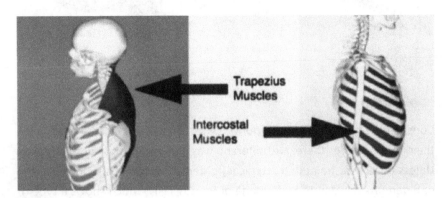

Diagrams 11-16
The Trapezius Muscles
Left: Trapezius muscles of the upper back and top of shoulder.
Right: Intercostal (rib cage) muscles.
Source: *Wikipedia Commons*

Chapter 59

Conscious Control Over Normally Unconscious Muscle Groups

Some athletic demonstrations are so amazing that they appear to defy common understanding of the physics of force, speed, and body mechanics. Examples of this kind of extraordinary ability can be observed in some of the more spectacular knock out punches thrown by world-famous boxer Muhammad Ali. [16] In some of the more remarkable examples, Ali was seen to floor an opponent with what seemed like little more than a light punch.

This is not an argument for, or against, the existence of an unseen internal energy that might contribute to the apparent superhuman ability of an exceptional athlete. Instead, this part of the discussion focuses on the use of subtler bio-mechanical factors that might contribute to what is sometimes described in terms of "internal energy" in an athletic contest. One aspect of this discussion addresses the athlete's ability to gain conscious control over normally unconscious muscle groups.

Photos 11-17
Shoulder-Trapezius Compared to Ribcage-Intercostal Punching
Left: A typical upper shoulder-based punch.

Right: A punch incorporating the intercostal/ rib cage muscles. Note the incorporation of the abdominal muscles in the right photo.

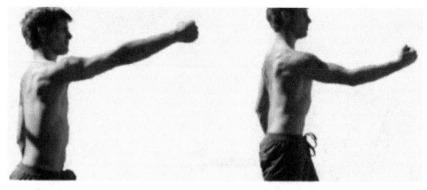

Consider the typical cross body punch. Based on the way an athlete engages their musculature, there are different ways to throw this kind of strike. Unless otherwise trained, the typical fighter's punch tends to look like the one demonstrated in the left image of Photos 11-17, which shows a type of upper shoulder / fulcrum-based strike. This relies primarily on striking force delivered from the trapezius muscles of the upper back and shoulders.

Although there is no doubt that this type of upper back and shoulder muscle use can be effective, there is another, less commonly trained set of muscle groups that can add to striking power, ball throwing, and other athletic skills. This group, as illustrated in the second image, incorporates more of the ribcage (intercostal) muscles. Although the natural athlete will often employ intercostal muscles unconsciously, it is rare that they are specifically addressed in training.

Diagrams 11-16 compares the trapezius at the top of the upper back to the intercostal muscles between the ribs. When consciously activated, use of the intercostals allows for more sophisticated application of power than is achieved by relying mostly on the muscles of the trapezius in the upper shoulder and back.

Note that it is perhaps an over-simplification to say that only one set of muscles initiates the kind of bio-mechanical changes that are described in this chapter. Muscles are never used in isolation, and when it comes to athletic performance, any set of muscles addressed in training form part of a constellation of integrated muscle systems. For example, while the intercostals are the focus of the present discussion, related muscles of the transversus abdominis, rectus abdominis, external oblique muscles, and internal oblique muscles are also recruited for what is a coordinated effort.

With an increase in conscious control over normally unconscious muscle groups, as is often the case when intercostals are consciously applied, an athlete gains the potential for using more nuanced technical skills. This is possible because conscious control over the nine sets of intercostal muscles allows one to adapt instantly and make slight modifications to the course and direction of a strike or technique.

An additional benefit of learning to use the intercostal muscles in this way is the decreased susceptibility to injury to the rotator cuff. [17] By contrast, when the ribcage is only minimally involved in the movement of the arms and shoulder, the rotator cuff is overly relied upon for strength and motion. With over-reliance on the rotator cuff, force and stress become less evenly distributed among various muscle groups, which tends to strain or tear tissue, especially the tendons, due to the amount of force being exerted as a result of the demands of athletic performance (risk of injury applies to the supraspinatus on top of the joint when elevating the arm). In contrast, when the muscles of the ribcage are more active and involved, the teres minor and subscapularis handle the burden of movement and transmit stress through the shoulder blade, which connects to the spine and ribcage. Thus, learning to incorporate the intercostal / ribcage muscles is not only safer, but also increases speed, flexibility, and power!

The Intercostals and the Boxer

A few years ago, I was working with a boxer at the gym of a very seasoned and highly knowledgeable boxing coach. The old coach had worked with many famous boxers over the course of his 50+ years in the sport, but one day, when I was at his gym working with a mid-20s boxing student, he stopped and stared in amazement as we practiced a set of striking patterns on the heavy bag. I was working to get the aspiring fighter to employ his intercostal muscles against the bag target; the training goal was to add, by accessing specific intercostal sequences, variations in the angles from which the boxer could present power against the target. In my mind, as a coach, this was all just basic training. However, I was struck by the old pro's sudden intense interest in what we were working on, and stunned when he remarked, "I've never seen that taught before."

Could this be true? Although some of the best boxers apply this bio-mechanical technique unconsciously, was it possible that such an experienced coach really had never seen specifically-targeted, intercostal muscle-based strike training? To me, the old pro's comments illustrated how sometimes even the most experienced trainers teach their sport in the same old way that was taught to them. In too many cases, the ritualized pattern of instruction is passed from generation to generation with little innovation. It seems that nowhere along the old pro's line of extensive training experience had someone asked, "Is it possible that intercostal-abdominal muscle sequences could produce a more powerful or different kind of punch?" Very curious.

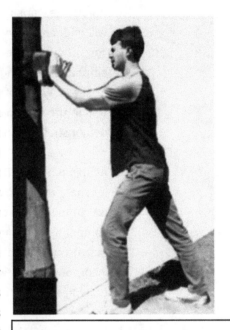

Photo 11-18

Training the Intercostal Muscles

The "wall training" exercise involves using <u>only</u> the slightest amount of pressure necessary to hold a lightweight object against a stable structure, such as a tree or wall, with the outer edge of slightly cupped hands.

In this photo, the practitioner holds a target pad against a palm tree. The holding force of very light contact, without a lean, develops tensile strength that courses through the entire body. In practice, the goal is to keep the object in place with just enough pressure so that it won't drop. Start by holding the position for two minutes and then gradually working up to fifteen or twenty minutes. Important: the practitioner's center line should be either forward or to the rear of center, but <u>not balanced in a 50-50 weight distribution</u>

Link to "Wall Training" Video

https://youtu.be/1ggOtkipzZ8

or

https://chiarts.com/11-19

Box 11-19

More Conscious Control Over the Intercostal / Ribcage Muscles

An athlete's ability to increase conscious control over the ribcage muscles will offer an advantage in any sport. One of the best ways to develop willful control over these muscles is to add exercises to your training routine that emphasize holding the intercostal muscles in static stress positions. One of these types of exercises, called "wall training" (performed against a tree in the example shown), is illustrated in Photos 11-18. A link to a video demonstrating the practice can be viewed from the link in Box 11-19.

At this juncture, it may be enlightening for athletes and athletic trainers if I share a personal story highlighting the value of "wall training." When I was in my late forties, and before suffering a catastrophic injury, I was very competitive with my senior students. Up to that point, few of them could match my skill in sparring. However, that changed when a group of us incorporated the "wall training" method during a special series of advanced training sessions that took place over a two-month period.

Practicing together for those two months, we gradually increased the duration of our practice from 10 to 25 minutes. At the end of the period, I witnessed the single most dramatic improvement in student performance of my teaching career. For the first time, my senior students were able to equal, or even best me, in our sparring and ground-fighting contests. However, surprisingly, this newfound skill did not manifest the same way in everyone. For example, one very slight student in his early 20s, with barely a flick of the arm, was able to uproot and shoot me five to seven feet across the room at will, while another student was able to easily control me on the mat. For me, the results of our informal experiment were gratifying proof of the exceptional power that stress training of the intercostals could awaken.

Since that discovery, "wall training" has continued to be a major component of my athletic coaching, and has been applied to Olympic hopefuls, MMA fighters, and aspiring professional golfers. I never cease to marvel at the benefits.

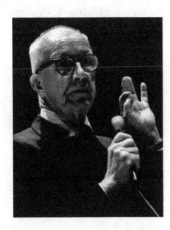

Photo 11-20
Buckminster Fuller
American architect, systems theorist,
author, designer, and inventor

Source: *Wikipedia Commons*;
Photo attributed to Dan Lindsay

Chapter 60

Tensegrity, Body Mechanics, and Subtle Energy

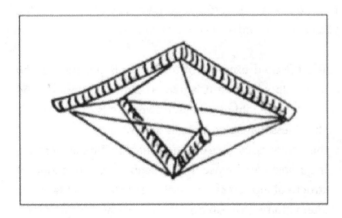

Diagram 11-21

A Tensegrity Structure

A basic cell from a tensegrity mast shown here illustrates the principle
of how two solids (compressive elements) are stacked on top of each
other and held in place by tensional elements.

From D.L. Robbie, MD., "Tensional Forces in the Human Body"

*T*his chapter seeks to understand whether a particular configuration of body support might contribute to the definition of "internal energy." The system of support under consideration is known as *tensegrity*, a term invented by the famous architect Buckminster Fuller (Photo 11-20) to describe how certain structures bear weight. A *tensegruous* structure, like the one illustrated in Diagram 11-21, bears weight through a configuration that alternates tensional (flexible) with strut (compressive) elements.

In this chapter, we apply some of the principles of tensegrity to an analysis of the structural support system of the human body; an example being the way normally unconscious muscles can be consciously triggered to improve athletic performance. Other aspects are speculative, such as the theory that the acupuncture meridian system, when tensegruous, promotes a more balanced bio-electrical field and thus produces less "noise." * In this way, the structure, like the configuration of an antenna network, creates a more efficient arrangement and results in enhanced performance.

* "Reduction of noise" pertains to a model of "internal energy in the martial arts" that was introduced in Section VIII

Body Support and Tensegrity

Applied to the human body, tensegrity defines the optimal bio-physical system as interconnected, springy, and resilient. Within the human frame, tensegrity consists of a mix of tensional elements such as fascia, ligaments, and tendons, as well as compressive elements of the bones that act as "struts." When tensegruous, the structure's response can be compared to the flexible recovery of a palm tree under the force of wind.

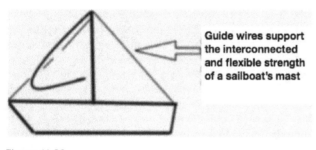

Guide wires support the interconnected and flexible strength of a sailboat's mast

Figure 11-22
Principles of Tensegrity Represented in
Support of a Sailboat's Mast

The oft-cited example of tensegrity is the functioning of a sailboat's mast (Diagram 11-22) as it supports and bears the weight of its sails. However, it is not the mast's sturdiness that holds the sails upright and thereby resists the tremendous force of wind acting on the sails. Instead, the principle of tensegrity describes how this kind of structural support can be explained in terms of the mast's interaction with flexible elements, such as the boat's stays (forestay, backstay, and shrouds). Together, they create an effective system to spread out, and cooperatively share, the force acting against the structure.

Applied to the human body, tensegrity explains how the spine, via "soft tissue" fascia elements, such as ligaments and tendons, work in concert with hard strut elements (bones) of the skeleton. These allow the body to bear weight and yet maintain a fluid interaction with gravity. The synchrony between these two types of interacting support mechanisms — flexible and rigid— is important for three reasons. First, in terms of structural support, the fascia function as guy lines; in the body's myofascial system, stress received through fascial elements provides an overall piezoelectric response. *Piezoelectric* has to do with the way certain structures in the body, such as fascia, tendons, and bones, much like crystals, generate an electrical charge when they are stimulated by pressure or stress. This function not only contributes to the body's measurable bioenergetic field, but, as will be discussed later, also provides more clues to the nature of the body's "energy" system. [18]

Second, the tensegrity model helps describe the body's ability to heal structural injuries when proper alignment displaces extreme stress or trauma away from a concentrated area, such as the spine. This synchronic interaction allows the body to function as an integrated support-healing system. Third, the principle applies to more advanced athletic abilities, as the athlete who fully realizes the potential of the tensegruous structure is then able to engage increasingly subtle levels of interconnected and highly refined force.

The description of tensegrity principles as applied to the human spine was proposed by D.L. Robbie, MD. In his 1977 paper, Robbie explained how the principles described by Fuller apply to human physiology, arguing that the vertebrae of the spinal column, in concert with flexible elements such as fascia, ligaments, and tendons, act as discontinuous tensional elements. In the proposed model, force, and the expression of power, alternate with compressive and flexible elements that work together to form the body's continuous tensional system. Robbie's theory is supported by analysis of the spinal vertebrae, which are not designed to support significant weight, but rather to function as attachment points so that the ligaments and tendons around the spine are able to lift each vertebra off the one below it.

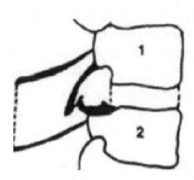

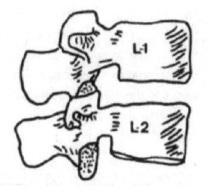

Schematic Diagrams of an Intervertebral Joint between the First and Second Lumbar Vertebrae

As Robbie explains, these drawings illustrate the structure and support of the first and second lumbar vertebrae (Figs 1, 2). Note that the upper tip of the superior articular process of L-2 is situated higher than the lower tip of the inferior articular process of L-1 … The connective tissue forms a sling by which the inferior articular process of L-1 is suspended from the superior articular process of L-2. If we now expand our view to include both intervertebral joints between L-1 and L-2, we see that the weight of L-1 is being supported by L-2 by means of a tensional rather than a compressional force."

From D.L. Robbie, MD. [26]

Robbie Figure 1

Diagrams 11-23
Robbie Figure 1. This linear diagram illustrates how vertebral body one is suspended over the vertebral body two by the tensional properties of the connective tissue as opposed to the compressional properties of the vertebral bodies.

Robbie Figure 2

Robbie Figure 2. This is an actual drawing of L-1 and L-2, showing the relationship between the inferior articular process of L-1 and the superior articular process of L-2.

Akin to the flexible support structures of dome tents and sailboat masts, the body does not rely on a single, dominant "post" (e.g., the spinal column) to lift and move against the forces of gravity. It functions as an integrated system, involving stretchy tendon and fascia "wires" being integrated with rigid structures — principally the bones — that act as "struts" (Diagrams 11-23). Together, these work cooperatively to lift, move, and bear weight. [19]

In regard to the human body, the following definition of a tensegrity structure is provided by James Oschman, PhD:

> [*Tensegrity* in the human body is] characterized by a continuous tensional network (tendons) connected by a discontinuous set of compressive elements (struts). A tensegrity structure forms a stable yet dynamic system that interacts efficiently and resiliently with forces acting upon it. [20]

The two sections below describe tensegrity as it applies to the body's energy and structural support systems. Part A examines how tensegrity relates to the body's bio-energetic fields, while Part B describes an exercise designed to trigger normally unconscious tensegrity responses in the body.

Part A

Tensegrity and Body-Mind "Energy"

The tensegrity model provides three more clues that suggest the body functions as an integrated bio-mechanical and bio-energetic whole. The first clue has to do with bio-mechanical efficiency, the second clue is how proportional and balanced movement influences the body's subtle energy field, and the third clue is related to how the piezoelectric properties of the integrated fascia *connective tissue matrix* contribute to the body's subtle energy field.

Tensegrity and Bio-mechanical Efficiency

With optimal postural alignment and efficient movement, there is less stress on the system. This translates into less wasted movement and optimized function, reflected by balanced body suspension and movement.

Tensegrity and Bio-fields

This part of our discussion of tensegrity focuses on the nature of human physiology as an as an electromagnetic, or electromagnetic-like, "energy system." It suggests that "energy practices," like *qigong* and energetic yoga, may function as two-way sending and receiving antenna systems. ** However, when considered in the context of tensegrity, the model provides a new way to reflect on the meaning of electrically conductive and piezoelectric aspects of the myofascial network function.

** The embedded nature of the body's meridians as an antenna system
is described in Section II, and is addressed again in Section XII.

In this light, the piezoelectric nature of the myofascial meridians suggests that they may interact with the body as a tensegruous structure. It has been proposed that the meridians function in response to stress placed along the body's myofascial / meridian system, which, if true, means that targeted stress applied to the meridians will generate at least some measurable changes in the body's bioelectrical fields.

When it comes to learning to direct this kind of subtle stress along these channels, a practitioner of yoga, *t'ai-chi, qigong,* and similar practices gradually becomes aware of these piezoelectric corridors that run throughout the body. In their practices, they search for a certain tug in their postures, or tingling of current, associated with an exercise. These are activated through posture, breath, and intention, which merge with the practice. In this way, these types of practices can be thought of as disciplines concerned with *consciously* directing stress to specific areas (myofascial tracks) of the body. Through attention directed to those myofascial lines, the practitioner learns to "tune" the input and output of the body's bio-electrical antenna grid. These might well be the practices that can lead a practitioner to state of *coherence.*

Small stresses to the body's embedded piezoelectric systems generate a variety of electrical field patterns. Aside from the healthful benefits to the body related to these field patterns, they also form (depending on the skill of the practitioner) either as more or less ordered electromagnetic (EM) wave patterns. The **ordering** of wave patterns is an important part of William Tiller's hypothesis that "movements of a particular body part give rise to two emitted EM wave patterns." [21] As Tiller explains:

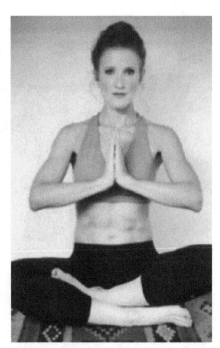

> The body can be thought of as a type of transmitting / receiving antenna. Incoming EM waves of a particular frequency range will stimulate movement of the appropriately sized body part, either by direct EM-coupling or by piezoelectric transduction to sound-coupling. If there are no correlations between the movements of the various sized body parts, there is no integration in the system and the outflowing radiation has no pattern … The greater the degree of correlated movements between different sized body parts, the more pattern-like is the total emission, the greater is its information content and the more integrated is the system. [22]

Photo 11-24
Activating Tensegrity Principles in the Practice of Yoga or Meditation Increases Coherence

A Model of Mastery?

It is intriguing to think about the body as a piezoelectric network; the implications of which become even more profound when one lays the tensegrity network over the piezoelectric myofascial meridian grid. This combined modeling allows us to speculate over a new way to study yoga, *t'ai-chi,* and other practices in the context of their optimal antenna signal functioning (Photo 11-24). In this light, one style of movement, or twist of the body, might be better correlated with the principles of tensegrity and access to the piezoelectric grid than others.

In this context, a movement, posture, or yogic pose can be evaluated based on the degree to which it is tensegruous. Because of the way tensegrity interacts with the body's built-in piezoelectric antenna network, it stands to reason that *every* movement — every twist of the arm or stretch of the back — may have an *ideal* correlated movement when matched with the opposing aspect of the body. This suggests that increased *coherence,* meaning less "noise" and more internal order, provides a new definition of mastery in "mind-body" practices. Whether through yoga, meditation, *t'ai-chi,* sitting, conscious breathing, or walking, as one *purposefully* attends to the piezoelectric resistance and hum of the myofascial meridians, one is led increasingly to the reduction of "noise" and increased *coherence.*

However, learning to gain conscious control over the placement of gentle myofascial stress through the body in order to optimally stimulate the overlays between tensegrity and piezoelectric coherence is not easy. It requires disciplined attention to learn the secrets of activating the body's embedded meridian myofascial network.

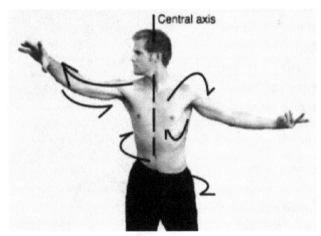

Central axis

While one aspect of the embedded array is physical, another is mental. Due to their nature, directed attention also plays a role in the optimal activation of the meridian structure. Demonstrating the relationship between energy and form, consider that when a practitioner of *t'ai-chi* or hatha yoga practices with one hand stretched high and the other one low, this stimulates a very specific EM field pattern. However, focused attention to those aspects of the body will also induce changes to the "energy field" of the body.

Diagram 11-25
Baguazhang as a Tensegrity-Based and Bio-energetically Balanced Exercise Exercise / practice with lines of force and counter-force. Movement is counter balanced along the body's central axis. This example is a movement from baguazhang.

As one applies these principles to the body, the practitioner will notice that different styles of stretching and posturing will affect the perception of the energy field in and around the body in different ways. For example, one might notice a slightly different sensation from a posture like the one just described, compared to one where both hands are resting on the knees.

Tensegrity and Subtle Energy in Physical Disciplines

Applied to athletic performance, tensegrity provides more clues to the meaning of internal energy. Since the question of more vs. less efficient movement of the body relates to the meaning of "internal energy," a closer look at the relationship between *tensegrity* and internal energy is warranted.

Based on the previous discussion, not only one's movement, but also stances and fighting postures, may be described as being either more or less efficient. In the context of the present discussion, this relates to the degree of *tensegrity*.

This principle is especially applicable to the so-called "energetic" martial arts, such as *t'ai-chi, aikido,* and *baguazhang.* It appears that, at least in their idealized form, and without necessarily being consciously aware of the implications of the principles they developed, that the founders of these systems had an intuitive understanding of the body as a tensegruous structure. In this light, force-counterforce movement that extends outward from a vertical centerline characterizes these arts, with *baguazhang* serving as a particularly good test case when assessing these principles in terms of force-counterforce in relation to the tensegrity model. As suggested by the figure shown in Diagram 11-25, a practice like this provides a blueprint for a tensegruous approach to the internal and meditative movement arts.

Part B

Tensegrity and Unconscious Muscle Groups

Another aspect of tensegrity applies to the unconscious support of the body by accessory muscles. This section introduces a game-changing technique for the training of athletes, and the principle is also useful as an adjunctive therapy for many types of musculoskeletal pain. The technique is called *tensegrity-block training* (TBT), and it aims to accomplish two outcomes. First, it teaches one to recognize <u>unconscious</u> muscle choices that the body makes in terms of support, and second, it is useful as a training device to help the practitioner learn to trigger those normally unconscious muscle groups in a *conscious* way.

For the last twenty-five years, my students and I have worked with the following technique as a regular part of our curriculum. It has also been presented during international seminars and has always been well-received (typical examples of practitioners and their reported experience with the training is included in Boxes 11-26, 11-29, and 11-30). As a training protocol for contact sports and martial arts, TBT teaches the practitioner to acquire more refined muscle control, as well as a superior level of performance I refer to as "athletic connection" (that will be defined shortly).

> While performing the "block exercise" I almost instantaneously feel *hua jing* / tingling sensations in my hands and forearms, which indicates that I am internally connected. I'm hoping this will speed up the recovery of my chronic lower back, shoulder, and neck pain.
>
> —Naveen, United Kingdom

Box 11-26

A similar exercise that can be compared with TBT is *zhan zhuang* (站桩), a "standing practice" found in Chinese *qigong* / internal martial arts, which involves the practitioner learning to "stand still as a tree." [23] Similar methods, sometimes referred to as "post standing," have been included in many styles of Chinese martial arts since ancient times. As a method, TBT is distinguished by the way a practitioner first identifies and then gradually learns to trigger normally unconscious muscle groups for the support and movement of the body. One of our martial art program graduates, an accomplished martial artist and medical doctor, shares his experience with the TBT technique:

> As a martial artist of over 20 years' experience and a career scientist, the platform test that Shrfu Bracy introduced to me during one of our sessions was quite extraordinary. By merely standing on a place of "perceived danger" (i.e. platform), the body automatically achieves an advanced level of connection. The body's posture changes from a tense and forceful stance to a more relaxed but powerful posture that is able to neutralize and repel attackers with the ease of motion and light effort reminiscent of the old internal masters. Step off the platform for a few moments, and those same attackers whom earlier were being thrown with mere touches now requires additional strength, effort, and struggle to repel. Apparently, when the body senses danger (the instability of the platform, possibility of falling off) it acts by recruiting accessory muscles throughout the body to increase its stability and power. This entire process occurs on a subconscious level because there is only the subtlest sensation of physical change when stepping onto a platform; often it is the dramatic improvement in effortless power and connection, which reveals the change. Be it a natural physiologic response, a primitive survival reflex, or the proper flow of "chi," I remain perplexed as to the exact mechanism of this phenomenon. The goal, nevertheless, for the internal martial artist is to be able to sustain this level of power and connection without the benefit of the platform.

> Tony C. Ho, MD

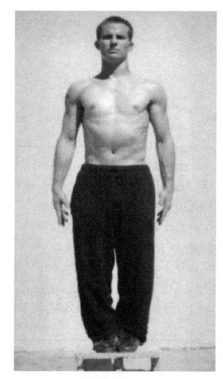

Photo 11-27
"Tensegrity - Block Training"

A video demonstrations of Block-Tensegrity Training and "athletic connection" can be viewed at

https://www.youtube.com/watch?v=9U4p_B3xe48

or

https://chiarts.com/11-28

Box 11-28

As demonstrated in Photo 11-27, TBT requires the practitioner to remain still, but relaxed, while standing on an elevated platform. Correct, upright posture is important during the practice, since slumping or hunching can interfere with the benefits. The raised platform does not need to be very high, but it must be just high enough to induce a *slight feeling of danger*. That is the experience necessary to trigger an unconscious body response related to wiry athleticism and "athletic connection." In this way, the raised platform gets your body's attention.

Block training as a therapy for "widows hump"

Characterized by its bent over posture, the "widow's hump" or "dowager's hump," primarily affects older women. The condition is often associated with weakening or fracturing of the bones of the upper back.

One 63-year-old woman reports her experiences with Tensegrity-Block Training as a treatment for the Widow's Hump in the following way:

"A few years ago, I became aware of my hunched-over widow's hump. One day, my daughter was visiting and was on my case about my back starting to look like a bent-over old lady. I was horrified. I didn't know what I could possibly do about it. Thank the Lord that my friend, John, taught me about Block Training. I didn't want to LOOK LIKE A BENT OVER OLD WOMAN IN MY ELDER YEARS!

"John brought a concrete block from his studio for me to practice on. At first, I was very faithful to the practice. Sometimes now I forget and get a little lazy — and it really starts to show if I miss a week. But after the first three months, the shape of my back began to change. Guess what? My eyesight and memory started to improve along with my back. Maybe it's coincidence, but I even started to remember my dreams. All in all, it took months of daily work before I noticed a big difference in my life — all from the Block Training! And even better when, about six months later, my sharp-eyed daughter next came to visit she exclaimed: 'Mom! Your back looks better. What have you been doing?' Until I told her, she had no idea that I've been doing this new exercise. Sometimes I forget, but overall I try to practice Block Training daily."

—Camille, 63 years young

Box 11-29

When standing on a raised platform, the body will unconsciously choose to pay more attention. In this way, formerly passive muscles are activated, which results in a stronger and more "athletically connected" body status. It is a simple trick that takes the body out of an unconscious laziness, which explains the rule I developed to illustrate the principle:

The body prefers the path of least effort, unless a tiger is chasing it.

The slight feeling of danger perceived by the body in response to standing on a raised platform is the "tiger" in the rule. Thus, the perception of danger, even the slightest amount, unconsciously triggers the body to activate a more complete range of accessory muscles. This results in more springy, wiry, and "connected" power.

For most individuals, *immediately* upon beginning their training on the elevated platform, there is a change in the way their body unconsciously supports itself. Although the body will seem to relax and feel looser, at the same time, it will become stronger and more "athletically connected."

Definition:

Athletic connection is the *ability to present effective and stable power* in context of a loose, wiry athletic state. It is not strength that is as if muscle groups are tense and resisting a force. Although appearing "loose" and without apparent tension, the "athletic connection" phenomenon presents when a strike or other movement meets a target. The skill manifests as a special kind of power which, no doubt, is part of the secret of "soft power" in the internal martial arts, but is also seen in other forms of athletics.

In such a relaxed and loose physical state, it is as if the body has decided to drop all unnecessary tension and adopt a primal wiriness out of necessity, and for most individuals, the practice allows them to experience a new category of relaxed power. However, this is not a tense, muscle-locked kind of power, but power through looseness directed at an impact point (see Athletic Connection test explanation and examples below). In most cases, the practitioner can demonstrate a looser and more connected kind of "soft" power while on the platform. This is the phenomenon that I refer to as "athletic connection." In nearly all cases, individuals practicing TBT, even for the first time, are noticeably stronger and more effective while they are on the raised platform. Next comes the ultimate challenge. For most individuals, try as they might, the instant they step off the elevated platform, they immediately lose their newfound athletic strength and connection. The challenge is to be able to recreate the wiry athletic connection, consciously, and without the aid of the raised platform.

As noted earlier, in *most* cases (about 95 percent of individuals), students quickly gain and just as quickly lose their new-found strength and athletic connection as they step on or off the training platform. The few exceptions were, for the most part, individuals who were serious surfers and rock climbers. Often, those individuals show little or no difference in their athletic connection whether on or off the raised platform. I believe that they, by default, naturally "suspend" their bodies, regardless of the environment.

I just had to write you because I purchased the body structure video and laughed at how simple the concept of standing on a cinder block and tricking the body to link the muscle so to speak. I was laughing and smiling all evening. Tomorrow I too will be on an elevated surface. Thanks.

Myron (www.chi-arts.com on-line customer)

Box 11-30

Studying the Body's Subtle Cues While on the Raised Platform

The body presents very subtle cues when on the raised platform, and the practitioner needs to pay attention to them. They are an invaluable part of being able to induce the new-found "athletic connection" state at will. Although extremely subtle, cues that might be observed by the practitioner include the flushing of one's hands or the dropping of the shoulders while on the raised platform. Later, the practitioner will rely on the triggering of those cues while *off* the raised platform to initiate those formerly unconscious choices.

With practice, the use of those cues as "triggers" allows the practitioner to fully engage an athletic springy-connectedness at will. For most of us who are not "naturals," this can take a while, and even with regular practice. It normally takes weeks, or even months, to develop conscious control over the body's "suspended" response when off the training device. At first, daily practice on the block (or another raised platform) is essential. Time and regular practice are necessary for the practitioner to gain enough skill to be able to instantly identify those subtle cues associated with this kind of body "suspension." The list presented in Box 11-31 includes the steps to develop a *tensegrity support habit*.

Five Steps to Developing a New *Tensegrity* Body Support Habit

1. Learn the feeling of your body's unconscious *tensegrity* support.

2. Identify the subtle cues associated with your body's triggering of an unconscious and superior connection.

3. Learn to induce cues consciously as triggers.

4. Learn to induce superior *tensegrity* at will.

5. Generalize the feeling of *tensegrity* throughout your normal day.

Box 11-31

Discovering Unconscious Tensegrity

The story of how I discovered and developed TBT explains the underlying principles of tensegrity. For more than three decades, I operated training centers along the southern California coast, so, inevitably, our studio's membership included a fair number of surfers. Observing that some students were more naturally "connected" than others, it seemed that a high percentage of those more natural practitioners were surfers. I wondered if there could be a link between the water sport and their superior "connected" and "springy" athletic ability.

Figure 11-32
Chinese Character for Song

The Flow State

As with those earlier examples, the "athletic connection" triggered by the TBT exercise also refers to a special relaxed, loose, yet connected power that can be accessed by the athlete. However, this is a special state of being that can only be actuated when one surrenders and becomes completely immersed in the task. Mihaly Csíkszentmihályi calls it the "flow state," [24] and it provides still more clues to the meaning of "soft" power in the martial arts and contact sports.

Although these forms of martial arts are sometimes said to be relaxed, or "soft," one must ask *why?* What is this "softness," and what makes it different from other kinds of athletic activities? In many respects, this kind of "soft" power is no different from the power expressed in other pugilistic forms. However, regardless of whether they are described as "soft" or "relaxed," this category of power is no different from examples found in baseball, basketball, and many other endeavors.

What characterizes many top tier athletes in their chosen sports is an ability to apply highly focused tension through *a relaxed body*. Thus, when the term "softening" is applied to *t'ai-chi* and related arts, on one level, this seems to be a contradictory notion. It might seem paradoxical that something "soft" and "relaxed" could simultaneously be powerful and effective. However, from a bio-mechanical viewpoint, the "softening" of *t'ai-chi* and other internal arts is no "softer" than the action of a loose spring-release-like throwing arm of a highly skilled baseball pitcher. † What does make the internal martial arts *distinctive*, though, is their approach to training, which incorporate a special kind of relaxation as the basis of their practice.

> † Note that an example of tensional strength in the martial arts, applied through a loose and relaxed body, can be viewed via the link provided in Box 11-33.

The *Song-Peng* Continuum

Confusion over the issue of "softening" starts to dissipate when one considers the special type of body mechanics inherent in these "internal" martial arts. In martial arts such as *t'ai-chi* and *baguazhang*, the contradiction is at least partly explained through the interaction of two central principles known as *song* (鬆) and *peng* (掤).

Illustrated in Figure 11-32, the phonetic *"song"* forms the bottom half of the character for *song*. The top is a semantic, meaning the appearance of long hair about the shoulders. Although *song* is often translated as "relaxed," in martial arts such as *t'ai-chi*, this idea of "relaxed-ness" is often over-applied, which sometimes results in the practitioner acquiring a "soggy noodle"

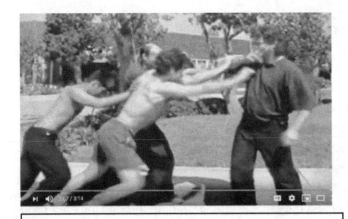

Link to Video Demonstrating Tensional Strength applied through a Relaxed Body. The Song-Peng Continuum

https://www.youtube.com/watch?v=j2D5chPv26k

or

https://chiarts.com/11-33

Box 11-33

style of practice with no, or at least very limited, martial value. In contrast, and as demonstrated in the video that can be accessed from the link in Box 11-33, to be useful when one is in close contact with an opponent, akin to the pro baseball pitcher, one must simultaneously master the ability to direct tensional lines of force within the body. Access to this kind of skill is dependent on one's ability to gain control over the continuum of tensional forces in the body.

The model of a continuum of tensional forces involves myofascial lines overlaid on a relaxed frame. In this light, it is suggested that a more complete picture of internal martial arts includes *song*, or "relaxed-ness," as only *part* of a continuum. The other part of the proposed continuum includes the principle of a "repellent force," described in *t'ai-chi* literature as *peng*, or, *pengjin* (掤勁).

The *song-peng* continuum can be imagined as expressing the tenacity of young, healthy bamboo that springs back into position after being pushed out of shape. As used here, *song-peng* refers to a variable, yet tensional, strength that can be accessed by a person who is in a tensegruous state. The practitioner who embodies a range of highly focused, springy power through specific myofascial lines learns to apply the tensional line of concentrated force to an exact point where it meets the opponent. This model coincides with eighteenth-century martial arts master Chang Naizhou's (萇乃周) teachings on training the *qi* by combining softness with hardness, and the importance of "focusing the body's energy to a single point." (Section VIII). [25]

The *song-peng* continuum is expressed when resilient tensional force is delivered through a strike, throw, or other technique. However, mastery of variable tension *song-peng* force under stress presents an arduous and perplexing challenge for the internal martial artist. Again, this may be compared to the explosive baseball-throw release from the mound of a major league baseball pitcher. Significantly, the most advanced levels of performance in most sports cannot be attained without the total integration of the athlete's ability to express graduated tensional skill along the *song-peng* continuum. The most "natural" athletes, from boxers to basketball players, learn to harness the variable tensile strength through the *song-peng* power continuum, and especially under the stressful conditions of contact sports.

Returning to the development of the TBT, while operating martial arts schools close to the California coast, I became fascinated by the way a few individuals were able to quickly apply that elusive *song-peng* principle to their martial arts practice. For the most part, these were young athletes who could be physically loose and yet powerful.

Again, since many of those "naturals" were surfers, I first thought that their ability to activate their springy power must be related to their sport. I reasoned that surfers could more easily "get" this normally difficult principle because of the way they trained themselves to move and balance on the most unstable of training platforms: a lightweight floating object on top of moving water. I reasoned that their *song-peng* skill must somehow be related to the sport's requirement for maintaining balance and directing force on a highly unstable base. I decided to test the theory.

In the mid 1990s, near the entrance to our martial art studio, there was a short, unstable wall that served to separate the classroom from the lobby. As an attempt to imitate the surfer's unstable platform, I had asked various students to stand and practice on the little wall. Remarkably, under this condition, both seasoned surfers and non-surfers instantly increased their loose, wiry athletic connection. Everyone who tried out the short wall *immediately* increased their athletic strength and fluidity, evidenced by how they could generate more power in strikes from shorter distances and easily push away mock opponents who attacked them while they were standing on the dividing wall. Standing on the unstable platform, they increased their "athletic connection," while at the same time releasing their shoulder tension. However, for most, they immediately reverted to their old habits as soon as they stepped off the wall and attempted to interact with opponents.

It appeared that we were onto something, and further experimentation brought a surprising result. Although the average student would immediately lose power and connection when stepping off the wobbly platform and onto the level floor, if, instead, they stepped from the unstable wall onto one of the office desks a foot or so away, the superior athletic connection principle would be maintained, *even without the wobbly platform*. This meant that the superior athletic connection wasn't triggered by the wobbly platform, but a *raised* platform. We observed that when a student stepped on top, and near to the edge, of an adjacent office desk, they experienced the same improved strength and connection that the unstable platform had triggered.

Testing the theory under various conditions with countless individuals, we found that in most cases a high-elevation platform, such as the top of a desk, wasn't necessary. The same type of superior performance could be duplicated by standing on a platform only a few inches off the ground, and, for most individuals, the use of a cinder block, such as the one shown in Photo 11-27, was sufficient.

We discovered that the mysterious springy-connectedness could be induced so long as a slight bit of perceived danger was present, and after much trial and error, five to six inches off the ground seems to be the magic distance. Under this condition, the practitioner's unconscious body-mind *paid attention*. Thus, the rule that explains this phenomenon might be expressed as: *The body prefers the path of least effort, unless a tiger is chasing it.*

TBT Step by Step

Note: If you are balance challenged in any way, do not attempt the exercise without someone assisting you.

- Step onto the raised platform.

- Direct your focus to a point in the distance. Focusing on a tree or other natural object is better than looking at a wall. Stand straight and comfortable. Do not lock your knees.

- Slightly stretch your fingers apart as you focus on the target — this helps you carry the stretchy-springy *song-peng* feeling through your entire body.

- Begin by practicing a few minutes at a time. Gradually increase your time on the block to ten or fifteen minutes.

- Observe the feeling of warmth in your hands and other signals associated with your body relaxing into the springy-tensegrity state. These are the type of signals that you will be learning to replicate at will in order to create the experience.

- Follow the instructions for developing a new habit in Box 3-27.

Photo 11-34

Intermediate – Advanced TBT

Photo shows a student in a suspended-tensegrity posture practicing xingyiquan''s "splitting strike" on a log

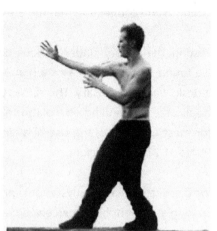

A video of a student practicing martial arts on a log as a form of moving suspension-tensegrity

training can be viewed at

https://youtu.be/ Gw4CmfeRjBY

or,

https://chiarts.com/11-36

Box 11-35

Intermediate and Advanced Levels of Training

Intermediate and advanced levels of practice incorporate athletic connection principles while in motion. An example of TBT in motion is shown in Photo 11-34. The photo is of a practitioner moving on a raised platform, in this case, a repurposed telephone pole. A link to a video of the practice is included in Box 11-35.

Testing for "Athletic Connection"

The "athletic connection test" is not a test of strength or the ability to resist force. It is designed to determine whether the person performing the test is "athletically connected" at the point of target impact. Here, "connection" refers to the ability to exhibit connected power, and the potential to express connected power, through a relaxed body. Note: The lower photo is an example of an incorrect test, and not a test of athletic connection, as the testing person's body weight is aligning into the test subject's body, which would not be a test of "response," but rather a test of adaptive strength that challenges the subject to change and repel the tester's changing weight and strength).

Block-Tensegrity Training — Contributions to a Bio-Tensegrity Model

In recent years, a substantial volume of work describing how bio-tensegrity principles apply to the human body and athletics has been published. Subsequently, a tremendous amount of discussion on the topic is now available on the web. Prominent among these contributions are those by Stephen M. Levin, MD, whose articles, presentations of *biotensegrity* models, and published papers are available through the website: http://biotensegrity.com. Resources there include papers on topics such as the dynamics of pelvic mechanics, the tensegrity model for spine mechanics, and the importance of soft tissue structural support of the body.

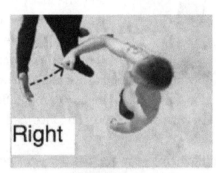
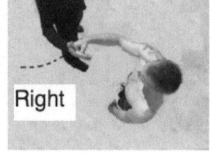
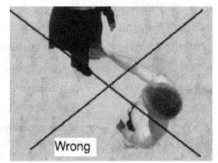

Diagram Series 11-36
Athletic Connection Test

The TBT protocol described in this chapter contributes to the discussion of bio-tensegrity in two ways: first, it provides a simple way to identify and test for unconscious preferences that break, or *denature,* the body's natural tensegrity. Second, it provides a method for teaching individuals to re-establish their own natural tensegrity. This observation of how to correct otherwise unconscious preferences has important implications for both the training of athletes and the application of TBT as an adjunctive therapy for patients suffering from musculoskeletal pain.

The terms "broken" or "interrupted" tensegrity are sometimes used by adherents of bio-tensegrity models to describe serious or pathological conditions, or those normally associated with the "natural" process of aging. In contrast, observations of individuals who engaged in TBT, and particularly those described in the "athletic connection test," reveal how "broken tensegrity" in both athletes and non-athletes is more prevalent than generally realized. These observations suggest that most of us make unconscious decisions to interrupt the body's natural tensegrity, which becomes "denatured" by an unchallenging environment comprised of level floors and walkways, resulting in patterns of "broken" tensegrity.

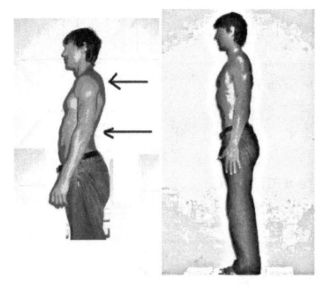

Passive vs. Active Support of the Body

Unless corrected, the body's unconscious preference is to become passive. This tendency influences most people to break their natural tensegrity in favor of allowing the body to fall into a posture requiring the least effort. This is not a judgment on the human's inherent laziness, but likely an unconscious instinct to conserve energy. However, because most of us live in flat and level "denatured" environments, this tendency is heightened, and the body is often inadequately supported. For most of our lives, and particularly as we age, our bodies increasingly prefer to "hang out," and, unless this is consciously corrected, we will inevitably favor positions / postures that require less effort. For example, our necks hang forward and tend to lock into unnatural orientations associated with "normal" aging. Likewise, other parts of our once youthful, spring-like bodies begin to sag.

Diagrams 11-37
Passive vs. Active Support of the Body
The arrows in the left photo show the typical profile of a collapsed body, with major fulcrums indicated at the upper back/neck and lower-mid back. In contrast, the right photo demonstrates a natural "suspension" of the body.

There are two ways that this negative tendency can be corrected. One is through the environment, as a person living most of their time in a more natural environment will tend to ambulate in a springier and more interactive way with nature and her obstacles (Diagram 11-38). Balancing on rocks in the forest forces the body to lift and balance, while stepping into a hollow in the ground causes the foot to initiate a more robust adaptive response. In contrast, the unconscious tendency toward "laziness" is observed when the elbow can rest on a table, or when we drop back into our soft chairs and allow the body to slouch.

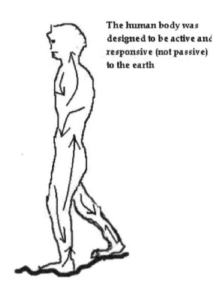

The human body was designed to be active and responsive (not passive) to the earth

In these last examples, nature's design is thwarted, and, although not normally causing a health problem, like the frog that sat in gradually warming water, the danger isn't readily noticed until it's too late. When a maladaptive posture pattern persists over a long period, problems resulting from dysfunction appear, such as a widow's hump or extreme forward inclination of the neck. In the case of persistent bad posture, long-term dysfunction produces negative health consequences and limits an individual's natural athletic potential.

Diagram 11-38
The Body's Active Responses
How tensional forces interact together and are distributed throughout the body

Denaturing

The *natural*, integrated, springy-support system of the human frame supports athletic performance and is an important part of rehabilitation after a physical injury. However, as illustrated in the left image of Diagrams 11-37, the human body, when removed from the constant variability of natural terrain, tends to fall into lazy positions that require less effort. The image on the left shows an example of "least effort," with the head falling forward, compensated by the "sway back," whereas the image on the right illustrates the more ideal form of body support.

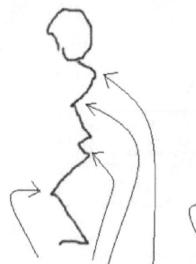 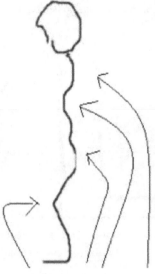

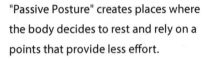

"Passive Posture" creates places where the body decides to rest and rely on a points that provide less effort.

An "Active Posture" creates suspension against the earth. This kind of resistance / interaction stretches muscles and opens "energy channels."

Diagrams 11-39
Passive vs. Active Support of the Body

The figure on the right in Diagrams 11-39 represents the tensegruous structure expressed in the human frame. It is a symbolic representation of the body's connective tissue matrix, which is designed to *interact, flex, and adapt* to a constantly changing terrain. However, as suggested by the figure on the left in Diagrams 11-39, aberrations in the body's natural upright support occur when the body is removed from the constant variability of the uneven natural terrain. Under artificially level conditions, instead of proper fascia support, the body unconsciously prefers orientations that require the least amount of effort.

The second way to correct the body's tendencies toward laziness is to change one's *preferences*. Psychologically speaking, this category belongs to a subset of study called behavior therapy, and the process of changing habits is expressed through a principle known as *positive reinforcement*. Positive reinforcement takes place when behavior (whether conscious or unconscious) is met with positive consequences (reward); the rule that applies is that behavior tends to be repeated when reinforced by rewards. To apply this method in the area of posture correction, the trick is to learn to experience the corrected posture with a feeling of *enjoyment*. Since behavior, when matched with a favorable outcome, tends to be repeated, the feeling of a correctly suspended body frame becomes enjoyable, and this acts as a type of positive reinforcement or reward.

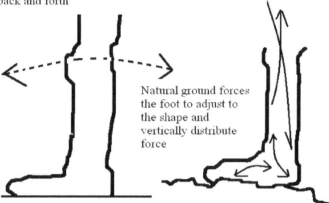

On flat and level ground, the body becomes lazy and unconsciously tends to rock back and forth

Natural ground forces the foot to adjust to the shape and vertically distribute force

Comparisons of foot shape and consequent lines of Force
Flat and level compared to natural ground

Diagram 11-40
The Interaction of the Knee
with Natural Versus Paved Terrain

As a final example, fulcrums and rest points in the body replace fascia stretch and support, and this denaturing occurs when movement requires less effort. It is *easier*, for example (see Diagram 11-40), if instead of engaging the abductor and adductor muscles of the leg, the knee joint takes on increasing stress as it operates as a fulcrum and works out of proper balance with the total musculature of the body. In many cases, the cumulative effect of this habit leads to knee problems years down the road.

Smile. Even though you don't feel like it, the mere act of smiling repetitively helps to interrupt mood disorders and strengthen the brain's neural ability to maintain a positive outlook on life. And even if you fake a smile, other people will respond to you with greater generosity and kindness. To my knowledge, the only religion to incorporate smiling into a spiritual practice is Buddhism. For example, Thich Nhat Hanh suggests that we do "smiling meditation" whenever we have a spare moment during the day.

— Neuroscientist Andrew Newberg, MD

Chapter 61

The Power of the Smile

A Simple Trick to a More Integrated Body

*T*his chapter describes a simple trick for developing a more integrated and "athletically connected" body. These changes, activated through the simple act of smiling, can be seen instantly, and they affect the entire body.

It may sound strange, but the practice of smiling enhances athletic ability in a surprising way. I discovered the strange relationship between smiling, athletic performance, and physical therapy while working with patients suffering from chronic neck and shoulder pain.

One day, I was training a particularly tense and "locked up" martial arts and internal energy client with some "standing practices" (Section VIII, Chapter 43). It seemed that there was no way to get this physically and emotionally rigid middle-aged businessman to relax for more than a fraction of a second, which was an issue because the foundation of my meditation and martial arts teaching requires a kind of springy relaxation called *song* or *song-peng*. The client was so tense that it seemed miraculous he could move at all.

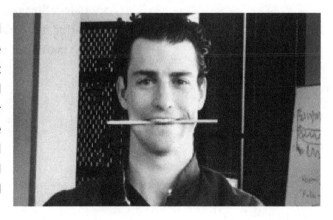

Photo 11-41
Training with Chopsticks

My challenge was to get this habitually tense client to relax *somehow*, even if only for a few moments, so that he could experience the feeling of "soft" movement. I already had an intuitive understanding of the relationship between smiling, relaxation, and athletic performance, and I would later come to understand these in terms of the relationships between tense facial muscles, particularly of the jaw, and how a tense jaw also causes /maintains tension in the neck and shoulder muscles. While working with the client during standing practice, the more I tried to get him to relax, the more tense he became. Every attempt to get the man to surrender his tension and characteristic frown was useless.

The practice of "standing" involves holding a posture very still for 12 minutes or longer. When performed correctly, tension gradually releases in the neck, shoulder, and back. However, this client was unable to relax, and held on to his tension as if his very life depended on it. Encouraging clients to smile usually helps them to release tension faster, but in his case, trying to get the tense client to smile was useless.

When he really tried, the client could affect a smile for a half a second, but then his face would immediately return to its habitual frown. Determined to find a way for him to maintain his "smile" a little longer, and then, in turn, get his body to relax, I grabbed a pen off the front desk and asked him to hold the device in his mouth. It worked! Not only did the pen break his habitual patterns, but with the pen in his mouth, he was able to mobilize more power, move more fluidly, and easily maintain that earlier described wiry state of "athletic connection."

Intrigued by the implications of "grubby pen-smile technique," I began to experiment with the newfound training method with both groups and individuals. Substituting the random pen on the desk for a more sanitary alternative, students and instructors alike began to use disposable wooden chopsticks in many classes. Everyone noticed an improvement, and the practice soon became popular. Both students and the present author experienced faster release of tense shoulder and neck muscles, as well as improved ability to express that elusive relaxed springy internal martial art power. Thereafter, the trick helped many students with their sore backs and shoulders; the practice continued to gain popularity, and our group members requested more "chopstick training." I am sure that for a time we became the largest martial art school purchaser of disposable chopsticks in the West.

Conclusion to Section XI

The Confluence of Energy, Posture, and Bio-mechanics

Although a clear definition of "internal energy" is not yet available, many of the benefits associated with strong internal energy seem indistinguishable from the influences of posture and advanced body mechanics. In some examples, benefits attributed to "strong internal energy" could well be said to be merely a function of bio-physical mechanics and one's ability to control normally unconscious muscle groups in a conscious way. Other attributes related to "internal energy" can be described in terms of posture and the way one interacts with the forces of gravity. In these examples, the influence of "postural practices" leads the practitioner to increased confidence, clearer thinking, and brain detoxification. Significantly, all these benefits are associated with a high degree of "internal energy."

The common denominator uniting all the principles presented in this chapter suggests that a relationship exists among what is identified as "internal energy" or "internal power," efficient bio-mechanics, and the correct support of the human frame. In the pursuit of a meaningful definition of "internal energy," beyond the nebulous *life energy*, it is also necessary to consider the interaction between improved posture, efficient bio-mechanics, and related physiological factors contributing to the status of a person with "strong internal energy."

Consider the earlier presentation of *qigong* as a *stillness practice*. That example involved holding the head very still and in the proper position for several minutes. After a few minutes of holding the position, most practitioners notice positive mental and emotional changes. The recent scientific discovery of the brain's connection to the lymphatic system, in a way beyond that which was previously understood, suggests that a "qigong" or "meditation" practice that involves holding the head in this way may contribute to improved brain function associated with the proper flow of lymph (a detoxification process). Thus, this kind of exercise, based on holding the head upright and still, promotes a positive attitude and improved concentration.

As science considers increasingly subtle aspects of human physiology, the lines between healthful "energy training" and beneficial physiological practices will no doubt continue to merge. The value of many of the exercises in the present section were once regarded by practitioners to be "circulating the *qi* energy" or "aligning the body's energy channels." These same practices can now also be understood in terms of the proper maintenance of the human frame, which in turn promotes proper blood and nerve-support functions.

In much the same way, physiological principles can sometimes explain a top athlete's ability to exhibit exceptional prowess. For example, the role of vertical posture might, at least in some cases, explain phenomena understood in Asian martial arts in terms of the flow of internal energy. In this light, many of the demonstrations by masters such as Cheng Man-ching and Morihei Ueshiba might be explained, not only in terms of their expression of internal power, *qi*, or *ki*, but also their physical posture and bio-mechanics. These are exemplary models of the relationship between "energy" and "form."

As a final comment, it is noteworthy that many ancient energetic-meditation and prayer practices emphasized the importance of posture. The point is demonstrated in Tibetan Lama Dudjom Rinpoche's instructions to his disciples to pay attention to their posture, so that "the channels" will be held straight and the "wind-energy" will thereby be "unobstructed." Emphasizing the relationship between mind, *subtle energy,* and physical posture, the Rinpoche explains that only then can "the mind rest in its natural, unaltered flow." Another example describing the relationship between posture and subtle energy is found in the core practices of the Taoist alchemist-meditators. They, too, believed that their erect posture was an important precondition for transmuting coarse *jing* energy into subtle *shen*, or "spiritual" energy, a principle later adopted as the cornerstone of *t'ai-chi* instruction.

Endnotes

1   https://brighamhealthhub.org/spine/that-headache-may-be-a-pain-in-the-neck

2   http://newsroom.uvahealth.com/about/news-room/missing-link-found-between-brain-immune-system-with-profound-disease-implications

3 http://www.feeltheqi.com/articles/rc-lymph.htm

4 http://newsroom.uvahealth.com/about/news-room/missing-link-found-between-brain-immune-system-with-profound-disease-implications

5   http://newsroom.uvahealth.com/about/news-room/missing-link-found-between-brain-immune-system-with-profound-disease-implications

6 Goldthwait, J.E., et al., "The conservation of human energy: A plea for a broader outlook in the practice of medicine," *Rocky mountain medical journal*, 19 (Oct) 1934.

7 Oschman, James, *Energy medicine, the scientific basis*. pp. 147-148.

8 Goldthwait, J.E., et al., "The conservation of human energy: A plea for a broader outlook in the practice of medicine," *Rocky mountain medical journal,* 19 (Oct):341-350.

9 Broadbent, Elizabeth, Nair, Shwetha, et al, "Do slumped and upright postures affect stress responses? A randomized trial," *Health psychology*, Vol 34(6), Jun 2015, pp. 632-641.

10 Broadbent, Elizabeth, Nair, Shwetha, et al., "Do slumped and upright postures affect stress responses? A randomized trial," *Health psychology,* Vol 34(6), Jun 2015, pp. 632-641.

11 https://en.wikipedia.org/wiki/Anderson_Silva

12 Illustrations by Sergio Verdeza based on photographs presented in other works and by other authors. Bottom right image based on photo presented in Robert Smith's *Chinese Boxing: Masters and Methods*.

13 As a neurotransmitter, serotonin helps to relay messages from one area of the brain to another. Because of the widespread distribution throughout the brain, it is believed to influence a variety of psychological and body functions. Of the approximately 40 million brain cells, most are influenced either directly or indirectly by serotonin. This includes brain cells related to mood, sexual desire and function, appetite, sleep, memory and learning, temperature regulation, and some social behavior. Source: Web MD http://www.webmd.com/depression/features/serotonin

14 Merton, Thomas, (translator), *The way of Chuang Tzu*, New Horizons Press, 1969 p. 60.

15 Ware (translator), Ko Hung, *The pao pu tzu of Ko Hung.*

16 https://www.youtube.com/watch?v=C_fEIVwjrew

17 The rotator cuff is considered a "soft tissue joint" made up of the four muscles that surround the shoulder: *infraspinatus, teres minor, supraspinatus, subscapulatus.*

18 https://en.wikipedia.org/wiki/Piezoelectricity

19 Robbie, 6:45-48.

20 Oschman, James L., *Energy Medicine: The scientific basis*, Churchill Livingstone, Harcourt Publishers Ltd, 2000 p. 153.

21 Tiller, William, *Science and human transformation: Subtle energies, intentionality, and consciousness*. Pavior, p. 107.

22 Tiller

23 Wile, Douglas, *The art of the bedchamber: The Chinese sexual yoga classics, including women's solo meditation texts,* State University of New York (1992), p. 351.

24 Defined as "the mental state operation in which a person performing an activity is fully immersed in a feeling of energized focus, full involvement, and enjoyment in the process of the activity. In essence, flow is characterized by complete absorption in what one does, and a resulting loss in one's sense of space and time."

https://en.wikipedia.org/wiki/Flow_(psychology)

25 Wile, Douglas, *Lost t'ai-chi classics from the late Ch'ing dynasty*, State University of New York, 1996, p.79.

26 Robbie D.L. 1977 "Tensional forces in the human body," *Orthopedic review* 6: 47.

Section XII
Speculation and Dimensional Stuff

Physics is often stranger than science fiction, and I think science fiction takes its cues from physics: higher dimensions, wormholes, the warping of space and time, stuff like that.

— Michio Kaku

Section XII

Speculation and Dimensional Stuff

Introduction to Section XII

Speculation and Dimensional Stuff

*I*s it possible that a testable definition of *qi*, prana, and "internal energy" by other names is so elusive, and the phenomenon so resistant to measurement, because the "life force" operates, at least partially, beyond the boundaries of our known reality? This section details a new way to think about and explore the meaning of internal energy. It is based on the notion that the *qi* of Chinese *qigong* and martial arts masters, the *prana* of the yogi, and the *lung-wind* of the Tibetan meditator function the way they do because these forms of what we refer to as "energy" actually represent the practitioner's ability to interact with another dimension or dimensions.

To accomplish this task, this section includes speculation on alternative models of bio-physics. If even partially true, these models will begin to explain how the power of intention interacts with both the physical body and the physical world beyond one's physical demarcations. If, one day, the aphorisms that the "mind influences the body" and "our thoughts contribute to our reality" are proven correct, then the models presented below will contribute to explanations of the *life force*, <u>not</u> in terms of belief or magic, but concrete science.

At that time, there will be a more clearly understood science of mind as it relates to the meaning of "energy." Simultaneously, a broader understanding of bio-physics will include an expanded knowledge of how one's intention influences the electromagnetic (EM) and EM-like energy spheres that surround the body, which in turn allow us to access other dimensions.

The speculation put forward here describes interactions between electromagnetic and electromagnetic-like energies, such as "near reactive fields," presumed to surround the body, and the *ether*. In the pages that follow, these interactions are sometimes described in the context of a particular modality; for instance, acupuncture or non-contact healing. However, it should be noted that the principles discussed in one modality are assumed to have a wider application in other "energetic technologies," such as energetic healing, *qigong*, energetic meditation, and so on. Thus, a given example should not be thought of as representing only that particular modality, but as representing a more universal application.

These proposals are presented through two interwoven themes. The first is a new way to conceptualize the meaning of subtle energies based on suggestions by leading scientists in the field. Those ideas include the notion that subtle forces operate ***through*** an ***intersection*** between known dimensional and measurable attributes, and another yet-to-be-measured dimension or dimensions.

The second theme concerns new ways of accessing and working with "internal energy" on an "other-dimensional" basis. For my students, clients, and in my own practice, the methods discussed here have been revolutionary. Our experiences with the described training methods continue to provide testimony to the powerful results one can achieve by working with these hypothesized cross-dimensional electromagnetic-like interactions.

The approaches that follow increase the healing power of acupuncture and energetic bodywork. They enhance one's experience of subtle energy accessed through yoga, *qigong*, and meditation, and offer new ways to investigate the meaning of internal energy in the martial arts. Note that many of the assertions that follow are highly speculative, and so the reader is encouraged to consider whatever they find useful and ignore the rest.

Chapter 62

Alternative Explanations

*T*he preceding pages have stressed that, to date, there is no testable definition of internal energy. This means that any and all alternative definitions remain open for consideration, even the most novel and unorthodox. If some of these new ways to think about "internal energy" are even partially correct, then the methods described below to explore those suggestions signal a sea change in the way we think about and practice energetic meditation, healing, and martial arts, such as *t'ai-chi* [1] and aikido.

Why, you ask? Because those methods look at the body's energetic system quite differently in comparison with conventional viewpoints. Most striking among these is how a person's "energy" is explained not as an "internal force," but in terms of a **relationship** between the body's built-in energetic infrastructure and another yet-to-be-measured dimension(s). In other words, internal energy is not explained as something the practitioner manages *within* the confines of the physical body, but rather through cross-dimensional and *magnetic-like* interactions.

This, what might be classified as an "interaction model," is different from most others. For example, in many *qigong* practices, the practitioner is taught to "cultivate" and "store" life's subtle energy, whereas the interaction model deemphasizes the importance of "gathering," "cultivating," and "storing" one's internal energy. However, these newly proposed methods do share some important similarities with other approaches, such as *t'ai-chi*, energetic meditation, and many styles of yoga, where **sensitivity to sensations** remains the cornerstone of practice. Sensitivity brings awareness; awareness links mind and intention to sensations. Awareness and attention to sensations can trigger the cross-dimensional "energetic" experiences that relate to one's mastery of the *life force*.

The psycho-biological foundation of this investigation into "internal energy" is based on working with the body's energetic infrastructure. In this context, infrastructure refers to the body's acupuncture meridian system, based on the idea that the "channels" are not imaginary energy lines, but in fact physical structures. According to Myers and Dorsher, the meridians consist of myofascial tracks of piezoelectric fibers* that are not only important because of their ability to convert physical stress into electricity, but also because of their antenna function. Furthermore, consistent with the ideas proposed by

Dr. William Tiller, they function as the body's flexible, piezoelectric antenna "suit."

* Introduced in Section II

A New Look at the Meridian-Channels

Earlier chapters have described known attributes of the acupuncture meridians, such as their ability to conduct electrical current. This property provides an important clue as to the force, or influence, we might call internal energy. However, it is problematic that, after thousands of research studies conducted by scientists throughout the world and over many decades, there is not yet a testable model to explain how the "energy" of acupuncture works for healing and other purposes. Scientists cannot yet explain why acupuncture, and related healing arts, sometimes works so effectively.

The quandary is reflected in David Eisenberg's experiences as a medical exchange student in China. His first-hand account includes his description of an encounter with a woman on a bus in Beijing, who suffered an attack of numbing paralysis in her legs. Subsequently, Eisenberg accompanied the woman to be treated by a traditional physician, where he observed the individual receive a simple acupuncture treatment. Soon afterward, she recovered both sensation and the ability to walk. According to Eisenberg, there is no Western medical model or known scientific explanation that might account for how the woman healed and regained her ability to walk so quickly. [2]

This is one of many examples of the kind of frustration researchers experience as they seek answers to explain the healing powers of acupuncture and energetic medicine. The challenging search for acupuncture's underlying mechanism is highlighted by remarks on the subject by UCLA acupuncture researcher David Bressler. A report, delivered after several years of his research team's investigation into the technique, included the remarkable statement: "The mechanism [of] acupuncture remains unknown." [3] More recently, the National Institute of Health published a similar declaration on the nature of the acupuncture meridians: "The definition and characterization of these [meridian] structures remain elusive." [4]

Despite considerable efforts to uncover the mechanism that might provide a meaningful explanation of acupuncture points and theory, a workable definition of how the modality functions remains largely hidden. Thus, an entirely new model is necessary to enable researchers to investigate the mechanism. The ideal framework would be one that offers a one-day testable definition of "internal energy" as a measurable force by currently available instruments.

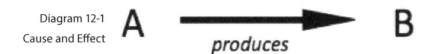

Diagram 12-1
Cause and Effect

Interaction and Relationship vs. Cause and Effect

Consider whether energetic methods, such as non-contact healing, might be explained in terms of cause and effect (Diagram 12-1). The proposal was previously put forward in Section IV, as a possible explanation for a human-directed healing force. There, we considered suggestions by some researchers that the effects of *qi* / internal energy can be accounted for by electromagnetic or infrared emissions from the hands of a skilled healer.

Applied as an explanation for energetic healing, this example of cause and effect would apply as follows: an invisible force is emitted by a practitioner → the invisible force influences a target (a patient) → the patient receives measurable benefits. These assertions are extraordinary, and, if true, suggest that human-directed electromagnetic / infrared emissions act as a *force of nature*. This is a remarkable claim, which therefore requires remarkable supporting evidence.

As covered earlier, there are some issues with proposals that suggest *qi* / internal energy can be measured by currently available instruments. One theory advanced by Akira Seto, PhD and Chikaaki Kusaka, MD proposed that the electromagnetic fields they measured from non-contact healers represented examples of purposefully emitted *qi* or *ki* energy. [5] However, they concluded that only a small percentage of the known healers they studied were able to emit an anomalously large electromagnetic field. In light of this observation, it is instructive to take a closer look at the subjects in the Seto and Kusaka investigation. [6]

How important is it that only a handful — three of the 37, or about 12 percent — of the "known" healers in the Seto-Kusaka study could emit the impressive and measurable electromagnetic field? Keep in mind that those 37 individuals were not randomly chosen, but selected because they, as the researchers describe them, were "known to be able to emit the healing force." [7]

Results like those obtained in the Seto-Kusaka study suggest one of two conclusions: first, that either the mysterious healing force is truly evidenced through the emission of electromagnetic energy, and that only 12 percent of "known healers" were able to emit healing energy. If true, this means that the remaining individuals had no energetic healing ability, despite being "known healers" ahead of their selection for the study. The second possible conclusion is that the meaning of consciously-directed healing energy is something beyond what can be detected and measured as electromagnetic energy.

Extra-Dimensional Explanations?

In Section IV, it was also described how a healer's electromagnetic field emissions, like those observed by Seto and Kusaka, might not be causal, but correlational. If true, this would mean that the remarkable observed phenomena, where some individuals were able to emit an extraordinarily large electromagnetic field, may not necessarily represent the emission of *qi* or internal energy *per se*. Instead, extraneous electromagnetic field emissions may be related to the way *some* individuals learn to *interact* with *something else*. Among the possible candidates to explain this unknown, or *x-factor*, is the possibility of an entirely new explanation, and, perhaps, even an extra-dimensional one.

If extra-dimensionality is part of the explanation for what we call energetic healing, it would mean that a healer's ability to project a healing influence may not be due to the *extension* **of a measurable energetic force** *per se*. Instead, the effect might be attributed to the healer's ability to mediate an **interaction** between the patient and the healing source. If this were true, it would mean that the measured EM field radiations, such as those observed by Seto, would represent a particular individual's way of interacting with *something else*.

If such a proposition is even partly true, it would suggest that an entirely new way of thinking about "energetic healing" is warranted. To summarize, the investigation of these ideas encourages us to think about whether the *key* to understanding energetic healing might not lay in the practitioner's consciously directed *force* or *energy*. Instead, the more likely explanation would be found through the way an individual learns to interact and "dance" with that *something else*.

If such a theory proves accurate, it would mean that phenomena we call "energy," *qi*, *prana*, etc., might not be best thought of as an energetic reserve that is developed within, or directed through, the practitioner. In its place, the new model suggests that the healer's ability refers to the management of a special kind of *interaction*.

However, to appreciate the "interaction hypothesis" fully, another point needs to be brought into the discussion. A potential issue is whether or not intention — here referring to intention research in the West — might belong to the category of "internal energy." Earlier chapters cited William Tiller's study of the power of intention to influence a physical target, and relevant to the present point is how an individual who, relying on focused intention, and without physical contact — for example, as demonstrated in Tiller's gas-discharge device study — was documented as being able to initiate a physical response in the experimental device (Section VII). These observations are relevant to the "energy" question because, as Tiller reports, that kind of consciously-directed influence was effected by a practitioner *even while isolated within the boundaries of a Faraday cage*. [8]

The results obtained in Tiller's gas-discharge device experiments are crucial to the suggestions that follow, due principally to the electromagnetic shielding afforded by a Faraday cage. This is because, in those experiments, a human emitted **electromagnetic field** could not have caused the device to register an electrostatic charge. This means that either the power of intention to influence the external physical environment observed in those experiments is in a class completely separate from *qi* and internal energy, or that the enigmatic force, however it will eventually be described, is not exclusively dependent on a person's ability to emit an electromagnetic field. In that case, then, the individual's ability to extend non-physical and non-electromagnetic influence would be an important aspect of the new model. In other words, if "internal energy" is of the same class of "forces" studied in Tiller's intention experiments, then the phenomena we refer to as *qi / ki / prana* and so forth is **not electromagnetic**, but points to the involvement of a form of "energy," "information," or "interaction" on another level that functions beyond the normally understood electromagnetic spectrum. This point supports the earlier suggestion that the electromagnetic field radiations emitted by some individuals, although correlational, may not be causal.

Chapter 63

Other-Dimension Possibilities

*F*or many of us, two concepts that will be particularly difficult to grasp are the idea that we may function in a sea of multiple interacting dimensions, and how the way that we consciously or unconsciously interact with these other dimensions may not only have a direct influence on our physical health, but also our access to optimal power and potential. In the foreword to Tiller's *Science and Human Transformation*, Ernest F. Pecci, MD describes the difficulty in attempting to grasp the significance of such an invisible parallel dimension:

> Our eyes can visualize only 3-dimensional configurations while remaining oblivious to the panoply of subliminal energies from other dimensionalities interwoven into a flowing pattern. Our left brain attempts to analyze the isolated fragments it can perceive and constructs beliefs to make sense of and to add predictability to these observations. [9]

Although we cannot yet measure the other-dimensional aspects of the theory through mathematical proofs, physicists tell us that they exist. For practitioners of energetic arts like *t'ai-chi*, energetic meditation, and *qigong*, these theories are potentially important because they include definitions of "energetic practices" that increase their effectiveness by incorporating extra-dimensional modeling beyond our normal "reference frame" (RF).

To restate, the cross-dimensional model that is described here does not rely exclusively on the notion that a practitioner transmits an invisible "energy." Instead, the new model incorporates the notion of a practitioner not as a "projector," but instead as an intermediary, who is able to orchestrate a cross-dimensional "relationship."

An example of this kind of relationship is found in the beliefs of the Hawaiian shamans, or *kahuna*. They believe that it is not the power of the *kahuna* that brings about healing, but their ability to create a relationship between the patient and *mana* that realizes the desired effect. Applied to "energetic modalities," such as acupuncture and energetic healing, although these techniques might appear as though their results can be described in terms of cause and effect, they might be more accurately understood as a cross-dimensional exchange of *information*.

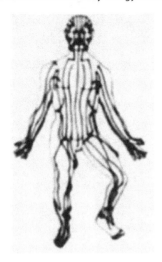

Figure 12-2
Tiller's Model of the Body's Meridian
System as an Antenna Array
Although presented in Section II,
the image is repeated here for the
convenience of the reader.
Source: William Tiller, Science and
Human Transformation [20]

As an introduction to the new model, let's take a closer look at those physical structures within the body that would allow for a cross-dimensional interaction. First, an antenna system is necessary that would allow for the transfer of cross-dimensional information.

The Embedded Antenna Array

Section II introduced Tiller's proposal that acupuncture points and meridians may function as an embedded antenna array. There, it was proposed that these structures, because of their antenna function, link the physical body with an "other dimensional" aspect that, for now, will be referred to as the *ether*.

For the mind-body to engage and manage those cross-dimensional interactions, the embedded network must be piezoelectric. This means that, similar to the way crystals react, physical stress placed upon the structure induces an electrical charge, and the resulting voltage field that forms around the human antenna mimics the way that simple dipole antennas function. For the purposes of the model introduced here, the most efficient antenna network would consist of a flexible network and, like meridians, be located on the surface of the body.

Based on the physical location of the surface meridians, those "antenna structures" are perfectly situated to engage what might be considered the cloud-like grid, or aura, that surrounds the body. Accordingly, the antenna structures serve to emit two distinct fields of radiation, one near and the other distant. Included among the basic roles of these fields would be the ability to sense danger. However, their function also includes the sending and receiving of various types of information.

For example, more advanced antenna functions are believed to be associated with inspiration; they also serve as conveyances of spiritual experiences and function to connect a person psychically to others. Because of their piezoelectric nature, presumably these structures would be more responsive to some activities than others. For example, the stretchy tension associated with yoga and *qigong* may more readily activate these structures than passive states.

As proposed by Tiller, those antenna structures interface between the physical and the non-physical dimensions, operating in the interstitial space between the physically solid and the etheric. Because of their link to mind and intention, the antennae are more responsive to certain kinds of mental activities, such as daydreaming. [10] Likewise, deep thought, prayer, meditation, reflection, and walks in nature are, either alone or when combined with one another, examples of activities that stimulate activity within those embedded cross-dimensional networks. These kinds of activities would not only provide the individual with insight and guidance on deep levels, but also challenge the "normal" A → B cause and effect perception of events.

These concepts merge as elements of Tiller's model of the meridians and acupuncture points as an embedded antenna array. They represent the interaction between the physical points / meridians on the body's surface and "something else" beyond measurement. Let us take a closer look at how the body's embedded antenna is theorized to work:

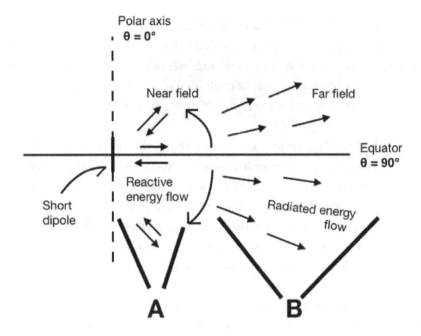

Diagram 12-3
Tiller's Schematic of Near (Reactive) and Distant (Radiated) Energy Fields
The illustration shows the radiated field pattern from an acupuncture point and meridian perspective. Note that field demarcations A and B are the author's and not part of Tiller's original diagram. Originally presented in Section IV, the diagram it is presented again for the convenience of the reader.
(Schematic modeled from one presented by William A. Tiller in *Science and Human Transformation*)

As illustrated by Diagram 12-2, the model of the meridians functioning as an embedded antenna array was introduced in Section II. That proposition included the notion that the meridians operate as an elaborate two-way sending-receiving network, akin to the function of a simple dipole antenna (Diagram 12-3). Thus, like the function of such an antenna, they are believed to emit two distinct fields of subtle radiation. This is an important point, since the suggestions that follow are based on these "radiated fields" and our ability to moderate our interactions with them.

Dipole antennas, the simplest type of antenna, do not work because they appear as a piece of wire that sticks up into the air. Their operation depends on a fluctuating voltage in the wire that generates an electrical field around the structure. Keep in mind that it is the *field*, and not the wire, that allows it to function as an antenna.

The proposed model suggests that humans likewise have a bifurcated electrical-like field that radiate from the meridians. Like AM or FM radio signals, these fields move around and through us. However, for the most part, EM and, especially, EM-like fields remain invisible and undetectable. In some applications that relate to what might be called energetic technologies, the undetectable part has to do with RF.

Let us take a closer look at how the acupuncture meridians function as an embedded antenna grid that allows an individual to interact with those other dimensions. Tiller describes the embedded network:

> All humans (and probably all vertebrates) contain a rudimentary acupuncture meridian / chakra system and have their own Qi / prana pump that, via focused intention, can at least metastably raise the local EM [electromagnetic] gauge symmetry of their surrounding space and thus, can produce healings of great variety. [11]

Tiller's parallel dimension model is radical. It suggests an expansion of presently accepted biophysics to include the notion that an individual's etheric, intentional, and emotional representation extends beyond the confines of the physical body as normally perceived. Here, we are introduced to some of the elements of the body's "antenna system:"

> My views of this antenna system are 1) The primary structural elements of this antenna system are located at the etheric substance level rather than at the physical substance level in order to explain the lack of major histological difference between [acupuncture points] and surrounding tissue. 2) Subtle energy wave flow along the etheric meridians yields a transduced flow of magnetic vectors potential, A, waves along the physical locus of these meridian channels. [12]

Although this paragraph is very dense, the points become more accessible when unpacked. Tiller proposes a model of the body's energy system, which, as part of its antenna array function, relies on the interaction between the meridian and another dimensional field he calls the ***etheric substance level.***

Near and Far Radiated Fields

According to the model proposed by Tiller, the embedded antenna array meridian network possesses both sending and receiving capabilities. In other words, functioning like a simple dipole antenna, they both send and receive information. One of the operations of the "antenna function" would be to pick up and interpret the emotional states of other individuals, especially those with whom we are physically near or emotionally close. This not only explains functions like energetic healing, but also how these antennae also generate their own energy fields that radiate around our bodies. They may be the mechanism that provides for our intuition and "gut feelings."

The distinction between the two fields, and our respective interactions with them, may account for different aspects of what is normally referred to as "internal energy." The primary distinction between them is the **near reactive field** and the **distal radiating field**; the near field explains what psychics sometimes describe as the "close to skin" human aura. More importantly, the model implicitly offers a new explanation for the underlying mechanism of acupuncture, as well as other "energy" technologies. At this juncture, it is important to emphasize that the antenna function — and this gets into the extra-dimensional component of the theory — is "located at the *etheric* level rather than the substance level." [13]

The other part of the theory that continues to stretch physics as presently understood is that one's consciousness becomes entangled within these fields. Representing the interstitial planes between the tangible and intangible, entanglement allows for an individual's intention to extend outward. This is a crucial point, since it heralds a future when physics will be able to explain how intention and consciousness act upon the physical world.

The piezoelectric nature of the acupuncture meridian network provides a new way to think about practices such as *qigong* and hatha yoga. The network, composed of piezoelectric fibers — because of the way tensional stress converts physical stress into an electrical charge — is believed to be more "charged" following consciousness-related practices such yoga, *qigong, t'ai-chi,* and meditation. Posture and, for most of us, consciously-directed tension through those postures, provide a certain amount of stretchy stimulation that is inherent in these practices. [14] This kind of stimulation is believed to activate the antenna function of the embedded network, and, because of its central role in the theory, a closer look at the radiated fields of the embedded antenna network is warranted.

Consider the field (Demarcation A in Diagram 12-3) that Tiller describes as the near, or *reactive field*, lying about an inch or so around the body:

> Subtle levels of substance exist in the body, and they give rise to radiation emission in much the same manner that physical substance generates EM emissions. Likewise, just as the physical body has major antenna systems associated with it, the etheric body and our more subtle bodies have special antenna systems associated with them. Thus, each of these antenna systems is expected to have a transduced A-Field correlate manifest at the physical level, and its near field radiation pattern will be a standing wave field or auric field representation of the subtle body. [15]

Tiller's description of a "standing wave" surrounding the body is the best explanation for the near skin surface *aura*.

The Near Field or *Aura*

Like the sixteenth-century Swiss physician Paracelsus, for centuries, mystics, psychics, and spiritual teachers have described a glowing field of light surrounding the human body. This chapter considers the "near field" as a way of understanding the meaning of that "light."

Psychic and intuitive Barbara Brennan describes the near field as the layer or "state" between energy and matter. As Brennan explains, the inner layer / state "is composed of tiny energy lines that act like a sparkling web of light beams, similar to the lines on a television screen." [16] Brennan refers to the "energy" field surrounding the human body as the *etheric* body, which, she explains, "consists of a definite structure of lines of force, or energy matrix, upon which the physical matter of the body tissues is shaped and anchored." According to Brennan, "The physical tissues exist as such only because of the vital field behind them; that is, the field, is prior to, not a result of, the physical body." [17]

> The web-like structure of the etheric body is in constant motion. To clairvoyant vision, sparks of bluish-white light move along its energy lines throughout the entire dense physical body. The etheric body extends from one quarter to two inches beyond the physical body, pulsating at about 15-20 cycles per minute. [18]

Continuing her description of the *etheric body*, Brennan writes that the field acts as the "missing link" between biology, physical medicine, and psychotherapy. It's the "place where all the emotions, thoughts, memories, and behavior patterns we discuss so endlessly in therapy are located. They're not just suspended somewhere in our imaginations, but they are located in time and space. Thoughts and emotions move between people in time and space through the human energy field. [19]

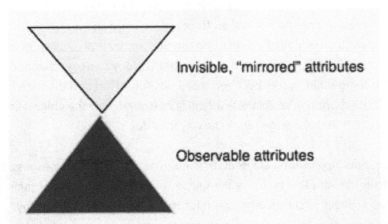

Diagram 12-4
Observed and Invisible Mirrored Attributes

Chapter 64

Mirroring

*T*his aspect of the new way to think about the meaning of "internal energy" and "energetic technologies" is based on a principle known as *mirroring*. Represented by the two opposing triangles shown in Diagram 12-4, mirroring suggests that a yet-to-be-measured EM-like field exists in a "parallel" dimension to our own. Although not yet measurable, because of a theorized mirrored relationship to conventionally understood electromagnetism, the action and properties of the unmeasured EM-like energy can be estimated as following the rules that one would apply to conventional EM phenomena.

The two images in Diagrams 12-5 illustrate the interaction between the *sanjiao*, or "Triple Warmer," acupuncture meridian and the near "radiated" "auric" field that is theorized as running outside and parallel to the meridian. While the upper of the two images shows the portion of the meridian that travels along the outside of the arm, the lower image shows the radiated "energy" of the acupuncture point and meridian system outside the surface of the skin.

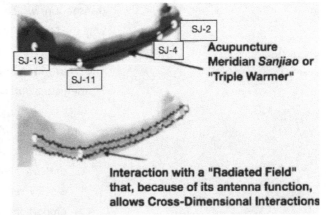

Interaction with a "Radiated Field" that, because of its antenna function, allows Cross-Dimensional Interactions

Diagrams 12-5
An Example of an Acupuncture
Meridian and "Mirrored"
System of the Ether

The new model suggests that, although the action of the associated points along the meridian cannot be explained by the physical acupoints on the surface of the skin, their function may be explained by features associated with the <u>EM-like</u> energy that may run parallel to the meridian outside of the body, which is generated by the near field.

The *Mirroring* Explanation

The piezoelectric strands of fascial webs. A "parallel," but invisible, energy system from another dimension. The electric spark that initiates between these two lines of "energy" when their forces consolidate and merge in just the right way. Like magnetic fields of opposing positive sides of two magnets as they approach each other, could the hum of the body's energy channels act as the charge that sparks between these two (observed and theorized) pathways? Furthermore, could these *interactions* explain how the enigmatic forces we call "internal energy" work the way they do?

The new model incorporates elements of mind, intention, and consciousness. Thus, if true, it means that how one thinks about and practices "tuning" their "field" has a direct effect on what we refer to as the individual's "energy." Although many of us intuitively feel a relationship exists between intangible elements, such as thoughts, emotions, intention, and one's energy field, so far, there is very little in the way of a scientific framework that might describe the mechanism(s) for how these are linked. That may soon change.

Hidden in plain sight. If this proposal is viable, it proffers not only a model of what might one day be accepted as a scientific explanation for energetic healing arts such as acupuncture, but also a model for understanding "energy" technologies in all their forms, from the *qi* of the *t'ai-chi* master and energetic healer to the *lung-wind* of the Tibetan meditator. More importantly, not only does this model portend a new mind / body energy-physics, it also promises practical principles for us to become more powerful and effective today!

The core of the new model is how to think about the subtle electromagnetic-like energy fields that we emanate. The explanation for "energy" offered here is based on the notion that a mirrored interaction exists between the observable and electromagnetic forces beyond measurement. This transaction, which at present is beyond measurement, would also explain why the "energy" question is so elusive and defies quantification.

The mirroring principle is said to have been originated by Hermes Trismegistus: *that which is below reflects that which is above.* Pecci explains:

> The law of correspondence between all things small and large is attributed to Hermes Trismegistus, the architect of the Great Pyramid: "That which is below reflects that which is above." This applies not only to geometric proportions and form but also to the harmonic relationships between one fixed point and another. [21]

As a possible explanation for the mechanism underlying acupuncture, mirroring suggests that some classes of measurable phenomena, such as the physical structures of acupuncture points and meridians, represent only the surface level of the phenomenon. Since the known attributes of points and meridians alone do not contain enough data to explain the therapeutic benefits, the knowledge gap is presumed to be populated by information from the theorized mirror aspect.

We suggest that the missing, or mirrored, interactions and data offer a more complete understanding of the phenomenon, because the "missing" components exist in the other "parallel" dimensional fields. Accordingly, although invisible, aspects beyond our observable dimension, or RF, nonetheless make up a large part of our psycho-emotional, spiritual, and energetic lives. In other words, we are multi-dimensional beings, but most of us don't know it.

This model may hold the ultimate secrets to empowerment and healing. This is because those of us engaged in energetic practices can make our disciplines more powerful when we learn to work with the totality of the mind-body energy system. A closer look at some aspects of these other-dimensions is warranted.

The *Ether*

By way of brief introduction, *ether* (Box 12-6) represents a subtle field that exists in a dimension separate from the physical body. Tiller suggests that human consciousness, and in particular, focused intention [22] and emotion, interact with physical matter through closely paired relationships with "parallel" phenomena. These parallel systems include EM and EM-like energies that are associated with conventional electromagnetism.

> *Ether* (also *aether*) From archaic physics, a very rarefied and highly elastic substance formerly believed to permeate all space, including the interstices between the particles of matter, and to be the medium whose vibrations constituted light and other electromagnetic radiation.
>
> New Oxford American Dictionary

Box 12-6

If the theory holds, the close equivalent to electromagnetism is speculated to be a key component to subtle energy forces, such as *qi*, *ki*, or internal energy. In his model of an expanded physics, Tiller often relies on the construct of the invisible etheric field, which for the moment one might think of as surrounding the body. Other researchers, as well as many psychics, also describe what, for most of us at least, remains the invisible field of the *ether*.

It is conceivable that such a working model for "energy" might explain, for example, why the mechanism of acupuncture is resistant to measurement. If we indeed swim in a parallel dimension of energy, like fish in the water, the medium that supports the fish remains invisible to detection by the creature immersed within it.

If the new model of "energies" as *interactions* is valid, then not only through our eyes, but also through the devices we rely upon to measure our environment, we are like the fish thriving in the undetectable medium of water. As such, we, too, may be unable to perceive the subtle fields that surround and support us.

Reference Frame

Nature carefully hides its greatest secrets. A *reference frame* (RF) refers to assumptions we make about reality. From our RF, we construct knowledge of our physical world, and it also serves as the foundation that researchers rely upon in their investigations of phenomena. However, RFs change. For example, before there was an understanding that infections resulted from microorganisms, [23] the accepted medical theory was that they occcured from *miasma*, or "bad air." Thus, the "germ" theory proposed by Girolamo Fracastoro and Marcus von Plenciz (in 1546 and 1762, respectively) was long regarded as not worthy of consideration by their peers. As a result, scientists and doctors were, for a long while, delayed from understanding the progression of disease.

However, our present RF, in the realm of physics, cannot account for the influence of subtle forces, like prayer, intention, and consciousness. Where electromagnetism can be measured, the *qi* of the Chinese, the *prana* of the Indians, and the *mana* of the Hawaiian shaman is not yet measurable, or at least not with currently available instruments. The aspects of our normally perceptible physical reality, *and the assumptions we make about it*, whether experientially or through available instrumentation, relates to what Tiller refers to as our current RF. Represented by the dark, lower triangle in Diagram 12-4, this represents the observable side of the "mirrored" model. Tiller proposes an expanded physics to explain phenomena represented by the clear triangle, which symbolizes the underlying mechanism that is a counter-balance to the dark triangle. According to the proposed model, the invisible triangle actuates subtle energy "technologies," such as acupuncture and energetic healing.

When it comes to human-directed, non-physical influence, the mirrored aspects of the known RF are theorized to account also for demonstrations where *intention* has been shown to influence the physical world. This category of experience belongs to an expanded reference frame, or RF 2. Tiller introduces the reasoning for an expanded RF in a white paper:

> It is time to help the quantum mechanical (QM) paradigm to expand significantly beyond what it presently is! As presently formulated mathematically, quantum mechanics is a very precise theory whose reference frame (RF) of mathematics is a four-dimensional spacetime-only RF within the classical electric particle velocity limits from zero to the velocity of electromagnetic (EM) light, c, in physical vacuum, and involving the four fundamental forces discovered by establishment science to date of (1) gravity (2) Maxwellian electromagnetism (3) the long-range nuclear force and (4) the short-range nuclear force. This

theory has been remarkably successful for particle physics, small atoms, molecules, and photons. However, many of the outcomes from today's experiments are requiring weirder and weirder explanations. This is a clear sign that the present conceptual framework of quantum mechanics has reached the limits of its useful modeling capabilities. [24]

Tiller is stating the need for an expanded physics that will accommodate subtle forces, such as human non-physical influence, into its modeling.

Chapter 65

Your Radiated Energy and *Transduction*

$\mathcal{F}$or practical purposes, the *mirroring theorem* suggests that we all, usually on an unconscious level, "tune into" and interact with what might be referred to as a parallel dimension.

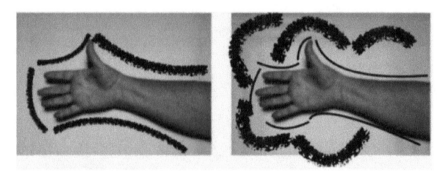

Diagrams 12-7

Images of Energy Fields around the Hand of a Very Experienced Energy Practitioner

Left image is of the "normal" close reactive auric field. Right image illustrates how the energy fields surrounding the hand changed when the practitioner intended to interact with a "spiritual" or "divine" source.

Acting as an invisible gravity field that can stir our hearts, the pull toward a transpersonal field — referred to by terms such as the *Tao*, the invisible sacred, or a universal intelligence — may explain the attraction that draws many of us to prayer, meditation, yoga, energetic healing, and other mind-body practices, but why is this so?

An expansion of the mass → energy to include consciousness provides a new framework to investigate the mystery of energy, *qi, prana*, and the implications of these for a spiritual practice. In terms of the mind-body energy field, the invisible part of the pyramid relationships (Diagram 12-4) represents one's interaction with the presumed EM-like energies that respond to the way one thinks, meditates, and reflects. Domains such as thoughts, emotions, and intention are normally considered intangible and seemingly impossible to observe. However, the new model suggests a way to study these kinds of influences in a relatively more concrete way.

We are what our thoughts have made us; so, take care about what you think. Words are secondary. Thoughts live; they travel far.

Swami Vivekananda

The proposed model describes how insubstantial elements, such as intention, might interact with the close reactive, or aura, field of energy near the body. The basic rule: how we think about, and interact with, the subtle fields around the body influences the near reactive (aura) field. Allow me to give some examples.

When one is consumed with the limited "self" — the endless drama, fears, and need for self-satisfaction — the "energy" of the close reactive / auric field is constrained, and the psychic appearance of these two different types of energy fields surrounding an individual becomes quite different.

Consider the images presented in Diagrams 12-7. The left image shows the "normal" energy (near reactive field) pattern around a person's hand; the field that can be felt by most people and which, in my experience, anyone with an open mind can learn to see for themselves. The right image demonstrates how the near radiation field changes and expands when the individual is reflecting on connecting with a divine, spiritual, or transpersonal source.[25] Also, note the additional line that appears near the surface of the hand and arm in the right image.

With an experienced meditator, that close line appears when the "normal" near reactive field, typically an inch ¼-inch ½, expands when one is engaged in transpersonal thoughts, prayer, or meditation. I interpret these observations to mean that a person seeking to develop their "energy" cannot neglect what might be referred to as a spiritual component. However, no one can tell you what that *spiritual component* means. Each person has to figure that out for themselves.

道可道非常道. 名可名非常名

Tao k'o Tao, fei ch'ang Tao; Ming k'o ming fei ch'ang ming
The Tao that can be described is not the true Tao;
the name that can be named is not the true name.

— Opening lines of the *Tao Te Ching*

Another clue is revealed when reflecting on the nature of the subtle energy fields that are theorized to surround the body. Consider the descriptions by the mystics now, as in ancient times, of the subtle energy fields that are said to encapsulate, and emanate from, living creatures. Previous chapters have included citations by a number of early scientists, such as Reichenbach, who strongly argued for the existence of these subtle fields. Reichenbach, among other early scientists, believed that the vital energy surrounding living things could be perceived by the sensitives (psychics) he employed in his research.

Although there is increasing evidence that fields like these exist, they may not act as a natural force *per se*. However, they do provide meaning for terms like *qi, prana,* and our understanding of "internal energy" in other ways.

In this light, one might think about these emitted / enveloping *auric* fields as Tiller suggests, radiations akin to those of a simple dipole antenna. With a little practice, and openness to the experience, most people can feel these "energy fields" that surround the body, and many can learn to perceive them visually. In this model, these near reactive fields are suggested to function as the medium between emotions, thoughts, belief, and physical matter. In this way, they represent the effluence of intention and consciousness to extend outward. Thus, they are the candidates for the mechanism that will one day explain how our mind and intention interact with the physical world.

The amorphous "energy" clouds that surround the body, whether perceived in a tactile way, or visually, or both, are sometimes described as the "energy" of *qi* or *prana*. However, this explanation may be too simplistic. It may not be quite accurate to equate these fields as an "energetic" force with, for example, the *qi* of the healer or *qigong* master. Instead, the palpable fields and their visual representations experienced by practitioners are more likely the intermediate "antenna emissions" communication sending / receiving system. A more complete understanding of the enigmatic force called *qi, ki,* or *prana* requires an additional layer of interaction through a principle known as *transduction*.

Transduction

Transduction refers to the conversion of energy from one form to another, such as heat to electricity, and vice versa.[26] However, in Tiller's model, the principle is extrapolated to provide a tentative definition of "energy work." In this usage, Tiller suggests transduction to account for the transference of subtle energy from a "theorized etheric domain" to the physical dimension, or current reference frame. In this context, transduction provides another way to look at the meaning of "energy experiences" on several levels. For example, this principle explains how some "energetic" healers are able to generate an exceptionally large bio-electric field.[27]

Transduction suggests a mechanism to explain how some kinds of "energetic" interactions defy explanation; one dramatic case of what appears to be an example of the transduction of "energy" between etheric and observable realms was shared in the Introduction. In the narrative about the welt that appeared on my classmate's hand when our teacher applied non-physical acupuncture, or *transduction* — the transfer of "energy" or *information* from the etheric to our normally perceived dimensional realm (RF) — we are provided with a working explanation. This is the case because no known "energy" could explain the appearance of the welt without physical contact.

Accordingly, the model holds that "energy" transduced from another dimension and produced the pulsing red mound on my classmate's hand.

In a published study that describes anomalous electrical emissions by Therapeutic Touch (TT) healers,[28] Tiller suggests that this same kind of transduction could explain the electrical energy effects observed by the scientists who conducted the study. Commenting on the study by E.F. Green, Anomalous Electrostatic Phenomena in *Exceptional Subjects*,[29] Tiller writes:

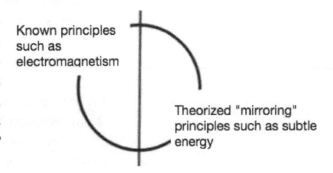

Known principles such as electromagnetism

Theorized "mirroring" principles such as subtle energy

Diagram 12-8
Known vs. Theoretical

> It appears from the data. . . . that the training and practice involved in TT develops in the healer a somewhat automatic internal power buildup at subtle levels of the body that discharges periodically and generates a very large electrical voltage pulse in the physical body.[30][31]

Tiller provides more insight into the meaning of transduction in the context of an individual's ability to express subtle energy, which:

> Starts from a hypothesized level of subtle substance in the healer's body and ends at a measurable level of electrical substance in the healer's body.[32]

Here, Tiller again refers to the subtle "etheric" substance theorized to exist in a parallel realm beyond presently accepted mainstream physics. Due to *transduction, information* contained in the *etheric field* converts into measurable electrical radiation. What Tiller calls the *etheric field* is the most likely storage place or capacitor[33] for what we might call "energetic residue" (my words).

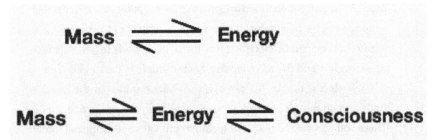

Diagrams 12-9
Conventional Mass-Energy Equation Compared with Tiller's Expanded Mass-Energy-Consciousness Equation

Expansion of the Mass-Energy Equation

In response to the currently accepted Mass-Energy equation illustrated in the top part of Diagram 12-9, Tiller suggests that this be expanded to include *consciousness*, as shown in the lower equation. Expansion of the Mass-Energy equation in this way would recognize the faculty of human consciousness and intention as a force of nature. The new paradigm accommodates the results observed in Tiller's experiments and other similar studies of human intention, such as those observed by Grad in the 1960s.**

** Grad's research was discussed in Section X

The centerpiece of the Tiller hypothesis is the suggestion that the Mass-Energy equation be expanded to include human mental-emotional-intentional influence(s). As presently understood, the mass $\rightarrow$ energy equation describes an exchange between energy and matter; in other words, how matter converts to energy, and energy converts to matter. As illustrated in Diagram 12-9, Tiller proposes an expansion of the core physics formula to include consciousness. The inclusion of consciousness as part of the mass $\rightarrow$ energy equation would recognize the role of human intention interacting with physical matter. [34] If accepted, this model of *consciousness* would also contribute to our understanding of the actions attributed to the powers of *qi, prana,* and internal energy.

Model for an Expanded Physics of Subtle (Internal) Energy

Referring again to Tiller's comments on the large electromagnetic bursts generated by some TT practitioners, and expanding on a quote presented earlier, Tiller introduces us to a new and speculative physics:

> The theoretical model proposed to account for this remarkable voltage phenomenon is a transduced field effect, which starts from a hypothesized level of subtle substance in the healer's body and ends at a measurable level of electrical substance in the healer's body. The underlying physical signal is thought to be a magnetic vector potential pulse. From conventional electro-dynamics, such a pulse always generates a bipolar electric field pulse in the immediate vicinity of the source. This, in turn, acts on nearby electrolytes of the physical body to generate first an expanding and then a collapsing electric dipole in the physical body. It is this electric dipole that gives rise to voltage signals in the healer's body and on the copper walls [where the experiment was conducted]. These voltages are the readily detectable correlates of the original subtle energy pulse which is hypothetically associated with the intention to heal. [35]

The above paragraph is extremely dense, and it is useful to consider some of these statements separately. This represents Tiller's comments on the observed attributes of TT healers, where large, anomalous "voltage signals" were recorded both on the healer's body and on the copper walls near the subjects in the laboratory. In suggesting an explanation for how the anomalous signals might have been generated, of particular relevance is the phenomenon Tiller refers to as the "hypothesized level of substance," a concept he develops in his later work describing acupuncture point and meridian theory. If the hypothesized level of substance does exist, and if one individual is able to access this hypothesized substance, it means that **we all** have the potential to do the same.

Tiller suggests that a human can interact with "other dimensions." Significant to the present discussion, this particular kind of *interaction* may account for at least some types of what are normally referred to as "energetic" phenomena. Among these is the earlier introduced principle of transduction that purports to explain how "energy" in the form of *information* transfers from a separate "theoretical dimension or substance" to our current dimensional RF.

Borrowed from conventional physics, transduction is proposed as the mechanism to explain how a practitioner (e.g., energetic healer) is able to transfer, or *transduce*, "energy." In this case, transduction is postulated to occur in the form of a "subtle energy pulse" that transduces (converts / transfers) from a <u>theorized subtle</u> dimension to the <u>physical plane</u>. A closer look at the meaning of transduction is presented in the first part of his statement:

> The theoretical model proposed to account for this remarkable
> voltage phenomenon is a transduced field effect.

As introduced earlier, a transducer converts energy, or "signal," from one form to another; for example, as in converting mechanical energy into electrical energy and vice versa. Here, Tiller extrapolates the process to explain how "subtle energy" from an unspecified domain might convert into a measurable voltage at the physical level. Tiller is suggesting that since there is no known source for this "energy" that we *can* identify, it therefore must be accounted for as being transduced from a "hypothesized level of substance."

Coherence and the Meridians as an Antenna Array

An important aspect of Tiller's model has to do with the function of the earlier described acupuncture meridian-grid system that overlays the human frame (Figure 12-3). In the proposed model, the meridian network plays key roles that may lead to a viable understanding of "internal energy." Thus, a closer look at the meridians is warranted.

The meridians possess the necessary requirements to provide basic antenna functions. If they indeed do function as antennae, this would imply that the human antenna array, like all antenna arrays, can be arranged to function either more or less optimally. Applied to the human body, the optimal functioning of the antenna system is related to the particular individual's degree of *coherence*. This portion of the present chapter considers the meaning of coherence and the role it plays in the human antenna grid network. The following points are proposed:

- The meridian antenna system allows consciousness and intent to interact with the physical world.

- When optimally functional or coherent, the meridian system provides the necessary psychic infrastructure to fulfill functions related to advanced thought, consciousness, and, in some cases, extraordinary creative inspiration.

- Directly working with the embedded antenna array can enhance and add new meaning to one's ability to work with "energy" modalities.

At its most basic level, the antenna array alerts us to danger. It is the source of our "gut feelings," speaking through the voice that says, "Don't go down that alley" or "A certain person is trying to cheat you." Sometimes, the myofascial piezoelectric network really needs to get our attention. When that happens, our hair stands on end. The meridians communicate to us through those "gut" feelings.

However, when the embedded antenna system is engaged through deep thought or reflection, it is proposed it begins to function more actively as the interface between the physical and the etheric planes. When this happens, it becomes the medium that accesses inspiration, participates in the mystic's connection to the divine, and manifests super creativity.

As the embedded antenna array takes on meaning beyond alerting us to danger, the embedded array receives, interacts with, and extends information on a deeply unconscious level. When honed with intention and an empowering personal practice, the human dipole antenna myofascial network shifts to awaken mind and body potential in new ways.

By way of review, the proposed model of the meridian /embedded antenna system is based on the notion that the network functions as a two-direction information sending and receiving (infrastructure + radiated field) system. This means that information not only comes in, but also goes out through this medium. Importantly, it is not the antennae themselves, but rather the presumed voltage field-like radiations that surround the antenna, and *our mind-body interactions* with them, that presume to explain the experience referred to as "internal energy." Later, the meaning of these fields and their voltage field-like fluctuations will be discussed in their role as "internal energy," covering a range of contexts from energetic healing to contact sports.

Because of their piezoelectric nature, when paired with practices involving consciousness and intent, and then actuated with gentle stretching associated with yoga, energetic meditation, *qigong*, or *t'ai-chi*, the embedded antenna network awakens as a tool to allow greater access to those enigmatic subtle forces described as "internal energy." At that stage, the meridian grid network begins to function in ways that are responsive to the individual's degree of coherence or internal order. [36]

On the physical level, yogic stretching, as well as some approaches to "energy technologies," such as *qigong*, are based on stimulating tension-release patterns, which physically "tunes" the meridians / myofascial channels. The key is to hone these kinds of practices with just the right amount of tensional pressure to stimulate the meridian channel. In this regard, tensional forces applied to the meridian channels should be neither too slack, nor too tense. [37] Thus, practices like these, especially when performed in a calm and centered way, awaken the piezoelectric meridian grid as a tool to increase immune system function, while simultaneously developing tools that promote increased consciousness.

Other than physical stimulation of the meridians, because of the presumed comingling of intention and consciousness, the piezoelectric grid is believed to be responsive to certain types of mental activity more than others. For example, meditation, prayer, and emotional self-management are thought to represent the kinds of mental activities that more readily interface with the myofascial meridian antenna system.

Chapter 66

Strange Explorations

Note: As first presented in Section III, *qi*, *prana*, or "energy" sensing exercises, like those described here, are proposed to function through the body's embedded antenna receiving-transmission networks. As described here, these are proposed to allow one's *intention* to extend outward. Thus, it is STRONGLY RECOMMENDED that before engaging any type of "energy sensitivity" exercise, the practitioner first prepare themselves by prayer, or setting the intention, to interact with and be guided by a positive or benevolent source. This is believed to protect the individual during these kinds of practices.

Play and Experiment with the Near Reactive Field

*P*ractical exercises apply to learning to attend to, and work with, the near and far reactive fields. Learning to become sensitive to one's near reactive aura field, and incorporating sensations associated with the subtle fields in and around the body with one's "energy" work, improves one's skill in energetic practices, from *qigong* to yoga, to energetic meditation and more.

The exercises in this chapter are called "strange explorations." They are designed to increase one's awareness of the same subtle radiated fields around the body that have been the subject of the present section. Particular attention is directed to sensations one experiences during practice. These exercises are designed to build the practitioner's confidence in attending to the amorphous "energy work" that takes place via the interplay between EM and EM-like sensations, that exist in the interstitial "energetic" ebb and flow within and around the body. These exercises / experiments / explorations demonstrate how one's attention and intention can interact with the magnetic and magnetic-like sensations through three domains.

The first domain is the body's "hard-wired" meridian network. As discussed earlier, piezoelectric structures form the body's subtle energy grid and promote simple dipole antenna-like functions. The second domain is the near reactive field, which is associated with the aura. In normal, healthy individuals, it is most often somewhat static and lying between an inch ¼ to an inch ½ from the body's surface. The third domain is the source of electromagnetic-like energy, which exists in what Tiller describes as an "other-dimensional" space separate from the body.

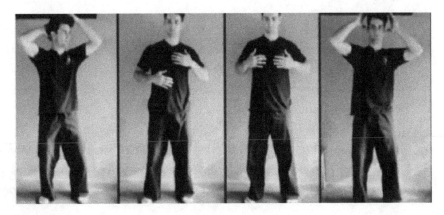

Photos 12-10

"Massaging," and Interacting with, the Near Reactive Field

This exercise is designed to familiarize oneself with sensations associated with the near field aura.

Strange Explorations 1

Encounters with the Near Reactive Field

The easiest way for a person to familiarize themselves with the near reactive field is to feel and interact with it. The more real it appears, the easier it will be to work with, and a great way to effect this is through performing a kind of "massage." A basic aura massage is shown in the examples provided in Photos 12-10, and a video of the practice can be viewed from the link in Box 12-11.

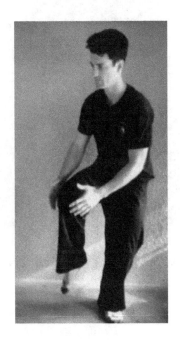

Box 12-11
"Massaging" the Near Reactive Field
Video link to on-line library:

https://youtu.be/KbUs20yo4uE
or
https://chiarts.com/12-11

Near Field Energetic Massage

Begin by touching the auric / near reactive field very lightly. If you can't feel it at first, try imagining that you are trying to make contact with an extremely thin and delicate spider's web that is suspended just over an inch from your body; your goal is to interact with the web without breaking it. During this exercise, make no contact with your physical body. If you are new to this kind of practice, at first you might not feel anything special at all. In that case, just imagine that you are feeling and interacting with it. Through regular practice, one's experience of the field becomes increasingly palpable and "real."

During the practice, explore the tactile sensations associated with the near reactive field. Start by feeling for the near field that radiates off the arm, and then try to sense the feeling of the radiating field at other places about your body. See if you can feel the field near your shoulders, and then the head, and so forth.

As you gain confidence in your ability to sense and interact with the near reactive field, continue to pay attention to the sensations associated with it. Those sensations are the keys to mastery of your mind-body energy fields.

As you explore the sensations associated with the near reactive field, pay close attention to the changes you notice in the boundaries of the field. Continue to explore the limits of the field, observing your thoughts and feelings as you do, and noting which of these affects the field and makes it expand or shrink.

As you gain confidence with the practice, notice the limits surrounding your body and how they increase or decrease as you go about your day. Notice how positive emotions, such as trust and love, expand the boarders of the field, and how negative emotions, such as fear or anger, constrict the boundaries.

If you are new to this kind of practice and can't seem to feel the near reactive field right away, don't be discouraged. It is helpful for newcomers to the exercise to *imagine* that they are feeling the near reactive field. Through regular practice, one's experience of the field becomes increasingly palpable and "real."

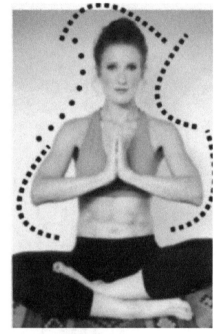

Diagram 12-12
Intention, Meditation, and the Body's Energy Fields

Strange Explorations 2

An Experimental Model of Energetic Meditation

While practicing energetic meditation, contemplation, or prayer, experiment with placing awareness beyond the limits of the physical body.

The second strange exploration looks at the interaction between one's awareness and the subtle radiation fields around the body, as they change shape and vary in density during meditation. This exercise is designed for someone who is already familiar with sensations associated with the subtle field that surrounds the body.

Start by sitting quietly, while engaging in meditation or contemplation as you normally would, and then place your attention on the feeling of the near reactive field. Intend to perceive the boundary outside of your physical body, observing how the near reactive field changes in response to your attention.

As suggested by the dotted lines around the meditator shown in Diagram 12-12, the near reactive field is never static; it constantly changes shape and density around the body. Sometimes it will feel as though it extends outward, and at other times it will be perceived as being barely beyond the body's surface. As with the previous exercise, as you gain confidence in your ability to feel and interact with the subtle reactive field around your body, you will be able to observe how the field changes and responds to your thoughts and emotions. If you have a religious or spiritual practice, try incorporating it into the exercise.

For more experienced practitioners, a variation of the exercise is to study how breathing can be integrated with the shape, feeling, and density of the field. Try this "strange exploration" by imagining that, as you slowly breathe in, your breath effuses outward from the pores of your skin and pushes against the near field boundary beyond the body's surface. Start by focusing on the area of the heart and intend to extend the field outward. Next, try other areas, such as the front of the face or back of the neck, before eventually trying to "breathe" outward through the surface of your entire body. Most practitioners find this especially enjoyable and calming. In each example, the goal is to develop a palpable sensation of the "breath" interacting with the near field surrounding the body.

After you develop confidence in your ability to sense the energy merging with breath and then effusing outward, try a more advanced variation. For this step, you will need to be familiar with surface aspects of one or more meridians. In Diagram 12-13, the image shows the surface aspect of the large intestine channel (LI). This exploration is related to the intentional triggering of meridians and points that was described in Section III.

By way of review, focused attention can stimulate acupuncture points or meridians. Initiate the practice by assuming a posture that creates the feeling of a deep stretchy sensation along the channel you are working with; you can achieve this by experimenting with placing your arm away from your body. You are looking for the meridian line being stretched, but it must be able to be relaxed at the same time, as meridians are stimulated by that perfect balance of tension and relaxation.

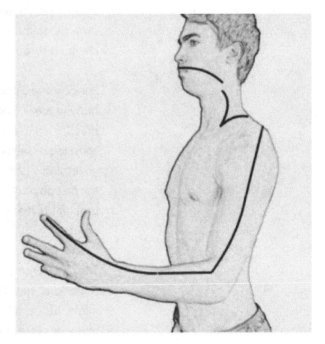

Diagram 12-13
Major Portion of the Surface Aspect of
the Large Intestine Meridian

This represents a yogic practice that creates sensations you identify with "energy" along the large intestine meridian. After you feel a slight stretchy sensation along the channel, begin the practice by intending to effuse the breath outward into, and beyond, the physical meridian. The intention should be directed with the inhalation.

In the practice illustrated in Diagram 12-13, intend that the large intestine meridian of the forearms effuse energy outward into the near reactive

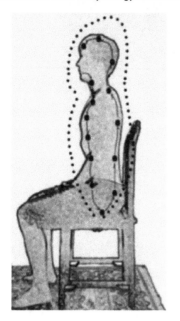

Diagram 12-14
The Perception of Channel Flow without Physical Connections

field. This has proven to be such a valuable exercise that I ask my advanced students to become familiar with the basic acupuncture meridian lines in order to facilitate this aspect of their training.

When perfected, the sensation associated with the practice will be as though one's breath interacts with the sensation of "energy fields" around the body.

Strange Explorations 3

The Perception of "Energy" Flow During Energetic Meditation

Section V included an overview of various forms of energetic meditation. As with some of the examples cited there, since ancient times, meditators have reported the experience of "energy" moving through areas of the body that have no physiological explanation. This "strange exploration" proposes a new way to investigate these kinds of experiences, with a good example to be seen in the practice of orbital meditation. The exercise focuses on the flow of energy along the back and front channels, respectively known as the "conception" (任) and "governing" (督) vessels. Consider the accounts by energetic meditators that included reports of "energy" channels running from the tailbone, through the perineum, and then into connecting energy channels through the genitals (Diagram 12-14).

For centuries, practitioners have described the flow of energy through the body in areas that have no anatomical correspondence. Orbital meditation practice is a useful case in point, as an important part of the practice involves conscious control over the flow of energy between the lowest point of the governing vessel (midway between the tip of the coccyx and the anus) and the first point of the conception vessel located at the perineum. The obvious problem is that there is no direct physical structure that connects the two points.

Thus, it is interesting to consider that, in light of practitioners' reports of sensations traveling through these two locations, that those sensations might be explained, not in terms of a direct connection, but instead, in terms of sensations associated with the near reactive field. Such modeling might provide at least one explanation for the reported "current" that travels between those locations, since the proposed model suggests that sensations may interchange between physical structures, such as the spine, and that near reactive field properties, but are simultaneously perceived by the practitioner as forming a continuous pathway.

This alternative explanation for the "flow of energy" through the body is suggested by the dotted lines that surround the meditator shown in Diagram 12-14.

As suggested by the illustration, the perceived "flow of energy" might not be those sensations directed through known anatomical structures, but instead those of the near reactive field, which, from the viewpoint of the energetic meditator, blend with the experience of energy flow through known physical locations. In other words, subtle energy pathways outside the normally understood ones might interact with the physical structures to such a degree that, at times, it is impossible for the practitioner to distinguish sensations generated by the near reactive field from sensations associated with the physical myofascial structures of the channels.

Strange Explorations 4

The Near Reactive Field as an *Information* Containing Medium

After Section IV introduced *information theory*, Section VIII expanded on it to include a model for "internal energy in the martial arts." Now, Strange Exploration 4 suggests a mechanism that might one day explain the "physics" *of information*.

One way of investigating the nature of the near reactive field as an information containing medium relates to the principle of cross-body energetic relationships, referred to as the *wai san he*, or "outer three relationships (OTR)," which was covered in Section III.

Wai San He and Cross-Body Energy Relationships

This strange exploration considers whether the near reactive field might function as an "information containing" medium. If so, it would provide a template for studying the mechanism for *wai san he* / outer three relationships, or "holographic" principles, used in acupuncture, energetic healing, bodywork, and the energetic martial arts.

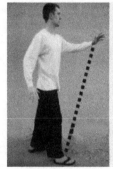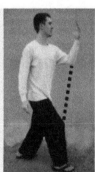

Diagram 12-15
Studying Energetic Cross Relationships

This strange exploration integrates principles from several areas that were previously discussed. Principal among these are the holographic theory of acupuncture presented in Section II, and the *wai san he* (外 三 合), or cross-body magnetic resonance theory, and related exercises that were covered in Section III.

The *wai san he*, or outer three relationships / holographic aspects of the proposal, describe how some aspects of the body seem to magnetically / energetically relate to others. An example of this is the way in which a certain aspect of the body can be experienced as having "energetic" relationships with other parts. As was illustrated in Section III, and presented again in the first image of Diagrams 12-15, the exercise depicted demonstrates how the wrist on one side of the body, when placed in just the right position, can trigger the experience of electromagnetic / energetic resonance with the ankle on the other side of the body.

Although no scientific theory is yet available to explain this phenomenon, the principle is described throughout the TCM literature. An example is found in an article published in the *American Journal of Acupuncture*, where R.A. Dale informs us that "Every part of the body can function as an energetic reflection of the body as a whole, both diagnostically and therapeutically," and that for half a century, "investigations by many researchers back the validity of [these] microsystems." [38]

Information theory, combined with near field modeling, provides insight into the nature of these relationships, complementing the model proposed by Tiller to explain the efficacy of acupuncture and the meridians. In the same way that Tiller suggests that their function can be understood by their relationship to the radiated near reactive field, the proposed extrapolation is based on the notion that "cloud-like" storage and communicative properties are contained in the near reactive "aura" field that surrounds the body.

The field described by Tiller would consist of a mix of measurable EM and EM-like emissions. For this expanded model, the metaphor of the "cloud" is borrowed from the computer / cell phone function that most of us are now familiar with. We may be aware of the functions and storage capabilities that take place within our devices, and many of us are familiar with something known as the "cloud," which, despite not part of the device, our technology interacts with.

For most of us, the "cloud" remains amorphous, but nevertheless, we still rely on it to provide data to our local smart phone or computer. This strange exploration asks the question: could the amorphous field that Tiller presumes to surround the body, like the amorphous field that our electronic communication devices interact with, exchange data to such an extent that its functions include a mechanism to explain the body's *wai san he / holographic* operations?

If true, this would mean that there is an "energetic" field around us that contains *information*. The model suggests that the holographic relationships, such as those described by Dale, explain humans as being more holographic than many researchers and therapists realize.

Examples of the OTR that were previously described are found in the way the wrist relates energetically to the ankle, the elbow to the knee, and the shoulder to the hip. In the first image of Diagrams 12-15, the practitioner demonstrates sensing and working with the feeling of these energetic relationships by placing the wrist into alignment with the opposite ankle; the second image illustrates the same energetic relationship between the elbow and knee. In Section III, the reader was invited to explore the "magnetic" nature of these relationships for themselves.

The technique can be practiced by holding your hand out away from the body in different positions, while intending to establish cross-body energetic-magnetic feelings. When one gets the particular placement-relationship just right, the practitioner will feel sensations such as buzzing or warmth at targeted areas of the body (Section III also included a link to a video that demonstrates these relationships).

This proposed *cloud*-energetic relationship model may provide support for why and how *anti-entropic* (meaning health promoting, anti-aging, or therapeutic) *information* might be triggered by certain techniques. It might also explain how specific postures might induce other reflexive reactions in the body. For example, the cloud-information model presents a rationale for why a treatment to the right wrist contributes to the healing response of the left ankle; the right elbow to the left knee, and so on. The thesis is supported by the descriptions of "holographic" relationships. †

> † Such as those exemplified in the Tung acupuncture system described
> by Dr. Henry McCain and discussed in Section II.

In this light, it is useful to reflect again on some of Henry McCain's comments that were included in Section II. There, in describing the nature of these "holistic relationships," McCain explains how this type of clinical knowledge is not based on the foundational TCM canons, nor on an analysis of the diagrams that illustrate the acupuncture meridian network, but on "family" knowledge that is passed from one generation to the next. As described by McCain, this kind of knowledge represents collective experience, and thus the inheritance of a particular family system.

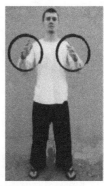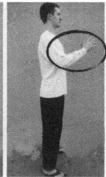

Diagram 12-16
"Energy Fields" Surrounding the Body:
Start with the Arms
This exercise expands on the
suggestion that "energy" exists in a
transduced space separate from the
physical body.

Strange Explorations 5

Playing with the Cross-Dimensional Nature of the Near Reactive Field

The ideas presented in this strange exploration may have profound implications for practitioners of arts like energetic meditation, *qigong*, and other forms of "energy work." The exercises were developed from three propositions:

1. Sensations that we identify as "energy" may actually be experiences of either the near reactive *auric* field and / or the interaction of this field with a cross-dimension (expanded RF) source.

2. The medium for a cross-dimensional interaction is (for the most part) ‡ the near reactive field.

3. The near reactive field is responsive to intent. Qigong and other "energetic techniques" become more powerful when the practitioner extends their intention into the near reactive field, just beyond the limits of the physical body.

‡ The present section focuses on the near reactive field, with limited consideration of the distal field.

The exercises that follow are designed to further allow the practitioner to become sensitive to the subtle energy fields that can be thought of as surrounding the body.

Consider the exercise illustrated in Diagram 12-16. As the practitioner slowly moves his extended arms, he is also careful to extend his awareness an inch or so in all direction (360 degrees) around the arms and hands. The practice involves imagining that the limits of your body extend beyond your physical demarcations.

Try this exercise for yourself by first imagining that you can feel and move your arms with the awareness of the near reactive field. In other words, when your arms change position, imagine that you are simultaneously interacting with the invisible near reactive field. When correctly performed, the feeling will be as if you have a layer of very light jelly in contact with your body.

For most individuals, with a little practice, one's imagination of these fields becomes increasingly less necessary, as the ability to perceive the physical perception of "energy" around the body becomes increasingly palpable. The more "real" the experience, the less imagination is required.

Note, that since illustrations like those shown in Diagrams 12-16 are two-dimensional, it is impossible to convey the three-dimensional nature of the experience through the medium of two-dimensional print. When trying these for yourself, imagine the "energy" moving around your arms as being present 360 degrees. The goal is for the practitioner to experience sensations of "energy" on the inside and outside / top and underside of the arm simultaneously.

Once the practitioner is successful with the first exercise, they are then freer to experiment with how intention might interact with sensations associated with the near reactive field.

Once you are confident working with sensations associated with the near reactive field, try extending the feeling of energy external to, and around, other aspects of the body as you apply the protocol to your practice of yoga, *t'ai-chi*, or *qigong*. Variations of the practice, shown in Diagrams 12-17, demonstrate the practitioner learning to "get in touch" with sensations associated with the near reactive field in front and behind the body.

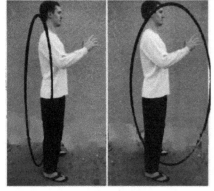

Diagrams 12-17
Integrating Movement with Front and
Back Near Reactive Fields

Strange Explorations 6

Magnetic Energy Fields in Advanced Martial Arts Application

Inner and Outer Expressions of the Mind-Body Magnetic Fields

Warning: The examples provided in this section are extremely dangerous and can result in serious injury to the practitioner. The principles discussed and demonstrated here are performed by a highly trained expert; they are presented for research and discussion purposes only. Do not attempt these demonstrations without many years of training and guidance by a qualified expert.

This is the strangest of the "strange explorations," and the most difficult to describe. I had mixed feelings about whether to include this material in the present work, because I do not completely understand it myself. Thus, the following discussion includes some guesswork regarding what I believe takes place in this category of advanced practice, and combines elements from Sections III, IV, and VIII. Material from Section III involves the practitioner's sense of electrical and electrical-like sensations within their body, while material expanded from Sections IV and VIII relates to the practitioner's conscious extension of *disruptive information*.

The basis of the model is the notion that, at advanced levels, a practitioner can generate and control sensations within the body that appear as electromagnetic or electromagnetic-like. As will be described in a moment, when "externalized" against an opponent, they allow the transfer of *disruptive information*.

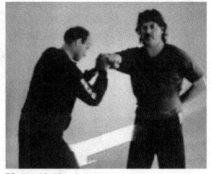

Photo 12-18

Can Practitioner-directed Magnetic Fields Neutralize the Opponent's Force?

Section VIII included discussion of how neutralization of an opponent's force might be explainable not in terms of the skilled practitioner's ability to transmit a willfully directed force *per se*, but rather as the ability to transmit *disruptive information*. It also considers how *information*, acting through the medium of an extremely subtle (EM + EM-like) influence, could enhance an expert martial artist's skill through *disruptive information* that can destabilize and / or weaken the opponent. Taken together, the model proposes to explain how what appears as only a minute amount of force or contact against an opponent can still be effective in close combat.

Please note carefully the advisory message that precedes this strange exploration. The examples and demonstrations included here are for research and discussion purposes only. They are very advanced and dangerous and should not be attempted by anyone who has not been properly prepared over many years and supervised by a qualified master.

To present a demonstration of the kind shown in Photo 12-18, and viewable through the video link included in Box 12-19, the performer must accomplish several steps in quick succession. First, the practitioner attains the requisite mental state. Second, he becomes sensitive to, induces, and begins working

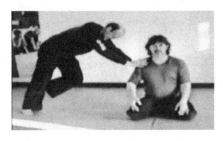

Video Link: Magnetic Fields and Disruptive Information against an Opponent

https://www.youtube.com/watch?v=KLqhOiQcerg
or
https://chiarts.com/12-19

Box 12-19

with the body's lower abdominal energy fields. Third, the practitioner must intend the body's "energy fields" to interact with the opponent. The resulting experience can be very intense, and what follows is my interpretation of these strange and, at times, unsettling experiences.

As previously noted, an important part of the experience relates to the practitioner being able to attend to sensations in the lower abdomen. These feelings may initially appear as warmth, either with or without pressure. However, at more advanced levels, they will appear as the play of magnetic fields within the lower abdomen.

At advanced levels of practice, the practitioner will experience sensations that feel like moving electromagnetic forces in the lower abdomen, and my interpretation of these is that the energy vortexes of the lower abdomen have become very dynamic. In the accompanying video of the demonstrations, accessible via the link in Box 12-19, I refer to these sensations as "the floating *dan tian*." [39]

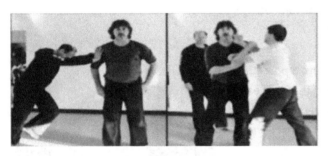

Photos 12-20
Disruptive Energy Fields Applied to Training Partners
Applying the magnetic field to multiple attackers

When applying the energy fields against an opponent, the most conspicuous experience for the practitioner is that of effortlessness. Performed correctly, it seems that regardless of how much physical force the attacker applies, in the practitioner's experience, the encounter involves no more than the most minimal pressure being placed against their body. An experience like this seems to defy normally accepted rules of force and mechanics, and thus, is difficult to put into words. My interpretation of the phenomenon is that when it is applied against an opponent, some unknown influence — presumably *information* — interrupts the opponent's ability to use his strength and body mechanics effectively. When performing these demonstrations against assistants, I felt only the most minimal physical force on my body. The experience was simultaneously strange and fascinating (examples of this kind are presented in Photos 12-18 and 12-20, and a video of the demonstration can be viewed from the link provided in Box 12-19).

When performed correctly against an opponent, the lightest contact appears to interrupt and weaken their physical integrity. I've applied the principle during many demonstrations, and on a few occasions, actual close combat. When applied against an adversary attempting to move or push me, although there is only the sense of minimal, if any, force on my body, other cues act as guides that tell me I'm performing the technique properly. Prominent among these are strange sensations within the body, the most noticeable being the heightened sense of moving and swirling magnetic field vortexes within the lower abdomen.

Although some martial arts bio-mechanics involving "neutralizing force" are also part of the technique, * in the examples shown in the video, these physical actions alone do not seem to fully explain the experience of "lightness" against an aggressor. In applying the principle, I physically relax all unnecessary tension and hold the intention to engage those subtle energy vortexes in the lower abdomen. I intend to effuse them outward, and then allow them to interact with the opponent. This is one of the reasons that, for me, the *disruptive information* model is the best explanation for this kind of technique.

*A video introduction to neutralizing force for martial art application can be viewed at https://youtu.be/EoxDalBYAfA

The demonstration of this category of skill against an adversary occurs in two steps. First, one simultaneously relaxes all unnecessary physical attention and attends to the practiced feelings of electromagnetic-like sensations in the lower abdomen. Second, the practitioner applies trained skills against an opponent in a relaxed [40] way. With the exception of specific tensional lines along relevant myofascial and meridian channels, all unnecessary physical and mental tension continues to be relaxed as the opponent(s) is engaged. By this process, select tensional lines are directed through relevant meridians to join with technique. However, the expression can be neither too hard, nor too soft, consistent with a principle introduced in Section VII known as *gangrou xiangji* (刚柔相济), or "hard and soft complementing each other."

My impression of this kind of practice is that when in contact with an opponent, the technique generates a "magnetic field" — most probably related to the phenomenon that Tiller describes as a magnetic vector potential pulse — that allows *disruptive information* to interact with, and influence, the opponent. It is speculated that this initiates the emission of a weakening, or destabilizing, influence.

When the full implications of aether science become known to humanity at large, a very significant paradigm shift will be necessary.[41]

Chapter 67

Alternatives to Cause and Effect

*C*ause and effect are fundamental to the way science explains phenomena. For example, sunlight causes a photosynthesis response in plants, which leads to an increase in chlorophyll, which in turn leads to plant growth. As with this example, the cause and effect model will always remain core to the way events are predicted and how our knowledge of the physical world increases. However, intangible elements, such as "consciousness" and our ability to interact with "other dimensions," challenge the normally accepted cause and effect paradigm. Currently, these ambiguous influences cannot be quantified, nor their influence accurately and reliably measured.

Consider Dr. Grad's studies documenting the influence of intention on plant growth; ** those demonstrations are examples of phenomena that seem to suspend, or lay outside of, the normally accepted rules of cause and effect. Thus, at this juncture, one could ask: What alternatives to cause and effect might be available?

**Discussed in Section X

Some alternative models have previously been proposed, the most prominent among them being one provided by the renowned psychiatrist and philosopher Carl Jung. Expressed through the principle of *synchronicity*, Jung forwards an alternative view in the form of a set of dynamics he refers to as "the simultaneous occurrence of mutually influencing events." In his introduction to Helmut Wilhelm's translation of the *I Ching*, [42] Jung defines *synchronicity*:

> This assumption involves a certain curious principle that I have termed synchronicity, a concept that formulates a point of view diametrically opposed to that of causality. Since the latter is a merely statistical truth and not absolute, it is a sort of working hypothesis of how events evolve one out of another, whereas synchronicity takes the coincidence of events in space and time as meaning something more than mere chance, namely, a peculiar interdependence of objective events among themselves as well as with the subjective (psychic) states of the observer or observers.

> The ancient Chinese mind contemplates the cosmos in a way comparable to that of the modern physicist, who cannot deny that his model of

the world is a decidedly psychophysical structure. The microphysical event includes the observer just as much as the reality underlying the *I Ching* comprises subjective, i.e., psychic conditions in the totality of the momentary situation. Just as causality describes the sequence of events, so synchronicity to the Chinese mind deals with the coincidence of events. The causal point of view tells us a dramatic story about how D came into existence: it took its origin from C, which existed before D, and C in its turn had a father, B, etc. The synchronistic view, on the other hand, tries to produce an equally meaningful picture of coincidence. How does it happen that A′, B′, C′, D′, etc., appear all in the same moment and in the same place? It happens in the first place because the physical events A′ and B′ are of the same quality as the psychic events C′ and D′, and further because all are the exponents of one and the same momentary situation. [43]

Jung's alternative to cause and effect might well begin to explain what is sometimes referred to as a chance encounter. The principle suggests the workings of a subtle physics that begins to explain how, at least some of the time, events transpire. It is the experience of a person who, while engaged in problem-solving, when all seems lost, nevertheless continues to move toward finding a solution. Out of the blue, the solution presents itself when least expected. Most of us have had this kind of experience.

In light of Jung's theory of synchronicity, our most powerful engagement with other dimensions takes place when the body and mind operate harmoniously. Under these conditions, our unconscious mind works in the background, where it is most free to engage *information* from multiple dimensions, and problems are solved without our conscious involvement. This view speaks to the intelligence of the mind being far greater, and also much more intimately involved in aspects of our lives, than we are consciously aware.

Our relationship to the "other-dimensional" through the lens of synchronicity might well explain how, through a "chance encounter," a person meets one's true love. In ancient Arabic alchemy, the principle is expressed through the term *maktub,* meaning "it is written." On the surface, this expression describes the way events seem to fall into place as happenstance, but it might also point to an alternative physics beyond cause and effect. Evidence of this alternative way of interacting with the world presents itself when a person takes a new route, turns the corner, and "just happens" to meet the love of their life. Although the logical mind argues that occurrences like these are only chance, the heart may be a bit wiser than the brain in these matters. It understands events like these as destiny or fate, or what the Chinese refer to as *yuan-fen* (缘分), or *hung-hsien* (紅線), "the red thread," which has secretly connected the lovers since the time of their birth. [44] Such is the new physics of an "other-dimensional" reality, which incorporates an expansion of presently understood laws of cause and effect.

The principle of synchronicity might also apply to the highest and most profound examples of martial arts prowess, or, for that matter, the highest caliber of athletic performances in sport or other disciplines. It has always struck me that a true master moves against their opponents as a flow of effortlessness; in these examples, the expert seems to proceed in accordance with laws outside of time and space. Such a demonstration becomes an "other-dimensional dance," representing the true definition of mastery as expressed through the highly-skilled performer, who gracefully steps to a tune that only they can hear.

Such perfect harmony is exemplified in the skill demonstrated by *Aikido's* founding master, Morihei Ueshiba. † In that example, the master's effortless skill in subduing his attackers depended on no more than the minimal expenditure of physical effort. Observing the high level of performance exhibited in those demonstrations, the observer is left with the impression that Ueshiba was so immersed in his smiling-joy-in-the-moment that it seems as though he might not have been consciously aware of whatever skillful technique he employed.

† Examples of which were included in Section VIII

Could Ueshiba's performances be evidence of a great master's ability to move seamlessly between our normally perceived dimension and a higher one? Might such uncanny skill be explained by the gifted person's ability to move gracefully within a framework that is visible only to the initiated? In the Preface to Tiller's *Science and Human Transformation*, Pecci describes the interaction between known and unseen dimensions in terms of a perfectly ordered lattice framework:

> Energies not available to everyday consciousness form the field in which all observed activity takes place. It is a multidimensional field, described by Dr. Tiller as a perfectly ordered lattice framework, a microscopic pattern of complex, geometrically harmonic grids filling in all of space free from the limitations of time-space, where cause and effect is only an illusion, and where "accidents" or randomness cannot exist. [45]

In the context of such a proposal, some of the more cryptic statements by masters, such as Ueshiba, begin to make sense. Another story about Ueshiba involves one particular demonstration, and the master's subsequent comments on it. The demonstration took place after some of his students asked him about the ninja skill of invisibility. Ueshiba's first response to his disciples' expressed interest in Japan's legendary assassins was to tell them that they "had been watching too many movies," but then a moment later, his playful side took over. "Grab your swords and sticks," he told his students, "and I'll give you a real demonstration of *ninjutsu*." [46]

Obeying their master's instructions, the group of ten or so students, wooden swords in hand, surrounded Ueshiba in the center of the *dojo*. However, when they attacked, their wooden swords were unable to find him. As they attacked, their only impression was the sense of a swoosh of air, as the teacher somehow vanished. Miraculously, Ueshiba, reappeared twenty feet away, standing halfway up the second story, from where he yelled at his students, "Over here, over here!" [47]

The master's stunning demonstration had only whetted the students' appetites; they wanted more. However, Ueshiba refused their requests to perform additional "tricks," admonishing them by asking, "Are you trying to kill me just to entertain yourselves? Each time one performs such techniques, his lifespan is reduced five to ten years." [48] It appears that Ueshiba's ability to access this subtle physics of the other-dimension was physically and emotionally taxing.

Conclusion to Section XII

*T*he "speculations" advanced in this section are based on an alternative way of examining the meaning of "internal energy." As in *qigong* and energetic meditation, sometimes these energetic forces are consciously directed, whereas at other times, as described in the TCM traditions, our bodies unconsciously manage and balance these forces. In either scenario, the alternative models of subtle / internal energy that have been presented here do not describe the phenomenon as being a projected force, nor an energy field lying dormant within the body, waiting to be awakened. Instead, the energetic forces are seen, at least partly, as an interaction between dimensions.

Many of the concepts covered here are based on, or extrapolated from, theories proposed by Dr. William Tiller, and chief among them is the notion that human consciousness and intention can act as a natural, causal force. If true, one day physicists may accept this statement as fundamental, rather than rejecting it as heretical to the laws governing scientific inquiry.

Another argument put forward in this section is the notion that acupuncture points and meridians, through their antenna functions, exchange information through electromagnetic and electromagnetic-like interactions. However, if such a model is even partially correct, then those expanded physical laws that account for their function open an avenue of investigation beyond the orthodox science of acupuncture. Those models simultaneously offer a framework from which to construct the mathematics of non-contact healing, energetic meditation, the healing power of *qigong*, and perhaps, in rare examples, even internal energy in the martial arts. To summarize, these "speculations" represent a particular way of looking at the body's myofascial meridian network, asking if it is indeed possible that the meridians hold the keys to unlocking many secrets.

The meridians speak their own language, communicating not through words, but through the locution of vibration. When the myofascial meridians begin to buzz and hum, they become the mechanism through which one's intention can cross the presumed boundary separating the subjective and intangible from the physically real. If one day these theories prove correct, then the myofascial lines, and in particular the antenna voltage-regulation-like emissions they generate, are the vehicle that allows our thoughts to interact with, and at times influence, the physical world.

In the context of yoga or meditation, the hum of the meridians electrifies the life force. Through meditation, it allows one to view otherwise hidden worlds, and when expressed through *qigong*, the buzz of the energy channels enlivens the body's energy structures, thereby invigorating the organs and restoring health and youthfulness.

The more one engages with their myofascial meridian system, the more they reveal. Stretch the meridians in yoga, align them in meditation, and the glands of the endocrine system will light up. When electrified and charged as a daily habit, they sometimes induce the nectar of youth that belies one's years; actuate them in the flowing piezo-electric dance of *t'ai-chi* or *bagua*, and they'll whisper their secrets. By the same token, ignore them, let your body slump, and the mind-body system will trend toward collapse.

Their language is like no other, their communication is piezoelectric, and their language forms from the buzzing-hum that communicates and establishes connections throughout the body's physical, energetic, hormonal, and emotional systems. Some meridian secrets address the physical support of the body, while others activate tools that increase awareness and promote the advancement of one's consciousness. Like layers of an onion, their secrets are revealed little by little, in small ways; their first secret having to do with efficient and anti-aging support for the body.

At their most basic level, the myofascial meridians provide soft tissue lifting support for the human frame. This is important as an anti-aging principle, as many contributors toward premature aging are, along with a decrease of one's power in general, related to the lack of optimal support of the human frame. In that example, the stretchy-elastic springiness of the meridians is functioning less than optimally, and, in such a scenario, instead of springy support, aspects of the body are allowed to sag to levels of least resistance.

Due to the insidious nature of aging, as well as the body's unconscious preference for the path of least effort, fulcrums and "rest points" gradually replace active support of the body. Like the story of a frog sitting in a slowly-warming pot of water, the head tends to fall to the point of least effort, the shoulders slump instead of lift, and the optimal position of the spinal nerves that feed the heart and other organs assume positions and operations that are less than ideal.

More active myofascial meridian support is evidenced in the bounciness of the young, healthy athlete. It is expressed in the person who walks with a "spring" in their step, and it reveals itself in the firmness of one's skin, particularly in the face and neck. Together, these contribute to how the person is perceived to age.

However, if Tiller's suggestions about the nature of the meridian network are correct, then full activation of the acupuncture meridian-myofascial network serves as the gateway to even more profound secrets. This means that the stretchy piezoelectric meridians not only define the acupuncture lines, but also serve as an embedded antenna that emits two distinct fields of radiation. As mentioned earlier, these fields are believed to be the medium that allows us to interact in subtle, mostly unconscious ways with the proposed *ether* of another dimension.

Tiller's contention that the acupuncture meridian system functions as an embedded antenna network is paradigm-changing. It describes an infrastructure that includes an expansion of physics which might one day explain the ability to interface with "another dimension." In this pursuit, the myofascial meridian networks are the laboratory in which to test and experiment with the meaning of human potential, and the possibility that human consciousness can interact with physical matter.

Afterword to Section XII

Can Spiritual Knowledge be Transferred via an Energetic Interaction?

*I*s it possible that, like the tuning of a piano, a great master can "tune" the energy fields of a disciple? Might a transduced field effect function as a mechanism to explain how consciousness, or advanced spiritual knowledge, might transfer from master to disciple? In the East, and particularly within the spiritual traditions of India, it is held that spiritual influence or knowledge can be converted into subtle "energy" that can be transmitted from master to disciple. In the Hindu religion, the principle is described as the transfer of *shakti*, or "spiritual energy," which is consciously directed from master to disciple to initiate *siddhi*, the supernatural powers derived from spiritual practice. [49]

For the same reason, some spiritual traditions, especially those of India and Tibet, hold the belief that merely being in the presence of a holy man or woman has a positive, growth-promoting influence on the individual's subtle energy and consciousness fields. For example, in the spiritual traditions of India, the *auric* influence of a holy person is described as being transferable through their radiant *shakti*. Padma Aon Prakash describes *shakti* as the "creative power of life-force energy — the flow that connects your body, mind, and soul." [50] In some cases, the radiant *shakti* of an advanced teacher can be so strong that those in the presence of the master experience mind-altering states. "Often, *bhaktas*, spiritual seekers who focus on devotion, love, and surrender as their practice, have experiences of powerful bliss and spiritual ecstasy, even to the extent as if they were drunk." [51]

The notion that one person can energetically influence another in a spiritual way has its corollary in the West, where some extraordinary individuals have been described as emitting a "light" or "radiant energy." An example is found in the Christian Gnostic traditions, where an association was said to exist between the attainment of advanced spiritual understanding and the experience of *light*. Writing on the subject, Luke Myers informs us that the early Christian Gnostic sect believed that radiant light was emitted by a person with advanced spiritual understanding. [52]

Adapting the model of transduction as a way of explaining how *shakti* transfers *siddhi* to a disciple, the transfer of "energy" from *guru* to disciple involves the spiritual teacher acting as a "frequency transducer." Thus, the holy man would conceivably access "higher" etheric frequencies and, through transduction, re-processes these into a lower frequency that the student is capable of resonating with. This speculation suggests that once the frequency is reduced to a level that the student is capable of handling, the guru acts as a tuning fork, which influences the student to "vibrate" at a higher harmonic of their potential frequency. [53]

Endnotes

1 As described in the introductory pages, although the majority of the present work relies on *pinyin* style Romanization, there are a few exceptions. Examples of transliterations used in the present chapter that uses the Wade-Giles Romanization include *t'ai chi,* and the opening lines to the *Tao Te Ching.*

2 Eisenberg, David, MD, "The woman on a bus," in *Encounters with qi: Exploring Chinese medicine*, Norton and Co, New York, 1995.

3 Bressler, David and Kroening, Richard, "Three essential factors in effective acupuncture therapy," American Journal of Chinese Medicine, Vol. 4, No. 1, 1976, p. 81.

4 NIH Consensus Statement. 1997. Acupuncture. Bethesda, MD: NIH. 15: 1–34 5.

5 Seto, et al., "Detection of extraordinary large bio-magnetic field strength," *Journal of acupuncture and electro-therapy research,* Vol. 17, pp. 75-94

6 Seto

7 Ibid.

8 A Faraday cage, named after nineteenth-century scientist Michael Faraday, consists of a mesh of electrical conducting material, which inhibits the transference of electromagnetic signals.

9 Pecci, Ernest, Foreword to William Tiller's, *Science and human transformation: Subtle energies, intentionality and consciousness.* Pavior Publishing, Walnut Creek, 1997, p. xvii

10 Because daydreaming tends to be associated with relaxation and non-linear thinking.

11 Tiller, William, *Science and human transformation: Subtle energies, intentionality and consciousness.* Pavior Publishing, Walnut Creek, 1997 p. 93

12 Tiller, p. 119

13 Ibid., p. 120

14 The exceptions are the more "natural" among us, who unconsciously direct more optimally efficient tensional forces through their body.

15 Ibid., p. 128

16 Brennan, Barbara, *Hands of light*, Batam Books, 1987, p. 49

17 Brennan, p. 49

18 Ibid.

19 Ibid.

20 Tiller, William, *Science and human transformation: Subtle energies, intentionality and consciousness.* Pavior Publishing, Walnut Creek, 1997

21 Pecci, Earnest F, From the Foreword, Tiller, William, *Human transformation: Subtle energies, intentionality, and consciousness*, p. XVII

22 Here referring to "intention," as in the intention research discussed in Section IX.

23 "Germ theory was proposed by Girolamo Fracastoro in 1546 and expanded upon by Marcus von Plenciz in 1762." https://en.wikipedia.org/wiki/Germ_theory_of_disease

24 William A. Tiller, Ph.D. and Walter E. Dibble, Jr., Ph.D. "Why the last century's quantum mechanics (QM) is irrelevant in a duplex, reciprocal subspace, reference frame for our cognitive world," White Paper #XXXIX.

25 Note, the expanded energy field is that of an experienced meditator. It is not yet clear whether the same kind of changes are exhibited in a person without regular "energetic practice," prayer, or similar transpersonal practices.

26 Here, using the derivative of transducer: a device that changes power from one system in another form. Source: Merriam Webster online dictionary.

27 For example, such as those described in Dr. Seto's study cited in Section IV, and in the later described study of Therapeutic Touch practitioners.

28 Therapeutic Touch (T.T.) is an "energy healing" system developed by Dora Kunz and Dolores Krieger in the 1970s.

29 E.F. Green, et al., "Anomalous electrostatic phenomena in exceptional subjects," *Subtle energies*, 1993; 2:69.

30 "This voltage pulse is measured via both an ear electrode and a nearby very large copper-wall electrode. When the healer is intentionally healing, these internal voltage surges increase in both frequency and magnitude. The subject studied here generated 15 anomalous surges during one 30-minute healing session." Tiller, William, "Towards explaining anomalously large body voltage surges on exceptional subjects: Part I: The electrostatic approximation," *Journal of scientific exploration*, Vol. 9, No. 3, 1995, p. 2.

31 Tiller, William, "Towards explaining anomalously large body voltage surges on exceptional subjects: Part I: The electrostatic approximation," *Journal of scientific exploration*, Vol. 9, No. 3, pp. 33 1-350, 1995.

32 Tiller

33 A capacitor is a device capable of storing an electric charge.

34 Tiller, William, *Science and human transformation: Subtle energies, intentionality and consciousness.* Pavior Publishing, Walnut Creek, 1997, pp. 63-68.

35 Tiller, William, et al., "Towards explaining anomalously large body voltage surges on exceptional subjects Part I: The electrostatic approximation," *Journal of scientific exploration*, Vol. 9, No. 3, pp. 331-350, 1995.

36 Here referring to "internal order," resulting from the synchronization of biological rhythms, as discussed in Sections VII and IX.

37 There are rare exceptions to this "not too relaxed, not too tense" approach to training, where one's mind and intention is so emphasized, and in this regard, so strong, that the body might appear extremely soft and relaxed, yet somehow, effective skill can still be manifested. Likewise, on the other end of the continuum, there are practitioners who emphasize extreme tension during *qigong* practice. I personally have never seen overall positive outcomes in this kind of practice, and I have been asked to intervene in some cases where a practitioner's tensional practice produced dangerous health consequences for the individual.

38 Dale RA. "The systems, holograms, and theory of micro-acupuncture." *American journal of acupuncture*, 1999; 27(3/4): 207-42.

39 The *dan tian* was described in earlier chapters as the "energy center" of the lower abdomen associated with Taoist yoga, *t'ai-chi*, and other schools of internal martial arts and meditation.

40 However, not overly relaxed. The correct amount of physical tension, applied in this way, was described in Section XI as belonging to the *song-peng* continuum.

41 Quote from http://divinecosmos.com/index.php/start-here/books-free-online/19-the-science-ofoneness/80-the-science-of-oneness-chapter-02-the-aether-is-pure-conscious-oneness

42 The *I Ching* (also written *Yijing*), or "Book of Changes," is an ancient Chinese classic revered by both Taoists and Confucianists. From the subject's Wikipedia entry: "The core of the *I Ching* is a Western Zhou divination text called the *Changes of Zhou* (周易 *Zhōu yì*). Various modern scholars suggest dates ranging between the tenth and fourth centuries BCE for the assembly of the text in approximately its current form." From https://en.wikipedia.org/wiki/I_Ching

43 Jung, Carl, from the Introduction to Helmut Wilhelm's, *I Ching*, Pantheon Books, 1950.

44 The notion of the "red thread" is closely connected with *yuan-fen* and is often said in the same breath. It connects lovers who are destined to meet. It gets shorter and shorter as they grow up, until it's so short they meet face-to-face and fall in love.

45 From the Foreword by Ernest F. Pecci, MD, Tiller, William, *Science and human transformation: Subtle energies, intentionality, and consciousness*. Pavior Publishing, Walnut Creek, 1997, p. xv.

46 Stevens, John, Aikido: *The way of harmony*, Shambala, Boston, MA 1984 p. 11.

47 Stevens

48 Ibid.

49 See http://en.wikipedia.org/wiki/Siddhi

50 Prakasha, Padma Aon, *The power of shakti: 18 pathways to ignite the energy of the divine woman,* Simon and Shuster, 2009, p. xiii

51 http://guruslight.blogspot.com/2013/07/radiant-saint-and-ordinary-saint.html

52 Myers, Luke, Gnostic visions: Uncovering the greatest secret of the ancient world, iUniverse, 2011, p .45.

53 Thanks to Frank van Gieson for his suggestion of *shakti* as a model, and his contribution of the original text in this paragraph.

<u>Conclusion</u>

In this study, we have considered the meaning of "internal energy" in the context of numerous traditions. We examined the martial power that the *t'ai-chi* master knows as *qi,* the energy that the *aikido* practitioner refers to as *ki,* and the spiritual force of *lung-wind* that is the focus of the Tibetan *tantric* practitioner. Other sections looked at the *shakti, prana,* and *kundalini* traditions that originated on the Indian subcontinent. We also noted the healing abilities of the non-contact healer and the experience of "energy" as heat or pressure within the body. We have described similarities between the descriptions of the life force found in these traditions and what the indigenous North American shaman calls *manitou,* the Hawaiian *kahuna* knows as *mana,* and the subtle influence that some Western investigators refer to as *information.*

One's experience of life energy is multifaceted; it can be physical, mental, emotional, spiritual, or a combination of all of these. Thus, the discussion of "internal energy" depends on the context. It can be a force for healing the self or others, a training method to aid and awaken one's spiritual development, or a powerful weapon that can be employed in contact sports and martial arts.

One's personal experience of "energy" can be subjectively electrical or objectively warm. For the practitioner of Taoist, *hatha,* and other yogas, the ability to unify one's movement with *prana,* breath, *qi,* or *ki* defines mastery. In those systems, one's psycho-emotional connection to the energetic sensation can advance consciousness, and in many examples, the practitioner's experience with the life force can be life-changing. However, interaction with the enigmatic "energy" can, at times, be unsettling, and, in rare cases, even psychologically dangerous.

As a spiritual force, one's interaction with "internal energy" can initiate the flowering of personal mystical experience. Examples are found in the *manitou* of the indigenous North American shaman, as well as the *mana* that is revered by the Hawaiian *kahuna.* In traditions such as those, mastery of the life force requires the practitioner to focus attention inward. Another example is in the practice of Taoist *neidan* yoga, where the practitioner works with the power of breath, mixes this resource with physical yoga and intention, and then directs these toward gaining conscious control over the body's most subtle rhythms. This demonstrates the goal of the Taoist yogi: first to gain control over the movement of internal *nei qi* (內氣) within the body, and then to transmute the coarse aspects of one's *jing qi* (精氣) into rarified essence, or *shen* (神), which represents the quintessence of the individual.

Earlier, some comparisons were made between the internal experience of the Taoist energetic meditator and the tantric practitioner of Tibetan Buddhism. Among those parallels is the manifestation of palpable yogic inner heat that the *tantric* initiates call *tummo*. One of the Six Yogas of the eleventh-century teacher Naropa, the practice of *tummo* can be undertaken by an initiated tantric disciple while in the deepest state of meditation. Here, the initiate has dedicated their life to observing and mastering the flow of *lung*-wind (ཚ) moving through the body's invisible tsa (ས) energy channels. However, an experience like this is not limited to the traditions of Tibet, as practitioners of Taoist mediation and yoga traditions report similar experiences. These, too, involve sensations of heat in the body, and, in some cases, what appear to be channels along the center axis of the body, identical to those associated with *tantric* practice.

Some traditions are less concerned with the flow of energy within the body, and instead focus on the movement of the life force *outside and around* the body. In China, from ancient times and continuing to the present, the study of energy in the environment has been the specialty of the *feng shui* master. At some point in ancient China, a person observed that when objects in a room were arranged harmoniously, their order could induce calm in those who entered. This observation gave birth to *feng shui,* the art of "wind and water" (風水). Thus, *feng shui* evolved as a discipline concerned with attention to the movement of unseen forces in the environment, which, like invisible rivers of wind, flow not only through passes and around trees, but also through windows and doorways.

The belief, found in Eastern traditions, that an invisible force can influence health, power, and well-being has its Western parallel. Diogenes of Apollonia provides the earliest description of the body's energetic force in Western literature. In the fifth century BCE, he taught his disciples that the life force travels within the body and along the spine from the genitals to the brain.

In some cultures, there are those who believe that a resonance exists in the balance of energy between the individual, the social group, and the natural world. The Chinese Taoists held that the state of subtle energy maintained by a social group could influence the natural order. Thus, when society was in harmony with the natural order, things went well. However, by the same token, when natural laws are ignored, the tripartite realms of heaven, man, and earth tend to break down. The most revered text of the Taoists, the *Tao Te Ching,* teaches that when the Tao is present in the world, it portends gentle rain to fall, but when the principles of the natural order are ignored, warhorses are bred outside the city. Generally, not a good sign.

More recently, some scientists have begun to investigate the possibility that non-physical, human-directed influence might act as a *force of nature.* The scientist Carl von Reichenbach proposed such a notion in the early nineteenth-century. However, he was unable to convince his colleagues of the physical reality of the force he called *Od*, or *odic force*, after the Norse god Odin. At the dawn of the twentieth century, Sir William Crookes, another scientist and member of the Royal Society, wrote about the existence of an invisible force, but again, his colleagues remained unconvinced.

In the 1950s, the noted physician William Reich so strongly believed in the existence of an invisible healing force that he constructed devices to treat patients with concentrated doses of the revitalizing force he called *orgone*. No doubt, Dr. Reich's interests influenced Bernard Grad's research a decade later. In the 1960s, Grad became the first to use modern scientific methods and controls to document the power of human non-physical influence to affect the growth rate of plants.

Sometimes, researchers of Chinese-style, non-contact healing describe two kinds of *qi*, labeling these as (+) positive, growth promoting, and (-) negative, or disruptive energy. Since the late 1950s, the Chinese government has encouraged studies investigating the proposal that *qi* masters could emit a healing force. Studies of this style of non-contact healing energy are currently being conducted in some Chinese hospitals and research centers. Although results supporting the theory forwarded by Chinese scientists have thus far failed to be confirmed by Western investigators, the inclusion of this kind of inquiry as an acceptable area of research is encouraging. It is a sign that the current scientific paradigm denying the ability of human will to act on the physical world is being increasingly challenged.

Since the ascendancy of the British empiricists, the experience of the Chinese energetic master, like the shaman, has been relegated to the veiled world of the mystic and the dragon-filled shadows of children's stories and myths. Currently, the arts and sciences of human–directed, non-physical influence are not widely acknowledged because of the current scientific paradigm, which states that a well-designed experiment should be free of human (emotion, intentional, etc.) influence. However, we live in a time when that old paradigm is increasingly being challenged to the point that it may soon be expanded to include the forces of consciousness and intent. Ernest F. Pecci describes the current Western scientific paradigm, here referred to as "the old perspective:"

> The old perspective is perhaps best exemplified by the accepted scientific framework wherein everything in the world obeys purely objective laws with no influence arising from human consciousness or human intentionality. [1]

What is Internal Energy?

Before any meaningful definition of internal energy can be formulated, the right questions must first be asked. This is an arduous task, since, at this juncture, there are too many different "starting point" definitions of internal energy, and together these pose a challenge to the possibility of asking the right questions. Moreover, a succinct, one-sentence definition of internal / subtle energy is elusive, since so many factors contribute to the meaning of the life force. Some of the factors addressed in the preceding pages range from one's mental attitude, heart electrophysiology, posture, social support network, expectation, and belief. A complete discussion of internal energy is indeed daunting.

Some clues to the nature of internal energy are contained in the ancient beliefs of the native Hawaiians. In their culture, a shaman with strong enough *mana*, or spiritual force called *ka 'ike huna*, is believed to be able to influence nature and events. However, the study of subtle human-directed influence no longer belongs exclusively to the domain of the shaman. Presently, scientists, under strict laboratory conditions, are documenting the power of trained individuals to consciously direct non-physical influence, with Dr. William Tiller's gas-discharge device experiment in particular seeming to support the notion that human *intention* acts as a force of nature. Tiller's experiment is an example of an exceptionally well-designed, controlled, and replicable study that suggests that an individual is able to non-physically induce an electrostatic charge in a device designed to respond to human intention. This is only one example of the kind of power of intention research now being undertaken.

When internal energy is more clearly defined by science, it will no doubt be found to be closely related to the expression of human will and potential. Eventually, that yet-to-be-measured *x-factor* will be shown as intertwining with our thoughts, emotions, and physical bodies. It is probable that internal energy, when more completely understood, will be accepted as the link between an individual's mind, body, spirit and, quite possibly, other dimensions. When this happens, the current paradigm defining human will and non-physical influence as separate from the environment will be replaced by a new understanding of the way human will, thought, and intention are intimately linked through subtle strands of "energy" with the environment.

However, the awakening of latent power can be expressed only through an awakened individual. Here, awakening refers to a person who has learned to synchronize their rhythms. Whether *t'ai-chi* master or yogi, their art reaches maturity when they learn to become aware of, and consciously manage, their subtle biological rhythms.

Three Categories

The human being's interaction with what is called subtle or internal energy can be divided into three categories. The first of these is unconscious, and has to do with the balance of subtle energy in the body's energy channels. This category highlights the search for homeostasis, as it addresses the flow of life force within the body and its contribution to the maintenance of the physical frame and organs. In the context of traditional energetic medicine, this aspect of unconscious energy is represented by the acupuncture meridians and the traditional diagrams of the body's energy lines.

Category I

Category I also includes traditional medicine's description of the transformation of life energy in the body. An example of this is the relationship between blood and *qi*, which in TCM is said to be "paired." Other examples of normally unconscious life energy processes include descriptions of the liver as "responsible for the smooth flow of *qi*," and the role of the kidneys to "store essence." These are attempts to explain the normally unconscious processes of the body's *qi* energy economy that can be influenced through acupuncture, massage and / or herbal prescriptions.

In summary, the central purpose of traditional energetic medicine is the restoration of harmony, or balance, of the body's "energy systems." Ancient therapies, many of which are still in use today, rely on these understandings of the body's energy system to treat illness. Therapies falling within this category are based on the notion that disease forms from disharmony between these unconsciously managed systems. In traditional Chinese medicine, disharmonies are classified by conditions such as *excess, deficiency, heat, cold, external, internal, yin* or *yang*. In addition to interventions like acupuncture or massage, Category I also relies on herbal formulae to restore harmony to the body's energetic system.

Category II

The second category has to do with mastery of "energetic" systems within the body that, although unconscious for most of us, through sufficient training and dedication can be accessed and manipulated by talented individuals. This category focuses on the skill and discipline related to perception and conscious control over subtle cues within the body. Through yoga, meditation, and internal energy practices such as *t'ai-chi ch'üan* and *qigong*, or through methods like those employed in *tantric* energy practices, this category involves learning to master the flow of energy within the body. Other examples of Category II control over the body's subtle energy include Taoist energetic practices, such as "microcosmic orbit" meditation. In both Chinese alchemy and Tibetan *tantric* systems, mastery involves control over the flow of subtle energies within the human frame, and especially those that flow along the spinal corridor. The primary concern of many systems, including those just mentioned, is manipulation of the magnetic and powerful sexual energy of the lower torso. Through transmutation, this rarified force is then raised along the spine to the brain, a practice believed by its proponents to initiate both advanced consciousness and psychic powers.

Categories II and III utilize a variety of methods for manipulating internal energy, including yogic posture and breathing techniques that direct targeted pressure to specific areas of the body. In addition, these practices feature mental techniques that allow us to become sensitive to the body's "energy centers" and the flow of "energy." These categories include the advanced meditator who possesses the ability to observe the inner workings of the mind and body, and thereby influence one's normally unconscious nervous system.

Category III

The final category is the most controversial, as it relates to the topic of non-contact, or energetic, influence on an external object or another person. Psychokinesis — the ability to move an object without making physical contact — belongs to this category, as does non-contact healing such as was exhibited by the *qigong* master in China, who can annihilate bacteria in a Petri dish. This category also includes demonstrations of internal energy in the martial arts, as well as applications of acupuncture or massage amplified by "energy" transfer from the practitioner; examples related to claims that a yet-to-be-defined and willfully directed "energy" can influence another person.

Diagram C-1
Biological Harmony + Intention

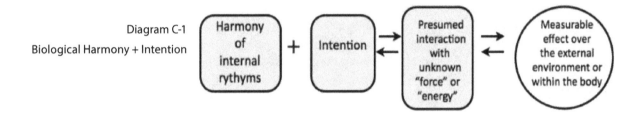

Intention

Intention is the cornerstone of Categories II and III. Increasingly lending itself to scientific scrutiny, intention (represented in the second box of Diagram C-1) is believed by both traditional practitioners and investigators to be the key that unlocks one's ability to influence control over "internal energy," which in turn extends an influence on the environment or another person.

One aspect of a tentative definition of internal energy can be characterized in terms of efficiency. More efficiency equals more internal energy, while less efficiency equals less. Efficiency represents a number of attributes that come together just right, one aspect of which is psychological and relates to the principle that how a person thinks influences the body. Thoughts are powerful; they have an immediate impact on the nervous system and other physiological systems. Thus, practicing in a way that fosters good mental habits is a discipline that contributes toward efficiency. It is a discipline that manifests first as habit, before later becoming one's whole way of life. It is important to remember this, since the mind-body also responds to negative thoughts in the form of persistent anger and judgment by becoming more tense and generating more stress response and inflammation.

Another aspect of efficiency has to do with the relative biomechanical balance of the body, with an example of this being the influence of proper suspension of the head above the shoulders. This aspect of biomechanical efficiency not only influences the blood and cerebrospinal fluid transport between the upper spine and brain, but, simultaneously, also the relative coherence of the individual's subtle energy.

In this light, it is helpful for us to remember that a chronic headache or neck pain related to bad posture is more than just the experience of inconvenient discomfort. It is the body telling us that something is awry and in need of attention.

As has been suggested by numerous sources, cross-culturally and from ancient times to the present, there is another subtle and powerful aspect of that *x-factor* life energy. This aspect is an effluence of a subtle magnetic-like field that can allow our hearts and souls to extend influence outward. The Chinese healing masters and martial artists know it as *qi,* while the indigenous people of the American northeast called it *manitou.* For centuries, like the sixteenth-century Swiss physician Paracelsus, mystics, psychics, and spiritual teachers have described a glowing field of light surrounding the human body. Modern scientists, like Tiller and Gerber, called the magnetic-like interactions between mind, intention, emotions, posture, and the meridian system the *ether,* theorizing that it represents our ability to influence the physical world by psychic force.

Before the formula describing how consciousness is linked to internal energy can be written down, we must learn a bit more from the yogi sitting high in the Himalayas; we need to listen closely to what the yogi, monk, and spiritual recluse tell us about how to unlock the powers of the mind and the potential of focused intent. Of the things we learn, calm and centeredness will be among the more important lessons. This is based on the fact that the common denominator in each tradition, whether in the pursuit of "energy," internal power, *qi,* or *prana,* is that the master practitioner is one who has learned to function as the eye of a hurricane, with calm center, and who embodies *calmness in the heart of movement, which is the secret of all power.*

However, before one can tune their internal order to synchrony, there must be the purposefully directed, deep experience of inner peace. For most of us, this ability does not spontaneously appear, it has to be worked at. Conscious calmness brings order to our biological rhythms, which in turn increases *coherence.*

Pay attention. Practices that bring one into *coherence* are simple, but they must be exercised carefully and daily. Pay attention to them to touch the magic of internal energy. Ignore them, and the harmony that connects one to the life force will weaken, allowing chaos to easily take the upper hand.

Coherence is brought about by focusing on one's inner rhythms, such as the inward and outward rhythm of the breath. For some, it begins when attention is paid to the heartbeat, while for others it is the result of a *choice* to minimize negative thoughts and emotions. For others, coherence is initiated when attention is paid to one's steps upon the earth. There is no shortage of methods by which practitioners can discover this state for themselves.

Long ago, some Chinese sages left humanity's caravan routes as they sought to find the Tao in places far removed from society's distractions. Common to many seekers then, as now, they began a journey to attain greater coherence, brought about by their resolving to prioritize attention not to the external world, but to their interior.

Regardless of the culture, time, or practice, becoming more coherent always involves a decision to focus not on the world of advertising, to-do lists, and the latest social media update, but instead *choosing* to prioritize one's inner life. From the balance point of coherence, a person moves harmoniously with one's natural rhythms, new power is discovered, and stress associated with formerly overactive amygdala — the brain's fight or flight center — is minimized. Simultaneously, the problem-solving portions of the brain become more active, and synchronistic, creative solutions appear out of nowhere.

Information

Preceding chapters have speculated that at least some aspects of internal or subtle energy may not turn out to be a form of "energy" at all, but rather, *information*. Information might more aptly begin to explain the unseen communication and *magnetism* between two young lovers as they sit close together, stare into each other's eyes, and energetically merge through their shared trance. On one level, their experience of mutual ecstasy can be explained in terms of the effects of endorphins excited by secreted pheromones, however, at the same time, another interaction contributes to their trance state: the exchange of invisible *information*. In this context, information, operating through their overlapping energetic fields, contributes to bonding and promotes deeper communication, as the two lovers make their unspoken pacts with infinity.

While some aspects of the invisible communication between the young lovers are measurable, others are not. We can predict with certainty that while in their trance-like state, the blood serum of each will show increased levels of life-enhancing hormones. We can also predict that other blood variables will show a marked decrease in the stress hormone cortisol, and that their biological rhythms will have become *entrained*.

As a by-product of their experience of ecstasy, we know that on multiple levels, the biological systems of these young lovers will have become harmonious, both within themselves and in synchrony with each other. With this comes increased exchange of *information* that is beyond words, and with the exchange of information comes deeper bonding, and with more bonding comes more information.

When a clearer understanding of internal energy is available, it will be simultaneously explained from a variety of viewpoints. One of these will be as a *subtle energy matrix*, and another will be as the conveyor of *intelligence* between the body's life support, emotional, and survival systems; these will then be recognized as an additional aspect of physiology. Then, the contributing factors that awaken one's internal energy and internal power will be understood as a constellation of perspectives that will include physical as well as mental / emotional factors that contribute to their definition, among which will be posture and the relationship between energy and form expressed in Dudjom Rinpoche's words: "If the body is held straight, the wind-energy will be unobstructed."

Of the numerous factors contributing to a person's access to abundant internal energy, the most important are the mental habits one develops as a response to challenge. By becoming a little more balanced and centered, one simultaneously develops the habit of not easily giving up power to fear, anger, and fight or flight reactions. With attention to this kind of mental practice, one discovers that just a little more mental / emotional space is created. This kind of space gives one room to engage problems with creative, problem-solving brain centers and, on occassion, sparks that magical synchronicity of events beyond words.

> ... there are no problems,
> only solution
> John Lennon

Training the brain not to automatically, and instantly, react with fear-protective responses while the individual is under stress takes practice. Before an *aikido* master can throw an opponent in a real attack, and while expending no more than the most minimal physical effort, many years are spent mastering calmness, as along with the mastery of the technical art, attention is also directed to the practitioner's internal state. This is an example of a martial art where learning to induce relaxation as a conscious act is essential. When paired with study, the practiced release of stress and tension is at least as important as technique, and perhaps, even more so. This observation speaks to the notion that the expression of real power derives from learning to become the eye of the hurricane. When translated into practice, although the threatening winds swirl around you, you stay unaffected and calm. That is a challenging but worthwhile goal.

In the 1960s, I read about how the Chinese believed that a person's martial arts power could be enhanced by *qi* energy, and it was this that sparked my quest to learn everything I could about this mysterious force. However, at that time, information of substantive value was difficult to find. Back then, as now, written sources often provided little more than a few lines elucidating the meaning of the *life force*.

In the late-1970s, I told my first martial arts instructor about my plans to go to China and learn more about the *qi* life force, and he replied by telling me two things that proved incorrect. First, that no Chinese *sifu* (master) would ever accept a non-Chinese student, and second, that an energetic force called *qi* wasn't real. A few years later, I was in Taiwan studying with three masters, and in the years since, I have been accepted as an "inner-door" initiated disciple by *kung fu* families in both Taiwan and Mainland China, where I witnessed some amazing demonstrations of the *life force*. Over the subsequent decades, I have continued my research into the meaning of *qi*.

Internal energy, whether referred to as *qi, ki, prana, lung*, or any other term is real. However, a precise definition of the life force remains elusive. This is probably because "it" is not *one thing*, but the aggregate of many. Some aspects of this enigmatic force may never be fully understood, since they are linked to unquantifiable features of what make us human, including consciousness, will, and intent. The relative strength or weakness of that mysterious force is partly influenced by posture, and it is enhanced through positivity. When full, its potential is associated with healthy heart factors, and its expression is tied to the optimal functioning of the nervous system. It possesses the potential to influence the individual, and by extension, the world. When expressed through the practice of intentionality and coherence, it can, and does, change things for the better.

Endnotes

1 Ernest F. Pecci, MD, From the Forward to Tiller, William, *Science and Human Transformation*

Appendix A
Five Elements and Personality

This appendix provides supplementary information on the five-element theory as it applies to the seasons and personality. As described in TCM literature, every individual, for better or worse, has a kind of resonance with a particular "season," which makes them especially sensitive to those conditions. The below diagram illustrates those correspondences:

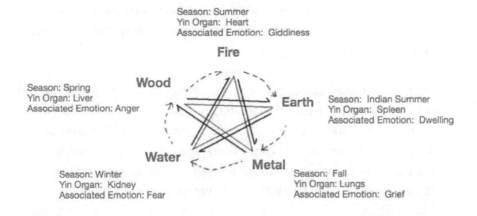

Diagram A-1

The Five-Elements with Corresponding Season and Personality Types

As illustrated in Diagram A-1, an individual whose personality is associated with the spring season is known as "wood type." Similarly, a person who is more sensitive / reactive to summer is "fire type," one who resonates with the early fall / Indian summer is "earth type," the fall is "metal type," and winter is "water type."

According to an individual's sensitivity/ reactivity to a particular season, emotional balance should be carefully monitored and managed during that period.

Note: TCM therapy almost always includes a constellation of treatment approaches which often include the selection of several points. The acupuncture point treatment and "interventions" presented in this section are for discussion purposes and intended to introduce the subject in a general way. Those discussions should not be used in lieu of proper diagnosis and treatment by a qualified practitioner.

Liver Personality

The liver personality is associated with the wood element and is most sensitive to the spring season. Accordingly, and especially during the spring, this personality type can be easily angered. Demonstrating the resonance between personality, season, and visceral organ, the liver of this personality type is more reactive during the spring.

Positive attributes associated with this personality type are drive and determination. The resonance-vibration of spring / wood is reflected in the new sprouts of grass that, in the springtime, have the "will" to push up and through the tiniest cracks in concrete. In human terms, this corresponds to the person who has the willpower to overcome challenges and give birth to new creations. The dark side of the liver personality is anger, and those individuals who are sensitive to the spring resonance can be particularly susceptible to fits of extreme anger in the springtime, a reaction that can be exacerbated by alcohol.

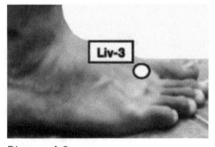

Diagram A-2

The Liver 3 (Liv-3) Acupuncture Point

The Liver 3 (Liv-3) Acupuncture Point

In terms of physical health, the liver personality, especially during the springtime and when "out of balance," may experience tension or heat at the right mid-torso, where the liver is located. Illustrated in Diagram A-2, a traditional treatment for liver excess includes acupuncture or acupressure to Liver 3 (Liv-3), located in the web between the big and second toe. In TCM theory, treating this point "calms" the liver; in most cases, anger will subside, and emotional balance be restored. Often, the release of tension in the patient suffering from "liver heat" can be observed moments after receiving treatment. When the liver is "out of balance," and self-directed pressure to the point is applied, the location becomes highly reactive, and thus you will know when you've hit the right spot.

Heart Personality

When one is excessively joyful, the spirit scatters and can no longer be stored

— The *Lingshu*

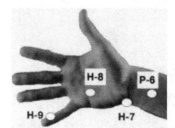

Diagram A-3

Select Acupuncture Points of the Hand and Forearm

Pericardium 6 (P-6), Heart 7 (H-7), Heart 8 (H-8), and Heart 9 (H-9)

The heart personality is associated with the fire element and is most sensitive to the summer season. The summer personality tends to be subject to "excessive joy" or giddiness; the positive result of this being that the person tends to be especially loving and compassionate. However, especially during the summer, the person with this personality can be influenced by the seasonal energy, which can manifest as a tendency to engage in shallow, constant chatter.

Any of these behaviors can harm the heart, especially during the summer. As traditionally described, the heart personality feels that it cannot exist alone and needs "fuel" provided by others. For the fire personality, the most reactive time of year is mid-summer, which brings the maximum expression of *yang* energy. The danger in this kind of "excess joy" is that it can lead to heart-related issues, such as sleep disorders, palpitations, anxiety and panic attacks.

Shown in Diagram A-3, Heart 7 (H-7 in Diagram 2-4) and Pericardium 6 (P-6), stimulation of these points produces a calming effect. Heart 8 (H-8) is useful when in distress.

Spleen Personality

The spleen personality is associated with the earth element and is thus most reactive to the season of late summer / early fall. In TCM theory, the spleen works with the stomach to digest food, and it is the nature of the spleen personality to digest things emotionally over and over. Accordingly, a person with "earth personality" tends toward obsessive ideation, especially during the "reactive season." Obsession, or "excessive dwelling," is said to be harmful to the spleen.

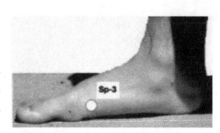

Diagram A-4

Acupuncture Point Spleen 3 (Sp-3)

A positive aspect of this personality type is the ability to "chew things down" and get to the essence of an issue. Imbalance of the spleen presents as loose stools, diarrhea, and pale lips. Acupuncture point Spleen 3 (Diagram 2-5) can help calm the excessive activity of the spleen. In severe cases, a palpable area of tension can be found on the posterior and left-side of the torso, in the area of the spleen organ.

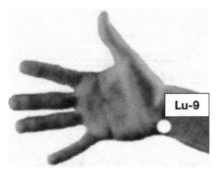

Diagram A-5

Lung 9 (Lu-9) The Lung "Source Point"

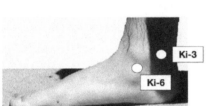

Diagram A-6

**Acupuncture Points Kidney 6 (Ki-6)
and Kidney 3 (Ki-3)**

Lung Personality

The lung personality is associated with the metal element and is most reactive to the "season" of late fall / early winter. During this period, the lung personality type can easily be moved to grief, and excessive indulgence in this emotion can harm the lungs. From the viewpoint of TCM, the lungs' role is to direct the dispersal and dissension of *qi* energy. When out of balance, the lung personality tends toward domineering and authoritarian attitudes.

The lung is tasked with maintaining a boundary between the inner and the outer world; the inner environment needs to be protected by a clear boundary which both defends and defines the person. When healthy, that boundary is both flexible and responsive. Positive and abundant lung energy manifests as strong physical vitality and a strong, clear voice.

Following TCM principles, there are several types of lung problems, with the most common being lung *qi* deficiency and lung *yin* deficiency. Lung *qi* deficiency syndrome is characterized by shortness of breath and fatigue, while lung *yin* deficiency is in the category of endogenous disease and is associated with chronic grief and / or sadness, accompanied by dry cough and a dry, red, often peeling tongue.

Under care of a traditional TCM practitioner, a constellation of points will be selected that typically includes the lung "source point," Lung 9, which "tonifies" the lung and Kidney 6 (Ki-6) to support lung *yin*.

Kidney Personality

The kidney personality is associated with the water element and is most reactive to the season of winter. This personality tends toward fear, which, when chronic, harms the kidney. According to TCM, the kidneys are responsible for the endocrine and hormonal system, and they are also closely related to the adrenal glands. Since the kidney is related to the water element, sustained cold can damage the organ. Symptoms of kidney imbalance usually include water retention, together with joint and back pain. Points Kidney 6 is one of the points that is used to balance kidney energy.

Appendix B

Entrained Pulse Training (EPT)

This appendix provides a more detailed discussion of the Entrained Pulse Training (EPT) protocol introduced in Section VII. EPT is a modern variation of neiguan "inner yoga" and was developed to induce entrainment — the ordering of one's biological rhythms.

EPT is based on one's ability to pay attention to the heartbeat and distal pulse at various locations throughout the body. In this way, the power of attention interacts with, and synchronizes, one's biological rhythms. EPT functions as a biofeedback technique with three principal actions. First, attending to the profusion of blood through arterial vessels tends to bring other bodily rhythms into "phase," or synchrony. Second, concentrating on the pulse at a specific area of the body can induce relaxation at the targeted location. Third, learning to become aware of the pulse during sitting or moving meditation practices helps quiet the mind.

Review of Initial Training

The basics of the EPT protocol include:

- Directing mental awareness to the heartbeat and pulse to induce relaxation.

- Learning to detect the heartbeat, first through the relaxed palms, and later through mental attention.

- Learning to detect the pulse at distal locations throughout the body.

- Inducing entrainment by paying attention to the time delay between the heartbeat and arrival of the pulse at targeted location, such as the hands or abdomen.

More advanced practice of the technique is available to practitioners who have attained proficiency in the basic levels. More advanced levels include:

- The ability to mentally attend to the heartbeat and pulse at distal locations while sitting.

- Attending to the heartbeat and pulse while in conversation.

- Attending to these while standing.

- While walking or moving about.

- While engaged in athletic training.

- While engaged in competitive athletics.

Notes for more Advanced EPT Practice

Sitting Practice

Practice at this level involves attuning to the same signals associated with pulse and the profusion of blood through the arteries, but with the added influence of gravity. Start by sitting relaxed in a chair and apply the EPT protocol described in Section III.

Following the same protocol described for the basic level, begin by attending to the heartbeat in the center of the chest. Next, learn to sense and focus on the pulse at distal locations, such as the abdomen or feet. Success at this stage requires patience and regular practice.

Attending to the Pulse while Engaged in Conversation

Learning to become aware of the pulse and entraining one's biological rhythms during conversation brings several benefits; the practice is especially valuable for dealing with stress during difficult workplace interactions. For example, when attending to the pulse transit while speaking, the cadence of one's speech will change, and the voice often deepens. Regular practice of the technique brings calmness under stress, and often causes other people to respond to the synchrony of your rhythms. In other words, a sense of "flow" and "harmony" is created between individuals. In some cases, the results will seem magical.

During the practice, you may notice that your timing changes and new pauses appear as your bodily rhythms synchronize. As you become more "in sync" with those you converse with, you will be able to communicate more effectively. Pay attention under these conditions; your heart has become in sync with your brain. Those who have studied the technique report that even their phone conversations go more smoothly when they engage it.

How it Works

The ability to practice EPT during conversation takes dedication and patience. At first, the practitioner will be able to attend to the pulse at distal locations for only a few moments at a time, but with practice, the time in the entrained state during conversation can be extended; the key is to identify the "background feeling" associated with the distal pulse. As part of my practice, I focus on feelings in the body that go along with awareness of the heartbeat and distal pulse. I pay attention to things like the relaxation of the chest or flushing of the hands or feet. These act as cues that are easier to observe when, due to stress, observations of the pulse at distal locations are less obtainable. This is an example of how "background" signals can induce entrainment under difficult circumstances.

While Standing, Moving, and for More Advanced Practice

EPT can be practiced while standing, whether as a formal meditation (e.g., "standing practice") or as a personal "secret" self-cultivation technique. An example of this sort of secret practice might be applied while in a grocery store queue, where EPT practice will allow you to maximize those queuing experiences. In the same manner, the technique dramatically improves one's yoga, *t'ai-chi*, or other internal martial arts. This is because of the technique's ability to relax unnecessary tension and clear the way for the natural tendency to synchronize one's movement with those subtle biological rhythms.

As noted in Section III, EPT has become the cornerstone of practice for many of my martial arts students and other clients. Most of our association students develop their own version of the technique, which they regularly apply to the practice of t'ai-chi and related arts. Some of the more advanced athletes even apply the technique to their running. One client reported: "When using it, I feel that I can run forever."

Bibliography

Adams, Jad, "Blake's big toe" A review of *Why Mrs. Blake cried: William Blake* and *the sexual basis of spiritual vision,* The Guardian/Books Saturday 1 April 2006

Allen, Paula Gunn, from the introduction to Ingo Swann's *Psychic sexuality,* Panta Rei, [Crossroads Press digital edition]

Avila, Elena, *Woman who glows in the dark: A curandera reveals traditional Aztec secrets of physical and spiritual health,* Penguin Putnam, New York, 2000

Baker, Ian A., *The Dalai Lama's secret temple: Tantric wall paintings from Tibet,* Thomas & Hudson, NY, 2000

Basil, Johnston Basil, *The manitous: The spiritual world of the Ojibway,* New York Harper Collins

Becker, Robert, *The body electric: Electromagnetism and the foundation of life,* William Morrow & Co, 1985

Bentov, I., *Stalking the wild pendulum: On mechanics of consciousness* New York: Dutton, 1977

Bi Yongsheng, *Chinese Qigong Outgoing-Qi Therapy.* Shandong Science and Technology Press, 1997

Blofeld, John, *Taoism: The road to Immortality,* Shambhala, Boston, 1978

Blofeld, John, *The secret and sublime: Taoist mysteries and magic,* Penguin Group 1973

Bracy, John, *Ba gua: Hidden knowledge in the Taoist internal martial art,* North Atlantic Books, 1998

Bracy, John, "Internal Energy in the Martial Arts," *Qi: The journal of traditional health and fitness,* Summer 2002. www.qi-journal.com

Brennan, Barbara, *Hands of light,* Batam Books, 1987

Bressler, David and Kroening, Richard, "Three essential factors in effective acupuncture therapy," *American journal of Chinese medicine,* Vol. 4, No. 1, 1976

Broadbent, Elizabeth, Nair, Shwetha, et al., "Do slumped and upright postures affect stress responses? A randomized trial," *Health psychology,* Vol 34(6), Jun 2015

Bruce Greyson in "Some neuropsychological correlates of the physio-kundalini syndrome," *The journal of transpersonal psychology,* Vol. 32, No. 2, 2000

Burton Watson (translator) *Chuang Tzu: The basic writings,* Columbia University Press, 1965

Carfagno, Farrar Straus and Giroux, New York, 1973 Original manuscript, *Die Entdeckung des Orgons, Erster Teil: Die Function des Orgasmus,* Copyright © 1968 by Mary Boyd Higgins as Trustee of the Wilhelm Reich Infant Trust Fund

Chang, Stephen T., *The complete system of self-healing internal exercises,* Tao Publishing, San Francisco, 1986

Chang, Steven, *The complete book of acupuncture,* Celestial Arts, 1976

Chao Pi-ch'en, originally titled *The Secrets of Cultivating Essential Nature and Eternal Life,* from the introduction to Lu Kuan Yu's *Taoist yoga: Alchemy & immortality,* Samuel Weiser, Inc. 1973

Cho, Philip S., "Ritual and the occult in Chinese medicine and religious healing: The development of zhuyou exorcism" (January 1, 2005). *Dissertations available from ProQuest.* Paper AAI3197659 http://repository.upenn.edu/dissertations/AAI3197659

Chuang Tzu (Zhuangzi) as cited by Kohn, Livia, "Taoist insight meditation," *Taoist meditation and longevity techniques,* University of Michigan Center for Chinese Studies, 1989

Chun-Ri Li, et al, "Effects of acupuncture at taixi acupoint (KI3) on kidney proteome," *The American journal of Chinese medicine,* Vol. 39

Cibot, *Memories concernant l'histoire, les sciences les arts de Chinois,* 1779

Cohen, Dayan E, "Neuroplasticity subserving motor skill learning." *Neuron.* 2011 Nov 3; 72(3):443-54. As cited by Danielle S. Basset, et al, in "A network neuroscience of human learning: Potential to inform quantitative theories of brain and behavior," *Trends Cogn Sci.* 2017 April; 21(4): 250–264.

Coopersmith, Jennifer, *Energy, the subtle concept: The discovery of Feynman's blocks from Leibniz to Einstein,* Oxford University Press, 2010.

Curran, James, "Huangdi neijing," *British journal of medicine,* 2008 Apr 5; 336(7647)

Dale RA. "The systems, holograms, and theory of micro-acupuncture." *American journal of acupuncture,* 1999; 27(3/4)

Dass, Ram, et al., *Miracle of love: Stories about Neem Karoli Baba,* E. P. Dutton: New York. 1979

Davis, Devra Lee, "The history and sociology of the scientific study of acupuncture," *American journal of Chinese Medicine,* Vol. 3, no. 1 1975

DeMarco, Michael A., "The origin & evolution of taijiquan," *Journal of Asian martial arts,* 1992

Despeux, Catherine, "Gymnastics: the ancient tradition," *Taoist meditation and longevity techniques,* University of Michigan Center for Chinese Studies, 1989

Diamond, John, MD, *Life energy: Using the meridians to unlock the power of your emotions,* Athena Books, Paragon House, NY, 1990

Ding Li, *Acupuncture meridian and acupuncture points.* China Books & Periodicals, Inc., 1992

Dorsher, Peter, MD, "Myofascial meridians as anatomical evidence of acupuncture channels," *Medical acupuncture,* Vol. 21, No. 2, 2009

Dowman Keith, *Masters of mahamudra*, State University of New York, 1986

Dunning, Trish (Editor), *Complementary therapies and management of diabetes and vascular medicine*, John Wiley and Sons, Ltd, 2006

E.F. Green, et al., "Anomalous electrostatic phenomena in exceptional subjects," Subtle Energies, 1993; 2

Eisenberg, David, MD, "Energy fields, meridians, chi and device technology," *Energy medicine in China: Defining a research strategy. Noetic Sciences Review*, Spring 1990

Eisenberg, David, MD, *Encounters with qi: Exploring Chinese medicine*, Norton & Norton, New York, NY, 1985

Feng, Lida, et al., *Proceedings of the first annual meeting of the Beijing qigong scientific research society*, Beijing, China, 1981

Fleet, Thurman, DC, *Rays of the dawn: Natural laws of the body, mind, and soul*, Concept therapy Institute, San Antonio, TX 2000

Gerber, Richard, MD, in *A practical guide to vibrational medicine*. Quill, An Imprint of Harper Collins Publications, 2001

Gerber, Richard, *Vibrational medicine*, Bear & Co., Rochester, VT, 2001

Gluck, Jay, *Zen combat*, Ballentine Books, 1962 (1976 edition)

Goldfield, Rose Taylor from the forward to Gyamtso, Khenpo Tsultrim, *Training the wisdom body*, Shambhala Publications, 2013 Boston, MA.

Goldthwait, J.E., et al., "The conservation of human energy: A plea for a broader outlook in the practice of medicine," *Rocky mountain medical journal*, 19 (Oct) 1934

Gori, L, "Ear acupuncture in European traditional medicine," *Evidence-based complementary and alternative medicine.* 2007 Sep:4

Greyson, Bruce, MD, "Some neuropsychological correlates of the physio-kundalini syndrome," *The journal of transpersonal psychology*, 2000, Vol. 32, No. 2

Gu, Hansen and Lin Housheng, "Preliminary experimental results of the investigation on the materialistic basis of 'therapy of qi mobilization' in qi gong." *Ziran Zachi (The nature Journal/ Chinese)* 1:12

Hawkins, David, MD, *Power vs. force: The hidden determinants of human behavior*, Hay House, 1995

Heikkila, Timo and Jiong, Li (translators) "Wang Xiang–Zai discusses the essence of combat science," *Shibao* Newspaper, Beijing, 1940

Hintz, Kenneth, et al., "Bio-energy definitions and research guidelines," *Alternative therapies in health and medicine.* May/June 2003

Hoare, Philip, "Some very unreasonable erotic practices," A review of Marsha Keith Schuchard, *Why Mrs. Blake cried: William Blake* and *the sexual basis of spiritual vision*, printed in *The Telegraph*, April 30, 2006

Holmes, Keikobad, "Using acupoint heart 7: An anatomical approach," *Medical acupuncture*, June 2009

Hsi Lai, *The sexual teachings of the white tigress: Secrets of female Taoist masters*, Destiny Books, Rochester, VT 2001

Human Rights Watch "Crackdown on Falun Gong," (Appendix III) *Dangerous minds: Political psychiatry in China today and its origins in the Mao era*. Published by Human Rights Watch and Geneva Initiative on Psychiatry. August 2002.

Ishida Hidemi, "Body and mind: The Chinese perspective," Livia Kohn (Editor) *Taoist meditation and longevity techniques,* Center for Chinese Studies, University of Michigan, 1989

ITOH Tomoko, SHEN Zaiwen ITOH[2] Yasuhiro, TAMURA Akira and ASAYAMA Masami, "The effects of wai qi on rats under stress based on urinary excretion measurements of catecholamines," *Journal of international society of life information science, Vol.*18, No.2, September 2000 [Proceedings of The Tenth Symposium of Life Information Science]

Jung, Carl, from the Introduction to Helmut Wilhelm's, *I Ching,* Pantheon Books, 1950

Kamada T., et al., "Power spectral analysis of heart rate variability in type As and type Bs in mental workload," *Journal of psychosomatic medicine*, 1992;54

Keeney, Bradford, *Shaking medicine: The healing power*, Destiny Books, VT. 2007

Kennedy, Brian, *Chinese martial arts training manuals: A historical survey*, North Atlantic Books, Berkley, 2005

Kohn, Livia, "Guarding the one: Concentrative meditation in Taoism," *Taoist meditation and longevity techniques,* Center for Chinese Studies, The University of Michigan, 1989

Kollai, M, "Cardiac vagal tone in generalized anxiety disorder," *British Journal of Psychiatry*, 1992;161

Krishna, Gopi, *Kundalini: Empowering human evolution: selected writings of Gopi Krishna, Paragon* House; Revised edition, 1996

Krishna, Gopi, *Kundalini: The evolutionary energy in man*, Shambala, Boston, 1997

Krishna, Gopi, *Living with Kundalini*, Shambhala, Boston, 1993

Krishna, Gopi, *The biological basis of religion and genius*, New York, Harper & Row, 1972

Lama Yeshe, *The bliss of inner fire: Heart practice of the six yogas of Naropa*, Wisdom publications, Sommerville, MA 1998

Langevin HM, YANDOW, JA, "Relationship of acupuncture points and meridians to connective tissue planes," Anat Rec. 2002

Lee, et al., "Endorphin release: A possible mechanism of acupuncture analgesia," *Comparative medicine, east and west*, Vol. vi., no. 1. pp. 57-60, 1978

Lee, M.S., et al, "Is there any energy transfer during acupuncture?" *American journal of Chinese medicine,* 2005

Li Ding, *Acupuncture, meridian theory and acupuncture points*, China Books & Periodicals, Inc.; Beijing: Foreign Languages Press, 1992

Lindquist, A, et al., "Heart rate variability, cardiac mechanics, and subjectively evaluated stress during simulator flight." *Aviation and Space Environmental Medicine* 1983; 54

Lipton, B.H., K.G. Bench, et al [1991], "Microvessel endothelial cell trans-differentiation phenotypic characterization." *Differentiation* 46:117-133

Lipton, Bruce, The *biology of belief: Unleashing the power of consciousness, matter, & miracles*, Hay House, 2016

Lowenthal, Wolfe, *There are no secrets: Professor Cheng Man-Ching*, North Atlantic Books, Berkeley, 1991

Lu K'uan Yu (Charles Luk), *Taoist yoga & immortality*, Samuel Weiser, Inc., York Beach, ME 1973

Lu K'uan Yu (translator), Chao Pi-ch'en, (*The secrets of cultivating essential nature and eternal life)* from *Taoist yoga alchemy and immortality*, Samuel Weiser, York Beach, ME, 1973

Lu, Gwei-Djen & Joseph Needham, *Celestial lancets: A history and rationale of acupuncture and moxibustion*, Cambridge University Press, 1980

Maciocia, Giovanni, *The foundations of Chinese medicine: A comprehensive text for acupuncturists and herbalists*, Second Edition Churchhill Livingstone, 2005

Mackall CL, Punt JA, Morgan P, Farr AG, Gress RE., "Thymic function in young/old chimeras: Substantial thymic T cell regenerative capacity despite irreversible age-associated thymic involution." Eur J Immunol. 1998;28

Mackenzie, Vicki, *Cave in the snow: On the life of Tenzin Palmo*, Bloomsburg Publishing, London. 1998

Mann, Felix, *Acupuncture*, New York: Random House   As cited by Davis, Devra Lee, *American journal of Chinese medicine*, Vo 3, No. 1, pp. 5-26, 1975

Markides, Kyriacos C., *The magus of Strovolos: The extraordinary world of a spiritual healer*, Penguin Books, London, 1985

McCann, Henry, "A Practical Guide to Tung's Acupuncture," *Journal of Chinese Medicine*, February 2006

McCann, Henry, "Tung's acupuncture: An introduction to a classical lineage of acupuncture." *The journal of Chinese medicine*, Feb 2006

McEvilley, C., *The shape of ancient thought: Comparative studies in Greek and Indian philosophies*, Allworth Press, New York, 2002

McTaggart, L., *The intention experiment: Using your thoughts to change your life and the world*, Free Press: Simon and Shuster, NY

Melzack R. and Wall, P.D., "On the nature of cutaneous sensory mechanism," *Brain*, 1962 Jun;85:331-56

Merton, Thomas (translator), *The way of Chuang Tzu*, New Horizons Press, 1969

Miller, James, "Chinese sexual yoga and the way of immortality," adapted from the translation by Paul R. Goldin, "The cultural and religious background of sexual vampirism in ancient China," *Theology and sexuality* 12(3): 285-308. Sage Publications, London, 2006

Miura, Kunio, "The revival of qi," *Taoist meditation and longevity techniques,* edited by Livia Kohn, Center for Chinese Studies, University of Michigan, 1989

Mullin, Glen, *Readings on the six yogas of Naropa*, Snow Lion Publications, 1997

Myers, Luke, *Gnostic visions: Uncovering the greatest secret of the ancient world*, iUniverse 2011

Myers, Thomas W., *Anatomy trains: Myofascial meridians for manual and movement therapists*, Elsevier, Ltd., 2009

Myss, Carolyn, *Anatomy of the spirit: The seven stages of power and healing*, Three Rivers Press, 1997

Nathan Sivin (Editor), From the Introduction, Needham, Joseph, *Science and civilization in China*, Vol. 6, Cambridge University Press, 1983

Needham, Joseph (translator), *Thai hsi ken chih yao chueh (Instructions on the Essentials of Understanding Embryonic Respiration)* Anonymous, Tang or Sung dynasty (618-1126 CE), as cited in *Science and civilization in China*, Vol 5, Cambridge University Press, 1983

Needham, Joseph (translator), passage from *Chih kua' chi* ("Pointing the Way Home to Life Eternal"), part of a collection of Taoist treatises called the *Tao Tsang (Daozang)*

Needham, Joseph (translator), *Tung Chung*-Shu *Chhun Chhiu Fan Lu, Science and civilization in China*, Vol. 2, Cambridge University Press, 1983

Needham, Joseph (translator), Excerpts from the *San Kuo Chih (Romance of the three kingdoms),* the biography of surgeon Hua Tho, *Science and civilization in China*, Vol. 5 1983

Needham, Joseph (translator), *Lü shih chhun chhiu*, as cited in *Science and civilization in China*, Cambridge University Press, Vol. 6, 1983

Needham, Joseph (translator), *Hsiu chen pi* or *"Esoteric Instruction on the regeneration of the primary vitalities,"* as translated by Joseph Needham, *Science and civilization in China*, Cambridge University Press, 1983

Needham, Joseph, *Clerks and craftsmen in China and the west*. Cambridge: University Press, 1970

Needham, Joseph, *Science and civilization in China*, Vol. 2, Cambridge University Press, 1983

Needham, Joseph, *Science and civilization in China:* Vol. 5, *Chemistry and Chemical Technology Spagyrical Discovery and Invention Physiological Alchemy*, Cambridge University Press, 1983

Needham, Joseph, *Science and civilization in China*, Vol. 6, Cambridge University Press, 1983

Newberg, Andrew MD, *How God changes your brain: Breakthrough findings from a leading neuroscientist.* Ballantine Books, NY, 2010

Ni, Maoshing (translator), *Yellow emperor's classic of medicine, A new translation of the neijing suwen with commentary,* Shambhala, Boston 1995

NIH Consensus Statement. 1997. Acupuncture. Bethesda, MD: NIH. 15

NMJ Contributors, "An evidence-based review of qigong by the National Standard Research Collaboration," *National Medicine Journal,* May 2010, Vol. 2, Issue 5

Norbu, Chögyal Namkhai, *The Crystal and the way of light: Sutra, tantra, and dzogchen,* Shambhala, Snow Lion Publications, 2000, p. 124

O'Byrne, F.D., (Translator and author of the Introduction) *Reichenbach's letters on od and magnetism: Published for the first time in English, with extracts from his own works, so as to make a complete presentation of the odic theory.* London, 1952

O'Connoer, J. and Bensky, D., "A summary of research concerning the effects of acupuncture," *American journal of Chinese medicine,* 3:377-394, 1975. As cited in Milovanovic, Miomir, et al., "Mental stimulation of acupuncture point zusanli (St-36) for rise of leukocyte count: Psychopuncture." *Comparative medicine east and west,* Vol. VI. No. 4

Omura, Y., "Anatomical relationship between traditional acupuncture point ST 36 and Omura's ST 36 (True ST 36) with their therapeutic effects: 1) inhibition of cancer cell division by markedly lowering cancer cell telomere while increasing normal cell telomere, 2) improving circulatory disturbances, with reduction of abnormal increase in high triglyceride, L-homocystein, CRP, or cardiac troponin I & T in blood by the stimulation of Omura's ST 36--Part 1." *Journal of acupuncture and electrotherapy Research,* 2007

Omura, Y., "Connections found between each meridian (heart, stomach, triple burner, etc.) and organ representation area of corresponding internal organs in each side of the cerebral cortex; release of common neurotransmitters and hormones unique to each meridian and corresponding acupuncture point and internal organ after acupuncture, electrical stimulation, mechanical stimulation (including shiatsu), soft laser stimulation or qi gong," *Journal of acupuncture and electrotherapy research,* 1989

Omura, Y., "Application of intensified (+) qi gong energy, (-) electrical field, (S) magnetic field, electrical pulses (1-2 pulses/sec), strong shiatsu massage or acupuncture on the accurate organ representation areas of the hands to improve circulation and enhance drug uptake in pathological organs: clinical applications with special emphasis on the " chlamydia-(lyme)-uric acid syndrome" and "chlamydia-(cytomegalovirus)-uric acid syndrome". *Acupuncture and electrotherapy research* 1995 Jan-Mar;20(1):21-72

Omura, Y., et al., "Unique changes found on the qi gong master's and patient's body during qi gong treatment; their relationships to certain meridians & acupuncture points and the re-creation of therapeutic Qi Gong states by children & adults." *Journal of acupuncture and electrotherapy research* 1989;14(1):61-89

Oschman, James, *Energetic medicine: The scientific basis,* Churchill Livingstone, 2000

Pabst, M., "The tattoos of the Tyrolean iceman: a light microscopical, ultrastructural and element analytical study," *J. archaeological science,* Vol 36, Issue 10, October 2009

Patrol Rinpoche, *Words of my perfect teacher,* Vistaar publications, New deli, India, 2004

Peacher, William G. MD, "Adverse reactions, contraindications and complications of acupuncture and moxibustion," *American journal of Chinese medicine,* Vol. 3, No. 1, 1975

Pearl, Bill, *Keys to the inner universe: World's best built man*, Typecraft, Inc., Pasadena, 1979

Pecci, Ernest P., From the introduction to Tiller, William, *Science and human transformation: Subtle energies, intentionality, and consciousness,*

Pavior Books, 1997, p.x

Prakasha, Padma Aon, Prakasha, Padma Aon, *The power of shakti: 18 pathways to ignite the energy of the divine woman,* Simon and Shuster, 2009, p. xiii

Purves D, Augustine GJ, Fitzpatrick D, et al., editors., *Neuroscience.* 2nd edition, Sunderland, 2000

Raghavendra, BR et al, "Voluntary heart rate reduction following yoga using different strategies," *Int J Yoga.* 2013 Jan-Jun; 6(1)

Rajagopalan, Krishnaswamy, *A brief history of physical education in India* (New Edition), Author House, 2014

Reich, William, *Function of the orgasm,* Translated from the German by Vincent R., Archives of the Orgone Institute

Reichmanis, et al., "Electrical correlates of acupuncture points." *IEEE transactions on biomedical engineering.* 1975. 22 (November)

Reichmanis, M, et al., "D.C. skin conductance variation and acupuncture loci," The *American journal of Chinese medicine,* Vol. 4, Issue 1, 1976

Robbie D.L. 1977, "Tensional forces in the human body," *Orthopedic review* 6: 47

Robinet, Isabelle, "Original contributions of *nei tan,*" *Taoist meditation and longevity techniques,* Livia Kohn (editor), University of Michigan Center for Chinese Studies, 1989

Rossi, Ernest, *The psychobiology of mind-body healing: New concepts of therapeutic hypnosis* (Revised Edition), W.W. Norton, 1993

Roth, Harold, *Original tao: Inward training (Nei-yeh) and the foundations of mysticism,* Columbia University Press, 1999

Roth, Harold, (translator) *Tao yeh,* as cited in *Original tao: Inward training (Nei-yeh) and the foundations of mysticism,* Columbia University Press, 1999

Sancier, K.M., "Medical applications of qigong and emitted qi on humans, animals, cell cultures, and plants: review of selected scientific research." *American journal of acupuncture,* Vol. 19, No. 4

The Search for Mind-Body Energy: Meditation, Medicine & Martial Arts

Sawai, Kenichi, *Taiki-ken: The essence of kung fu*, Japan publications, 1976

Schlitz, M. PhD, "Distant healing intention: Definitions and evolving guidelines for laboratory studies," *Alternative therapies in health and medicine. May/June 2003*. Vol. 9. No. 3.

Seidel, Anna, "A Taoist immortal of the Ming dynasty," *Self and society in Ming thought,* New York: Columbia University Press, 1970

Seto, A., et al. "Detection of extraordinary large biomagnetic field strength from the human hand," *Acupuncture and Electro-Therapeutics Research International Journal,* 1992, 17:75-94

Singer Dh, Martin, e al., "Lower heart rate variability and sudden cardiac death." *J Electrocardial,* 1998

Sivin, Nathan, "On the word 'Taoist' as a source of perplexity. With special reference to the relations of science and religion in traditional China," *History of religions,* Vol. 17, No. 3/4, Current Perspectives in the Study of Chinese Religions (Feb. - May (1978)

Smith, Robert, *Hsing-I: Chinese mind-body boxing,* North Atlantic Books, 1974

Smith, Suzzy, *ESP and hypnosis,* Excel Press, iUniverse, Lincoln, NE

Religious daoism, Stanford encyclopedia of philosophy, Aug 2016

Stein, Diane, *Essential psychic healing: A complete guide to healing yourself, healing others, and healing the earth.* Google e Book

Steiner, Rudolf, *Knowledge of higher worlds,* Rudolph Steiner Press, 2013

Stevens, John, *The philosophy of Aikido,* Kodansha America, New York, 2001

Swann, Ingo, *Psychic Sexuality: The bio-psychic "anatomy" of sexual energies,* Panta Rei/Crossroads Press, 1998/2014

Talbot, Brian, "Schuchard's Swedenborg," *The new philosophy,* July-December 2007

Telesford, Qawi K, et al, *Neuroimage,* 2016 Nov 15; 142: 198–210

Thai-chhing tao yin yang shhg ching (Manual of Nourishing the Life-Force by Physical Exercises and Self-Massage). From the *Mawangdui* tomb as cited by Needham, Joseph, *Science and civilization in China,* Cambridge University Press, 1983 Vol. 3

Thayer, JF, et al., "Autonomic characteristics of generalized anxiety disorder and worry," *Journal of sociology and biological psychology.* 1995; 37

Thondup, Tulku, *Incarnation: The history and mysticism of the tulku tradition of Tibet,* Shambala Publications, 2011

Tianjun Liu, Xiao Mei Qiang, *Chinese medical qigong* (Google eBook). Singing Dragon, May 28, 2013

Tiller, William, *Science and human transformation: Subtle energies, intentionality, and consciousness,* p. x, Pavior Books, 1997

Tiller, William, "Towards explaining anomalously large body voltage surges on exceptional subjects: Part I: The electrostatic approximation," *Journal of scientific exploration,* Vol. 9, No. 3, 1995

Helms, J., as cited by William Tiller, *Acupuncture energetics: A clinical approach for physicians,* Medical Acupuncture Publishers, Berkley, CA 1995

Tiller, William, et al, "Cardiac coherence: A new, non-invasive measure of autonomic nervous system order," *Alternative therapies,* Vol. 2:1 1996

Tiller, William, PhD, et al., *Some science adventures with real magic,* Pavior Publishing, Walnut Creek, CA 2005

Timo Heikkila and Li Jiong, (translators) "Wang Xiang–Zai discusses the essence of combat science," *Shibao* Newspaper, Beijing, 1940

Tsenshap, Kirti, *Principles of Buddhist Tantra,* Wisdom Publications, Somerville, MA

Upledger, John, D.O., *Your inner physician and you,* North Atlantic Books, Berkley, 1997

Veith, Ilza (translator), *Yellow emperor's classic of medicine, A new translation of the neijing suwen with commentary,* University of California Press, Oakland, 1975

Veith, Ilza (translator), *The Yellow emperor's classic of internal medicine, University* of California Press, Berkley, 1949

Voigt, John, "The man who invented 'qigong'" *Qi: Journal of Traditional Eastern Health and Fitness,* Autumn 2013

Waley, Arthur, *The nine songs,* Forgotten books, 2014

Waley, Arthur, *The way and its power: Lao Tzu's tao te ching,* Grove Press, 1958

Walsch, Neale Donald, *Conversations with God,* Penguin Putman, Inc., New York, NY

Wang and Wu, *The history of Chinese medicine.* Originally published by the National Quarantine Service of Shanghai, 1936. Reprinted by Southern Materials Center, Inc, Taipei, 1977

Ware, James R., *Alchemy, medicine, and religion in the China of A.D. 320: the nei p'ien of Ko Hung (Pao-p'u tzu),* Cambridge, MA and London, 1966

Watts, Allen, *Tao: The watercourse way,* Pantheon Books, 1975

Wayne Jonas and Jeffrey Wayne, *Essentials of complementary and alternative medicine,* Lippincott Williams & Wilkins, 1999

Weiqiao, Jiang, *Quiet sitting with master Yinshi,* as cited by Miura, Kunio, "The revival of qi," *Taoist meditation and longevity techniques,* University of Michigan Center for Chinese Studies, 1989

Wile, Douglas (translator), *Annals of the state of Wu,* as cited in *T'ai-chi's Ancestors: The making of an internal art,* Sweet Chi Press, 1999

Wile, Douglas (translator), Selected portion of Li Yi-Yu's, *Song of the essence of t'ai-chi chüan*

Wile, Douglas, "Fighting words: Four new document finds reignite old debates in taijiquan historiography," *Martial arts studies* 4, 2016

Wile, Douglas, *Art of the bedchamber: The Chinese sexual Yoga classics including women's solo meditation texts:* State University of New York, 1992

Wile, Douglas, *Lost t'ai-chi classics from the late ch'ing dynasty,* State University of New York, 1996

Wile, Douglas, *T'ai-chi's ancestors: The making of an internal martial art.* Sweet Ch'i Press, Brooklyn, New York, 1999

Wilhelm Reich, Archives of the Orgone Institute

William A. Tiller, PhD and Walter E. Dibble, Jr., PhD, "Why the last century's quantum mechanics (QM) is irrelevant in a duplex, reciprocal subspace, reference frame for our cognitive world," White Paper #XXXIX

Tiller, William, *Science and human transformation: Subtle energies, intentionality and consciousness.* Pavior Publishing, Walnut Creek, 1997

Wing, R.L., *The tao of power: Lao Tzu's classic guide to leadership, influence, and excellence,* Doubleday, NY 1986

Xin Yan, et al. 1999 Mat Res Innovat (1999) 2:349-359

Yang, Jwing-ming, *Qigong: The secret of youth*, YMAA publications, Boston, MCA 2000

Yangpönga, Gyalwa, *Secret map of the body: Visions of the human energy structure, Guarisco, Elio,* (translator/editor) Shang Shun Foundation, 2015

Yeragani, VK, et al., "Decreased HRV in panic disorder patients: a study of power-spectral analysis of heart rate," *Psychiatric research 1993; 46:89-103*

Yeragani, VK, et al., "Heart rate variability in patients with major depression." *Psychiatric research* 1991; 37:35-46 (As cited by Tiller in A., et al., "Cardiac Coherence: A new, noninvasive measure of autonomic nervous system order, *Alternative therapies,* 1996, Vol. 2, No. 1

Yeshe, Thubten, *The bliss of inner fire: Heart practice of the six yogas of naropa,* Simon and Schuster, 2005

Yuzo HIGUCHI, Yasunori KOTANI, Hironobu HIGUCHI, Yukiko MINEGISHI, Yukio TANAKA, Yong Chang YU, and Shinichiro MOMOSE, "Immune Changes during Cosmic Orbit Meditation of Qigong," *Journal of international society of life information science,* Vol.18, No.2, September 2000 [Procedures of the Tenth Symposium of Life Information Science] .

On-Line Video Library

Section II

Box 2-19
Working and Experiment with Exaggerated Foot Shape
https://youtu.be/6YQnKruUQEA
or, https://chiarts.com/2-19

Section III

Box 3-9
Working with Resonance
https://www.youtube.com/watch?v=vf8a6g1BtiU
or https://chiarts.com/3-9

Box 3-18
More Advanced Studies of Signal: Movement
A video of students in a class practicing these exercises can be viewed at
https://www.youtube.com/watch?v=TvTPffDs_Z4
or, https://chiarts.com/3-18

Box 3-23
Examples of *Wai San He:* The Outer Three Relationships
Outer training for martial arts and the study of the body energy matrix can be viewed at https://www.youtube.com/watch?v=s6FME9-B9gc
or, https://chiarts.com/3-23

Box 3-28
"Opening the Shoulder Joints" Training
A video showing the Opening the Shoulder Joints training can be viewed at the following link:
https://youtu.be/BqsNcrli1Rl
or, https://chiarts.com/3-28

Section VII

Box 7-5
Demonstrations of practitioners using entrainment during close combat practice http://youtu.be/uVhkCtUav4g
or, https://chiarts.com/7-5

Box 7-12
A video demonstration of Eight Diagram Palm's "Soft Hands" can be viewed at
https://www.youtube.com/watch?v=RRYS0fWDElU
or, https://chiarts.com/7-12

Box 7-13
A brief clip of Baguazhang "tiao da" practice in Beijing
https://youtu.be/1qpl1a4l8jA
or, https://chiarts.com/7-13

Box 7-14
The Two-Person routines Nanjing Central Martial Arts Academy, circa 1930 https://youtu.be/A1qrgVQXu_0
or, https://chiarts.com/7-14

Section XI

Box 11-19
"Wall Training"
https://youtu.be/1ggOtkipzZ8
or, https://chiarts.com/11-19

Box 11-28
Block-Tensegrity Training and "athletic connection"
https://www.youtube.com/watch?v=9U4p_B3xe48
or, https://chiarts.com/11-28

Box 11-33
Video Demonstrating Tensional Strength applied through a Relaxed Body.
The Song-Peng Continuum
https://www.youtube.com/watch?v=j2D5chPv26k
https://chiarts.com/11-33

Box 11-34
A video of a student practicing martial arts on a log as a form of moving suspension-tensegrity training
https://youtu.be/Gw4CmfeRjBY

Section XII

Box 12-11
"Massaging" the Near Reactive Field
https://youtu.be/KbUs20yo4uE
or, https://chiarts.com/12-11

Box 12-19
Magnetic Fields and Disruptive Information against an Opponent
https://youtu.be/KLqhOiQcerg
or, https://chiarts.com/12-19

A demonstration of "neutralizing force" for martial art application https://youtu.be/EoxDalBYAfA

Glossary of Chinese Terms and Phrases Appearing in this Work

Chinese Word or Phrase	Translation/ Meanin	*Pinyin*	Wade-Giles
an mo 按摩	massage	anmo	an-mo
an shen pao 安身炮	a xingyiquan martial arts form	anshenpao	an-shen-p'ao
baguazhang 八卦掌	"eight diagrams palm"; a Chinese internal martial art	baguazhang	pa-kua-chang
bai hui 百會	"hundred gatherings" (Du-20); acupuncture point at the top of the head	baihui	pai-hui
bu qi 布氣	"spreading the *qi*"	buqi	pu-ch'i
bi gu 辟穀	abstaining from grains	bigu	pi-ku
cai bu 採補	The Taoist practice of "absorbing energy"	caibu	ts'ai-pu
Cantongqi 參同契	oldest known book on Taoist alchemy	Cantongqi	Ts'an-t'ung-ch'i
ching jing 清靜	state of "clarity and quiescence"	chingjing	ch'ing-ching
cun 寸	an "acupuncture inch"	cun	t'sun
dan 丹	cinnabar; elixir of immortality	dan	tan
dan shi 丹室	alchemist's laboratory	danshi	tan-shih
dan tian 丹田	"field of cinnabar;" body energy center; lower abdomen	dantian	tan-t'ien
dao yin 導引	Taoist physical exercise; literally "guiding and pulling"	daoyin	tao-yin
de qi 得氣	the slightly achy sensation associated with acupuncture needling	deqi	te-ch'i

Chinese Word or Phrase	Translation/ Meaning	*Pinyin*	Wade-Giles
dong jin 懂勁	interpreting force	*dongjin*	*tong-chin*
du mai 督脈	energy channel that travels along the spine	*dumai*	*tu-mai*
wai qi liao fa 外气疗法	external energy healing	*waiqi liaofa*	*wai-ch'i liao-fa*
fang shi 方士	Taoist alchemists / geomancers, etc.	*fangshi*	*fang-shih*
fang shui 風水	Chinese geomancy	*fangshui*	*feng-shui*
fu 腑	the "hollow" organs in TCM	*fu*	*fu*
fu yue 服月	consuming moon influence	*fuyue*	*fu-yüeh*
jing luo 経絡	meridians / channels	*jingluo*	*ching-lo*
jen qi 真氣	true energy	*jenqi*	*chen-ch'i*
Huangdi neijing 黄帝内経	Yellow Emperor's Classic of Medicine	*Huangdi neijing*	*Huang-ti nei-ching*
gang rou xiang ji 刚柔相济	hard and soft complementing each other	*gangrou xiangji*	*kang-jou hsiang-chi*
gu qi 谷気	energy extracted from food through digestion	*guqi*	*ku-ch'i*
he gu 合谷	acupuncture point Li-4 (located in the webbing between the thumb and index finger)	*hegu*	*ho-ku*
ho dao 合道	mystical union with the Tao "mechanism of change"	*hedao*	*ho-tao*

Chinese Word or Phrase	Translation/ Meaning	*Pinyin*	Wade-Giles
hua ji 化機	"mechanism of change"	*huaji*	*hua-chi*
jing qi 精氣	sexual essence	*jingqi*	*ching-ch'i*
jing ye 精液	semen	*jingye*	*ching-ye*
jingzuo 静坐	Meditation / quiet sitting	*jingzuo*	*ching-zuo*
kong jin 空勁	empty force	*kongjin*	*k'ung-chin*
lien qi hua shen 鍊氣化神	transforminging the qi into spirit	*lienqi huashen*	*lian-ch'i hua-shen*
liu nei wai he 六内外合	six inner and outer relationships	*liuneiwaihe*	*liu-nei-wai-ho*
Mawangdui 馬王堆	Han Dynasty Tombs near Changsha	*Mawangdui*	*Ma-wang-tui*
ming 命	one's physical existence; the body in Taoist practices	*ming*	*ming*
nei jia quan 内家拳	internal martial arts	*neijiaquan*	*nei-chia ch'üan*
nei gong 内功	internal practices	*neigong*	*nei-kung*
nei qi 内氣	internal energy	*neiqi*	*nei-ch'i*
nei san he 内三合	inner three relationships	*neisanhe*	*nei-san-ho*
nei dan 内丹	inner elixir / inner alchemy	*neidan*	*nei-tan*
nei guan 内觀	meditation / passive yoga	*neiguan*	*nei-kuan*
nei shi 内視	a synonym for nei guan	*neishi*	*nei-shih*
peng / peng jin 掤/ 掤勁	repelling force	*pengjin*	*peng-chin*

Chinese Word or Phrase	Translation/ Meaning	*Pinyin*	Wade-Giles
pi mao 皮毛	superficial	*pimao*	*p'i-mao*
qi 氣	general term for "energy"	*qi*	*ch'i*
qigong 氣功	"energy practice"	*qigong*	*ch'i-kung*
ren mai 任脈	central energy channel running along the anterior of the body	*renmai*	*jen-mai*
rou shou 柔手	"soft hands" (a baguazhang partnering practice)	*roushou*	*jou-shou*
san bao 三寶	the "three treasures"	*sanbao*	*san-pao*
san yuan 三元	three primordial energies	*sanyuan*	*san-yüan*
san yuan qi 三元氣	three primordial energies	*sanyuanqi*	*san-yüan-ch'i*
shen men 神門	"spirit gate;" acupuncture point (H-7); located on the medial aspect of the wrist	*shenmen*	*shen-men*
shen 神	consciousness; spirit	*shen*	*shen*
shen ming 神明	a transcendental state	*shenming*	*shen-ming*
shouyi 守一	"guarding the one" (Taoist meditation practice)	*shouyi*	*shou-i*
shrfu 師父	Yale transliteration of shifu/ sifu; teacher" or "master"	*shifu*	*shih-fu*
sifu 師父	teacher / master	*shifu*	*shih-fu*
song 鬆	state of relaxation	*song*	*sung*
tai ji quan 太极拳	soft-style Chinese martial art	*taijiquan*	*t'ai-chi ch'üan*

Chinese Word or Phrase	Translation/ Meaning	*Pinyin*	Wade-Giles
tai yang 太阳	a meridian network; body's outermost defensive layer	*taiyang*	*t'ai-yang*
Tao 道	The primordial source, or "path"	*Dao*	*Tao*
Tao Te Ching 道德經	The Classic of the Way and its Power	*Daodejing*	*Tao Te Ching*
Te 德	primordial power; sometimes translated as "virtue"	*De*	*Te*
tiao da 調打	baguazhang two-man training routine	*tiaoda*	*tiao-ta*
wai qi 外氣	externally "emitted" qi	*waiqi*	*wai-ch'i*
wai san he 外三合	outer three relationships	*waisanhe*	*wai-san-ho*
wai dan 外丹	alchemical elixir of immortality	*waidan*	*wai-tan*
wai qi liao fa 外氣 疗法	non-contact projection of internal energy for healing	*waiqi liaofa*	*wai-ch'i liao-fa*
wei qi 衛氣	protective *qi*	*weiqi*	*wei-ch'i*
wei lü 尾闾	coccyx region	*weilü*	*wei-lü*
wu xing 五行	five elements; metal, wood, water, fire, earth	*wuxing*	*wu-hsing*
Wudang 武當	mountain range associated with Taoist centers and practices	*Wudang*	*Wu Tang*
xian 仙	immortal	*xian*	*hsien*
xiantian 先天	primordial / prenatal state	*xiantian*	*hsien-t'ien*

Chinese Word or Phrase	Translation/ Meaning	Pinyin	Wade-Giles
xin bao 心包	the pericardium region	xinbao	hsin-pao
xing 性	intrinsic nature; the mind in Taoist practices	xing	hsing
xing qi 行氣	circulating qi	xingqi	hsing-ch'i
yang sheng 養生	nurturing life; health practices	yangsheng	yang-sheng
xingyiquan 形意拳	one of the three internal martial arts	xingyiquan	hsing-i ch'üan
xue 穴	acupuncture point	xue	hsüeh
yang xin 養心	cultivating the mind	yangxin	yang-hsin
yang xing 養形	cultivating the body	yangxing	yang-hsing
Yijing/ I Ching 易經	Book of Changes	Yijing	I Ching
yin yang 陰陽	feminine and masculine cosmological principles	yinyang	yin-yang
ying qi 营気	nurturative energy	yingqi	ying-ch'i
yi quan 意拳	Mind / intention boxing	yiquan	i-ch'üan
yuan-fen 缘分	fate / destiny	yuanfen	yuan-fen
yuan qi 元気	primordial energy	yuanqi	yüan-ch'i
zhan zhuang 站椿	standing meditation/standing practices	zhangzhuang	chan-chuang
zhen dan tian 真丹田	true dantian	zhen tantian	chen tan-t'ien

Chinese Word or Phrase	Translation/ Meaning	*Pinyin*	Wade-Giles
zhen qi 真気	true energy	*zhenqi*	*chen-ch'i*
zhen ren 真人	an immortal	*zhenren*	*chen-jen*
zheng 正	straight, correct	*zheng*	*cheng*

INDEX

N

For more information on Chi-Arts services or to contact an instructor or health/ coaching professional trained in the Chi-Arts system, visit

www.chiarts.com

or write to

admin@chiarts.com

To send your comments, suggestions, or your personal mind-body energy stories to be included in future projects, write to:

bookfeedback@chiarts.com

John Bracy

Highly ranked in the Chinese internal martial arts traditions, John's first book was *Ba Gua: Hidden Knowledge in the Taoist Internal Martial Art*. He has devoted his life to martial arts and mind-body disciplines. In 1976, John founded what would become the Hsing Chen and Chi-Arts martial arts associations. John's study and teaching encompasses more than 45 years of experience in *ba gua zhang, yang style tai-chi ch'uan*, Yi family style internal shaolin, and *hsing-i ch'uan*. Admitted as a formal "inner door" disciple of two traditions, John was accepted by noted *ba gua* master Liu Xinghan at the founding place of the art in Beijing, China. The second admission involved the formerly secret Eight Diagram Society of Taiwan; in 1993 John received an eighth-degree instructor ranking from the Taiwan association. Other martial arts credentials include his being the first Westerner to receive a coaching license from the Beijing Full Contact Fighting Association in 1988.

The scope of John's experience and training extends beyond the martial to include healing and rehabilitation. That experience includes working with patients under the supervision of medical doctors where he specialized in developing prescriptive therapeutic exercises that incorporate *qigong (chi-kung)*, breathing, fascia manipulation, and intention exercises that produce remarkable results.

John is a master of spotting and correcting problematic biomechanical patterns. In this light, he has worked with many elite athletes to identify and correct their physical issues. Adding to that work and his training of martial artists and prize fighters, he has developed unique methods to teach athletes to harmonize and master their mind-body rhythms to awaken and optimize their potential.

CPSIA information can be obtained
at www.ICGtesting.com
Printed in the USA
BVHW010901070121
597127BV00008B/405

9 781913 479411